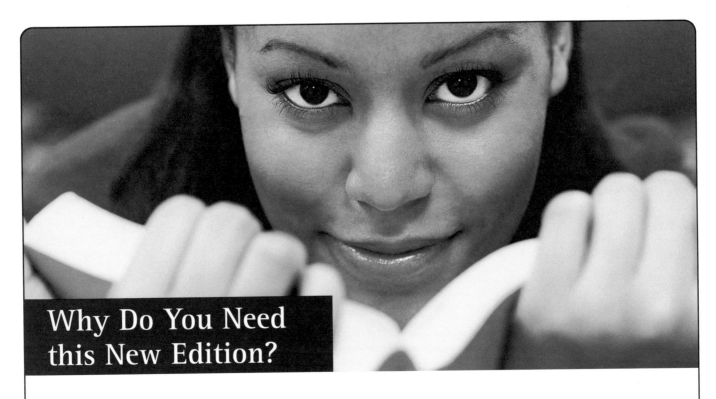

Why Do You Need this New Edition?

If you're wondering why you should buy this new edition of *Foundations of Behavioral Neuroscience*, here are several good reasons:

1 Neuroscience as a field evolves rapidly; new research methods are developed every year. The research reported in this edition reflects the enormous advances made in these research methods.

2 New research is published every year that advances our understanding of the physiology of behavior. This new edition describes research that has resulted in many new discoveries—for example, genes that control brain size, the action of acetaminophen, diffusion tensor imaging of fiber tracts, the gene responsible for congenital insensitivity to pain, the brain mechanisms involved in moral judgments, the effects of bariatric surgery on secretion of anorexic peptide, the role of the basal ganglia in nondeclarative learning, the causes of AIDS dementia complex, the possible role of vitamin D deficiency in development of schizophrenia, cleansing rituals as atonement for unethical behavior, the brain pathology in autistic disorder, and dozens of other studies.

3 This new edition features many entirely new topics that were not covered in previous editions, including, the role of sleep in procedural and declarative learning; the brain's REM-sleep flip-flop; the role of the ventromedial prefrontal cortex in reactions to violation of social norms; analysis of anorexic symptoms as response to starvation, leading to a new treatment for anorexia; identification of the visual word-form area; a reorganized section on anxiety disorders; the role of 5-HT transporters in PTSD; the role of the insular cortex in nicotine addiction; the importance of airway sensations in cigarette addiction; and many other topics.

4 The author has revised the existing art and prepared new art to illustrate research that is described for the first time in this edition. Dozens of new pieces of art have been developed and dozens of others have been revised. The result is a set of up-to-date, clear, consistent, and attractive illustrations.

Foundations of
Behavioral
Neuroscience

EIGHTH EDITION

Foundations of Behavioral Neuroscience

Neil R. Carlson
University of Massachusetts, Amherst

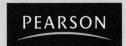

PEARSON

Boston | Columbus | Indianapolis | New York | San Francisco | Upper Saddle River
Amsterdam | Cape Town | Dubai | London | Madrid | Milan | Munich | Paris | Montreal | Toronto
Delhi | Mexico City | Sao Paulo | Sydney | Hong Kong | Seoul | Singapore | Taipei | Tokyo

Executive Editor: Susan Hartman
Editorial Assistant: Mary Lombard
Marketing Manager: Nicole Kunzmann
Marketing Assistant: Amanda Olweck
Production Editor: Karen Mason
Manufacturing Buyer: Debbie Rossi
Cover Administrator: Kristina Mose-Libon
Editorial Production and Composition Service: Modern Graphics
Photo Researcher: PoYee Oster

Photo credits appear on page 556, which constitutes an extension of the copyright page.

10 9 8 7 6 5 4 3 2 1   [CIN]   13 12 11 10 09

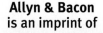

Allyn & Bacon
is an imprint of

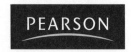

ISBN 10: 0-205-77608-6
ISBN 13: 978-0-205-77608-5

Brief Contents

Contents

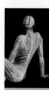

chapter 3
Structure of the Nervous System   56

chapter 4
Psychopharmacology   88

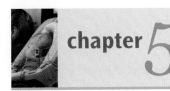

chapter 5

Methods and Strategies of Research   115

chapter 6

Vision   146

chapter 7
Audition, the Body Senses, and the Chemical Senses   177

chapter 8
Sleep and Biological Rhythms   212

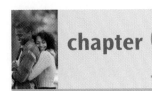

chapter 9

Reproductive Behavior 244

chapter 10

Emotion 275

chapter 11
Ingestive Behavior   301

chapter 12
Learning and Memory   336

chapter 13 · Human Communication 377

chapter 14 · Neurological Disorders 410

chapter 15   Schizophrenia, Affective Disorders, and Anxiety Disorders   442

chapter 16   Autistic, Attention-Deficit/Hyperactivity, Stress, and Substance Abuse Disorders   476

Preface

All my life I have wanted to know how things work. When I was a boy, I took apart alarm clocks, radios, my mother's sewing machine, and other interesting gadgets to see what was inside. Much to my parents' relief, I outgrew that habit (or at least got better at putting things back together), but my curiosity is still with me. Since my college days, I have been trying to find out all I can about the workings of the most intricate piece of machinery that we know of: the human brain.

The field of neuroscience research is a very busy and productive one today. A large number of scientists are trying to understand the physiology of behavior, using more and more advanced methods, yielding more and more interesting results. Their findings provide me with much to write about. I admire their dedication and hard work, and I thank them for giving me something to say. Without their efforts I could not have written this book.

I wrote the first edition of this book at the request of my colleagues who teach the course and wanted a briefer version of *Physiology of Behavior* with greater emphasis on research related to humans. The first part of this book is concerned with foundations: the history of the field, the structure and functions of neurons, neuroanatomy, psychopharmacology, and methods of research. The second part is concerned with inputs: the sensory systems. The third part deals with what might be called "motivated" behavior: sleep, reproduction, emotion, and ingestion. The fourth part deals with learning and verbal communication. The final part deals with neurological and mental disorders.

New to This Edition

Of course, all chapters in this book have been revised. My colleagues keep me busy by providing me with interesting research results to describe in my book.

The following lists include some of the information that is new to this edition:

New Research

- Genes that control brain size
- Action of acetaminophen
- Diffusion tensor imaging of fiber tracts
- Discovery of color "globs" in the visual association cortex
- Discovery of the gene responsible for congenital insensitivity to pain
- Revised section on neural control of maternal behavior
- Brain mechanisms of moral judgments
- Emotional judgments of body posture
- Bariatric surgery and secretion of anorexic peptide
- Role of the basal ganglia in nondeclarative learning
- Causes of AIDS dementia complex
- Possible role of vitamin D deficiency in development of schizophrenia

- Cleansing rituals as atonement for unethical behavior
- Brain pathology in autistic disorder

New Topics

- Evidence for fatty acid detectors in the tongue
- New section on the role of sleep in procedural and declarative learning
- Brain mechanisms of REM sleep: the REM flip-flop
- Role of the ventromedial prefrontal cortex in reactions to violation of social norms
- Role of the somatosensory system in emotional recognition and empathy
- Anorexic symptoms as a response to starvation
- New treatment for anorexia
- Transfer of memories from hippocampus to neocortex
- Identification of the visual word-form area
- Ketogenic diet and development of 2-DG trials for treatment of seizure disorders
- Brain-computer interfaces to operate computer-controlled devices
- Animal research on delivery of siRNA to treat Huntington's disease
- Reorganization of the section on anxiety disorders
- Role of 5-HT transporters in PTSD
- Role of the dorsal striatum in addictive behavior
- Role of the insular cortex in nicotine addiction
- New experimental drugs for treatment of addiction
- Role of airway sensations in cigarette addiction

Strategies for Learning

This theme of strategies for learning, which runs throughout the book, was created to help apply the research findings of behavioral neuroscience to daily life. For example, in Chapter 1 you will find a section called *Strategies for Learning* and in Chapter 5 a section called *Methods and Strategies of Research.* You will find that you are not faced with a bewildering list of research methods but instead are led through a set of hypothetical investigations organized the way that a research project might proceed. Each step in an investigation illustrates a particular procedure in the context in which it would be applied in an ongoing program.

The following sections in each chapter provide an overview of the chapter as well as a convenient review of the subjects covered.

- **Learning Objectives.** Each chapter begins with a list of Learning Objectives that also serve as the framework for the study guide that accompanies this text.

- **Prologue.** Each chapter opens with a Prologue that contains the description of an episode involving a neurological disorder or an issue in neuroscience.

- **Epilogue.** At the end of the chapter, an Epilogue resolves the issues raised in the prologue, discussing them in terms of what the reader has learned in the chapter, or it introduces a related topic.

- **Interim Summary.** An Interim Summary follows each major section of the book. The summaries not only provide useful reviews, but they also break each chapter into manageable chunks.

- **Thought Questions.** Most Interim Summaries are followed by Thought Questions. The questions provide students with an opportunity to think about what they have learned in the previous section.

- **Key Terms.** Definitions of Key Terms are printed in the margin on the page in the text where the terms are first discussed or on a facing page. For terms that might be difficult to pronounce, a pronunciation guide is included with the definition.

- **Key Concepts and Suggested Readings.** Each chapter ends with a Key Concepts section that provides a quick review and Suggested Readings that provide more information about the topics discussed in the chapter.

Pedagogically Sound Art

Jay Alexander, of I-Hua Graphics, prepared the illustrations in this book. Jay and I have been working together on my books for several years. I think the result of our collaboration is a set of clear, attractive, and pedagogically effective illustrations.

Supplements for Instructors

Several supplements are available for qualified instructors.

- **MyPsychKit (www.mypsychkit.com).** MyPsychKit, a new online resource, provides a wealth of study tools for students looking to clarify and deepen their understanding of the foundations of behavioral neuroscience. MyPsychKit includes animation modules on neurophysiology (*Neural Communication, The Action Potential, Synapses,* and *Postsynaptic Potentials*), neuroanatomy (*The Rotatable Brain, Brain Slices,* and *Meninges and CSF*), psychopharmacology, research methods, audition, memory, verbal communication, and autism. MyPsychKit also contains a set of self-scoring practice tests, interactive glossary flashcards, and access to Research Navigator, a resource that can help students with all parts of the research paper–writing process.

- **Instructor's Manual.** Written by John C. Churchwell, University of Utah, this manual provides a tool for classroom preparation and management. Each chapter includes an At-a-Glance Grid, with detailed pedagogical information linking to other available supplements, teaching objectives, lecture material, demonstrations and activities, and an updated list of video, media, suggested readings, and Web resources.

- **Test Bank.** Written by Paul Wellman, Texas A&M University, this resource contains questions that target key concepts. Each chapter has approximately 100 questions, including multiple choice, true/false, short answer, and essay—each with page references, difficulty rating, and type designation. A computerized version of the printed Test Bank is also available in Pearson MyTest, a powerful assessment generation program that helps instructors easily create and print quizzes and exams. Questions and tests can be authored online, allowing instructors ultimate flexibility and the ability to efficiently manage assessments anytime, anywhere. Instructors can easily access existing questions, edit, create, and store using simple drag and drop.

- **PowerPoint™ Presentation.** Created by Grant McLaren, Edinboro University of Pennsylvania, this interactive tool facilitates the development of lectures and the encouragement of classroom discussions by pairing key points covered in the chapters with images from the text.

- **Transparencies for Physiological Psychology.** The transparency package for Physiological Psychology contains approximately 100 full-color acetates of images found in Allyn & Bacon's major physiological psychology texts.

Supplements for Students

- **MyPsychKit (www.mypsychkit.com).** MyPsychKit, a new online resource, provides a wealth of study tools for students looking to clarify and deepen their understanding of the foundations of behavioral neuroscience. MyPsychKit includes animation modules on neurophysiology (*Neural Communication, The Action Potential, Synapses,* and *Postsynaptic Potentials*), neuroanatomy (*The Rotatable Brain, Brain Slices,* and *Meninges and CSF*), psychopharmacology, research methods, audition, memory, verbal communication, and autism. MyPsychKit also contains a set of self-scoring practice tests, interactive glossary flashcards, and access to Research Navigator, a resource that can help students with all parts of the research paper–writing process. Instructions on how to log onto MyPsychKit can be found at www.mypsychkit.com.

- **Study Guide.** Written by Heather Dickinson-Anson, University of California, Irvine, this workbook provides a framework for guiding study behavior, with questions organized according to learning objective, self tests, and crossword puzzles for each chapter. It promotes a thorough understanding of the principles of behavioral neuroscience through active participation in the learning process. An important part of learning about physiological psychology is acquiring a new vocabulary. The study guide contains a set of Concept Cards that will help with this task. Terms are printed on one side of these cards, and definitions are printed on the other.

- **Allyn & Bacon Physiological Psychology Study Site (www.abphysio.com).** Organized around key topics in the behavioral neuroscience course, the Allyn & Bacon Physiological Psychology Study Site features comprehensive practice tests, Web links, and flash cards of key terms presented in the text.

- **Study Card for Physiological Psychology.** Allyn & Bacon's Study Cards make studying easier, more efficient, and more enjoyable. Course information is distilled down to the basics, helping students quickly master the fundamentals, review a subject for understanding, or prepare for an exam.

In Conclusion

Trying to keep up with the rapid progress being made in neuroscience research poses a challenge for teachers and textbook writers. If a student simply memorizes what we believe at the time to be facts, he or she is left with knowledge that quickly becomes obsolete. In this book I have tried to provide enough background material and enough knowledge of basic physiological processes that the reader can revise what he or she has learned when research provides us with new information.

I designed this text to be interesting and informative. I have endeavored to provide a solid foundation for further study. Students who will not take subsequent courses in this or related fields should receive the satisfaction of a much better understanding of their own behavior. Also, they will have a greater appreciation for the forthcoming advances in medical practices related to disorders that affect a person's perception, mood, or behavior. I hope that people who read this book carefully will henceforth perceive human behavior in a new light.

Acknowledgments

Although I must accept the blame for any shortcomings of the book, I want to thank colleagues who helped me with the present edition of this book and the Tenth Edition of *Physiology of Behavior* by sending reprints of their work, suggesting topics that I should cover, sending photographs that have been reproduced in this book, and pointing out deficiencies in the previous edition. I thank the following reviewers for their comments on this edition:

Danny Benbassat, George Washington University
Robert Berks, Granite State College
Stacy Birch, SUNY College at Brockport
Melissa Burns-Cusato, Centre College
Patty Costello, Gustavus Adolphus College
Eleanor Downey, Lewis-Clark State College
Nukte Edguer, Brandon University
Edward Fox, Purdue University
David Ludden, Lindsey Wilson College
Donald Sweet, College of St. Catherine
Steve Weinert, Cuyamaca College

I also want to thank the people at Allyn & Bacon. Susan Hartman, my editor, provided assistance, support, and encouragement and Mary Lombard, editorial assistant, helped to gather comments and suggestions from colleagues who have read the book. Kara Kikel oversaw the production of the ancillary material: Study Guide, Instructor's Manual, Test Bank, and PowerPoint. Karen Mason, production editor, assembled the team that produced the book. Barbara Gracia demonstrated her masterful skills of organization in managing the book's production. She got everything done on time, despite an extremely tight schedule. Few people realize what a difficult, demanding, and time-consuming job a production editor has with a project such as this, with hundreds of illustrations and an author who tends to procrastinate—but I do, and I thank her for all she has done. Deidre Schaefer served as copy editor. She gave me the chance to fix my errors before anyone else saw them in print.

I must also thank my wife Mary for her support. Writing is a lonely pursuit, because one must be alone with one's thoughts for many hours of the day. I thank her for giving me the time to read, reflect, and write without feeling that I was neglecting her too much.

To the Reader

I hope that in reading this book you will come not only to learn more about the brain but also to appreciate it for the marvelous organ it is. The brain is wonderfully complex, and perhaps the most remarkable thing is that we are able to use it in our attempt to understand it.

While working on this book, I imagined myself talking with students, telling them interesting stories about the findings of clinicians and research scientists. Imagining your presence made the task of writing a little less lonely. I hope that the dialogue will continue. Please write to me and tell me what you like and dislike about the book. My e-mail address is nrc@psych.umass.edu. If you write to me, we can make the conversation a two-way exchange.

chapter 1

Origins of Behavioral Neuroscience

LEARNING OBJECTIVES

1. Describe the behavior of people with split brains and explain what study of this phenomenon contributes to our understanding of self-awareness.

2. Describe the goals of scientific research.

3. Describe the biological roots of behavioral neuroscience.

4. Describe the role of natural selection in the evolution of behavioral traits.

5. Describe the evolution of the human species.

6. Discuss the value of research with animals and ethical issues concerning their care.

7. Describe career opportunities in neuroscience.

8. Outline the strategies that will help you learn as much as possible from this book.

: PROLOGUE René's Inspiration

René, a lonely and intelligent young man of eighteen years, had secluded himself in Saint-Germain, a village to the west of Paris. He recently had suffered a nervous breakdown and chose the retreat to recover. Even before coming to Saint-Germain, he had heard of the fabulous royal gardens built for Henri IV and Marie de Médicis, and one sunny day he decided to visit them. The guard stopped him at the gate, but when he identified himself as a student at the King's School at La Flèche, he was permitted to enter. The gardens consisted of a series of six large terraces overlooking the Seine, planted in the symmetrical, orderly fashion so loved by the French. Grottoes were cut into the limestone hillside at the end of each terrace; René entered one of them. He heard eerie music accompanied by the gurgling of water but at first could see nothing in the darkness. As his eyes became accustomed to the gloom, he could make out a figure illuminated by a flickering torch. He approached the figure, which he soon recognized as that of a young woman. As he drew closer, he saw that she was actually a bronze statue of Diana, bathing in a pool of water. Suddenly, the Greek goddess fled and hid behind a bronze rosebush. As René pursued her, an imposing statue of Neptune rose in front of him, barring the way with his trident.

René was delighted. He had heard about the hydraulically operated mechanical organs and the moving statues, but he had not expected such realism. As he walked back toward the entrance to the grotto, he saw the plates buried in the ground that controlled the valves operating the machinery. He spent the rest of the afternoon wandering through the grottoes, listening to the music and being entertained by the statues.

During his stay in Saint-Germain, René visited the royal gardens again and again. He had been thinking about the relationship between the movements of animate and inanimate objects, which had concerned philosophers for some time. He thought he saw in the apparently purposeful, but obviously inanimate, movements of the statues an answer to some important questions about the relationship between the mind and the body. Even after he left Saint-Germain, René Descartes revisited the grottoes in his memory; he went so far as to name his daughter Francine after their designers, the Francini brothers of Florence.

The last frontier in this world—and perhaps the greatest one—lies within us. The human nervous system makes possible all that we can do, all that we can know, and all that we can experience. Its complexity is immense, and the task of studying it and understanding it dwarfs all previous explorations our species has undertaken.

One of the most universal of all human characteristics is curiosity. We want to explain what makes things happen. In ancient times, people believed that natural phenomena were caused by animating spirits. All moving objects—animals, the wind and tides, the sun, moon, and stars—were assumed to have spirits that caused them to move. For example, stones fell when they were dropped because their animating spirits wanted to be reunited with Mother Earth. As our ancestors became more sophisticated and learned more about nature, they abandoned this approach (which we call *animism*) in favor of physical explanations for inanimate moving objects—but they still used spirits to explain human behavior.

From the earliest historical times, people have believed that they possessed something intangible that animated them: a mind, a soul, or a spirit. This belief stems from the fact that each of us is aware of his or her own existence. When we think or act, we feel as though something inside us is thinking or deciding to act. But what is the nature of the human mind? We have physical bodies with muscles that move them and sensory organs such as eyes and ears that perceive information about the world around us. Within our bodies, the nervous system plays a central role, receiving information from the sensory organs and controlling the movements of the muscle—but what is the mind, and what role does it play? Does it *control* the nervous system? Is it a *part of* the nervous system? Is it physical and tangible, like the rest of the body, or is it a spirit that will always remain hidden?

Behavioral neuroscientists take an empirical and practical approach to the study of human nature. Most of us believe that the mind is a phenomenon produced by the workings of the nervous system. We believe that once we understand the workings of the human body—especially the workings of the nervous system—we will be able to explain how we perceive, how we think, how we remember, and

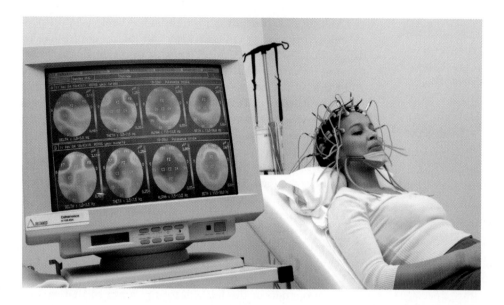

Scientists and engineers have developed research methods that enable neuroscientists to study activity of the human brain.

how we act. We will even be able to explain the nature of our own self-awareness. Of course, we are far from understanding the workings of the nervous system, so only time will tell whether this belief is justified.

Understanding Human Consciousness: A Physiological Approach

How can behavioral neuroscientists study human consciousness? First, let's define our terms. The word *consciousness* can be used to refer to a variety of concepts, including simple wakefulness. Thus, a researcher may write about an experiment using "conscious rats," referring to the fact that the rats were awake and not anesthetized. By *consciousness*, I am referring to something else: the fact that we humans are aware of—and can tell others about—our thoughts, perceptions, memories, and feelings.

We know that brain damage or drugs can profoundly affect consciousness. Because consciousness can be altered by changes in the structure or chemistry of the brain, we may hypothesize that consciousness is a physiological function, just as behavior is. We can even speculate about the origins of this self-awareness. Consciousness and the ability to communicate seem to go hand in hand. Our species, with its complex social structure and enormous capacity for learning, is well served by our ability to communicate: to express intentions to one another and to make requests of one another. Verbal communication makes cooperation possible and permits us to establish customs and laws of behavior. Perhaps the evolution of this ability is what has given rise to the phenomenon of consciousness. That is, our ability to send and receive messages with other people enables us to send and receive our own messages inside our own heads; in other words, to think and to be aware of our own existence. (See *Figure 1.1*.)

Split Brains

Studies of humans who have undergone a particular surgical procedure demonstrate dramatically how disconnecting parts of the brain that are involved with perceptions from parts involved with verbal behavior also disconnects them from consciousness. These results suggest that the parts of the brain involved in verbal behavior may be the ones responsible for consciousness.

FIGURE 1.1

Studying the Brain. Will the human brain ever completely understand its own workings? A sixteenth-century woodcut from the first edition of *De humani corporis fabrica (On the Workings of the Human Body)* by Andreas Vesalius.

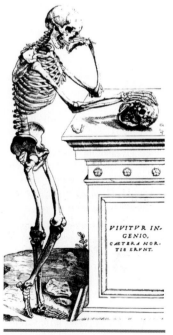

Courtesy of the National Library of Medicine.

FIGURE 1.2

The Split-Brain Operation. A "window" has been opened in the side of the brain so that we can see the corpus callosum being cut at the midline of the brain.

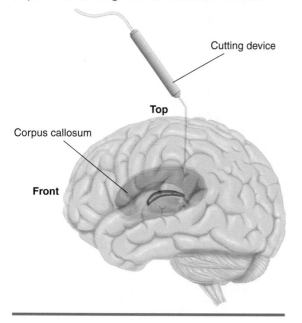

Cutting device

Top

Corpus callosum

Front

corpus callosum (*core pus ka* **low** *sum*) A large bundle of nerve fibers that connect corresponding parts of one side of the brain with those of the other.

split-brain operation Brain surgery that is occasionally performed to treat a form of epilepsy; the surgeon cuts the corpus callosum, which connects the two hemispheres of the brain.

cerebral hemispheres The two symmetrical halves of the brain; constitute the major part of the brain.

The surgical procedure is one that has been used for people with very severe epilepsy that cannot be controlled by drugs. In these people, nerve cells in one side of the brain become overactive, and the overactivity is transmitted to the other side of the brain by a structure called the corpus callosum. The **corpus callosum** is a large bundle of nerve fibers that connect corresponding parts of one side of the brain with those of the other. Both sides of the brain then engage in wild activity and stimulate each other, causing a generalized epileptic seizure. These seizures can occur many times each day, preventing the person from leading a normal life. Neurosurgeons discovered that cutting the corpus callosum (the **split-brain operation**) greatly reduced the frequency of the epileptic seizures.

Figure 1.2 shows a drawing of the split-brain operation. We see the brain being sliced down the middle, from front to back, dividing it into its two symmetrical halves. A "window" has been opened in the left side of the brain so that we can see the corpus callosum being cut by the neurosurgeon's special knife. (See *Figure 1.2*.)

Sperry (1966) and Gazzaniga and his associates (Gazzaniga and LeDoux, 1978; Gazzaniga, 2005) have studied these patients extensively. The largest part of the brain consists of two symmetrical parts, called the **cerebral hemispheres**, which receive sensory information from the opposite sides of the body. They also control movements of the opposite sides. The corpus callosum enables the two hemispheres to share information so that each side knows what the other side is perceiving and doing. After the split-brain operation is performed, the two hemispheres are disconnected and operate independently. Their sensory mechanisms, memories, and motor systems can no longer exchange information. The effects of these disconnections are not obvious to the casual observer, for the simple reason that only one hemisphere—in most people, the left—controls speech. The right hemisphere of an epileptic person with a split brain appears to be able to understand verbal instructions reasonably well, but it is incapable of producing speech.

Because only one side of the brain can talk about what it is experiencing, people who speak with a person with a split brain are conversing with only one hemisphere: the left. The operations of the right hemisphere are more difficult to detect. Even the patient's left hemisphere has to learn about the independent existence of the right hemisphere. One of the first things that these patients say they notice after the operation is that their left hand seems to have a "mind of its own." For example, patients may find themselves putting down a book held in the left hand, even if they have been reading it with great interest. This conflict occurs because the right hemisphere, which controls the left hand, cannot read and therefore finds the book boring. At other times, these patients surprise themselves by making obscene gestures (with the left hand) when they had not intended to. A psychologist once reported that a man with a split brain had attempted to beat his wife with one hand and protect her with the other. Did he *really* want to hurt her? Yes and no, I guess.

One exception to the crossed representation of sensory information is the olfactory system; that is, when a person sniffs a flower through the left nostril, only the left brain receives a sensation of the odor. Thus, if the right nostril of a patient with a split brain is closed, leaving only the left nostril open, the patient will be able to tell us what the odors are (Gordon and Sperry, 1969). However, if the odor enters the right nostril, the patient will say that he or she smells nothing when, in fact, the right brain *has* perceived the odor and *can* identify it. To show that this is so, we ask the patient to smell an odor with the right nostril and then reach for some objects that are hidden from view by a partition. If asked to use the left hand, controlled by the hemisphere that detected the smell, the patient will select the object that corresponds to the odor—a plastic flower for a floral odor, a toy fish for a fishy odor, a model tree for the odor of pine, and so forth. However, if asked to use the right hand, the patient fails the test because the right hand is connected to the left hemisphere, which did not smell the odor. (See *Figure 1.3*.)

The effects of cutting the corpus callosum reinforce the conclusion that we become conscious of something only if information about it is able to reach the parts of the brain responsible for verbal communication, which are located in the left hemisphere. If the information does not reach these parts of the brain, then that information does not reach the consciousness associated with these mechanisms. We still know very little about the physiology of consciousness, but studies of people with brain damage are beginning to provide us with some useful insights. This issue is discussed in later chapters.

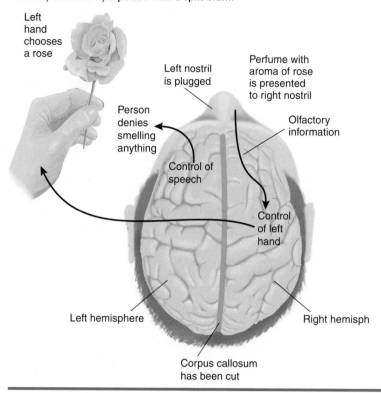

FIGURE 1.3

Smelling with a Split Brain.   An object is identified in response to an olfactory stimulus by a person with a split brain.

Left hand chooses a rose

Left nostril is plugged

Perfume with aroma of rose is presented to right nostril

Olfactory information

Person denies smelling anything

Control of speech

Control of left hand

Left hemisphere

Right hemisph

Corpus callosum has been cut

Interim Summary

Understanding Human Consciousness: A Psychological Approach

The concept of the mind has been with us for a long time—probably from the earliest history of our species. Modern science has concluded that the world consists of matter and energy and that what we call the mind can be explained by the same laws that govern all other natural phenomena. Studies of the functions of the human nervous system tend to support this position, as the specific example of the split brain shows. Brain damage, by disconnecting brain functions from the speech mechanisms in the left hemisphere, reveals that the mind does not have direct access to all brain functions.

When sensory information about a particular object is presented to the right hemisphere of a person who has had a split-brain operation, the person is not aware of the object but can, nevertheless, indicate by movements of the left hand that the object has been perceived. This phenomenon suggests that consciousness involves operations of the verbal mechanisms of the left hemisphere. Indeed, consciousness may be, in large part, a matter of our "talking to ourselves." Thus, once we understand the language functions of the brain, we may have gone a long way to understanding how the brain can be conscious of its own existence.

Thought Questions

1. Could a sufficiently large and complex computer ever be programmed to be aware of itself? Suppose that someone someday claims to have done just that. What kind of evidence would you need to prove or disprove this claim?

2. Clearly, the left hemisphere of a person with a split brain is conscious of the information it receives and of its own thoughts. It is not conscious of the mental processes of the right hemisphere. But is it possible that the right hemisphere is conscious too, but is just unable to talk to us? How could we possibly find out whether it is? Do you see some similarities between this issue and the one raised in the first question?

The Nature of Behavioral Neuroscience

The modern history of behavioral neuroscience has been written by psychologists who have combined the experimental methods of psychology with those of physiology and have applied them to the issues that concern all psychologists. Thus, we have studied perceptual processes, control of movement, sleep and waking, reproductive behaviors, ingestive behaviors, emotional behaviors, learning, and language. In recent years, we have begun to study the physiology of human pathological conditions, such as addictions and mental disorders.

The Goals of Research

The goal of all scientists is to explain the phenomena they study. But what do we mean by *explain*? Scientific explanation takes two forms: generalization and reduction. Most psychologists deal with **generalization**. They explain particular instances of behavior as examples of general laws, which they deduce from their experiments. For instance, most psychologists would explain a pathologically strong fear of dogs as an example of a particular form of learning called *classical conditioning*. Presumably, the person was frightened earlier in life by a dog. An unpleasant stimulus was paired with the sight of the animal (perhaps the person was knocked down by an exuberant dog or was attacked by a vicious one), and the subsequent sight of dogs evokes the earlier response: fear.

Most physiologists deal with **reduction**. They explain complex phenomena in terms of simpler ones. For example, they may explain the movement of a muscle in terms of the changes in the membranes of muscle cells, the entry of particular chemicals, and the interactions among protein molecules within these cells. By contrast, a molecular biologist would explain these events in terms of forces that bind various molecules together and cause various parts of the molecules to be attracted to one another. In turn, the job of an atomic physicist is to describe matter and energy themselves and to account for the various forces found in nature. Practitioners of each branch of science use reduction to call on sets of more elementary generalizations to explain the phenomena they study.

The task of the behavioral neuroscientist is to explain behavior in physiological terms—but behavioral neuroscientists cannot simply be reductionists. It is not enough to observe behaviors and correlate them with physiological events that occur at the same time. Identical behaviors may occur for different reasons and thus may be initiated by different physiological mechanisms. Therefore, we must understand "psychologically" why a particular behavior occurs before we can understand what physiological events made it occur.

Let me provide a specific example: Mice, like many other mammals, often build nests. Behavioral observations show that mice will build nests under two conditions: when the air temperature is low and when the animal is pregnant. A nonpregnant mouse will build a nest only if the weather is cool, whereas a pregnant mouse will build one regardless of the temperature. The same behavior occurs for different reasons. In fact, nest-building behavior is controlled by two different physiological mechanisms. Nest building can be studied as a behavior related to the process of temperature regulation, or it can be studied in the context of parental behavior.

generalization Type of scientific explanation; a general conclusion based on many observations of similar phenomena.

reduction Type of scientific explanation; a phenomenon is described in terms of the more elementary processes that underlie it.

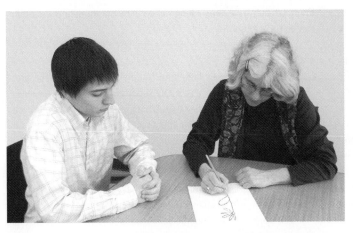

Studies of people with brain damage have given us insights into the brain mechanisms involved in language, perception, memory, and emotion.

In practice, the research efforts of behavioral neuroscientists involve both forms of explanation: generalization and reduction. Ideas for experiments are stimulated by the investigator's knowledge both of psychological generalizations about behavior and of physiological mechanisms. A good behavioral neuroscientist must therefore be both a good psychologist *and* a good physiologist.

Biological Roots of Behavioral Neuroscience

Study of (or speculations about) the physiology of behavior has its roots in antiquity. Because its movement is necessary for life and because emotions cause it to beat more strongly, many ancient cultures, including the Egyptian, Indian, and Chinese, considered the heart to be the seat of thought and emotions. The ancient Greeks did, too, but Hippocrates (460–370 B.C.) concluded that this role should be assigned to the brain.

Not all ancient Greek scholars agreed with Hippocrates. Aristotle did not; he thought the brain served to cool the passions of the heart. But Galen (A.D. 130–200), who had the greatest respect for Aristotle, concluded that Aristotle's role for the brain was "utterly absurd, since in that case Nature would not have placed the encephalon [brain] so far from the heart, . . . and she would not have attached the sources of all the senses [the sensory nerves] to it (Galen, 1968 translation, p. 387). Galen thought enough of the brain to dissect and study the brains of cattle, sheep, pigs, cats, dogs, weasels, monkeys, and apes (Finger, 1994).

René Descartes, a seventeenth-century French philosopher and mathematician, has been called the father of modern philosophy. Although he was not a biologist, his speculations about the roles of the mind and brain in the control of behavior provide a good starting point in the history of behavioral neuroscience. Descartes assumed that the world was a purely mechanical entity that, once having been set in motion by God, ran its course without divine interference. Thus, to understand the world, one had only to understand how it was constructed. To Descartes, animals were mechanical devices; their behavior was controlled by environmental stimuli. His view of the human body was much the same: It was a machine. As Descartes observed, some movements of the human body were automatic and involuntary. For example, if a person's finger touched a hot object, the arm would immediately withdraw from the source of stimulation. Reactions like this did not require participation of the mind; they occurred automatically. Descartes called these actions **reflexes** (from the Latin *reflectere*, "to bend back upon itself"). Energy coming from the outside source would be reflected back through the nervous system to the muscles, which would contract. The term is still in use today, but of course we explain the operation of a reflex differently.

Like most philosophers of his time, Descartes was a dualist; he believed that each person possesses a mind—a uniquely human attribute that is not subject to the laws of the universe. But his thinking differed from that of his predecessors in one important way: He was the first to suggest that a link exists between the human mind and its purely physical housing, the brain. He believed that the sense organs of the body supply the mind with information about what is happening in the environment, and that the mind, using this information, controls the movements of the body. In particular, he hypothesized that the interaction between mind and body takes place in the pineal body, a small organ situated on top of the brain stem, buried beneath the cerebral hemispheres. He noted that the brain contains hollow chambers (the *ventricles*) that are filled with fluid, and he believed that this fluid is under pressure. In his theory, when the mind decides to perform an action, it tilts the pineal body in a particular direction like a little joystick, causing pressurized fluid to flow from the brain into the appropriate set of nerves. This flow of fluid causes the same muscles to inflate and move. (See *Figure 1.4*.)

As we saw in the prologue, the young René Descartes was greatly impressed by the moving statues in the royal gardens (Jaynes, 1970). These devices served as models for

reflex An automatic, stereotyped movement produced as the direct result of a stimulus.

FIGURE 1.4

Decartes's Theory. A woodcut from *De homine* by René Descartes, published in 1662. Descartes believed that the "soul" (what we would today call the *mind*) controls the movements of the muscles through its influence on the pineal body. His explanation is modeled on the mechanism that animated statues in the royal gardens. According to his theory, the eyes sent visual information to the brain, where it could be examined by the soul. When the soul decided to act, it would tilt the pineal body (labeled H in the diagram), which would divert pressurized fluid through nerves to the appropriate muscles.

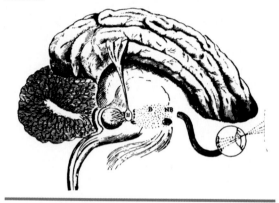

Courtesy of Historical Pictures Service, Chicago.

FIGURE 1.5

Johannes Müller (1801–1858).

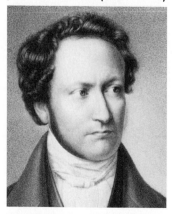

Courtesy of the National Library of Medicine.

Descartes in theorizing about how the body worked. The pressurized water of the moving statues was replaced by pressurized fluid in the ventricles; the pipes were replaced by nerves; the cylinders by muscles; and finally, the hidden valves by the pineal body. This story illustrates one of the first times that a technological device was used as a model for explaining how the nervous system works. In science, a **model** is a relatively simple system that works on known principles and is able to do at least some of the things that a more complex system can do. For example, when scientists discovered that elements of the nervous system communicate by means of electrical impulses, researchers developed models of the brain based upon telephone switchboards and, more recently, computers. Abstract models, which are completely mathematical in their properties, have also been developed.

Descartes's model was useful because, unlike purely philosophical speculations, it could be tested experimentally. In fact, it did not take long for biologists to prove that Descartes was wrong. For example, Luigi Galvani, a seventeenth-century Italian physiologist, found that electrical stimulation of a frog's nerve caused contraction of the muscle to which it was attached. Contraction occurred even when the nerve and muscle were detached from the rest of the body, so the ability of the muscle to contract and the ability of the nerve to send a message to the muscle were characteristics of these tissues themselves. Thus, the brain did not inflate muscles by directing pressurized fluid through the nerve. Galvani's experiment prompted others to study the nature of the message transmitted by the nerve and the means by which muscles contracted. The results of these efforts gave rise to an accumulation of knowledge about the physiology of behavior.

One of the most important figures in the development of experimental physiology was Johannes Müller, a nineteenth-century German physiologist. (See *Figure 1.5*.) Müller was a forceful advocate of the application of experimental techniques to physiology. Previously, the activities of most natural scientists were limited to observation and classification. Although these activities are essential, Müller insisted that major advances in our understanding of the workings of the body would be achieved only by experimentally removing or isolating animals' organs, testing their responses to various chemicals, and otherwise altering the environment to see how the organs responded. His most important contribution to the study of the physiology of behavior was his **doctrine of specific nerve energies**. Müller observed that although all nerves carry the same basic message, an electrical impulse, we perceive the messages of different nerves in different ways. For example, messages carried by the optic nerves produce sensations of visual images, and those carried by the auditory nerves produce sensations of sounds. How can different sensations arise from the same basic message?

The answer is that the messages occur in different channels. The portion of the brain that receives messages from the optic nerves interprets the activity as visual stimulation, even if the nerves are actually stimulated mechanically. (For example, when we rub our eyes, we see flashes of light.) Because different parts of the brain receive messages from different nerves, the brain must be functionally divided: Some parts perform some functions, while other parts perform others.

Müller's advocacy of experimentation and the logical deductions from his doctrine of specific nerve energies set the stage for performing experiments directly on the brain. Indeed, Pierre Flourens, a nineteenth-century French physiologist, did just that. Flourens removed various parts of animals' brains and observed their behavior. By seeing what the animal could no longer do, he could infer the function of the missing portion of the brain. This method is called **experimental ablation** (from the Latin *ablatus*, "carried away"). Flourens claimed to have discovered the regions of the brain that control heart rate and breathing, purposeful movements, and visual and auditory reflexes.

Soon after Flourens performed his experiments, Paul Broca, a French surgeon, applied the principle of experimental ablation to the human brain. Of course, he did not intentionally remove parts of human brains to see how they worked. Instead, he observed the behavior of people whose brains had been damaged by strokes. In 1861, he performed an autopsy on the brain of a man who had had a stroke that resulted in the loss of the ability to speak. Broca's observations led him to conclude that a portion of the cerebral cortex on the left side of the brain performs functions necessary for speech. (See *Figure 1.6*.) Other physicians soon obtained evidence supporting his conclusions. As you will learn in Chapter 13, the control of speech is not localized in a particular region of the brain. Indeed, speech requires many different functions, which are organized throughout the brain. Nonetheless, the method of experimental ablation remains important to our understanding of the brains of both humans and laboratory animals.

As mentioned earlier, Luigi Galvani used electricity to demonstrate that muscles contain the source of the energy that powers their contractions. In 1870, German physiologists Gustav Fritsch and Eduard Hitzig used electrical stimulation as a tool for understanding the physiology of the brain. They applied weak electrical current to the exposed surface of a dog's brain and observed the effects of the stimulation. They found that stimulation of different portions of a specific region of the brain caused contraction of specific muscles on the opposite side of the body. We now refer to this region as the *primary motor cortex*, and we know that nerve cells there communicate directly with those that cause muscular contractions. We also know that other regions of the brain communicate with the primary motor cortex and thus control behaviors. For example, the region that Broca found necessary for speech communicates with, and controls, the portion of the primary motor cortex that controls the muscles of the lips, tongue, and throat, which we use to speak.

One of the most brilliant contributors to nineteenth-century science was the German physicist and physiologist Hermann von Helmholtz. Helmholtz devised a mathematical formulation of the law of conservation of energy, invented the ophthalmoscope (used to examine the retina of the eye), devised an important and influential theory of color vision and color blindness, and studied audition, music, and many physiological processes. Although Helmholtz had studied under Müller, he opposed Müller's belief that human organs are endowed with a vital nonmaterial force that coordinates their operations. Helmholtz believed that all aspects of physiology are mechanistic, subject to experimental investigation.

Helmholtz was also the first scientist to attempt to measure the speed of conduction through nerves. Scientists had previously believed that such conduction was identical to the conduction that occurs in wires, traveling at approximately the speed of light, but Helmholtz found that neural conduction was much slower—only about 90 feet per second. This measurement proved that neural conduction was more than a simple electrical message, as we will see in Chapter 2.

Twentieth-century developments in experimental physiology include many important inventions, such as sensitive amplifiers to detect weak electrical signals, neurochemical techniques to analyze chemical changes within and between cells, and histological techniques to see cells and their constituents. Because these developments belong to the modern era, they are discussed in detail in subsequent chapters.

FIGURE 1.6

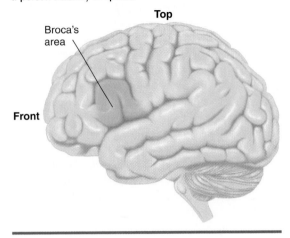

Broca's Area.   This region of the brain is named for French surgeon Paul Broca. Broca discovered that damage to a part of the left side of the brain disrupted a person's ability to speak.

Top

Broca's area

Front

model A mathematical or physical analogy for a physiological process; for example, computers have been used as models for various functions of the brain.

doctrine of specific nerve energies Müller's conclusion that because all nerve fibers carry the same type of message, sensory information must be specified by the particular nerve fibers that are active.

experimental ablation The research method in which the function of a part of the brain is inferred by observing the behaviors an animal can no longer perform after that part is damaged.

InterimSummary

The Nature of Behavioral Neuroscience

All scientists hope to explain natural phenomena. In this context, the term *explanation* has two basic meanings: generalization and reduction. Generalization refers to the classification of phenomena according to their essential features so that general laws can be formulated. For example, observing that gravitational attraction is related to the mass of two bodies and to the distance between them helps to explain the movement of planets. Reduction refers to the description of phenomena in terms of more basic physical processes. For example, gravitation can be explained in terms of forces and subatomic particles.

Behavioral neuroscientists use both generalization and reduction to explain behavior. In large part, generalizations use the traditional methods of psychology. Reduction explains behaviors in terms of physiological events that occur within the body—primarily within the nervous system. Thus, behavioral neuroscience builds upon the tradition of both experimental psychology and experimental physiology.

The behavioral neuroscience of today is rooted in important developments of the past. René Descartes proposed a model of the brain based on hydraulically activated statues. His model stimulated observations that produced important discoveries. The results of Galvani's experiments eventually led to an understanding of the nature of the message transmitted by nerves between the brain and the sensory organs and the muscles. Müller's doctrine of specific nerve energies paved the way for study of the functions of specific parts of the brain through the methods of experimental ablation and electrical stimulation.

Thought Questions

1. What is the value of studying the history of behavioral neuroscience? Is it a waste of time?
2. Suppose we studied just the latest research and ignored explanations that we now know to be incorrect. Would we be spending our time more profitably, or might we miss something?

FIGURE 1.7

Charles Darwin (1809–1882). Darwin's theory of evolution revolutionized biology and strongly influenced early psychologists.

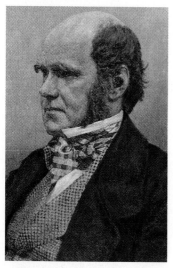

North Wind Picture Archives.

functionalism The principle that the best way to understand a biological phenomenon (a behavior or a physiological structure) is to try to understand its useful functions for the organism.

Natural Selection and Evolution

Müller's insistence that biology must be an experimental science provided the starting point for an important tradition. However, other biologists continued to observe, classify, and think about what they saw, and some of them arrived at valuable conclusions. The most important of these scientists was Charles Darwin. (See *Figure 1.7*.) Darwin formulated the principles of *natural selection* and *evolution*, which revolutionized biology.

Functionalism and the Inheritance of Traits

Darwin's theory emphasized that all of an organism's characteristics—its structure, its coloration, its behavior—have functional significance. For example, their strong talons and sharp beaks permit eagles to catch and eat prey. Most caterpillars that eat green leaves are themselves green, and their color makes it difficult for birds to see them against their usual background. Mother mice construct nests, which keep their offspring warm and out of harm's way. Obviously, the behavior itself is not inherited—how can it be? What *is* inherited is a brain that causes the behavior to occur. Thus, Darwin's theory gave rise to **functionalism**, a belief that characteristics of living organisms perform useful functions. So, to understand the physiological basis of various behaviors, we must first discover what these behaviors accomplish. We must therefore understand something about the natural history of the species being studied so that the behaviors can be seen in context.

To understand the workings of a complex piece of machinery, we should know what its functions are. This principle is just as true for a living organism as it is for a mechanical device. However, an important difference exists between machines and organisms: Machines have inventors who had a purpose when they designed them, whereas organisms are the result of a long series of accidents. Thus, strictly speaking, we cannot say that any physiological mechanisms of living organisms have a *purpose*, but they do have *functions*, and these we can try to determine. For example, the forelimbs shown in Figure 1.8 are adapted for different uses in different species of mammals. (See *Figure 1.8*.)

FIGURE 1.8

Bones of the Forelimb.   The figure shows the bones of (a) human, (b) bat, (c) whale, and (d) dog. Through the process of natural selection, these bones have been adapted to suit many different functions.

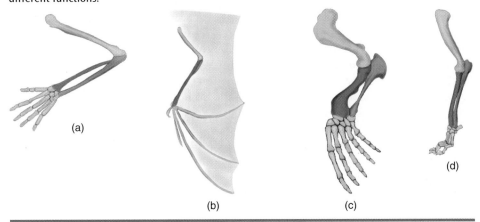

(a)

(b)   (c)

(d)

A good example of the functional analysis of an adaptive trait was demonstrated in an experiment by Blest (1957). Certain species of moths and butterflies have spots on their wings that resemble eyes—particularly the eyes of predators such as owls. (See *Figure 1.9.*) These insects normally rely on camouflage for protection; the backs of their wings, when folded, are colored like the bark of a tree. However, when a bird approaches, the insect's wings flip open, and the hidden eyespots are suddenly displayed. The bird then tends to fly away, rather than eat the insect. Blest performed an experiment to see whether the eyespots on a moth's or butterfly's wings really disturbed birds that saw them. He placed mealworms on different backgrounds and counted how many worms the birds ate. Indeed, when the worms were placed on a background that contained eyespots, the birds tended to avoid them.

Darwin formulated his theory of evolution to explain the means by which species acquired their adaptive characteristics. The cornerstone of this theory is the principle of **natural selection**. Darwin noted that members of a species were not all identical and that some of the differences they exhibited were inherited by their offspring. If an individual's characteristics permit it to reproduce more successfully, some of the individual's offspring will inherit the favorable characteristics and will themselves produce more offspring. As a result, the characteristics will become more prevalent in that species. He observed that animal breeders were able to develop strains that possessed particular traits by mating together only animals that possessed the desired traits. If *artificial selection*, controlled by animal breeders, could produce so many varieties of dogs, cats, and livestock, perhaps *natural selection* could be responsible for the development of species. Of course, it was the natural environment, not the hand of the animal breeder, that shaped the process of evolution.

Darwin and his fellow scientists knew nothing about the mechanism by which the principle of natural selection works. In fact, the principles of molecular genetics were not discovered until the middle of the twentieth century. Briefly, here is how the process works: Every sexually reproducing multicellular organism consists of a large number of cells, each of which contains chromosomes. Chromosomes are large, complex molecules that contain the recipes for producing the proteins that cells need to grow and to perform their functions. In essence, the chromosomes contain the blueprints for the construction (that is, the embryological development) of a particular member of a particular species. If the plans are altered, a different organism is produced.

The plans do get altered; mutations occur from time to time. **Mutations** that affect the development of offspring are accidental changes in the chromosomes of

FIGURE 1.9

The Owl Butterfly.   This butterfly displays its eyespots when approached by a bird. The bird usually will fly away.

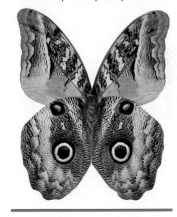

natural selection The process by which inherited traits that confer a selective advantage (increase an animal's likelihood to live and reproduce) become more prevalent in the population.

mutation A change in the genetic information contained in the chromosomes of sperms or eggs, which can be passed on to an organism's offspring; provides genetic variability.

sperms or eggs that join together and develop into new organisms. For example, cosmic radiation might strike a chromosome in a cell of an animal's testis or ovary, thus producing a mutation that affects that animal's offspring. Most mutations are deleterious; the offspring either fails to survive or survives with some sort of defect. However, a small percentage of mutations are beneficial and confer a **selective advantage** to the organism that possesses them. That is, the animal is more likely than other members of its species to live long enough to reproduce and hence to pass on its chromosomes to its own offspring. Many different kinds of traits can confer a selective advantage: resistance to a particular disease, the ability to digest new kinds of food, more effective weapons for defense or for procurement of prey, and even a more attractive appearance to members of the other sex (after all, one must reproduce in order to pass on one's chromosomes).

Naturally, the traits that can be altered by mutations are physical ones; chromosomes make proteins, which affect the structure and chemistry of cells. But the *effects* of these physical alterations can be seen in an animal's behavior. Thus, the process of natural selection can act on behavior indirectly. For example, if a particular mutation results in changes in the brain that cause a small animal to stop moving and freeze when it perceives a novel stimulus, that animal is more likely to escape undetected when a predator passes nearby. This tendency makes the animal more likely to survive and produce offspring, thus passing on its genes to future generations.

Other mutations are not immediately favorable, but because they do not put their possessors at a disadvantage, they are inherited by at least some members of the species. As a result of thousands of such mutations, the members of a particular species possess a variety of genes and are all at least somewhat different from one another. Variety is a definite advantage for a species. Different environments provide optimal habitats for different kinds of organisms. When the environment changes, species must adapt or run the risk of becoming extinct. If some members of the species possess assortments of genes that provide characteristics that permit them to adapt to the new environment, their offspring will survive, and the species will continue.

Evolution of the Human Species

To *evolve* means to develop gradually (from the Latin *evolvere*, "to unroll"). The process of **evolution** is a gradual change in the structure and physiology of plant and animal species as a result of natural selection. New species evolve when organisms develop novel characteristics that can take advantage of unexploited opportunities in the environment.

The first vertebrates to emerge from the sea—some 360 million years ago—were amphibians. In fact, amphibians have not entirely left the sea; they still lay their eggs in water, and the larvae that hatch from them have gills and only later transform into adults with air-breathing lungs. Seventy million years later, the first reptiles appeared. Reptiles had a considerable advantage over amphibians: Their eggs, enclosed in a shell just porous enough to permit the developing embryo to breathe, could be laid on land. Thus, reptiles could inhabit regions away from bodies of water, and they could bury their eggs where predators would be less likely to find them. Reptiles soon divided into three lines: the *anapsids*, the ancestors of today's turtles; the *diapsids*, the ancestors of dinosaurs, birds, lizards, crocodiles, and snakes; and the *synapsids*, the ancestors of today's mammals. One group of synapsids, the *therapsids*, became the dominant land animal during the Permian period. Then, about 248 million years ago, the end of the Permian period was marked by a mass extinction. Dust from a catastrophic series of volcanic eruptions in present-day Siberia darkened the sky, cooled the earth, and wiped out approximately 95 percent of all animal species. Among those that survived was a small therapsid known as a

selective advantage A characteristic of an organism that permits it to produce more than the average number of offspring of its species.

evolution A gradual change in the structure and physiology of plant and animal species—generally producing more complex organisms—as a result of natural selection.

cynodont—the direct ancestor of the mammal, which first appeared about 220 million years ago. (See *Figure 1.10*.)

Mammals (and the other warm-blooded animals, birds) were only a modest success for many millions of years. Dinosaurs ruled, and mammals had to remain small and inconspicuous to avoid the large variety of agile and voracious predators. Then, around 65 million years ago, another mass extinction occurred. An enormous meteorite struck the Yucatan peninsula of present-day Mexico, producing a cloud of dust that destroyed many species, including the dinosaurs. Small, nocturnal mammals survived the cold and dark because they were equipped with insulating fur and a mechanism for maintaining their body temperature. The void left by the extinction of so many large herbivores and carnivores provided the opportunity for mammals to expand into new ecological niches, and expand they did.

The climate of the early Cenozoic period, which followed the mass extinction at the end of the Cretaceous period, was much warmer than it is today. Tropical forests covered much of the land areas, and in these forests our most direct ancestors, the primates, evolved. The first primates, like the first mammals, were small and preyed

FIGURE 1.10

Evolution of Vertebrate Species

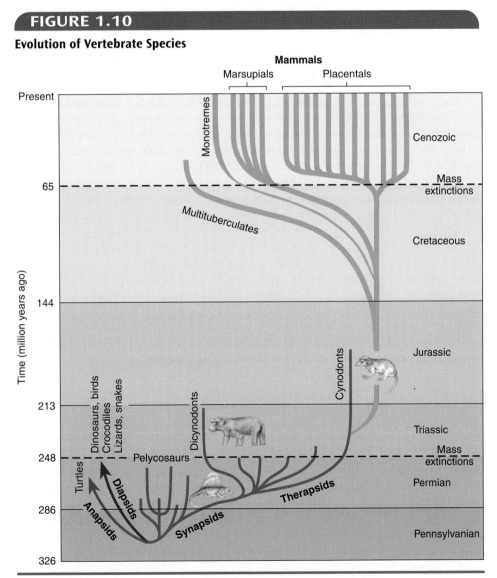

Adapted from Carroll, R. *Vertebrate Paleontology and Evolution*. New York: W. H. Freeman, 1988.

FIGURE 1.11

DNA Among Species of Hominids. This pyramid illustrates the percentage differences in DNA among the four major species of hominids.

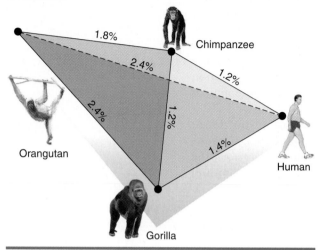

Redrawn from Lewin, R. *Human Evolution: An Illustrated Introduction.* Boston: Blackwell Scientific Publications, 1993. Reprinted with permission by Blackwell Science Ltd.

on insects and small cold-blooded vertebrates such as lizards and frogs. They had grasping hands that permitted them to climb about in small branches of the forest. Over time, larger species developed, with larger, forward-facing eyes (and the brains to analyze what the eyes saw), which facilitated arboreal locomotion and the capture of prey. As fruit-bearing plants evolved, primates began to exploit this energy-rich source of food, and the evolution of color vision enabled them to easily distinguish ripe and unripe fruit.

The first *hominids* (humanlike apes) appeared in Africa. They appeared not in dense tropical forests, but in drier woodlands and in the savanna—vast areas of grasslands studded with clumps of trees and populated by large herbivorous animals and the carnivores that preyed on them. Our fruit-eating ancestors continued to eat fruit, of course, but they evolved characteristics that enabled them to gather roots and tubers as well, to hunt and kill game, and to defend themselves against other predators. They made tools that could be used to hunt, produce clothing, and construct dwellings; they discovered the many uses of fire; they domesticated dogs, which greatly increased their ability to hunt and helped warn of attacks by predators; and they developed the ability to communicate symbolically, by means of spoken words.

Our closest living relatives—the only hominids besides ourselves who have survived—are the chimpanzees, gorillas, and orangutans. DNA analysis shows that genetically there is very little difference between these four species. For example, humans and chimpanzees share 98.8 percent of their DNA. (See *Figure 1.11*.)

The first hominid to leave Africa did so around 1.7 million years ago. This species, *Homo erectus* ("upright man"), scattered across Europe and Asia. One branch of *Homo erectus* appears to be the ancestor of *Homo neanderthalis*, which inhabited Western Europe between 120,000 and 30,000 years ago. Neanderthals resembled modern humans. They made tools out of stone and wood and discovered the use of fire. Our own species, *Homo sapiens*, evolved in East Africa around 100,000 years ago. They migrated to other parts of Africa, and out of Africa to Asia, Polynesia, Australia, Europe, and the Americas. They encountered the Neanderthals in Europe around 40,000 years ago and coexisted with them for approximately 10,000 years. Eventually, the Neanderthals disappeared—perhaps through interbreeding with *Homo sapiens*, perhaps through competition for resources. Scientists have not found evidence for warlike conflict between the two species.

Evolution of Large Brains

Our early humans ancestors possessed several characteristics that enabled them to compete with other species. Their agile hands enabled them to make and use tools. Their excellent color vision helped them to spot ripe fruit, game animals, and dangerous predators. Their mastery of fire enabled them to cook food, provide warmth, and frighten nocturnal predators. Their upright posture and bipedalism made it possible for them to walk long distances efficiently, with their eyes far enough from the ground to see long distances across the plains. Bipedalism also permitted them to carry tools and food with them, which meant that they could bring fruit, roots, and pieces of meat back to their tribe. Their linguistic abilities enabled them to combine the collective knowledge of all the members of the tribe, to make plans, to pass information on to subsequent generations, and to form complex civilizations that established their status as the dominant species. All of these characteristics required a larger brain.

A large brain requires a large skull, and an upright posture limits the size of a woman's birth canal. A newborn baby's head is about as large as it can be. As it is, the birth of a baby is much more arduous than the birth of mammals with proportionally smaller heads, including those of our closest primate relatives. Because a baby's brain is not large or complex enough to perform the physical and intellectual abilities of an adult, it must continue to grow after the baby is born. In fact, all mammals (and all birds, for that matter) require parental care for a period of time while the nervous system develops. The fact that young mammals (and, particularly, young humans) are guaranteed to be exposed to the adults who care for them means that a period of apprenticeship is possible. Consequently, the evolutionary process did not have to produce a brain that consisted solely of specialized circuits of nerve cells that performed specialized tasks. Instead, it could simply produce a larger brain with an abundance of neural circuits that could be modified by experience. Adults would nourish and protect their offspring and provide them with the skills they would need as adults. Some specialized circuits were necessary, of course (for example, those involved in analyzing the complex sounds we use for speech), but by and large, the brain is a general-purpose, programmable computer.

What types of genetic changes are required to produce a larger brain? This question will be addressed in greater detail in Chapter 3, but the most important principle appears to be a slowing of the process of maturation, allowing more time for growth. As we will see, the prenatal period of cell division in the brain is prolonged in humans, which results in a brain weighing an average of 350 g and containing approximately 100 billion neurons. After birth, the brain continues to grow. Production of new neurons almost ceases, but those that are already present grow and establish connections with each other, and other types of brain cells, which protect and support neurons, begin to proliferate. Not until late adolescence does the human brain reaches its adult size of approximately 1400 g—about four times the weight of a newborn's brain. This prolongation of maturation is known as **neoteny** (roughly translated as "extended youth"). The mature human head and brain retain some infantile characteristics, including their disproportionate size relative to the rest of the body. Figure 1.12 shows fetal and adult skulls of chimpanzees and humans. As you can see, the fetal skulls are much more similar than those of the adults. The grid lines show the pattern of growth, indicating much less change in the human skull from birth to adulthood. (See *Figure 1.12*.)

neoteny A slowing of the process of maturation, allowing more time for growth; an important factor in the development of large brains.

FIGURE 1.12

Neoteny in Evolution of the Human Skull.   The skulls of fetal humans and chimpanzees are much more similar than are those of the adults. The grid lines show the pattern of growth, indicating much less change in the human skull from birth to adulthood.

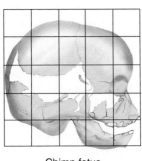
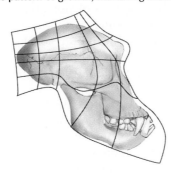
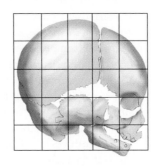
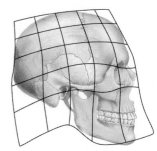

Chimp fetus   Chimp adult   Human fetus   Human adult

Redrawn from Lewin, R. *Human Evolution: An Illustrated Introduction*, 3rd ed. Boston: Blackwell Scientific Publications, 1993. Reprinted with permission by Blackwell Science Ltd.

InterimSummary

Natural Selection and Evolution

Darwin's theory of evolution, which was based on the concept of natural selection, provided an important contribution to modern behavioral neuroscience. The theory asserts that we must understand the functions performed by an organ or body part or by a behavior. Through random mutations, changes in an individual's genetic material cause different proteins to be produced, which results in the alteration of some physical characteristics. If the changes confer a selective advantage on the individual, the new genes will be transmitted to more and more members of the species. Even behaviors can evolve through the selective advantage of alterations in the structure of the nervous system.

Amphibians emerged from the sea 360 million years ago. One branch, the therapsids, became the dominant land animal until a catastrophic series of volcanic eruptions wiped out most animal species. A small therapsid, the cynodont, survived the disaster and became the ancestor of the mammals. The earliest mammals were small, nocturnal insectivores who lived in trees. They remained small and inconspicuous until the extinction of the dinosaurs, which occurred around 65 million years ago. The vacant ecological niches were quickly filled by mammals. Primates also began as small, nocturnal, tree-dwelling insectivores. Larger fruit-eating primates, with forward-facing eyes and larger brains, eventually evolved.

The first hominids appeared in Africa around 25 million years ago, eventually evolving into four major species: orangutans, gorillas, chimpanzees, and humans. Our ancestors acquired bipedalism around 3.7 million years ago and discovered toolmaking around 2.5 million years ago. The first hominids to leave Africa, *Homo erectus*, did so around 1.7 million years ago and scattered across Europe and Asia. *Homo neanderthalis* evolved in Western Europe, eventually to be replaced by *Homo sapiens*, which evolved in Africa around 100,000 years ago and spread throughout the world. By 30,000 years ago, *Homo sapiens* had replaced *Homo neanderthalis*.

The evolution of large brains made possible the development of toolmaking, fire building, and language, which in turn permitted the development of complex social structures. Large brains also provided a large memory capacity and the abilities to recognize patterns of events in the past and to plan for the future. Because an upright posture limits the size of a woman's birth canal and therefore the size of the head that passes through it, much of the brain's growth must take place after birth, which means that children require an extended period of parental care. This period of apprenticeship enabled the developing brain to be modified by experience.

Although human DNA differs from that of chimpanzees by only 1.2 percent, our brains are more than three times larger, which means that a small number of genes is responsible for the increase in the size of our brains. These genes appear to retard the events that stop brain development, resulting in a phenomenon known as neoteny.

Thought Questions

1. What useful functions are provided by the fact that a human can be self-aware? How was this trait selected for during the evolution of our species?
2. Are you surprised that the difference in the DNA of humans and chimpanzees is only 1.2 percent? How do you feel about this fact?
3. If our species continues to evolve, what kinds of changes do you think might occur?

Ethical Issues in Research with Animals

Most of the research described in this book involves experimentation on living animals. Any time we use another species of animals for our own purposes, we should be sure that what we are doing is both humane and worthwhile. I believe that a good case can be made that research on the physiology of behavior qualifies on both counts. Humane treatment is a matter of procedure. We know how to maintain laboratory animals in good health in comfortable, sanitary conditions. We know how to administer anesthetics and analgesics so that animals do not suffer during or after surgery, and we know how to prevent infections with proper surgical procedures and the use of antibiotics. Most industrially developed societies have very strict regulations about the care of animals and require approval of the experimental procedures used on them. There is no excuse for mistreating animals in our care. In fact, the vast majority of laboratory animals *are* treated humanely.

We use animals for many purposes. We eat their meat and eggs, and we drink their milk; we turn their hides into leather; we extract insulin and other hormones from their organs to treat people's diseases; we train them to do useful work on farms or to entertain us. Even having a pet is a form of exploitation; it is we—not they—who decide that they will live in our homes. The fact is, we have been using other animals throughout the history of our species.

Pet owning causes much more suffering among animals than scientific research does. As Miller (1983) notes, pet owners are not required to receive permission from a board of experts that includes a veterinarian to house their pets, nor are they subject to periodic inspections to be sure that their homes are clean and sanitary, that their pets have enough space to exercise properly, or that their pets' diets are appropriate. Scientific researchers are. Miller also notes that fifty times more dogs and cats are killed by humane societies each year because they have been abandoned by former pet owners than are used in scientific research.

If a person believes that it is wrong to use another animal in any way, regardless of the benefits to humans, there is nothing anyone can say to convince him or her of the value of scientific research with animals. For this person the issue is closed from the very beginning. Moral absolutes cannot be settled logically; like religious beliefs, they can be accepted or rejected, but they cannot be proved or disproved. My arguments in support of scientific research with animals are based on an evaluation of the benefits the research has to humans. (We should also remember that research with animals often helps *other animals*; procedures used by veterinarians, as well as those used by physicians, come from such research.)

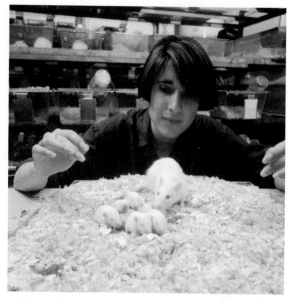

Unlike pet owners, scientists who use animals in their research must follow stringent regulations designed to ensure that the animals are properly cared for.

Before describing the advantages of research with animals, let me point out that the use of animals in research and teaching is a special target of animal rights activists. Nicholl and Russell (1990) examined twenty-one books written by such activists and counted the number of pages devoted to concern for different uses of animals. Next, they compared the relative concern the authors showed for these uses to the numbers of animals actually involved in each of these categories. The results indicate that the authors showed relatively little concern for animals used for food, hunting, or furs, or for those killed in pounds. In contrast, although only 0.3 percent of the animals are used for research and education, 63.3 percent of the pages were devoted to criticizing this use. In terms of pages per million animals used, the authors devoted 0.08 to food, 0.23 to hunting, 1.27 to furs, 1.44 to killing in pounds—and 53.2 to research and education. The authors showed 665 times more concern for research and education than for food and 231 times more than for hunting. Even the use of animals for furs (which consumes two-thirds as many animals as research and education) attracted 41.9 times less attention per animal.

The disproportionate amount of concern that animal rights activists show toward the use of animals in research and education is puzzling, particularly because this is the one *indispensable* use of animals. We *can* survive without eating animals, we *can* live without hunting, we *can* do without furs. But without using animals for research and for training future researchers, we *cannot* make progress in understanding and treating diseases. In not too many years, scientists probably will develop a vaccine that will prevent the further spread of AIDS. Some animal rights activists believe that preventing the deaths of laboratory animals in the pursuit of such a vaccine is a more worthy goal than preventing the deaths of millions of humans that will occur as a result of the disease if a vaccine is not found. Even diseases that we have already conquered would take new victims if drug companies could no longer use animals. If they were deprived of animals, these companies could no longer extract some of the hormones used to treat human diseases, and they could not prepare many of the vaccines that we now use to prevent them.

Our species is beset by medical, mental, and behavioral problems, many of which can be solved only through biological research. Let us consider some of the major neurological disorders. Strokes, caused by bleeding or occlusion of a blood vessel within the brain, often leave people partly paralyzed, unable to read, write, or converse with their friends and family. Basic research on the means by which nerve cells communicate with each other has led to important discoveries about the causes of the death of brain cells. This research was not directed toward a specific practical goal; the potential benefits actually came as a surprise to the investigators.

Experiments based on these results have shown that if a blood vessel leading to the brain is blocked for a few minutes, the part of the brain that is nourished by that vessel will die. However, the brain damage can be prevented by first administering a drug that interferes with a particular kind of neural communication. This research is important, because it may lead to medical treatments that can help to reduce the brain damage caused by strokes, however, it involves operating on a laboratory animal such as a rat and pinching off a blood vessel. (The animals are anesthetized, of course.) Some of the animals will sustain brain damage, and all will be killed so that their brains can be examined. However, you will probably agree that research like this is just as legitimate as using animals for food.

As you will learn later in this book, research with laboratory animals has produced important discoveries about the possible causes or potential treatments of neurological and mental disorders, including Parkinson's disease, schizophrenia, manic-depressive illness, anxiety disorders, obsessive-compulsive disorders, anorexia nervosa, obesity, and drug addictions. Although much progress has been made, these problems are still with us, and they cause much human suffering. Unless we continue our research with laboratory animals, the problems will not be solved. Some people have suggested that instead of using laboratory animals in our research, we could use tissue cultures or computers. Unfortunately, neither tissue cultures nor computers are substitutes for living organisms. We have no way to study behavioral problems such as addictions in tissue cultures, nor can we program a computer to simulate the workings of an animal's nervous system. (If we could, that would mean that we already had all the answers.)

This book will discuss some of the many important discoveries that have helped to reduce human suffering. For example, the discovery of a vaccine for polio, a serious disease of the nervous system, involved the use of rhesus monkeys. As you will learn in Chapter 4, Parkinson's disease, an incurable, progressive neurological disorder, has been treated for years with a drug called L-DOPA, discovered through animal research. Now, because of research with rats, mice, rabbits, and monkeys stimulated by the accidental poisoning of several young people with a contaminated batch of synthetic heroin, patients are being treated with a drug that may actually slow down the rate of brain degeneration. Researchers have hopes that a drug will be found to prevent the brain degeneration altogether.

The easiest way to justify research with animals is to point to actual and potential benefits to human health, as I have just done. However, we can also justify this research with a less-practical, but perhaps equally important, argument. One of the things that characterize our species is a quest for an understanding of our world. For example, astronomers study the universe and try to uncover its mysteries. Even if their discoveries never lead to practical benefits such as better drugs or faster methods of transportation, the fact that they enrich our understanding of the beginning and the fate of our universe justifies their efforts. The pursuit of knowledge is itself a worthwhile endeavor. Surely, the attempt to understand the universe within us—our nervous system, which is responsible for all that we are or can be—is also valuable.

Careers in Neuroscience

What is behavioral neuroscience, and what do behavioral neuroscientists do? By the time you finish this book, you will have as complete an answer as I can give to these questions, but perhaps it is worthwhile for me to describe the field and careers that are open to those who specialize in it before we begin our study in earnest.

Behavioral neuroscientists study all behavioral phenomena that can be observed in nonhuman animals. They attempt to understand the physiology of behavior: the role of the nervous system, interacting with the rest of the body (especially the endocrine system, which secretes hormones), in controlling behavior. They study such topics as sensory processes, sleep, emotional behavior, ingestive behavior, aggressive behavior, sexual behavior, parental behavior, and learning and memory. They also study animal models of disorders that afflict humans, such as anxiety, depression, obsessions and compulsions, phobias, psychosomatic illnesses, and schizophrenia.

Although the original name for the field described in this book was *physiological psychology*, several other terms are now in general use, such as *biological psychology*, *biopsychology*, *psychobiology*, and—the most common one—*behavioral neuroscience*. Most professional behavioral neuroscientists have received a Ph.D. from a graduate program in psychology or from an interdisciplinary program. (My own university awards a Ph.D. in neuroscience and behavior. The program includes faculty members from the departments of psychology, biology, biochemistry, and computer science.)

Behavioral neuroscience belongs to a larger field that is simply called *neuroscience*. Neuroscientists concern themselves with all aspects of the nervous system: its anatomy, chemistry, physiology, development, and functioning. The research of neuroscientists ranges from the study of molecular genetics to the study of social behavior. The field has grown enormously in the last few years; in 2009, the membership of the Society for Neuroscience was over thirty-eight thousand.

Most professional behavioral neuroscientists are employed by colleges and universities, where they are engaged in teaching and research. Others are employed by institutions devoted to research—for example, laboratories owned and operated by national governments or by private philanthropic organizations. A few work in industry, usually for pharmaceutical companies that are interested in assessing the effects of drugs on behavior. To become a professor or independent researcher, one must receive a doctorate—usually a Ph.D., although some people turn to research after receiving an M.D. Nowadays, most behavioral neuroscientists spend 2 years in a temporary postdoctoral position, working in the laboratory of a senior scientist to gain more research experience. During this time, they write articles describing their research findings and submit them for publication in scientific journals. These publications are an important factor in obtaining a permanent position.

Two other fields often overlap with that of behavioral neuroscience: *neurology* and *cognitive neuroscience*. Neurologists are physicians involved in the diagnosis and treatment of diseases of the nervous system. Most neurologists are solely involved in the practice of medicine, but a few engage in research devoted to advancing our understanding of the physiology of behavior. They study the behavior of people whose brains have been damaged by natural causes, using advanced brain-scanning devices to study the activity of various regions of the brain as a subject participates in various behaviors. Cognitive neuroscientists are scientists with a Ph.D. in psychology and specialized training in the principles and procedures of neurology—especially in the use of *functional imaging*, which permits them to measure activity of specific brain regions while people are engaging in various sensory, motor, or cognitive tasks. (Functional imaging is described in Chapter 5.)

Not all people who are engaged in neuroscience research have doctoral degrees. Many research technicians perform essential—and intellectually rewarding—services for the scientists with whom they work. Some of these technicians gain enough experience and education on the job to enable them to collaborate with their employers on their research projects rather than simply work for them.

behavioral neuroscientist (Also called *physiological psychologist*) A scientist who studies the physiology of behavior, primarily by performing physiological and behavioral experiments with laboratory animals.

InterimSummary

Ethical Issues in Research with Animals and Careers in Neuroscience

Research on the physiology of behavior necessarily involves the use of laboratory animals. It is incumbent on all scientists using these animals to see that they are housed comfortably and treated humanely, and laws have been enacted to ensure that they are. Such research has already produced many benefits to humankind and promises to continue to do so.

Behavioral neuroscience (originally called physiological psychology and also called biological psychology, biopsychology, and psychobiology) is a field devoted to our understanding of the physiology of behavior. Behavioral neuroscientists are allied with other scientists in the broader field of neuroscience. To pursue a career in behavioral neuroscience (or in the sister field of experimental neuropsychology), one must obtain a graduate degree and (usually) serve 2 years or more as a "postdoc"—a scientist pursuing further training.

Thought Question

Why do you think some people are apparently more upset about using animals for research and teaching than about using them for other purposes?

Strategies for Learning

The brain is a complicated organ. After all, it is responsible for all our abilities and all our complexities. Scientists have been studying this organ for a good many years and (especially in recent years) have been learning a lot about how it works. It is impossible to summarize this progress in a few simple sentences; therefore, this book contains a lot of information. I have tried to organize this information logically, telling you what you need to know in the order you need to know it. (After all, to understand some things, you need to understand other things first.) I have also tried to write as clearly as possible, making my examples as simple and as vivid as I can. Still, you cannot expect to master the information in this book by simply giving it a passive read; you will have to do some work.

Learning about the physiology of behavior involves much more than memorizing facts. Of course, there *are* facts to be memorized: names of parts of the nervous system, names of chemicals and drugs, scientific terms for particular phenomena and procedures used to investigate them, and so on. Still, the quest for information is nowhere near completed; we know only a small fraction of what we have to learn—and almost certainly, many of the "facts" that we now accept will someday be shown to be incorrect. If all you do is learn facts, where will you be when these facts are revised?

The antidote to obsolescence is knowledge of the process by which facts are obtained. In science, facts are the conclusions scientists make about their observations. If you learn only the conclusions, obsolescence is almost guaranteed. You will have to remember which conclusions are overturned and what the new conclusions are, and that kind of rote learning is hard to do. However, if you learn about the research strategies the scientists use, the observations they make, and the reasoning that leads to the conclusions, you will develop an understanding that is easily revised when new observations are made and new "facts" emerge. If you understand what lies behind the conclusions, then you can incorporate new information into what you already know and revise these conclusions yourself.

In recognition of these realities about learning, knowledge, and the scientific method, this book presents not just a collection of facts, but also a description of the procedures, experiments, and logical reasoning that scientists have used in their attempt to understand the physiology of behavior. If, in the interest of expediency, you focus on the conclusions and ignore the process that leads to them, you run the risk of acquiring information that will quickly become obsolete. On the other hand, if you try to understand the experiments and see how the conclusions follow from the results, you will acquire knowledge that lives and grows.

Now let me offer some practical advice about studying. You have been studying throughout your academic career, and you have undoubtedly learned some useful strategies along the way. Even if you have developed efficient and effective study skills, at least consider the possibility that there might be some ways to improve them.

If possible, the first reading of the assignment should be as uninterrupted as you can make it; that is, read the chapter without worrying much about remembering details. Next, after the first class meeting devoted to the topic, read the assignment again in earnest. Use a pen or pencil as you go, making notes. *Don't use a highlighter.* Sweeping the felt tip of a highlighter across some words on a page provides some instant gratification; you can even imagine that the highlighted words are somehow being transferred to your knowledge base. You have selected what is important, and when you review the reading assignment you have only to read the highlighted words. But this is an illusion.

Be active, not passive. Force yourself to write down whole words and phrases. The act of putting the information into your own words will not only give you something to study shortly before the next exam but also put something into your head (which is helpful at exam time). Using a highlighter puts off the learning until a later date; rephrasing the information in your own words starts the learning process *right then.*

A good way to get yourself to put the information into your own words (and thus into your own brain) is to answer the questions in the study guide. If you cannot answer a question, look up the answer in the book, *close the book*, and write the answer down. The phrase *close the book* is important. If you *copy* the answer, you will get very little out of the exercise. However, if you make yourself remember the information long enough to write it down, you have a good chance of remembering it later. The importance of the study guide is *not* to have a set of short answers in your own handwriting that you can study before the quiz. The behaviors that lead to long-term learning are doing enough thinking about the material to summarize it in your own words, then going through the mechanics of writing those words down.

Before you begin reading the next chapter, let me say a few things about the design of the book that might help you with your studies. The text and illustrations are integrated as closely as possible. In my experience, one of the most annoying aspects of reading some books is not knowing when to look at an illustration. Therefore, in this book you will find figure references in boldfaced italics (like this: ***Figure 5.6***), which means "stop reading and look at the figure." These references appear in locations I think will be optimal. If you look away from the text then, you will be assured that you will not be interrupting a line of reasoning in a crucial place and will not have to reread several sentences to get going again. You will find sections like this: "Figure 4.1 shows an alligator and a human. This alligator is certainly laid out in a linear fashion; we can draw a straight line that starts between its eyes and continues down the center of its spinal cord. (See ***Figure 4.1***.)" This particular example is a trivial one and will give you no problems no matter when you look at the figure, but in other cases the material is more complex, and you will have less trouble if you know what to look for before you stop reading and examine the illustration.

You will notice that some words in the text are *italicized* and others are printed in **boldface**. Italics mean one of two things: Either the word is being stressed for emphasis and is not a new term, or I am pointing out a new term that is not necessary for you to learn. On the other hand, a word in boldface is a new term that you should try to learn. Most of the boldfaced terms in the text are part of the vocabulary of behavioral neuroscience. Often, they will be used again in a later chapter. As an aid to your studying, definitions of these terms are printed in the margin of the page, along with pronunciation guides for those terms whose pronunciation is not obvious. In addition, a comprehensive index at the end of the book provides a list of terms and topics, with page references.

At the end of each major section (there are usually three to five of them in a chapter) you will find an *Interim Summary*, which provides a place for you to stop and think again about what you have just read to make sure that you understand the direction in which the discussion has gone. Many interim summaries are followed by some thought questions, which may serve to stimulate your thoughts about what you have learned and apply them to questions that have not yet been answered. Taken together, these sections provide a detailed summary of the information introduced in the chapter. My students tell me that they review the interim summaries just before taking a test.

Okay, the preliminaries are over. The next chapter starts with something you can sink your (metaphorical) teeth into: the structure and functions of neurons, the most important elements of the nervous system.

EPILOGUE   Models of Brain Functions

René Descartes had no way to study the operations of the nervous system. He did, however, understand how the statues in the Royal Gardens at Saint-Germain were powered and controlled, which led him to view the body as a complicated piece of plumbing. Many scientists have followed Descartes's example, using technological devices that were fashionable at the time to explain how the brain worked.

What motivates people to use artificial devices to explain the workings of the brain? The most important reason, I suppose, is that the brain is enormously complicated. Even the most complex human inventions are many times simpler than the brain, and because they have been designed and made by people, people can understand them. If an artificial device can do some of the things that the brain does, then perhaps both the brain and the device accomplish their tasks in the same way.

Most models of brain function developed in the last half of the twentieth century have been based on the modern, general-purpose digital computer. Actually, they have been based not on the computers themselves but on computer *programs*. Computers can be programmed to store any kind of information that can be coded in numbers or words, can solve any logical problem that can be explicitly described, and can compute any mathematical equations that can be written. Therefore, in principle at least, they can be programmed to do the things we do: perceive, remember, make deductions, solve problems.

The construction of computer programs that simulate human brain functions can help to clarify the nature of these functions. For instance, to construct a program and simulate, say, perception and classification of certain types of patterns, the investigator is forced to specify precisely what is required by the task of pattern perception. If the program fails to recognize the patterns, then the investigator knows that something is wrong with the model or with the way it has been implemented in the program. The investigator revises the model, tries again, and keeps working until it finally works (or until he or she gives up the task as being too ambitious).

Ideally, this task tells the investigator the kinds of processes the brain must perform. However, there is usually more than one way to accomplish a particular goal; critics of computer modeling have pointed out that it is possible to write a program that performs a task that the human brain performs and comes up with exactly the same results but does the task in an entirely different way. In fact, some say, given the way that computers work and what we know about the structure of the human brain, the computer program is *guaranteed* to work differently.

When we base a model of brain functions on a physical device with which we are familiar, we enjoy the advantage of being able to think concretely about something that is difficult to observe. However, if the brain does not work like a computer, then our models will not tell us very much about the brain. Such models are *constrained* ("restricted") by the computer metaphor; they will be able to do things only the way that computers can do them. If the brain can actually do some different sorts of things that computers cannot do, the models will never contain these features.

In fact, computers and brains are fundamentally different. Modern computers are *serial devices*; they work one step at a time. (*Serial*, from the Latin *sererei* "to join," refers to events that occur in order, one after the other.) Programs consist of a set of instructions stored in the computer's memory. The computer follows these instructions, one at a time. Because each of these steps takes time, a complicated program will take more time to execute. But we do some things extremely quickly that computers take a very long time to do. The best example is visual perception. We can recognize a complex figure about as quickly as a simple one; for example, it takes about the same amount of time to recognize a friend's face as it does to identify a simple triangle. The same is not true at all for a serial computer. A computer must "examine" the scene through an input device something like a video camera. Information about the brightness of each point of the picture must be converted into a number and stored in a memory location. Then the program examines each memory location, one at a time, and does calculations that determine the locations of

: PROLOGUE Unresponsive Muscles

Kathryn D. was getting desperate. All her life she had been healthy and active, eating wisely and keeping fit with sports and regular exercise. She went to her health club almost every day for a session of low-impact aerobics, followed by a swim. But several months ago, she began having trouble keeping up with her usual schedule. At first, she found herself getting tired toward the end of her aerobics class. Her arms, particularly, seemed to get heavy. Then when she entered the pool and started swimming, she found that it was hard to lift her arms over her head; she abandoned the crawl and the backstroke and did the sidestroke and breaststroke instead. She did not have any flulike symptoms, so she told herself that she needed more sleep and perhaps she should eat a little more.

Over the next few weeks, however, things only got worse. Aerobics classes were becoming an ordeal. Her instructor became concerned and suggested that Kathryn see her doctor. She did so, but he could find nothing wrong with her. She was not anemic, showed no signs of an infection, and seemed to be well nourished. He asked how things were going at work.

"Well, lately I've been under some pressure," she said. "The head of my department quit a few weeks ago, and I've taken over his job temporarily. I think I have a chance of getting the job permanently, but I feel as if my bosses are watching me to see whether I'm good enough for the job." Kathryn and her physician agreed that increased stress could be the cause of her problem. "I'd prefer not to give you any medication at this time," he said, "but if you don't feel better soon, we'll have a closer look at you."

She *did* feel better for a while, but then all of a sudden her symptoms got worse. She quit going to the health club and found that she even had difficulty finishing a day's work. She was certain that people were noticing that she was no longer her lively self, and she was afraid that her chances for the promotion were slipping away. One afternoon she tried to look up at the clock on the wall and realized that she could hardly see—her eyelids were drooping, and her head felt as if it weighed a hundred pounds. Just then, one of her supervisors came over to her desk, sat down, and asked her to fill him in on the progress she had been making on a new project. As she talked, she found herself getting weaker and weaker. Her jaw was getting tired, even her tongue was getting tired, and her voice was getting weaker. With a sudden feeling of fright she realized that the act of breathing seemed to take a lot of effort. She managed to finish the interview, but immediately afterwards, she packed up her briefcase and left for home, saying that she had a bad headache.

She telephoned her physician, who immediately arranged for her to go to the hospital to be seen by Dr. T., a neurologist. Dr. T. listened to a description of her symptoms and examined her briefly. She said to Kathryn, "I think I know what may be causing your symptoms. I'd like to give you an injection and watch your reaction." She gave some orders to the nurse, who left the room and came back with a syringe. Dr. T. took it, swabbed Kathryn's arm, and injected the drug. She started questioning Kathryn about her job. Kathryn answered slowly, her voice almost a whisper. As the questions continued, she realized that it was getting easier and easier to talk. She straightened her back and took a deep breath. Yes, she was sure. Her strength was returning! She stood up and raised her arms above her head. "Look," she said, her excitement growing. "I can do this again. I've got my strength back! What was that you gave me? Am I cured?"

(For an answer to her question, see p. 54.)

The brain is the organ that moves the muscles. That might sound simplistic, but ultimately, movement—or, more accurately, behavior—is the primary function of the nervous system. To make useful movements, the brain must know what is happening outside, in the environment. Thus, the body also contains cells that are specialized for detecting environmental events. Of course, complex animals such as we do not react automatically to events in our environment; our brains are flexible enough that we behave in different ways, according to present circumstances and those we experienced in the past. Besides perceiving and acting, we can remember and decide. All these abilities are made possible by the billions of cells found in the nervous system or controlled by them.

This chapter describes the structure and functions of the most important cells of the nervous system. Information, in the form of light, sound waves, odors, tastes, or contact with objects, is gathered from the environment by specialized cells called **sensory neurons**. Movements are accomplished by the contraction of muscles, which are controlled by **motor neurons**. (The term *motor* is used here in its original sense to refer to movement, not to a mechanical engine.) In between sensory neurons and motor neurons come the **interneurons**—neurons that lie entirely within the central nervous system. *Local interneurons* form circuits with

sensory neuron A neuron that detects changes in the external or internal environment and sends information about these changes to the central nervous system.

motor neuron A neuron located within the central nervous system that controls the contraction of a muscle or the secretion of a gland.

interneuron A neuron located entirely within the central nervous system.

nearby neurons and analyze small pieces of information. *Relay interneurons* connect circuits of local interneurons in one region of the brain with those in other regions. Through these connections, circuits of neurons throughout the brain perform functions essential to tasks such as perceiving, learning, remembering, deciding, and controlling complex behaviors. How many neurons are there in the human nervous system? The most common estimate is around 100 billion, but no one has counted them yet.

To understand how the nervous system controls behavior, we must first understand its parts—the cells that compose it. Because this chapter deals with cells, you need not be familiar with the structure of the nervous system, which is presented in Chapter 3. However, you need to know that the nervous system consists of two basic divisions: the central nervous system and the peripheral nervous system. The **central nervous system (CNS)** consists of the parts that are encased by the bones of the skull and spinal column: the brain and the spinal cord. The **peripheral nervous system (PNS)** is found outside these bones and consists of the nerves and most of the sensory organs.

Cells of the Nervous System

The first part of this chapter is devoted to a description of the most important cells of the nervous system—neurons and their supporting cells—and to the blood–brain barrier, which provides neurons in the central nervous system with chemical isolation from the rest of the body.

Neurons

Basic Structure

The neuron (nerve cell) is the information-processing and information-transmitting element of the nervous system. Neurons come in many shapes and varieties, according to the specialized jobs they perform. Most neurons have, in one form or another, the following four structures or regions: (1) cell body or soma; (2) dendrites; (3) axon; and (4) terminal buttons. (*MyPsychKit 2.1, Neurons and Supporting Cells*, illustrates the information presented in the following section.)

Soma   The **soma** (cell body) contains the nucleus and much of the machinery that provides for the life processes of the cell. (See *Figure 2.1.*) Its shape varies considerably in different kinds of neurons.

Dendrites   *Dendron* is the Greek word for tree, and the **dendrites** of the neuron look very much like trees. (See *Figure 2.1.*) Neurons "converse" with one another, and dendrites serve as important recipients of these messages. The messages that pass from neuron to neuron are transmitted across the **synapse**, a junction between the terminal buttons (described later) of the sending cell and a portion of the somatic or dendritic membrane of the receiving cell. (The word *synapse* derives from the Greek *sunaptein*, "to join together.") Communication at a synapse proceeds in one direction: from the terminal button to the membrane of the other cell. (Like many general rules, this one has some exceptions. As we will see in Chapter 4, some synapses pass information in both directions.)

Axon   The **axon** is a long, slender tube, often covered by a *myelin sheath*. (The myelin sheath is described later.) The axon carries information from the cell body to the terminal buttons. (See *Figure 2.1.*) The basic message it carries is called an *action potential*. This function is an important one and will be described in greater detail later in the chapter. For now, it suffices to say that an action potential is a brief electrical/chemical event that starts at the end of the axon next to the cell body and travels toward the terminal buttons. The action potential is like a brief pulse; in a given axon the action potential is always of the same size and duration. When it reaches a

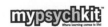

Animation 2.1
Neurons and Supporting Cells

central nervous system (CNS) The brain and spinal cord.

peripheral nervous system (PNS) The part of the nervous system outside the brain and spinal cord, including the nerves attached to the brain and spinal cord.

soma The cell body of a neuron, which contains the nucleus.

dendrite A branched, treelike structure attached to the soma of a neuron; receives information from the terminal buttons of other neurons.

synapse A junction between the terminal button of an axon and the membrane of another neuron.

axon The long, thin, cylindrical structure that conveys information from the soma of a neuron to its terminal buttons.

FIGURE 2.1

The Principal Parts of a Multipolar Neuron

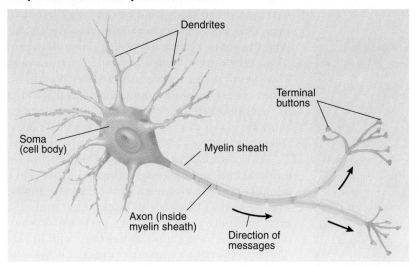

Dendrites

Terminal buttons

Soma (cell body)

Myelin sheath

Axon (inside myelin sheath)

Direction of messages

multipolar neuron A neuron with one axon and many dendrites attached to its soma.

bipolar neuron A neuron with one axon and one dendrite attached to its soma.

unipolar neuron A neuron with one axon attached to its soma; the axon divides, one branch receiving sensory information and the other sending the information into the central nervous system.

point where the axon branches, it splits but does not diminish in size. Each branch receives a *full-strength* action potential.

Like dendrites, axons and their branches come in different shapes. In fact, the three principal types of neurons are classified according to the way in which their axons and dendrites leave the soma. The neuron depicted in Figure 2.1 is the most common type found in the central nervous system; it is a **multipolar neuron**. In this type of neuron the somatic membrane gives rise to one axon but to the trunks of many dendritic trees. **Bipolar neurons** give rise to one axon and one dendritic tree, at opposite ends of the soma. (See *Figure 2.2a*.) Bipolar neurons are usually sensory; that is, their dendrites detect events occurring in the environment and communicate information about these events to the central nervous system.

The third type of nerve cell is the **unipolar neuron**. It has only one stalk, which leaves the soma and divides into two branches a short distance away. (See *Figure 2.2b*.) Unipolar neurons, like bipolar neurons, transmit sensory information from the environment to the CNS. The arborizations (treelike branches) outside the CNS are dendrites; the arborizations within the CNS end in terminal buttons. The dendrites of most unipolar neurons detect touch, temperature changes, and other sensory events that affect the skin. Other unipolar neurons detect events in our joints, muscles, and internal organs.

The CNS communicates with the rest of the body through nerves attached to the brain and to the spinal cord. Nerves are bundles of many thousands of individual fibers, all wrapped in a tough, protective membrane. Under a microscope, nerves look something like telephone cables, with their bundles of wires. (See *Figure 2.3*.) Like the individual wires in a telephone cable, nerve fibers transmit messages through the nerve, from a sense organ to the brain or from the brain to a muscle or gland.

FIGURE 2.2

Neurons.   Pictured here is (a) a bipolar neuron, primarily found in sensory systems (for example, vision and audition) and (b) a unipolar neuron, found in the somatosensory system (touch, pain, and the like).

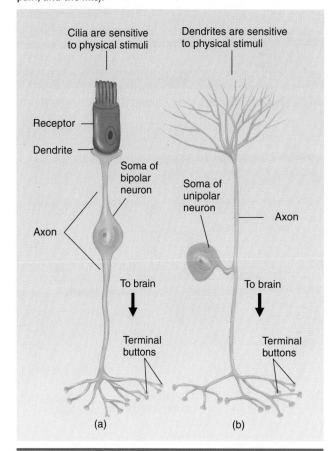

Cilia are sensitive to physical stimuli

Dendrites are sensitive to physical stimuli

Receptor

Dendrite

Soma of bipolar neuron

Soma of unipolar neuron

Axon

Axon

To brain

To brain

Terminal buttons

Terminal buttons

(a)

(b)

Nerves. A nerve consists of a sheath of tissue that encases a bundle of individual nerve fibers (also known as axons); BV = blood vessel; A = individual axons.

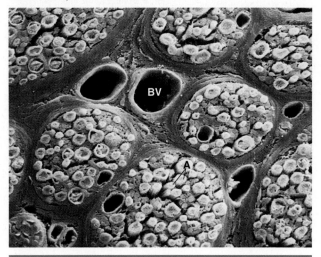

From *Tissues and Organs: A Text-Atlas of Scanning Electron Microscopy*, by Richard G. Kessel and Randy H. Kardon. Copyright © 1979 by W. H. Freeman and Co. Reprinted by permission of the authors.

terminal button The bud at the end of a branch of an axon; forms synapses with another neuron; sends information to that neuron.

neurotransmitter A chemical that is released by a terminal button; has an excitatory or inhibitory effect on another neuron.

Terminal Buttons Most axons divide and branch many times. At the ends of the twigs are found little knobs called **terminal buttons**. (Some neuroscientists prefer the original French word *bouton*, and others simply refer to them as *terminals*.) Terminal buttons have a very special function: When an action potential traveling down the axon reaches them, they secrete a chemical called a **neurotransmitter**. This chemical (there are many different ones in the CNS) either excites or inhibits the receiving cell and thus helps to determine whether an action potential occurs in its axon. Details of this process will be described later in this chapter.

An individual neuron receives information from the terminal buttons of axons of other neurons—and the terminal buttons of *its* axons form synapses with other neurons. A neuron may receive information from dozens or even hundreds of other neurons, each of which can form a large number of synaptic connections with it. Figure 2.4 illustrates the nature of these connections. As you can see, terminal buttons can form synapses on the membrane of the dendrites or the soma. (See *Figure 2.4.*)

Internal Structure

Figure 2.5 illustrates the internal structure of a typical multipolar neuron. (See *Figure 2.5.*) The **membrane** defines the boundary of the cell. It consists of a double layer of lipid (fatlike) molecules. Embedded in the membrane are a variety of protein molecules that have special functions. Some proteins detect substances outside the cell (such as hormones) and pass information about the presence of these substances to the interior of the cell. Other proteins control access to the interior of the cell, permitting some substances to enter but barring others. Still other proteins act as transporters, actively

An Overview of the Synaptic Connections Between Neurons. The arrows represent the directions of the flow of information.

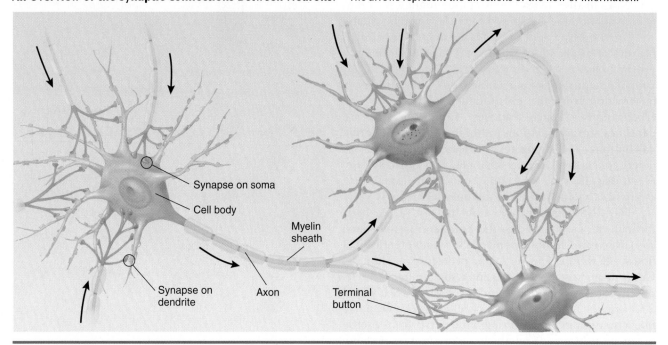

Synapse on soma

Cell body

Myelin sheath

Synapse on dendrite

Axon

Terminal button

carrying certain molecules into or out of the cell. Because the proteins that are found in the membrane of the neuron are especially important in the transmission of information, their characteristics will be discussed in greater detail later in this chapter.

The cell is filled with **cytoplasm**, a jellylike substance that contains small specialized structures, just as the body contains specialized organs. Among these structures are **mitochondria**, which break down nutrients such as glucose and provide the cell with energy to perform its functions. Mitochondria produce a chemical called **adenosine triphosphate (ATP)**, which can be used throughout the cell as an energy source. Many eons ago mitochondria were free-living organisms that came to "infect" larger cells. Because the mitochondria could extract energy more efficiently than their hosts, they became useful to them and eventually became a permanent part of them. Mitochondria still contain their own genetic information and multiply independently of the cells in which they live. We inherit our mitochondria from our mothers; fathers' sperms do not contribute any mitochondria to the ova they fertilize.

Deep inside the cell is the **nucleus** (from the Latin word for "nut"). The nucleus contains the chromosomes. **Chromosomes**, as you have probably already learned, consist of long strands of **deoxyribonucleic acid (DNA)**. The chromosomes have an important function: They contain the recipes for making proteins. Portions of the chromosomes, called **genes***, contain the recipes for individual proteins.

Proteins are important in cell functions. If a neuron grown in a tissue culture is exposed to a detergent, the lipid membrane and much of the interior of the cell dissolve away, leaving a matrix of insoluble strands of protein. This matrix, called the **cytoskeleton**, gives the neuron its shape. The cytoskeleton is made of various kinds of protein strands, linked to each other and forming a cohesive mass.

Besides providing structure, proteins serve as enzymes. **Enzymes** are the cell's marriage brokers or divorce judges: They cause particular molecules to join together or split apart. Thus, enzymes determine what gets made from the raw materials contained in the cell, and they determine which molecules remain intact.

Proteins are also involved in transporting substances within the cell. Axons can be extremely long, relative to their diameter and the size of the soma. For example, the longest axon in a human stretches from the foot to a region located in the base of the brain. Because terminal buttons need some items that can be produced only in the soma, there must be a system that can transport these items rapidly and efficiently through the axoplasm (that is, the cytoplasm of the axon). This system, **axoplasmic transport**, is an active process that propels substances from one end of the axon to the other. This transport is accomplished by long protein strands called **microtubules**, bundles of thirteen filaments arranged around a hollow core. Microtubules serve as railroad tracks, guiding the progress of the substances being transported. Movement from the soma to the terminal buttons is called *anterograde* axoplasmic transport. (*Antero-* means "toward the front.") *Retrograde* axoplasmic transport carries substances from the terminal buttons back to the soma. (*Retro-* means "toward the back.") Anterograde axoplasmic transport is remarkably fast: up to 500 mm per day. Retrograde axoplasmic transport is about

FIGURE 2.5

The Principal Internal Structures of a Multipolar Neuron

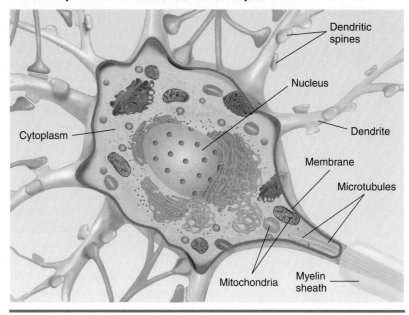

Dendritic spines

Nucleus

Cytoplasm

Dendrite

Membrane

Microtubules

Mitochondria

Myelin sheath

membrane A structure consisting principally of lipid molecules that defines the outer boundaries of a cell and also constitutes many of the cell organelles.

cytoplasm The viscous, semiliquid substance contained in the interior of a cell.

mitochondria An organelle that is responsible for extracting energy from nutrients.

adenosine triphosphate (ATP) (*ah deno seen*) A molecule of prime importance to cellular energy metabolism; its breakdown liberates energy.

nucleus A structure in the central region of a cell, containing the chromosomes.

chromosome A strand of DNA, with associated proteins, found in the nucleus; carries genetic information.

deoxyribonucleic acid (DNA) (*dee ox ee ry bo new clay ik*) A long, complex macromolecule consisting of two interconnected helical strands; along with associated proteins, strands of DNA constitute the chromosomes.

*Margin definitions for this and the following terms are on page 30.

half as fast. Energy for both forms of transport is supplied by ATP, produced by the mitochondria.

Supporting Cells

Neurons constitute only about half the volume of the CNS. The rest consists of a variety of supporting cells. Because neurons have a very high rate of metabolism but have no means of storing nutrients, they must constantly be supplied with nutrients and oxygen or they will quickly die. Thus, the role played by the cells that support and protect neurons is very important to our existence.

Glia

The most important supporting cells of the central nervous system are the *neuroglia*, or "nerve glue." **Glia** (also called *glial cells*) do indeed glue the CNS together, but they do much more than that. Neurons lead a very sheltered existence; they are buffered physically and chemically from the rest of the body by the glial cells. Glial cells surround neurons and hold them in place, controlling their supply of nutrients and some of the chemicals they need to exchange messages with other neurons; they insulate neurons from one another so that neural messages do not get scrambled; and they even act as housekeepers, destroying and removing the carcasses of neurons that are killed by disease or injury.

There are several types of glial cells, each of which plays a special role in the CNS. The three most important types are *astrocytes*, *oligodendrocytes*, and *microglia*. **Astrocyte** means "star cell," and this name accurately describes the shape of these cells. Astrocytes (or *astroglia*) provide physical support to neurons and clean up debris within the brain. They produce some chemicals that neurons need to fulfill their functions. They help to control the chemical composition of the fluid surrounding neurons by actively taking up or releasing substances whose concentrations must be kept within critical levels. Finally, astrocytes are involved in providing nourishment to neurons.

Some of the astrocyte's processes (the arms of the star) are wrapped around blood vessels. Other processes are wrapped around parts of neurons, so the somatic and dendritic membranes of neurons are largely surrounded by astrocytes. Evidence suggests that astrocytes receive nutrients from the capillaries, store them, and release them to neurons when needed (Tsacopoulos and Magistretti, 1996; Magistretti et al., 1999; Brown, Tekkök, and Ransom, 2003). Besides having a role in transporting chemicals to neurons, astrocytes serve as the matrix that holds neurons in place. These cells also surround and isolate synapses, limiting the dispersion of neurotransmitters that are released by the terminal buttons. (See *Figure 2.6*.)

When cells in the central nervous system die, certain kinds of astrocytes take up the task of cleaning away the debris. These cells are able to travel around the CNS; they extend and retract their processes (*pseudopodia*, or "false feet") and glide about the way amoebas do. When these astrocytes contact a piece of debris from a dead neuron, they push themselves against it, finally engulfing and digesting it. We call this process **phagocytosis** (*phagein*, "to eat"; *kutos*, "cell"). If there is a considerable amount of injured tissue to be cleaned up, astrocytes will divide and produce enough new cells to do the task. Once the dead tissue is broken down, a framework of astrocytes will be left to fill in the vacant area, and a specialized kind of astrocyte will form scar tissue, walling off the area.

The principal function of **oligodendrocytes** is to provide support to axons and to produce the **myelin sheath**, which insulates most axons from one another. (Very small axons are not myelinated and lack this sheath.) Myelin, 80 percent lipid and 20 percent protein, is produced by the oligodendrocytes in the form of a tube surrounding the axon. This tube does not form a continuous sheath; rather, it consists of a series of segments, each approximately 1 mm long, with a small (1–2 μm) portion of uncoated axon between the segments. (A *micrometer*, abbreviated μm, is one-millionth of a meter, or one-thousandth of a millimeter.) The bare portion of axon

gene The functional unit of the chromosome, which directs synthesis of one or more proteins. (See page 29.)

cytoskeleton Formed of microtubules and other protein fibers, linked to each other and forming a cohesive mass that gives a cell its shape. (See page 29.)

enzyme A molecule that controls a chemical reaction, combining two substances or breaking a substance into two parts. (See page 29.)

axoplasmic transport An active process by which substances are propelled along microtubules that run the length of the axon. (See page 29.)

microtubule (*my kro too byool*) A long strand of bundles of protein filaments arranged around a hollow core; part of the cytoskeleton and involved in transporting substances from place to place within the cell. (See page 29.)

glia (*glee ah*) The supporting cells of the central nervous system.

astrocyte A glial cell that provides support for neurons of the central nervous system, provides nutrients and other substances, and regulates the chemical composition of the extracellular fluid.

phagocytosis (*fagg o sy toe sis*) The process by which cells engulf and digest other cells or debris caused by cellular degeneration.

oligodendrocyte (*oh li go den droh site*) A type of glial cell in the central nervous system that forms myelin sheaths.

myelin sheath (*my a lin*) A sheath that surrounds axons and insulates them, preventing messages from spreading between adjacent axons.

FIGURE 2.6

Structure and Location of Astrocytes. The processes of astrocytes surround capillaries and neurons of the central nervous system.

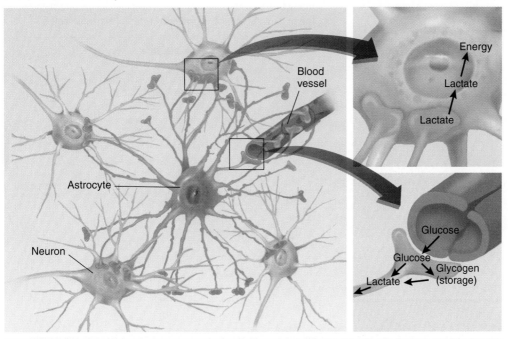

Blood vessel

Energy

Lactate

Lactate

Astrocyte

Neuron

Glucose

Glucose

Lactate

Glycogen (storage)

is called a **node of Ranvier**, after its discoverer. The myelinated axon, then, resembles a string of elongated beads. (Actually, the beads are *very much* elongated—their length is approximately eighty times their width.)

A given oligodendrocyte produces up to fifty segments of myelin. During the development of the CNS, oligodendrocytes form processes shaped something like canoe paddles. Each of these paddle-shaped processes then wraps itself many times around a segment of an axon and, while doing so, produces layers of myelin. Each paddle thus becomes a segment of an axon's myelin sheath. (See *Figures 2.7* and *2.8a*.)

As their name indicates, **microglia** are the smallest of the glial cells. Like some types of astrocytes, they act as phagocytes, engulfing and breaking down dead and dying neurons. In addition, they serve as one of the representatives of the immune system in the brain, protecting the brain from invading microorganisms. They are primarily responsible for the inflammatory reaction in response to brain damage.

Dr. C., a retired neurologist, had been afflicted with multiple sclerosis for more than two decades when she died of a heart attack. One evening, 23 years previously, she and her husband had had dinner at their favorite restaurant. As they were leaving, she stumbled and almost fell. Her husband joked, "Hey, honey, you shouldn't have had that last glass of wine." She smiled at his attempt at humor, but she knew better—her clumsiness wasn't brought on by the two glasses of wine she had drunk with dinner. She suddenly realized that she had been ignoring some symptoms that she should have recognized.

The next day, she consulted with one of her colleagues, who agreed that her own tentative diagnosis was probably correct: Her symptoms fit those of multiple sclerosis. She had experienced fleeting problems with double vision, she sometimes felt unsteady on her feet, and she occasionally noticed tingling sensations in her right hand. None of these symptoms was serious, and they lasted for only a short while, so she ignored them—or perhaps denied to herself that they were important.

A few weeks after Dr. C.'s death, a group of medical students and neurological residents gathered in an autopsy room at the medical school. Dr. D., the school's neuropathologist, displayed a

node of Ranvier (**raw** *vee ay*) A naked portion of a myelinated axon, between adjacent oligodendroglia or Schwann cells.

microglia The smallest of glial cells; act as phagocytes and protect the brain from invading microorganisms.

FIGURE 2.7

Oligodendrocyte.   An oligodendrocyte forms the myelin that surrounds many axons in the central nervous system. Each cell forms one segment of myelin for several adjacent axons.

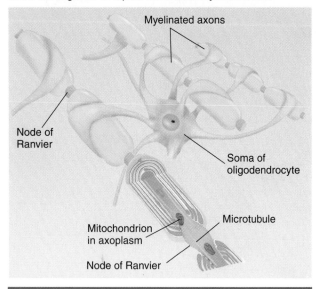

FIGURE 2.8

Formation of Myelin.   During development a process of an oligodendrocyte or an entire Schwann cell tightly wraps itself many times around an individual axon and forms one segment of the myelin sheath: (a) oligodendrocyte; (b) Schwann cell.

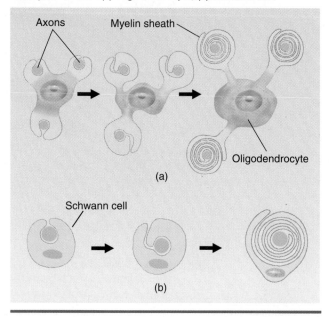

stainless-steel tray on which were lying a brain and a spinal cord. "These belonged to Dr. C.," he said. "Several years ago she donated her organs to the medical school." Everyone looked at the brain more intently, knowing that it had animated an esteemed clinician and teacher whom they all knew by reputation, if not personally. Dr. D. led his audience to a set of light boxes on the wall, to which several MRI scans had been clipped. He pointed out some white spots that appeared on one scan. "This scan clearly shows some white-matter lesions, but they are gone on the next one, taken 6 months later. And here is another one, but it's gone on the next scan. The immune system attacked the myelin sheaths in a particular region, and then glial cells cleaned up the debris. MRI doesn't show the lesions then, but the axons can no longer conduct their messages."

He picked up Dr. C.'s brain and cut it in several slices. He picked one up. "Here, see this?" He pointed out a spot of discoloration in a band of white matter. "This is a sclerotic plaque—a patch that feels harder than the surrounding tissue. There are many of them, located throughout the brain and spinal cord, which is why the disease is called multiple sclerosis." He picked up the spinal cord, felt along its length with his thumb and forefinger, and then stopped and said, "Yes, I can feel a plaque right here."

Dr. D. put the spinal cord down and said, "Who can tell me the etiology of this disorder?"

One of the students spoke up. "It's an autoimmune disease. The immune system gets sensitized to the body's own myelin protein and periodically attacks it, causing a variety of different neurological symptoms. Some say that a childhood viral illness somehow causes the immune system to start seeing the protein as foreign."

"That's right," said Dr. D. "The primary criterion for the diagnosis of multiple sclerosis is the presence of neurological symptoms disseminated in time and space. The symptoms don't all occur at once, and they can be caused only by damage to several different parts of the nervous system, which means that they can't be the result of a stroke."

Schwann cell   A cell in the peripheral nervous system that is wrapped around a myelinated axon, providing one segment of its myelin sheath.

Schwann Cells

In the central nervous system the oligodendrocytes support axons and produce myelin. In the peripheral nervous system the **Schwann cells** perform the same functions. Most axons in the PNS are myelinated. The myelin sheath occurs in segments, as it does in the CNS; each segment consists of a single Schwann cell, wrapped many times around the axon. In the CNS the oligodendrocytes grow a number of paddle-shaped processes that wrap around a number of axons. In the PNS a Schwann cell provides myelin for only one axon, and the entire Schwann cell—not merely a part of it—surrounds the axon. (See *Figure 2.8b*.)

There is an important difference between oligodendrocytes of the CNS and Schwann cells of the PNS: the chemical composition of the myelin protein they produce. The immune system of people with multiple sclerosis attacks only the myelin protein produced by oligodendrocytes; thus, the myelin of the peripheral nervous system is spared.

The Blood–Brain Barrier

Over 100 years ago, Paul Ehrlich discovered that if a blue dye is injected into an animal's bloodstream, all tissues except the brain and spinal cord will be tinted blue. However, if the same dye is injected into the fluid-filled ventricles of the brain, the blue color will spread throughout the CNS (Bradbury, 1979). This experiment demonstrates that a barrier exists between the blood and the fluid that surrounds the cells of the brain: the **blood–brain barrier**.

Some substances can cross the blood–brain barrier; others cannot. Thus, it is *selectively permeable* (from the Latin *per*, "through," and *meare*, "to pass"). In most of the body the cells that line the capillaries do not fit together absolutely tightly. Small gaps are found between them that permit the free exchange of most substances between the blood plasma and the fluid outside the capillaries that surrounds the cells of the body. In the central nervous system the capillaries lack these gaps; therefore, many substances cannot leave the blood. Thus, the walls of the capillaries in the brain constitute the blood–brain barrier. (See *Figure 2.9*.) Other substances must be actively transported through the capillary walls by special proteins. For example, glucose transporters bring the brain its fuel, and other transporters rid the brain of toxic waste products (Rubin and Staddon, 1999).

What is the function of the blood–brain barrier? As we will see, transmission of messages from place to place in the brain depends on a delicate balance between substances within neurons and in the extracellular fluid that surrounds them. If the composition of the extracellular fluid is changed even slightly, the transmission of these messages will be disrupted, which means that brain functions will be disrupted. The presence of the blood–brain barrier makes it easier to regulate the composition of this fluid. In addition, many of the foods that we eat contain chemicals that would interfere with the transmission of information between neurons. The blood–brain barrier prevents these chemicals from reaching the brain.

The blood–brain barrier is not uniform throughout the nervous system. In several places the barrier is relatively permeable, allowing substances that are excluded elsewhere to cross freely. For example, the **area postrema** is a part of the brain that controls vomiting. The blood–brain barrier is much weaker there, permitting neurons in this region to detect the presence of toxic substances in the blood. A poison that enters the circulatory system from the stomach can thus stimulate this area to initiate vomiting. If the organism is lucky, the poison can be expelled from the stomach before causing too much damage.

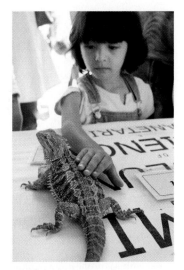

Touch, temperature changes, pain, and other sensory events that affect the skin are detected by the dendrites of unipolar neurons.

blood–brain barrier A semipermeable barrier between the blood and the brain produced by the cells in the walls of the brain's capillaries.

area postrema (*poss tree ma*) A region of the medulla where the blood–brain barrier is weak; poisons can be detected there and can initiate vomiting.

FIGURE 2.9

The Blood–Brain Barrier. This figure shows that (a) the cells that form the walls of the capillaries in the body outside the brain have gaps that permit the free passage of substances into and out of the blood and (b) the cells that form the walls of the capillaries in the brain are tightly joined.

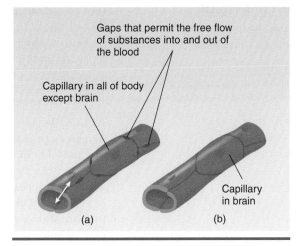

Gaps that permit the free flow of substances into and out of the blood

Capillary in all of body except brain

Capillary in brain

(a)   (b)

Interim Summary

Cells of the Nervous System

Neurons are the most important cells of the nervous system. The central nervous system (CNS) includes the brain and spinal cord; the peripheral nervous system (PNS) includes nerves and some sensory organs.

Neurons have four principal parts: dendrites, soma (cell body), axon, and terminal buttons. They communicate by means of synapses, junctions between the terminal buttons of one neuron and the somatic or dendritic membrane of another. When an action potential travels down an axon, its terminal buttons secrete a chemical that has either an excitatory or an inhibitory effect on the neurons with which they communicate. Ultimately, the effects of these excitatory and inhibitory synapses cause behavior, in the form of muscular contractions.

Neurons contain a quantity of clear cytoplasm, enclosed in a membrane. Embedded in the membrane are protein molecules that have special functions, such as the transport of particular substances into and out of the cell. The nucleus contains the genetic information—the recipes for the all the proteins that the body can make. Microtubules and other protein filaments compose the cytoskeleton and help to transport chemicals from place to place. Mitochondria serve as the location for most of the chemical reactions through which the cell extracts energy from nutrients.

Neurons are supported by the glial cells of the central nervous system and the supporting cells of the peripheral nervous system. In the CNS astrocytes provide support and nourishment, regulate the composition of the fluid that surrounds neurons, and remove debris and form scar tissue in the event of tissue damage. Microglia are phagocytes that serve as the representatives of the immune system. Oligodendrocytes form myelin, the substance that insulates axons, and also support unmyelinated axons. In the PNS, support and myelin are provided by the Schwann cells.

In most organs molecules freely diffuse between the blood within the capillaries that serve them and the extracellular fluid that bathes their cells. The molecules pass through gaps between the cells that line the capillaries. The walls of the capillaries of the CNS lack these gaps; consequently, fewer substances can enter or leave the brain across the blood–brain barrier.

Thought Question

The fact that the mitochondria in our cells were originally microorganisms that infected our very remote ancestors points out that evolution can involve interactions between two or more species. Many species have other organisms living inside them; in fact, the bacteria in our intestines are necessary for our good health. Some microorganisms can exchange genetic information, so adaptive mutations developed in one species can be adopted by another. Is it possible that some of the features of the cells of our nervous system were bequeathed to our ancestors by other species?

Communication Within a Neuron

This section describes the nature of communication *within* a neuron; the way an action potential is sent from the cell body down the axon to the terminal buttons, informing them to release some neurotransmitter. The details of synaptic transmission—the communication between neurons—will be described in the next section. As we will see in this section, an action potential consists of a series of alterations in the membrane of the axon that permit various substances to move between the interior of the axon and the fluid surrounding it. These exchanges produce electrical currents. (*MyPsychKit 2.2: The Action Potential*, illustrates the information presented in the following section.)

Animation 2.2
The Action Potential

Neural Communication: An Overview

Before I begin my discussion of the action potential, let's step back and see how neurons can interact to produce a useful behavior. We begin by examining a simple assembly of three neurons and a muscle that control a withdrawal reflex. In the next two figures (and in subsequent figures that illustrate simple neural circuits), multipolar neurons are depicted in shorthand fashion as several-sided stars. The points of these stars represent dendrites, and only one or two terminal buttons are shown at the end of the axon. The sensory neuron in this example detects painful stimuli. When its dendrites are stimulated by a noxious stimulus (such as contact with a hot object), it sends messages down the axon to the terminal buttons, which are located in the spinal cord. (You will recognize this cell as a unipolar neuron; see *Figure 2.10*.) The terminal buttons of the sensory neuron release a neurotransmitter that excites the interneuron, causing it to send messages down its axon. The terminal buttons of the interneuron release a neurotransmitter that excites the motor neuron, which sends messages down its axon. The axon of the motor neuron joins a nerve and travels to a muscle. When the terminal buttons of the motor neuron release their neurotransmitter, the muscle cells contract, causing the hand to move away from the hot object. (See *Figure 2.10*.)

So far, all of the synapses have had excitatory effects. Now let us complicate matters a bit to see the effect of inhibitory synapses. Suppose you have removed a hot casserole from the oven. As you start walking over to the table to put it down, the heat begins to penetrate the rather thin potholders you are using. The pain caused by the hot casserole triggers a withdrawal reflex that tends to make you drop it, yet you manage to keep hold of it long enough to get to the table and put it down. What prevented your withdrawal reflex from making you drop the casserole on the floor?

The pain from the hot casserole increases the activity of excitatory synapses on the motor neurons, which tends to cause the hand to pull away from the casserole. However, this excitation is counteracted by *inhibition*, supplied by another source: the brain. The brain contains neural circuits that recognize what a disaster it would be if you dropped the casserole on the floor. These neural circuits send information to the spinal cord that prevents the withdrawal reflex from making you drop the dish.

Figure 2.11 shows how this information reaches the spinal cord. As you can see, an axon from a neuron in the brain reaches the spinal cord, where its terminal buttons form synapses with an inhibitory interneuron. When the neuron in the brain becomes active, its terminal buttons excite this inhibitory interneuron. The interneuron releases an inhibitory neurotransmitter, which *decreases* the activity of the motor neuron, blocking the withdrawal reflex. This circuit provides an example of a contest between two competing tendencies: to drop the casserole and to hold onto it. (See *Figure 2.11*.)

Of course, reflexes are more complicated than this description, and the mechanisms that inhibit them are even more so. Thousands of neurons are involved in this process. The five neurons shown in Figure 2.11 represent many others: Dozens

FIGURE 2.10

A Withdrawal Reflex.   The figure shows a simple example of a useful function of the nervous system. The painful stimulus causes the hand to pull away from the hot iron.

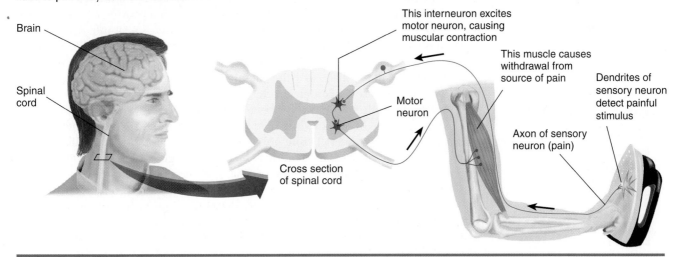

Brain

Spinal cord

Cross section of spinal cord

This interneuron excites motor neuron, causing muscular contraction

Motor neuron

This muscle causes withdrawal from source of pain

Dendrites of sensory neuron detect painful stimulus

Axon of sensory neuron (pain)

FIGURE 2.11

The Role of Inhibition. Inhibitory signals arising from the brain can prevent the withdrawal reflex from causing the person to drop the casserole.

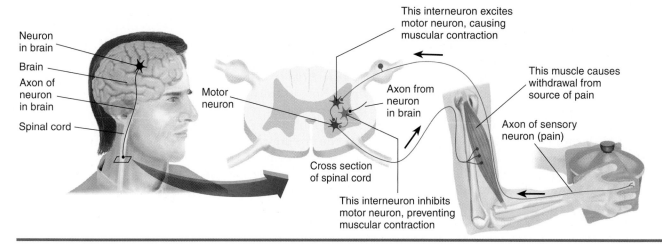

of sensory neurons detect the hot object, hundreds of interneurons are stimulated by their activity, hundreds of motor neurons produce the contraction—and thousands of neurons in the brain must become active if the reflex is to be inhibited, yet this simple model provides an overview of the process of neural communication, which is described in greater detail later in this chapter.

Measuring Electrical Potentials of Axons

Let's examine the nature of the message that is conducted along the axon. To do so, we obtain an axon that is large enough to work with. Fortunately, nature has provided the neuroscientist with the giant squid axon (the giant axon of a squid, not the axon of a giant squid!). This axon is about 0.5 mm in diameter, which is hundreds of times larger than the largest mammalian axon. (This large axon controls an emergency response: sudden contraction of the mantle, which squirts water through a jet and propels the squid away from a source of danger.) We place an isolated giant squid axon in a dish of seawater, in which it can exist for a day or two.

To measure the electrical charges generated by an axon, we will need to use a pair of electrodes. **Electrodes** are electrical conductors that provide a path for electricity to enter or leave a medium. One of the electrodes is a simple wire that we place in the seawater. The other one, which we use to record the message from the axon, has to be special. Because even a giant squid axon is rather small, we must use a tiny electrode that will record the membrane potential without damaging the axon. To do so, we use a microelectrode.

A **microelectrode** is simply a very small electrode, which can be made of metal or glass. In this case we will use one made of thin glass tubing, which is heated and drawn down to an exceedingly fine point, less than a thousandth of a millimeter in diameter. Because glass will not conduct electricity, the glass microelectrode is filled with a liquid that conducts electricity, such as a solution of potassium chloride.

We place the wire electrode in the seawater and insert the microelectrode into the axon. (See *Figure 2.12a*.) As soon as we do so, we discover that the inside of the axon is negatively charged with respect to the outside; the difference in charge being 70 mV (millivolts, or thousandths of a volt). Thus, the inside of the membrane is −70 mV. This electrical charge is called the **membrane potential**. The term

electrode A conductive medium that can be used to apply electrical stimulation or to record electrical potentials.

microelectrode A very fine electrode, generally used to record activity of individual neurons.

membrane potential The electrical charge across a cell membrane; the difference in electrical potential inside and outside the cell.

FIGURE 2.12

Measuring Electrical Charge.   The figure shows (a) a voltmeter detecting the charge across a membrane of an axon and (b) a light bulb detecting the charge across the terminals of a battery.

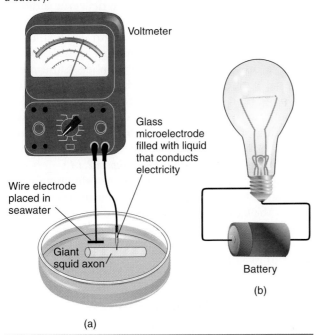

(a)

(b)

FIGURE 2.13

Studying the Axon.   The figure illustrates the means by which an axon can be stimulated while its membrane potential is being recorded.

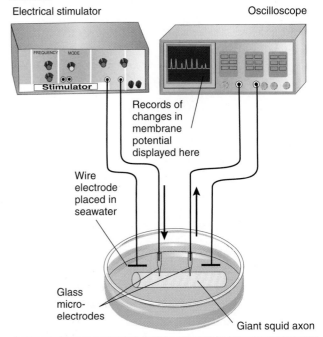

potential refers to a stored-up source of energy—in this case, electrical energy. For example, a flashlight battery that is not connected to an electrical circuit has a *potential* charge of 1.5 V between its terminals. If we connect a light bulb to the terminals, the potential energy is tapped and converted into radiant energy (light). (See ***Figure 2.12b.***) Similarly, if we connect our electrodes—one inside the axon and one outside it—to a very sensitive voltmeter, we will convert the potential energy to movement of the meter's needle. Of course, the potential electrical energy of the axonal membrane is very weak in comparison with that of a flashlight battery.

As we will see, the message that is conducted down the axon consists of a brief change in the membrane potential. However, this change occurs very rapidly—too rapidly for us to see if we were using a voltmeter. Therefore, to study the message, we will use an **oscilloscope**. This device, like a voltmeter, measures voltages, but it also produces a record of these voltages, graphing them as a function of time. These graphs are displayed on a screen, much like the one found in a television. The vertical axis represents voltage, and the horizontal axis represents time, going from left to right.

Once we insert our microelectrode into the axon, the oscilloscope draws a straight horizontal line at −70 mV, as long as the axon is not disturbed. This electrical charge across the membrane is called, quite appropriately, the **resting potential**. Now let us disturb the resting potential and see what happens. To do so, we will use another device: an electrical stimulator that allows us to alter the membrane potential at a specific location. (See ***Figure 2.13.***) The stimulator can pass current through another microelectrode that we have inserted into the axon. Because the inside of the axon is negative, a positive charge applied to the inside of the membrane produces a **depolarization**. That is, it takes away some of the electrical charge across the membrane near the electrode, reducing the membrane potential.

oscilloscope A laboratory instrument that is capable of displaying a graph of voltage as a function of time on the face of a cathode ray tube.

resting potential The membrane potential of a neuron when it is not being altered by excitatory or inhibitory postsynaptic potentials; approximately −70 mV in the giant squid axon.

depolarization Reduction (toward zero) of the membrane potential of a cell from its normal resting potential.

FIGURE 2.14

An Action Potential.   These results would be seen on an oscilloscope screen if depolarizing stimuli of varying intensities were delivered to the axon shown in Figure 2.13.

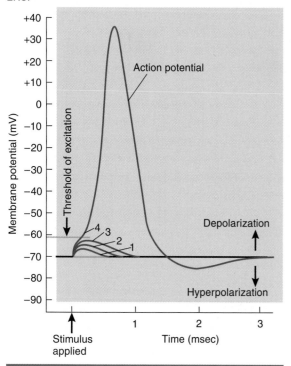

Let us see what happens to an axon when we artificially change the membrane potential at one point. Figure 2.14 shows a graph drawn by an oscilloscope that has been monitoring the effects of brief depolarizing stimuli. The graphs of the effects of these separate stimuli are superimposed on the same drawing so that we can compare them. We deliver a series of depolarizing stimuli, starting with a very weak stimulus (number 1) and gradually increasing their strength. Each stimulus briefly depolarizes the membrane potential a little more. Finally, after we present depolarization number 4, the membrane potential suddenly reverses itself, so that the inside becomes *positive* (and the outside becomes negative). The membrane potential quickly returns to normal, but first it overshoots the resting potential, becoming **hyperpolarized**—more polarized than normal—for a short time. The whole process takes about 2 msec (milliseconds). (See *Figure 2.14.*)

This phenomenon, a very rapid reversal of the membrane potential, is called the **action potential**. It constitutes the message carried by the axon from the cell body to the terminal buttons. The voltage level that triggers an action potential—which was achieved only by depolarizing shock number 4—is called the **threshold of excitation**.

The Membrane Potential: Balance of Two Forces

To understand what causes the action potential to occur, we must first understand the reasons for the existence of the membrane potential. As we will see, this electrical charge is the result of a balance between two opposing forces: diffusion and electrostatic pressure.

The Force of Diffusion

When a spoonful of sugar is poured carefully into a container of water, it settles to the bottom. After a time the sugar dissolves, but it remains close to the bottom of the container. After a much longer time (probably several days), the molecules of sugar distribute themselves evenly throughout the water, even if no one stirs the liquid. The process whereby molecules distribute themselves evenly throughout the medium in which they are dissolved is called **diffusion**.

When there are no forces or barriers to prevent them from doing so, molecules will diffuse from regions of high concentration to regions of low concentration. Molecules are constantly in motion, and their rate of movement is proportional to the temperature. Only at absolute zero [0 K (kelvin) = $-273.15°$C = $-459.7°$F] do molecules cease their random movement. At all other temperatures they move about, colliding and veering off in different directions, thus pushing one another away. The result of these collisions in the example of sugar and water is to force sugar molecules upward (and to force water molecules downward), away from the regions in which they are most concentrated.

The Force of Electrostatic Pressure

When some substances are dissolved in water, they split into two parts, each with an opposing electrical charge. Substances with this property are called **electrolytes**; the charged particles into which they decompose are called **ions**. Ions are of two basic types: *Cations* have a positive charge, and *anions* have a negative charge. For

hyperpolarization An increase in the membrane potential of a cell, relative to the normal resting potential.

action potential The brief electrical impulse that provides the basis for conduction of information along an axon.

threshold of excitation The value of the membrane potential that must be reached to produce an action potential.

diffusion Movement of molecules from regions of high concentration to regions of low concentration.

electrolyte An aqueous solution of a material that ionizes—namely, a soluble acid, base, or salt.

example, when sodium chloride (NaCl, table salt) is dissolved in water, many of the molecules split into sodium cations (Na^+) and chloride anions (Cl^-). (I find that the easiest way to keep the terms *cation* and *anion* straight is to think of the cation's plus sign as a cross and remember the superstition of a black *cat* crossing your path. A reader emailed another suggestion to me: "An ***anion* is *a n*egative *ion*.*")

As you have undoubtedly learned, particles with the same kind of charge repel each other (+ repels +, and − repels −), but particles with different charges are attracted to each other (+ and − attract). Thus, anions repel anions, cations repel cations, but anions and cations attract each other. The force exerted by this attraction or repulsion is called **electrostatic pressure**. Just as the force of diffusion moves molecules from regions of high concentration to regions of low concentration, electrostatic pressure moves ions from place to place: Cations are pushed away from regions with an excess of cations, and anions are pushed away from regions with an excess of anions.

Ions in the Extracellular and Intracellular Fluid

The fluid within cells (**intracellular fluid**) and the fluid surrounding them (**extracellular fluid**) contain different ions. The forces of diffusion and electrostatic pressure contributed by these ions give rise to the membrane potential. Because the membrane potential is produced by a balance between the forces of diffusion and electrostatic pressures, understanding what produces this potential requires that we know the concentration of the various ions in the extracellular and intracellular fluids.

There are several important ions in these fluids. I will discuss four of them here: organic anions (symbolized by A^-), chloride ions (Cl^-), sodium ions (Na^+), and potassium ions (K^+). The Latin words for sodium and potassium are *natrium* and *kalium*; hence, they are abbreviated *Na* and *K*, respectively. Organic anions—negatively charged proteins and intermediate products of the cell's metabolic processes—are found only in the intracellular fluid. Although the other three ions are found in both the intracellular and extracellular fluids, K^+ is found predominantly in the intracellular fluid, whereas Na^+ and Cl^- are found predominantly in the extracellular fluid. The sizes of the boxes in Figure 2.15 indicate the relative concentrations of these four ions. (See *Figure 2.15*.) The easiest way to remember which ion is found where is to recall that the fluid that surrounds our cells is similar to seawater, which is predominantly a solution of salt, NaCl. The primitive ancestors of our cells lived in the ocean; thus, the seawater was their extracellular fluid. Our extracellular fluid thus resembles seawater, produced and maintained by regulatory mechanisms that are described in Chapter 11.

Let's consider the ions in Figure 2.15, examining the forces of diffusion and electrostatic pressure exerted on each and reasoning why each is located where it is. A^-, the organic anion, is unable to pass through the membrane of the axon; therefore, although the presence of this ion within the cell contributes to the membrane potential, it is located where it is because the membrane is impermeable to it.

The potassium ion K^+ is concentrated within the axon; thus, the force of diffusion tends to push it out of the cell. However, the outside of the cell is charged positively with respect to the inside, so electrostatic pressure tends to force the cation inside. Thus, the two opposing forces balance, and potassium ions tend to remain where they are. (See *Figure 2.15*.)

The chloride ion Cl^- is in greatest concentration outside the axon. The force of diffusion pushes this ion inward. However, because the inside of the axon is negatively charged, electrostatic pressure pushes the anion outward. Again, two opposing forces balance each other. (See *Figure 2.15*.)

The sodium ion Na^+ is also in greatest concentration outside the axon, so it, like Cl^-, is pushed into the cell by the force of diffusion. However, unlike chloride, the sodium ion is *positively* charged, so electrostatic pressure does *not* prevent Na^+ from entering the cell; indeed, the negative charge inside the axon *attracts* Na^+. (See *Figure 2.15*.)

ion A charged molecule. *Cations* are positively charged, and *anions* are negatively charged.

electrostatic pressure The attractive force between atomic particles charged with opposite signs or the repulsive force between atomic particles charged with the same sign.

intracellular fluid The fluid contained within cells.

extracellular fluid Body fluids located outside of cells.

FIGURE 2.15

Control of the Membrane Potential.   The figure shows the relative concentration of some important ions inside and outside the neuron and the forces acting on them.

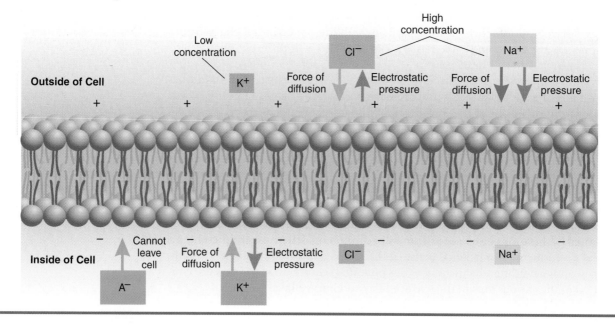

sodium–potassium transporter A protein found in the membrane of all cells that extrudes sodium ions from and transports potassium ions into the cell.

How can Na^+ remain in greatest concentration in the extracellular fluid, despite the fact that both forces (diffusion and electrostatic pressure) tend to push it inside? The answer is this: Another force continuously pushes Na^+ out of the axon. This force is provided by a large number of protein molecules embedded in the membrane, driven by energy provided by molecules of ATP produced by the mitochondria. These molecules, known as **sodium–potassium transporters**, exchange Na^+ for K^+, pushing three sodium ions out for every two potassium ions they push in. (See *Figure 2.16*.)

Because the membrane is not very permeable to Na^+, sodium–potassium transporters very effectively keep the intracellular concentration of Na^+ low. By transporting K^+ into the cell, they also increase the intracellular concentration of K^+ a small amount. The membrane is approximately 100 times more permeable to K^+ than to Na^+, so the increase is slight, but as we will see when we study the process of neural inhibition later in this chapter, it is very important. Sodium–potassium transporters use considerable energy: Up to 40 percent of a neuron's metabolic resources are used to operate them. Neurons, muscle cells, glia—in fact, most cells of the body—have sodium–potassium transporters in their membrane.

The Action Potential

As we saw, the forces of both diffusion and electrostatic pressure tend to push Na^+ into the cell. However, the membrane is not very permeable to this ion, and sodium–potassium

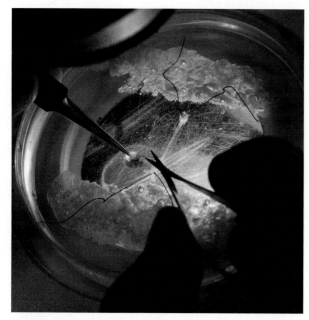

Using the giant axon of the squid, researchers discovered the nature of the message carried by axons.

transporters continuously pump out Na$^+$, keeping the intracellular level of Na$^+$ low. But imagine what would happen if the membrane suddenly became permeable to Na$^+$. The forces of diffusion and electrostatic pressure would cause Na$^+$ to rush into the cell. This sudden influx (inflow) of positively charged ions would drastically change the membrane potential. Indeed, experiments have shown that this mechanism is precisely what causes the action potential: A brief increase in the permeability of the membrane to Na$^+$ (allowing these ions to rush into the cell) is immediately followed by a transient increase in the permeability of the membrane to K$^+$ (allowing these ions to rush out of the cell). What is responsible for these transient increases in permeability?

We already saw that one type of protein molecule embedded in the membrane—the sodium–potassium transporter—actively pumps sodium ions out of the cell and pumps potassium ions into it. Another type of protein molecule provides an opening that permits ions to enter or leave the cells. These molecules provide **ion channels**, which contain passages ("pores") that can open or close. When an ion channel is open, a particular type of ion can flow through the pore and thus can enter or leave the cell. (See *Figure 2.17*.) Neural membranes contain many thousands of ion channels. For example, the giant squid axon contains several hundred sodium channels in each square micrometer of membrane. (There are one million square micrometers in a square millimeter; thus, a patch of axonal membrane the size of a lowercase letter "o" in this book would contain several hundred million sodium channels.) Each sodium channel can admit up to 100 million ions per second when it is open. Thus, the permeability of a membrane to a particular ion at a given moment is determined by the number of ion channels that are open.

The following numbered paragraphs describe the movements of ions through the membrane during the action potential. The numbers on the figure correspond to the numbers of the paragraphs that follow. (See *Figure 2.18*.)

ion channel A specialized protein molecule that permits specific ions to enter or leave cells.

FIGURE 2.16

A Sodium–Potassium Transporter, Situated in the Cell Membrane

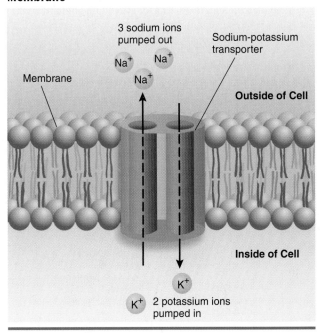

FIGURE 2.17

Ion Channels.   When ion channels are open, ions can pass through them, entering or leaving the cell.

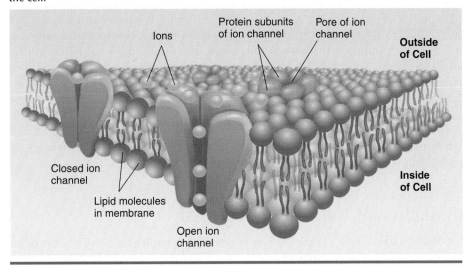

Ion Movements During the Action Potential.   The shaded box at the top shows the opening of sodium channels at the threshold of excitation, their refractory condition at the peak of the action potential, and their resetting when the membrane potential returns to normal.

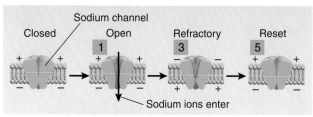

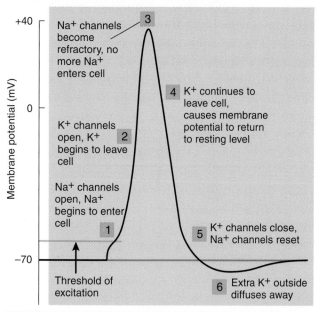

1. As soon as the threshold of excitation is reached, the sodium channels in the membrane open and Na$^+$ rushes in, propelled by the forces of diffusion and electrostatic pressure. The opening of these channels is triggered by reduction of the membrane potential (depolarization); they open at the point at which an action potential begins: the threshold of excitation. Because these channels are opened by changes in the membrane potential, they are called **voltage-dependent ion channels**. The influx of positively charged sodium ions produces a rapid change in the membrane potential, from -70 mV to $+40$ mV.

2. The membrane of the axon contains voltage-dependent potassium channels, but these channels are less sensitive than voltage-dependent sodium channels. That is, they require a greater level of depolarization before they begin to open. Thus, they begin to open later than the sodium channels.

3. About the time the action potential reaches its peak (in approximately 1 msec), the sodium channels become *refractory*—the channels become blocked and cannot open again until the membrane once more reaches the resting potential. At this time then, no more Na$^+$ can enter the cell.

4. By now, the voltage-dependent potassium channels in the membrane are open, letting K$^+$ ions move freely through the membrane. At this time, the inside of the axon is *positively* charged, so K$^+$ is driven out of the cell by diffusion and by electrostatic pressure. This outflow of cations causes the membrane potential to return toward its normal value. As it does so, the potassium channels begin to close again.

5. Once the membrane potential returns to normal, the sodium channels reset so that another depolarization can cause them to open again.

6. The membrane actually overshoots its resting value (-70 mV) and only gradually returns to normal as the potassium channels finally close. Eventually, sodium–potassium transporters remove the Na$^+$ ions that leaked in and retrieve the K$^+$ ions that leaked out.

Experiments have shown that an action potential temporarily increases the number of Na$^+$ ions inside the giant squid axon by 0.0003 percent. Although the concentration just inside the membrane is high, the total number of ions entering the cell is very small relative to the number already there. This means that on a short-term basis, sodium–potassium transporters are not very important. The few Na$^+$ ions that manage to leak in diffuse into the rest of the axoplasm, and the slight increase in Na$^+$ concentration is hardly noticeable. However, sodium–potassium transporters are important on a *long-term* basis. Without the activity of sodium–potassium transporters, the concentration of sodium ions in the axoplasm would eventually increase enough that the axon would no longer be able to function.

voltage-dependent ion channel An ion channel that opens or closes according to the value of the membrane potential.

Conduction of the Action Potential

Now that we have a basic understanding of the resting membrane potential and the production of the action potential, we can consider the movement of the message down the axon, or *conduction of the action potential.* To study this phenomenon, we again make use of the giant squid axon. We attach an electrical stimulator to an electrode at one end of the axon and place recording electrodes, attached to oscilloscopes, at different distances from the stimulating electrode. Then we apply a depolarizing stimulus to the end of the axon and trigger an action potential. We record the action potential from each of the electrodes, one after the other. Thus, we see that the action potential is conducted down the axon. As the action potential travels, it remains constant in size. (See *Figure 2.19.*)

This experiment establishes a basic law of axonal conduction: the **all-or-none law**. This law states that an action potential either occurs or does not occur, and once triggered, it is transmitted down the axon to its end. An action potential always remains the same size, without growing or diminishing. And when an action potential reaches a point where the axon branches, it splits but does not diminish in size. An axon will transmit an action potential in either direction, or even in both directions, if it is started in the middle of the axon's length. However, because action potentials in living animals always start at the end attached to the soma, axons normally carry one-way traffic.

As you know, the strength of a muscular contraction can vary from very weak to very forceful, and the strength of a stimulus can vary from barely detectable to very intense. We know that the occurrence of action potentials in axons controls the strength of muscular contractions and represents the intensity of a physical stimulus. But if the action potential is an all-or-none event, how can it represent information that can vary in a continuous fashion? The answer is simple: A single action potential is not the basic element of information; rather, variable information is represented by an axon's *rate of firing.* (In this context, *firing* refers to the production of action potentials.) A high rate of firing causes a strong muscular contraction, and a strong stimulus (such as a bright light) causes a high rate of firing in axons that serve the eyes. Thus, the all-or-none law is supplemented by the **rate law**. (See *Figure 2.20.*)

Recall that all but the smallest axons in mammalian nervous systems are myelinated; segments of the axons are covered by a myelin sheath produced by the oligodendrocytes of the CNS or the Schwann cells of the PNS. These segments are separated by portions of naked axon, the nodes of Ranvier. Conduction of an action potential in a myelinated axon is somewhat different from conduction in an unmyelinated axon.

Schwann cells and the oligodendrocytes of the CNS wrap tightly around the axon, leaving no measurable extracellular fluid between them and the axon. The

FIGURE 2.19

Conduction of the Action Potential.   When an action potential is triggered, its size remains undiminished as it travels down the axon. The speed of conduction can be calculated from the delay between the stimulus and the action potential.

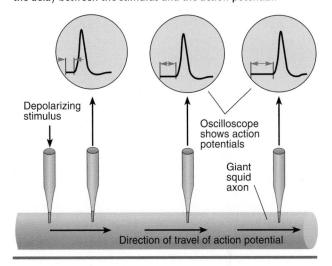

all-or-none law The principle that once an action potential is triggered in an axon, it is propagated, without decrement, to the end of the fiber.

rate law The principle that variations in the intensity of a stimulus or other information being transmitted in an axon are represented by variations in the rate at which that axon fires.

FIGURE 2.20

The Rate Law.   The strength of a stimulus is represented by the rate of firing of an axon. The size of each action potential is always constant.

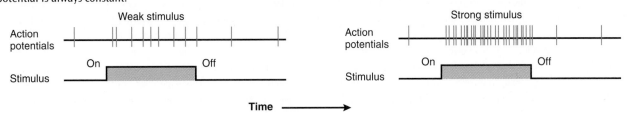

FIGURE 2.21

Saltatory Conduction. The figure shows propagation of an action potential down a myelinated axon.

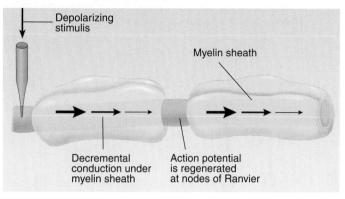

- Depolarizing stimulis
- Myelin sheath
- Decremental conduction under myelin sheath
- Action potential is regenerated at nodes of Ranvier

saltatory conduction Conduction of action potentials by myelinated axons. The action potential appears to jump from one node of Ranvier to the next.

only place where a myelinated axon comes into contact with the extracellular fluid is at a node of Ranvier, where the axon is naked. In the myelinated areas there can be no inward flow of Na^+ when the sodium channels open, because there *is* no extracellular sodium. The axon conducts the electrical disturbance from the action potential to the next node of Ranvier. The disturbance is conducted passively, the way an electrical signal is conducted through an insulated cable. The disturbance gets smaller as it passes down the axon, but it is still large enough to trigger a new action potential at the next node. (This decrease in the size of the disturbance is called *decremental conduction.*) The action potential gets retriggered, or repeated, at each node of Ranvier, and the electrical disturbance that results is conducted decrementally along the myelinated area to the next node. Transmission of this message, hopping from node to node, is called **saltatory conduction**, from the Latin *saltare*, "to dance." (See *Figure 2.21.*)

Saltatory conduction confers two advantages. The first is economic. Sodium ions enter axons during action potentials, and these ions must eventually be removed. Sodium–potassium transporters must be located along the entire length of unmyelinated axons because Na^+ enters everywhere. However, because Na^+ can enter myelinated axons only at the nodes of Ranvier, much less gets in, and consequently, much less has to be pumped out again. Therefore, myelinated axons expend much less energy to maintain their sodium balance.

The second advantage to myelin is speed. Conduction of an action potential is faster in a myelinated axon because the transmission between the nodes is very fast. Increased speed enables an animal to react faster and (undoubtedly) to think faster. One of the ways to increase the speed of conduction is to increase size. Because it is so large, the unmyelinated squid axon, with a diameter of 500 µm, achieves a conduction velocity of approximately 35 m/sec (meters per second). However, a myelinated cat axon achieves the same speed with a diameter of a mere 6 µm. The fastest myelinated axon, 20 µm in diameter, can conduct action potentials at a speedy 120 m/sec, or 432 km/h (kilometers per hour). At that speed a signal can get from one end of an axon to the other without much delay.

InterimSummary

Communication Within a Neuron

The withdrawal reflex illustrates how neurons can be connected to accomplish useful behaviors. The circuit responsible for this reflex consists of three sets of neurons: sensory neurons, interneurons, and motor neurons. The reflex can be suppressed when neurons in the brain activate inhibitory interneurons that form synapses with the motor neurons.

The message that is conducted down an axon is called an action potential. The membranes of all cells of the body are electrically charged, but only axons can produce action potentials. The resting membrane potential occurs because various ions are located in dif-

ferent concentrations in the fluid inside and outside the cell. The extracellular fluid (like seawater) is rich in Na^+ and Cl^-, and the intracellular fluid is rich in K^+ and various organic anions, designated as A^-.

The cell membrane is freely permeable to water, but its permeability to various ions—in particular, Na^+ and K^+—is regulated by ion channels. When the membrane potential is at its resting value (-70 mV), the voltage-dependent sodium and potassium channels are closed. The experiment with radioactive seawater showed us that some Na^+ continuously leaks into the axon but is

determined by the characteristics of the postsynaptic receptors—in particular, *by the particular type of ion channel they open.*

As Figure 2.27 shows, three major types of neurotransmitter-dependent ion channels are found in the postsynaptic membrane: sodium (Na^+), potassium (K^+), and chloride (Cl^-). Although the figure depicts only directly activated (ionotropic) ion channels, you should realize that many ion channels are activated indirectly, by metabotropic receptors coupled to G proteins.

The neurotransmitter-dependent sodium channel is the most important source of excitatory postsynaptic potentials. As we saw, sodium–potassium transporters keep sodium outside the cell, waiting for the forces of diffusion and electrostatic pressure to push it in. Obviously, when sodium channels are opened, the result is a depolarization—an **excitatory postsynaptic potential (EPSP)**. (See *Figure 2.27a.*)

We also saw that sodium–potassium transporters maintain a small surplus of potassium ions inside the cell. If potassium channels open, some of these cations will follow this gradient and leave the cell. Because K^+ is positively charged, its efflux will hyperpolarize the membrane, producing an **inhibitory postsynaptic potential (IPSP)**. (See *Figure 2.27b.*)

At many synapses inhibitory neurotransmitters open the chloride channels instead of (or in addition to) potassium channels. The effect of opening chloride channels depends on the membrane potential of the neuron. If the membrane is at the resting potential, nothing happens, because (as we saw earlier) the forces of diffusion and electrostatic pressure balance perfectly for the chloride ion. However, if the membrane potential has already been depolarized by the activity of excitatory synapses located nearby, then the opening of chloride channels will permit Cl^- to enter the cell. The influx of anions will bring the membrane potential back to its normal resting condition. Thus, the opening of chloride channels serves to neutralize EPSPs. (See *Figure 2.27c.*)

FIGURE 2.26

Metabotropic Receptors. When a molecule of neurotransmitter binds with a receptor, a second messenger is produced that opens nearby ion channels.

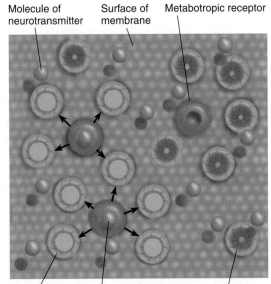

FIGURE 2.27

Ionic Movements During Postsynaptic Potentials

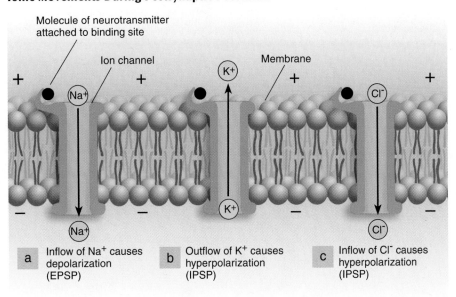

a Inflow of Na^+ causes depolarization (EPSP)
b Outflow of K^+ causes hyperpolarization (IPSP)
c Inflow of Cl^- causes hyperpolarization (IPSP)

excitatory postsynaptic potential (EPSP) An excitatory depolarization of the postsynaptic membrane of a synapse caused by the liberation of a neurotransmitter by the terminal button.

inhibitory postsynaptic potential (IPSP) An inhibitory hyperpolarization of the postsynaptic membrane of a synapse caused by the liberation of a neurotransmitter by the terminal button.

Termination of Postsynaptic Potentials

Postsynaptic potentials are brief depolarizations or hyperpolarizations caused by the activation of postsynaptic receptors with molecules of a neurotransmitter. They are kept brief by two mechanisms: reuptake and enzymatic deactivation.

The postsynaptic potentials produced by almost all neurotransmitters are terminated by **reuptake**. This process is simply an extremely rapid removal of neurotransmitter from the synaptic cleft by the terminal button. The neurotransmitter does not return in the vesicles that get pinched off the membrane of the terminal button. Instead, the membrane contains special transporter molecules that draw on the cell's energy reserves to force molecules of the neurotransmitter from the synaptic cleft directly into the cytoplasm—just as sodium–potassium transporters move Na^+ and K^+ across the membrane. When an action potential arrives, the terminal button releases a small amount of neurotransmitter into the synaptic cleft and then takes it back, giving the postsynaptic receptors only a brief exposure to the neurotransmitter. (See *Figure 2.28.*)

Enzymatic deactivation is accomplished by an enzyme that destroys molecules of the neurotransmitter. As far as we know, postsynaptic potentials are terminated in this way for only one neurotransmitter: **acetylcholine (ACh)**. Transmission at synapses on muscle fibers and at some synapses between neurons in the central nervous system is mediated by ACh. Postsynaptic potentials produced by ACh are short-lived because the postsynaptic membrane at these synapses contains an enzyme called **acetylcholinesterase (AChE)**. AChE destroys ACh by cleaving it into its constituents: choline and acetate. Because neither of these substances is capable of activating postsynaptic receptors, the postsynaptic potential is terminated once the molecules of ACh are broken apart. AChE is an extremely energetic destroyer of ACh; one molecule of AChE will chop apart more than 5000 molecules of ACh each second.

reuptake The reentry of a neurotransmitter just liberated by a terminal button back through its membrane, thus terminating the postsynaptic potential.

enzymatic deactivation The destruction of a neurotransmitter by an enzyme after its release—for example, the destruction of acetylcholine by acetylcholinesterase.

acetylcholine (ACh) (*a see tul koh leen*) A neurotransmitter found in the brain, spinal cord, and parts of the peripheral nervous system; responsible for muscular contraction.

acetylcholinesterase (AChE) (*a see tul koh lin ess ter ace*) The enzyme that destroys acetylcholine soon after it is liberated by the terminal buttons, thus terminating the postsynaptic potential.

FIGURE 2.28

Reuptake. Molecules of a neurotransmitter that has been released into the synaptic cleft are transported back into the terminal button.

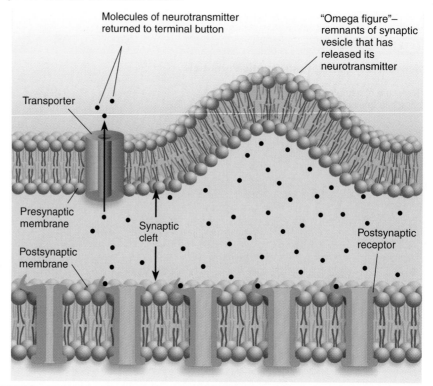

Effects of Postsynaptic Potentials: Neural Integration

We have seen how neurons are interconnected by means of synapses, how action potentials trigger the release of neurotransmitters, and how these chemicals initiate excitatory or inhibitory postsynaptic potentials. Excitatory postsynaptic potentials increase the likelihood that the postsynaptic neuron will fire; inhibitory postsynaptic potentials decrease this likelihood. (Remember, "firing" refers to the occurrence of an action potential.) Thus, the rate at which an axon fires is determined by the relative activity of the excitatory and inhibitory synapses on the soma and dendrites of that cell. If there are no active excitatory synapses or if the activity of inhibitory synapses is particularly high, that rate could be close to zero.

Let's look at the elements of this process. (*MyPsychKit 2.4, Postsynaptic Potentials*, illustrates the material presented in the rest of this chapter.) The interaction of the effects of excitatory and inhibitory synapses on a particular neuron is called **neural integration**. (*Integration* means "to make whole," in the sense of combining two or more functions.) Figure 2.29 illustrates the effects of excitatory and inhibitory synapses on a postsynaptic neuron. The left panel shows what happens when several excitatory synapses become active. The release of the neurotransmitter produces depolarizing EPSPs in the dendrites of the neuron. These EPSPs (represented in red) are then transmitted down the dendrites and across the soma to the *axon hillock* located at the base of the axon. If the depolarization is still strong enough when it reaches this point, the axon will fire. (See *Figure 2.29a.*)

Now let's consider what would happen if, at the same time, inhibitory synapses also become active. Inhibitory postsynaptic potentials are hyperpolarizing—they bring the membrane potential away from the threshold of excitation. Thus, they tend to cancel the effects of excitatory postsynaptic potentials. (See *Figure 2.29b.*)

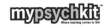

Animation 2.4
Postsynaptic Potentials

neural integration The process by which inhibitory and excitatory postsynaptic potentials summate and control the rate of firing of a neuron.

FIGURE 2.29

Neural Integration.   (a) If several excitatory synapses are active at the same time, the EPSPs they produce (shown in red) summate as they travel toward the axon, and the axon fires. (b) If several inhibitory synapses are active at the same time, the IPSPs they produce (shown in blue) diminish the size of the EPSPs and prevent the axon from firing.

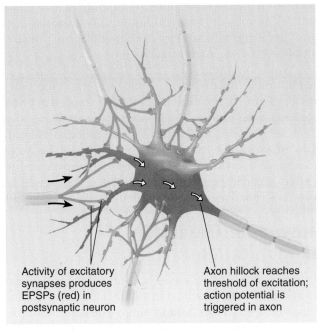

Activity of excitatory synapses produces EPSPs (red) in postsynaptic neuron

Axon hillock reaches threshold of excitation; action potential is triggered in axon

(a)

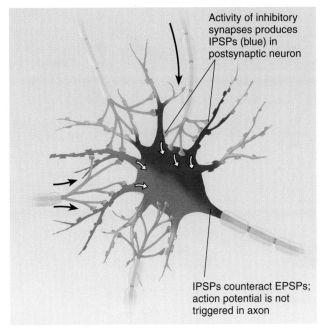

Activity of inhibitory synapses produces IPSPs (blue) in postsynaptic neuron

IPSPs counteract EPSPs; action potential is not triggered in axon

(b)

The rate at which a neuron fires is controlled by the relative activity of the excitatory and inhibitory synapses on its dendrites and soma. If the activity of excitatory synapses goes up, the rate of firing will go up. If the activity of inhibitory synapses goes up, the rate of firing will go down.

Autoreceptors

Postsynaptic receptors detect the presence of a neurotransmitter in the synaptic cleft and initiate excitatory or inhibitory postsynaptic potentials. But the postsynaptic membrane is not the only location of receptors that respond to neurotransmitters. Many neurons also possess receptors that respond to the neurotransmitter that *they themselves* release, called **autoreceptors**.

Autoreceptors can be located on the membrane of any part of the cell, but in this discussion we will consider those located on the terminal button. In most cases these autoreceptors do not control ion channels. Thus, when stimulated by a molecule of the neurotransmitter, autoreceptors do not produce changes in the membrane potential of the terminal button. Instead, they regulate internal processes, including the synthesis and release of the neurotransmitter. (As you may have guessed, autoreceptors are metabotropic; the control they exert on these processes is accomplished through G proteins and second messengers.) In most cases the effects of autoreceptor activation are inhibitory; that is, the presence of the neurotransmitter in the extracellular fluid in the vicinity of the neuron causes a decrease in the rate of synthesis or release of the neurotransmitter. Most investigators believe that autoreceptors are part of a regulatory system that controls the amount of neurotransmitter that is released. If too much is released, the autoreceptors inhibit both production and release; if not enough is released, the rates of production and release go up.

autoreceptor A receptor molecule located on a neuron that responds to the neurotransmitter released by that neuron.

presynaptic inhibition The action of a presynaptic terminal button in an axoaxonic synapse; reduces the amount of neurotransmitter released by the postsynaptic terminal button.

presynaptic facilitation The action of a presynaptic terminal button in an axoaxonic synapse; increases the amount of neurotransmitter released by the postsynaptic terminal button.

neuromodulator A naturally secreted substance that acts like a neurotransmitter except that it is not restricted to the synaptic cleft but diffuses through the extracellular fluid.

Axoaxonic Synapses

As we saw in Figure 2.22, the central nervous system contains three types of synapses. Activity of the first two types, axodendritic and axosomatic synapses, causes postsynaptic excitation or inhibition. The third type, axoaxonic synapses, does not contribute directly to neural integration. Instead, the activity of these synapses alter the amount of neurotransmitter released by the terminal buttons of the postsynaptic axon. They can produce presynaptic modulation: presynaptic inhibition or presynaptic facilitation.

As you know, the release of a neurotransmitter by a terminal button is initiated by an action potential. Normally, a particular terminal button releases a fixed amount of neurotransmitter each time an action potential arrives. However, the release of neurotransmitter can be modulated by the activity of axoaxonic synapses. If the activity of the axoaxonic synapse decreases the release of the neurotransmitter, the effect is called **presynaptic inhibition**. If it increases the release, it is called **presynaptic facilitation**. (See *Figure 2.30*.)

Nonsynaptic Chemical Communication

Neurotransmitters are released by terminal buttons of neurons and bind with receptors in the membrane of another cell located a very short distance away. The communication at each synapse is private. **Neuromodulators** are chemicals released by neurons that travel farther and are dispersed

FIGURE 2.30

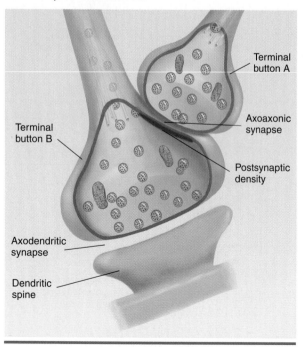

An Axoaxonic Synapse. The activity of terminal button A can increase or decrease the amount of neurotransmitter released by terminal button B.

Terminal button A

Axoaxonic synapse

Postsynaptic density

Terminal button B

Axodendritic synapse

Dendritic spine

more widely than are neurotransmitters. Most neuromodulators are **peptides**, chains of amino acids that are linked together by chemical attachments called *peptide bonds* (hence their name). Neuromodulators are secreted in larger amounts and diffuse for longer distances, modulating the activity of many neurons in a particular part of the brain. For example, neuromodulators affect general behavioral states such as vigilance, fearfulness, and sensitivity to pain. Chapter 4 discusses the most important neurotransmitters and neuromodulators.

Hormones are secreted by cells of **endocrine glands** (from the Greek *endo-*, "within," and *krinein*, "to secrete") or by cells located in various organs, such as the stomach, the intestines, the kidneys, and the brain. Cells that secrete hormones release these chemicals into the extracellular fluid. The hormones are then distributed to the rest of the body through the bloodstream. Hormones affect the activity of cells (including neurons) that contain specialized receptors located either on the surface of their membrane or deep within their nuclei. Cells that contain receptors for a particular hormone are referred to as **target cells** for that hormone; only these cells respond to its presence. Many neurons contain hormone receptors, and hormones are able to affect behavior by stimulating the receptors and changing the activity of these neurons. For example, a sex hormone, testosterone, increases the aggressiveness of most male mammals.

peptide A chain of amino acids joined together by peptide bonds. Most neuromodulators and some hormones consist of peptide molecules.

hormone A chemical substance that is released by an endocrine gland and that has effects on target cells in other organs.

endocrine gland A gland that liberates its secretions into the extracellular fluid around capillaries and hence into the bloodstream.

target cell The type of cell that contains receptors for a particular hormone and is affected by that hormone.

Interim Summary

Communication Between Neurons

Synapses consist of junctions between the terminal buttons of one neuron and the membrane of another neuron, a muscle cell, or a gland cell. When an action potential is transmitted down an axon, the terminal buttons at the end release a neurotransmitter, a chemical that produces either depolarizations (EPSPs) or hyperpolarizations (IPSPs) of the postsynaptic membrane. The rate of firing of the axon of the postsynaptic neuron is determined by the relative activity of the excitatory and inhibitory synapses on the membrane of its dendrites and soma—a phenomenon known as *neural integration*.

Terminal buttons contain synaptic vesicles, filled with molecules of the neurotransmitter. When an action potential reaches a terminal button, it causes the release of the neurotransmitter: Some of the synaptic vesicles fuse with the presynaptic membrane of the terminal button, break open, and release their contents into the synaptic cleft.

The activation of postsynaptic receptors by molecules of a neurotransmitter causes neurotransmitter-dependent ion channels to open, resulting in postsynaptic potentials. Ionotropic receptors contain ion channels, which are directly opened when a ligand attaches to the binding site. Metabotropic receptors are linked to G proteins, which, when activated, open ion channels—usually by producing a chemical called a second messenger.

The nature of the postsynaptic potential depends on the type of ion channel that is opened by the postsynaptic receptors at a particular synapse. Excitatory postsynaptic potentials occur when Na^+ enters the cell. Inhibitory postsynaptic potentials are produced when K^+ leaves the cell or Cl^- enters it

Postsynaptic potentials are normally brief. They are terminated by two means. The most common mechanism is reuptake: retrieval of molecules of the neurotransmitter from the synaptic cleft by means of transporters located in the presynaptic membrane, which transport the molecules back into the cytoplasm. Acetylcholine is deactivated by the enzyme acetylcholinesterase.

The presynaptic membrane, as well as the postsynaptic membrane, contains receptors that detect the presence of a neurotransmitter. Presynaptic receptors, also called autoreceptors, monitor the quantity of neurotransmitter that a neuron releases and, apparently, regulate the amount that is synthesized and released.

The presynaptic membrane, as well as the postsynaptic membrane, contains receptors that detect the presence of a neurotransmitter. Presynaptic receptors, also called autoreceptors, monitor the quantity of neurotransmitter that a neuron releases and apparently regulate the amount that is synthesized or released. Axoaxonic synapses produce presynaptic inhibition or presynaptic facilitation, reducing or enhancing the amount of neurotransmitter that is released.

Neuromodulators and hormones, like neurotransmitters, act on cells by attaching to the binding sites of receptors and initiating electrical or chemical changes in these cells. However, whereas the action of neurotransmitters is localized, neuromodulators and hormones have much more widespread effects.

Thought Questions

1. Why does synaptic transmission involve the release of chemicals? Direct electrical coupling of neurons is far simpler, so why do our neurons not use it more extensively? (A tiny percentage of synaptic connections in the human brain do use electrical coupling.) Normally, nature uses the simplest means possible to a given end, so there must be some advantages to chemical transmission. What do you think they are?

2. Consider the control of the withdrawal reflex illustrated in Figure 2.11. Could you design a circuit using electrical synapses that would accomplish the same tasks?

⁝ EPILOGUE Myasthenia Gravis

"Am I cured?" asked Kathryn.

Dr. T. smiled ruefully. "I wish it were so simple!" she said. "No, I'm afraid you aren't cured, but now we know what is causing your weakness. There *is* a treatment," she hastened to add, seeing Kathryn's disappointment. "You have a condition called *myasthenia gravis*. The injection I gave you lasts only for a few minutes, but I can give you some pills that have effects that last much longer." Indeed, as she was talking, Kathryn felt herself weakening, and she sat down again.

Myasthenia gravis was first described in 1672 by Thomas Willis, an English physician. The term literally means "grave muscle weakness." It is not a very common disorder, but most experts believe that many cases—much milder than Kathryn's, of course—go undiagnosed. Kathryn's disease involved her face, neck, arm, and trunk muscles, but sometimes only the eye muscles are involved. Before the 1930s, Kathryn would have become bedridden and almost certainly would have died within a few years, probably of pneumonia resulting from difficulty in breathing and coughing. Fortunately, Kathryn's future is not so bleak. The cause of myasthenia gravis is well understood, and it can be treated, if not cured.

The hallmark of myasthenia gravis is *fatigability*. That is, a patient has reasonable strength when rested but becomes very weak after moving for a little while. For many years, researchers have realized that the weakness occurs in the synapses on the muscles, not in the nervous system or the muscles themselves. In the late nineteenth century, a physician placed electrodes on the skin of a person with myasthenia gravis and electrically stimulated a nerve leading to a muscle. The muscle contracted each time he stimulated the nerve, but the contractions became progressively weaker. However, when he placed the electrodes above the muscle and stimulated it directly, the contractions showed no signs of fatigue. Later, with the development of techniques of electrical recording, researchers found that the action potentials in the nerves of people with myasthenia gravis were completely normal. If nerve conduction and muscular contraction were normal, then the problem had to lie in the synapses.

In 1934, Dr. Mary Walker remarked that the symptoms of myasthenia gravis resembled the effects of curare, a poison that blocks neural transmission at the synapses on muscles. The antidote for curare poisoning was a drug called *physostigmine*, which deactivates acetylcholinesterase (AChE). As you learned in this chapter, AChE is an enzyme that destroys the neurotransmitter acetylcholine (ACh) and terminates the postsynaptic potentials it produces. By deactivating AChE, physostigmine greatly increases and prolongs the effects of ACh on the postsynaptic membrane. Thus, it increases the strength of synaptic transmission at the synapses on muscles and reverses the effects of curare. (Chapter 4 will say more about both curare and physostigmine.)

Dr. Walker reasoned that if physostigmine reversed the effects of curare poisoning, perhaps it would also reverse the symptoms of myasthenia gravis. She tried it, and it did within a matter of a few minutes. Subsequently, pharmaceutical companies discovered drugs that could be taken orally and that produced longer-lasting effects. Nowadays, an injectable drug is used to make the diagnosis and an oral drug is used to treat it.

Researchers turned their efforts to understanding the cause of myasthenia gravis (MG). They discovered that MG is an *autoimmune disease*. Normally, the immune system protects us from infections by being alert for proteins that are present on invading microorganisms. The immune system produces antibodies that attack these foreign proteins, and the microorganisms are killed. However, sometimes the immune system makes a mistake and becomes sensitized against one of the proteins normally present in our bodies. As researchers have found, the blood of patients with MG contains antibodies against the protein that makes up acetylcholine receptors. Thus, myasthenia gravis is an autoimmune disease in which the immune system attacks and destroys many of the person's ACh receptors, which are necessary for synaptic transmission.

Recently, researchers have succeeded in developing an animal model of MG. An *animal model* is a disease that can be produced in laboratory animals and that closely resembles a human disease. The course of the disease can then be studied, and possible treatments or cures can be tested. In this case, the disease is produced by extracting ACh-receptor protein from electric rays (*Torpedo*) and injecting it into laboratory animals. The animals' immune systems become sensitized to the protein and develop antibodies that attack their own ACh receptors. The animals exhibit the same muscular fatigability shown by people with MG, and they become stronger after receiving an injection of a drug such as physostigmine.

One promising result that has emerged from studies with the animal model of MG is the finding that an animal's immune system can be *desensitized* so that it will not produce antibodies that destroy ACh receptors. If ACh-receptor proteins are modified and then injected into laboratory animals, their immune systems develop an antibody against the altered protein. This antibody does not attack the animals' own ACh receptors. Later, if they are given the pure ACh-receptor protein, they do *not* develop MG. Apparently, the pure protein is so similar to the one to which the animals were previously sensitized that the immune system does not bother to produce another antibody. Perhaps a vaccine can be developed that can be used to arrest MG in its early stages by inducing the person's immune system to produce the harmless antibody rather than the one that attacks acetylcholine receptors.

Even with the drugs that are available to physicians today, myasthenia gravis remains a serious disease. The drugs do not restore a person's strength to normal, and they can have serious side effects, but the progress made in the laboratory in recent years gives us hope for a brighter future for people like Kathryn.

Key Concepts

CELLS OF THE NERVOUS SYSTEM

1. Neurons have a soma, dendrites, an axon, and terminal buttons. Circuits of interconnected neurons are responsible for the functions performed by the nervous system. Neurons are supported by glia and by Schwann cells, which provide myelin sheaths, housekeeping services, and physical support. The blood–brain barrier helps to regulate the chemicals that reach the brain.

COMMUNICATION WITHIN A NEURON

2. The action potential occurs when the membrane potential of an axon reaches the threshold of excitation. Although the action potential is electrical, it is caused by the flow of sodium and potassium ions through voltage-dependent ion channels in the membrane. Saltatory conduction, which takes place in myelinated axons, is faster and more efficient than conduction in unmyelinated axons.

COMMUNICATION BETWEEN NEURONS

3. Neurons communicate by means of synapses, which enable the presynaptic neuron to produce excitatory or inhibitory effects on the postsynaptic neuron.

These effects increase or decrease the rate at which the axon of the postsynaptic neuron sends action potentials down to its terminal buttons.

4. When an action potential reaches the end of an axon, it causes some synaptic vesicles to release a neurotransmitter into the synaptic cleft. Molecules of the neurotransmitter attach themselves to receptors in the postsynaptic membrane.

5. When they become activated by molecules of the neurotransmitters, postsynaptic receptors produce either excitatory or inhibitory postsynaptic potentials by opening voltage-controlled sodium, potassium, or chloride ion channels.

6. The postsynaptic potential is terminated by the destruction of the neurotransmitter or by its reuptake into the terminal button.

7. Autoreceptors help to regulate the amount of neurotransmitter that is released.

8. Axoaxonic synapses consist of junctions between two terminal buttons. Release of neurotransmitter by the first terminal button increases or decreases the amount of neurotransmitter released by the second.

9. Neuromodulators and hormones have actions similar to those of neurotransmitters: They bind with and activate receptors on or in their target cells.

Suggested Readings

Aidley, D. J. *The Physiology of Excitable Cells*, 4th ed. Cambridge, England: Cambridge University Press, 1998.

Bean, B. P. The action potential in mammalian central neurons. *Nature Reviews: Neuroscience*, 2007, *8*, 451–465.

Cowan, W. M., Südhof, T. C., and Stevens, C. F. *Synapses*. Baltimore, MD: Johns Hopkins University Press, 2001.

Kandel, E. R., Schwartz, J. H., and Jessell, T. M. *Principles of Neural Science*, 4th ed. New York: McGraw-Hill, 2000.

Nicholls, J. G., Martin, A. R., Fuchs, P. A., and Wallace, B. G. *From Neuron to Brain*, 4th ed. Sunderland, MA: Sinauer, 2001.

Additional Resources

Visit www.mypsychkit.com for additional review and practice of the material covered in this chapter. Within MyPsychKit, you can take practice tests and receive a customized study plan to help you review. Dozens of animations, tutorials, and Web links are also available. You can even review using the interactive electronic version of this textbook. You will need to register for MyPsychKit. See www.mypsychkit.com for complete details.

chapter 3 : Structure of the Nervous System

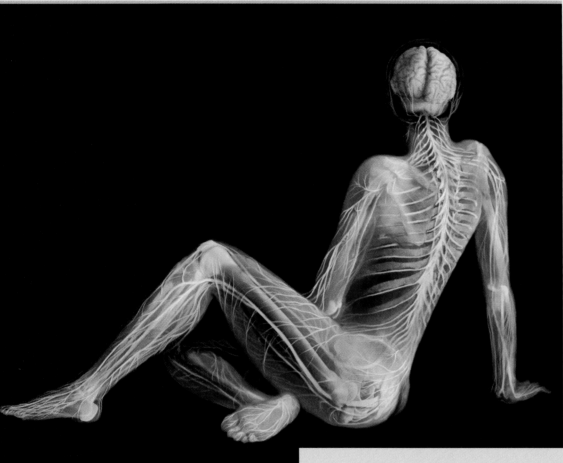

LEARNING OBJECTIVES

1. Describe the appearance of the brain and identify the terms used to indicate directions and planes of section.

2. Describe the divisions of the nervous system, the meninges, the ventricular system, and the production of cerebrospinal fluid and its flow through the brain.

3. Outline the development of the central nervous system.

4. Describe the telencephalon, one of the two major structures of the forebrain.

5. Describe the two major structures of the diencephalon.

6. Describe the major structures of the midbrain, the hindbrain, and the spinal cord.

7. Describe the peripheral nervous system, including the two divisions of the autonomic nervous system.

Miss S. was a 60-year-old woman with a history of high blood pressure, which was not responding well to the medication she was taking. One evening she was sitting in her reclining chair reading the newspaper when the phone rang. She got out of her chair and walked to the phone. As she did, she began feeling giddy and stopped to hold onto the kitchen table. She has no memory of what happened after that.

The next morning, a neighbor, who usually stopped by to have coffee with Miss S., found her lying on the floor, mumbling incoherently. The neighbor called an ambulance, which took Miss S. to a hospital.

Two days after her admission, I visited her in her room, along with a group of people being led by the chief of neurology. The neurological resident in charge of her case had already told us that she had had a stroke in the back part of the right side of the brain. He had attached a CT scan to an illuminated viewer mounted on the wall and had showed us a white spot caused by the accumulation of blood in a particular region of her brain. (You can look at the scan yourself if you like; it is shown in Figure 5.17.)

About a dozen of us entered Miss S.'s room. She was awake but seemed a little confused. The resident greeted her and asked how she was feeling. "Fine, I guess," she said. "I still don't know why I'm here."

"Can you see the other people in the room?"

"Why, sure."

"How many are there?"

She turned her head to the right and began counting. She stopped when she had counted the people at the foot of her bed. "Seven," she reported. "What about us?" asked a voice from the left of her bed. "What?" she said, looking at the people she had already counted. "Here, to your left. No, toward your left!" the voice repeated. Slowly, rather reluctantly, she began turning her head to the left. The voice kept insisting, and finally, she saw who was talking. "Oh," she said, "I guess there are more of you."

The resident approached the left side of her bed and touched her left arm. "What is this?" he asked. "Where?" she said. "Here," he answered, holding up her arm and moving it gently in front of her face.

"Oh, that's an arm."

"An arm? Whose arm?"

"I don't know. . . . I guess it must be yours."

"No, it's yours. Look, it's a part of you." He traced with his fingers from her arm to her shoulder.

"Well, if you say so," she said, still sounding unconvinced.

When we returned to the residents' lounge, the chief of neurology said that we had seen a classic example of unilateral neglect, caused by damage to a particular part of the brain. "I've seen many cases like this," he explained. "People can still perceive sensations from the left side of their body, but they just don't pay attention to them. A woman will put makeup on only the right side of her face, and a man will shave only half of his beard. When they put on a shirt or a coat, they will use their left hand to slip it over their right arm and shoulder, but then they'll just forget about their left arm and let the garment hang from one shoulder. They also don't look at things located toward the left or even the left halves of things. Once I saw a man who had just finished eating breakfast. He was sitting in his bed, with a tray in front of him. There was half of a pancake on his plate. 'Are you all done?' I asked. 'Sure,' he said. I turned the plate around so that the uneaten part was on his right. He gave a startled look and said, 'Where the hell did that come from?' "

The goal of neuroscience research is to understand how the brain works. To understand the results of this research, you must be acquainted with the basic structure of the nervous system. The number of terms introduced in this chapter is kept to a minimum (but as you will see, the minimum is still a rather large number). The MyPsychKit "Figures and Diagrams" exercise for this chapter will help you learn the names and locations of the major structures of the nervous system. (See *MyPsychKit, Figures and Diagrams.*) With the framework you will receive from this chapter and from MyPsychKit, you should have no trouble learning the material presented in subsequent chapters.

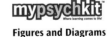

Figures and Diagrams

Basic Features of the Nervous System

Before beginning a description of the nervous system, I want to discuss the terms that are used to describe it. The gross anatomy of the brain was described long ago, and everything that could be seen without the aid of a microscope was given a name. Early anatomists named most brain structures according to their similarity to commonplace objects: amygdala, or "almond-shaped object"; hippocampus, or "sea horse"; genu, or "knee"; cortex, or "bark"; pons, or "bridge"; uncus, or "hook," to give a few examples. Throughout this book I will translate the names of anatomical terms as I introduce them, because the translation makes the terms more memorable. For example, knowing that *cortex* means "bark" (like the bark of a tree) will help you to remember that the cortex is the outer layer of the brain.

When describing features of a structure as complex as the brain, we need to use terms denoting directions. Directions in the nervous system are normally described relative to the **neuraxis**, an imaginary line drawn through the spinal cord up to the front of the brain. For simplicity's sake, let's consider an animal with a straight neuraxis. Figure 3.1 shows an alligator and two humans. This alligator is certainly laid out in a linear fashion; we can draw a straight line that starts between its eyes and continues down the center of its spinal cord. (See *Figure 3.1*.) The front end is **anterior**, and the tail is **posterior**. The terms **rostral** (toward the beak) and **caudal** (toward the tail) are also employed, especially when referring specifically to the brain. The top of the head and the back are part of the **dorsal** surface, while the **ventral** (front) surface faces the ground. (*Dorsum* means "back," and *ventrum* means "belly.") These directions are somewhat more complicated in the human; because we stand upright, our neuraxis bends, so the top of the head is perpendicular to the back. (You will also encounter the terms *superior* and *inferior*. In referring to the brain, these terms do not denote value judgments. *Superior* simply means "above," and *inferior* means "below." For example, the *superior colliculi* are located above the *inferior colliculi*.) The frontal views of both the alligator and the human illustrate the

---

FIGURE 3.1

Views of Alligator and Human.   These side and frontal views show the terms used to denote anatomical directions.

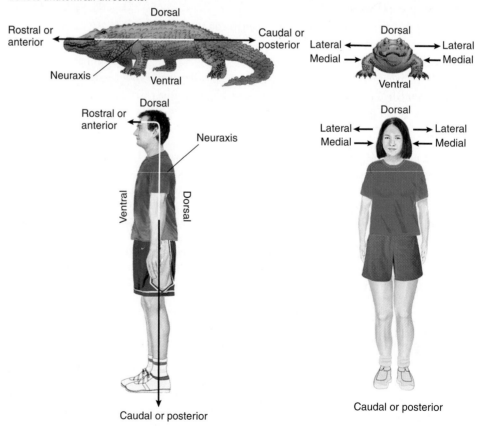

neuraxis An imaginary line drawn through the center of the length of the central nervous system, from the bottom of the spinal cord to the front of the forebrain.

anterior With respect to the central nervous system, located near or toward the head.

posterior With respect to the central nervous system, located near or toward the tail.

rostral "Toward the beak"; with respect to the central nervous system, in a direction along the neuraxis toward the front of the face.

caudal "Toward the tail"; with respect to the central nervous system, in a direction along the neuraxis away from the front of the face.

dorsal "Toward the back"; with respect to the central nervous system, in a direction perpendicular to the neuraxis toward the top of the head or the back.

ventral "Toward the belly"; with respect to the central nervous system, in a direction perpendicular to the neuraxis toward the bottom of the skull or the front surface of the body.

FIGURE 3.2

Brain Slices and Planes.   Planes of section as they pertain to the human central nervous system.

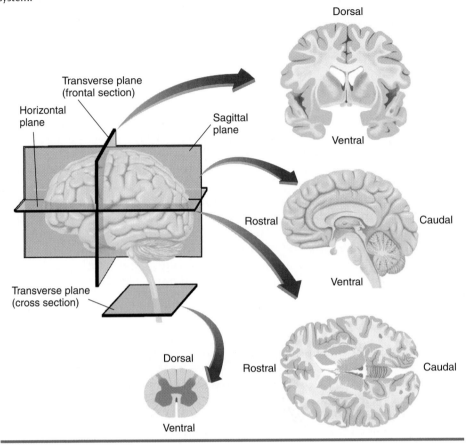

terms **lateral** and **medial**: toward the side and toward the midline, respectively. (See *Figure 3.1*.)

Two other useful terms are *ipsilateral* and *contralateral*. **Ipsilateral** refers to structures on the same side of the body. (*Ipsi* means "same.") If we say that the olfactory bulb sends axons to the *ipsilateral* hemisphere, we mean that the left olfactory bulb sends axons to the left hemisphere and the right olfactory bulb sends axons to the right hemisphere. **Contralateral** refers to structures on opposite sides of the body. If we say that a particular region of the left cerebral cortex controls movements of the *contralateral* hand, we mean that the region controls movements of the right hand.

To see what is in the nervous system, we have to cut it open; to be able to convey information about what we find, we slice it in a standard way. Figure 3.2 shows a human nervous system. We can slice the nervous system in three ways:

1. Transversely, like a salami, giving us **cross sections** (also known as **frontal sections** when referring to the brain)
2. Parallel to the ground, giving us **horizontal sections**
3. Perpendicular to the ground and parallel to the neuraxis, giving us **sagittal sections**. The **midsagittal plane** divides the brain into two symmetrical halves. The sagittal section in Figure 3.2 lies in the midsagittal plane.

Note that because of our upright posture, cross sections of the spinal cord are parallel to the ground. (See *Figure 3.2*.)

lateral Toward the side of the body, away from the middle.

medial Toward the middle of the body, away from the side.

ipsilateral Located on the same side of the body.

contralateral Located on the opposite side of the body.

cross section With respect to the central nervous system, a slice taken at right angles to the neuraxis.

frontal section A slice through the brain parallel to the forehead.

horizontal section A slice through the brain parallel to the ground.

sagittal section (*sadj i tul*) A slice through the brain parallel to the neuraxis and perpendicular to the ground.

midsagittal plane The plane through the neuraxis perpendicular to the ground; divides the brain into two symmetrical halves.

TABLE 3.1 The Major Divisions of the Nervous System	
Central Nervous System (CNS)	**Peripheral Nervous System (PNS)**
Brain	Nerves
Spinal cord	Peripheral ganglia

An Overview

The nervous system consists of the brain and spinal cord, which make up the *central nervous system* (*CNS*), and the cranial nerves, spinal nerves, and peripheral ganglia, which constitute the *peripheral nervous system* (*PNS*). The CNS is encased in bone: The brain is covered by the skull, and the spinal cord is encased by the vertebral column. (See *Table 3.1*.)

Figure 3.3 shows the relation of the brain and spinal cord to the rest of the body. Do not be concerned with unfamiliar labels on this figure; these structures will be described later. (See *Figure 3.3*.) The brain is a large mass of neurons, glia, and other supporting cells. It is the most protected organ of the body, encased in a tough, bony skull and floating in a pool of cerebrospinal fluid. The brain receives a copious supply of blood and is chemically guarded by the blood–brain barrier.

Meninges

The entire nervous system—brain, spinal cord, cranial and spinal nerves, and peripheral ganglia—is covered by tough connective tissue. The protective sheaths around the brain and spinal cord are referred to as the **meninges** (singular: *meninx*). The meninges consist of three layers, which are shown in Figure 3.3. The outer layer is thick, tough, and flexible but unstretchable; its name, **dura mater**, means "hard mother." The middle layer of the meninges, the **arachnoid membrane**, gets its name from the weblike appearance of the *arachnoid trabeculae* that protrude from it (from the Greek *arachne*, meaning "spider"; *trabecula* means "track"). The arachnoid membrane, soft and spongy, lies beneath the dura mater. Closely attached to the brain and spinal cord, and following every surface convolution, is the **pia mater** ("pious mother"). The smaller surface blood vessels of the brain and spinal cord are contained within this layer. Between the pia mater and the arachnoid membrane is a gap called the **subarachnoid space**. This space is filled with a liquid called **cerebrospinal fluid (CSF)**. (See *Figure 3.3*.)

The peripheral nervous system (PNS) is covered with two layers of meninges. The middle layer (arachnoid membrane), with its associated pool of CSF, covers only the brain and spinal cord. Outside the central nervous system, the outer and inner layers (dura mater and pia mater) fuse and form a sheath that covers the spinal and cranial nerves and the peripheral ganglia.

The Ventricular System and Production of Cerebrospinal Fluid

The brain is very soft and jellylike. The considerable weight of a human brain (approximately 1400 g), along with its delicate construction, necessitates that it be protected from shock. Fortunately, the brain is well protected. It floats in a bath of CSF contained within the subarachnoid space. Because the brain is completely immersed in liquid, its net weight is reduced to approximately 80 g; thus, pressure on the base of the brain is considerably diminished. The CSF surrounding the brain and spinal cord also reduces the shock to the central nervous system that would be caused by sudden head movement.

meninges (*singular:* **meninx**) (*men in jees*)   The three layers of tissue that encase the central nervous system: the dura mater, arachnoid membrane, and pia mater.

dura mater   The outermost of the meninges; tough and flexible.

arachnoid membrane (*a rak noyd*)   The middle layer of the meninges, located between the outer dura mater and inner pia mater.

pia mater   The layer of the meninges that clings to the surface of the brain; thin and delicate.

subarachnoid space   The fluid-filled space that cushions the brain; located between the arachnoid membrane and the pia mater.

cerebrospinal fluid (CSF)   A clear fluid, similar to blood plasma, that fills the ventricular system of the brain and the subarachnoid space surrounding the brain and spinal cord.

ventricle (*ven trik ul*)   One of the hollow spaces within the brain, filled with cerebrospinal fluid.

FIGURE 3.3

The Nervous System.   The figures show (a) the relation of the nervous system to the rest of the body, (b) detail of the meninges that cover the central nervous system, and (c) a closer view of the spinal cord and vertebrae.

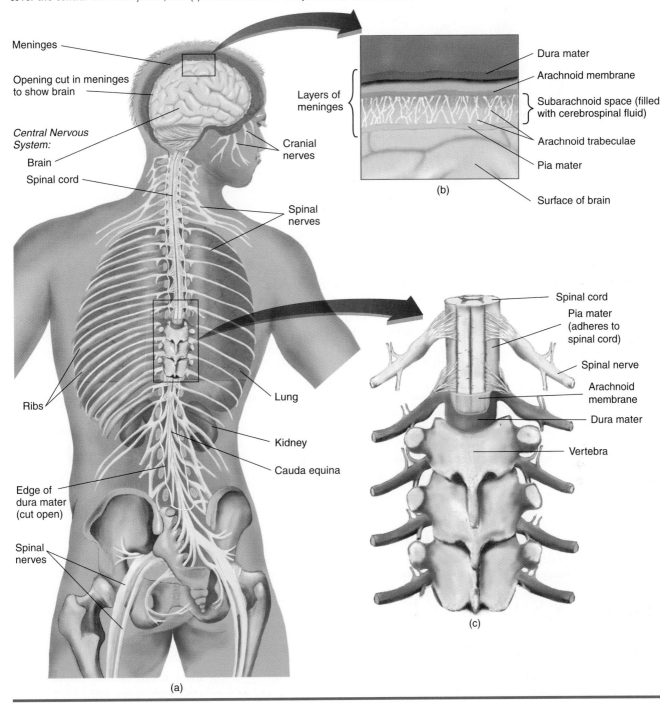

The brain contains a series of hollow, interconnected chambers called **ventricles** ("little bellies"), which are filled with CSF. (See *Figure 3.4.*) The largest chambers are the two **lateral ventricles**, which are connected to the **third ventricle**. The third ventricle is located at the midline of the brain; its walls divide the surrounding part of the brain into symmetrical halves. A bridge of neural tissue called the *massa intermedia* crosses through the middle of the third ventricle and serves as a convenient reference point. The **cerebral aqueduct**, a long tube, connects the

lateral ventricle One of the two ventricles located in the center of the telencephalon.

third ventricle The ventricle located in the center of the diencephalon.

cerebral aqueduct A narrow tube interconnecting the third and fourth ventricles of the brain, located in the center of the mesencephalon.

FIGURE 3.4

The Ventricular System of the Brain.   The figure shows (a) a lateral view of the left side of the brain and (b) a frontal view.

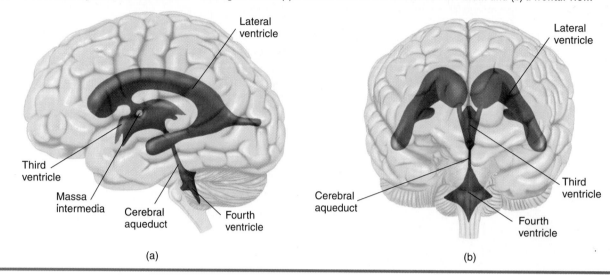

(a)   (b)

fourth ventricle The ventricle located between the cerebellum and the dorsal pons, in the center of the metencephalon.

choroid plexus The highly vascular tissue that protrudes into the ventricles and produces cerebrospinal fluid.

mypsychkit™
Where learning comes to life!

Animation 3.1
Meninges and CSF

third ventricle to the **fourth ventricle**. The lateral ventricles constitute the first and second ventricles, but they are never referred to as such. (See *Figure 3.4*.)

Cerebrospinal fluid is extracted from the blood and resembles blood plasma in its composition. It is manufactured by special tissue with an especially rich blood supply called the **choroid plexus**, which protrudes into all four of the ventricles. CSF is produced continuously; the total volume of CSF is approximately 125 ml, and the half-life (the time it takes for half of the CSF present in the ventricular system to be replaced by fresh fluid) is about 3 hours. Therefore, several times this amount is produced by the choroid plexus each day.

Cerebrospinal fluid is produced by the choroid plexus of the lateral ventricles and flows into the third ventricle. More CSF is produced by the choroid plexus located in this ventricle, which then flows through the cerebral aqueduct to the fourth ventricle, where still more CSF is produced. The CSF leaves the fourth ventricle through small openings that connect with the subarachnoid space surrounding the brain. The CSF then flows through the subarachnoid space around the central nervous system, where it is reabsorbed into the blood supply. (See *MyPsychKit 3.1, Meninges and CSF*.)

InterimSummary

Basic Features of the Nervous System

Anatomists have adopted a set of terms to describe the locations of parts of the body. *Anterior* is toward the head, *posterior* is toward the tail, *lateral* is toward the side, *medial* is toward the middle, *dorsal* is toward the back, and *ventral* is toward the front surface of the body. In the special case of the nervous system, *rostral* means toward the beak (or nose), and *caudal* means toward the tail. *Ipsilateral* means "same side," and *contralateral* means "other side." A cross section (or, in the case of the brain, a frontal section) slices the nervous system at right angles to the neuraxis, a horizontal section slices the brain parallel to the ground, and a sagittal section slices it perpendicular to the ground, parallel to the neuraxis.

The central nervous system (CNS) consists of the brain and spinal cord, and the peripheral nervous system (PNS) consists of the spinal and cranial nerves and peripheral ganglia. The CNS is covered with the meninges: dura mater, arachnoid membrane, and pia mater. The space under the arachnoid membrane is filled with cerebrospinal fluid (CSF), in which the brain floats. The PNS is covered with only the dura mater and pia mater. CSF is produced in the choroid plexus of the lateral, third, and fourth ventricles. It flows from the two lateral ventricles into the third ventricle, through the cerebral aqueduct into the fourth ventricle, then into the subarachnoid space, and finally back into the blood supply.

The Central Nervous System

Although the brain is exceedingly complicated, an understanding of the basic features of brain development makes it easier to learn and remember the location of the most important structures. With that end in mind, I introduce these features here in the context of development of the central nervous system. Two animations will help you learn and remember the structure of the brain. *MyPsychKit 3.2, The Rotatable Brain* is just what the title implies: a drawing of the human brain that you can rotate in three dimensions. You can choose whether to see some internal structures or see specialized regions of the cerebral cortex. *MyPsychKit 3.3, Brain Slices* is even more comprehensive. It consists of two sets of photographs of human brain slices, taken in the transverse (frontal) and horizontal planes. As you move the cursor across each slice, brain regions are outlined and their names appear. If you want to know how to pronounce these names, you can click on the region. You can also see magnified views of the slices and move them around by clicking and dragging. Finally, you can test yourself: The computer will present names of the regions shown in each slice, and you try to click on the correct region.

Development of the Central Nervous System

The central nervous system begins early in embryonic life as a hollow tube, and it maintains this basic shape even after it is fully developed. During development, parts of the tube elongate, pockets and folds form, and the tissue around the tube thickens until the brain reaches its final form.

An Overview of Brain Development

Development of the nervous system begins around the eighteenth day after conception. Part of the *ectoderm* (outer layer) of the back of the embryo thickens and forms a plate. The edges of this plate form ridges that curl toward each other along a longitudinal line, running in a rostral–caudal direction. By the twenty-first day these ridges touch each other and fuse together, forming a tube—the **neural tube**—that gives rise to the brain and spinal cord.

By the twenty-eighth day of development the neural tube is closed, and its rostral end has developed three interconnected chambers. These chambers become ventricles, and the tissue that surrounds them becomes the three major parts of the brain: the forebrain, the midbrain, and the hindbrain. (See *Figures 3.5a* and *3.5c.*) As development progresses, the rostral chamber (the forebrain) divides into three separate parts, which become the two lateral ventricles and the third ventricle. The region around the lateral ventricles becomes the telencephalon ("end brain"), and the region around the third ventricle becomes the diencephalon ("interbrain"). (See *Figures 3.5b* and *3.5d.*) In its final form, the chamber inside the midbrain (mesencephalon) becomes narrow, forming the cerebral aqueduct, and two structures develop in the hindbrain: the metencephalon ("afterbrain") and the myelencephalon ("marrowbrain"). (See *Figure 3.5e.*)

Table 3.2 summarizes the terms introduced here and mentions some of the major structures found in each part of the brain. The colors in the table match those in Figure 3.5. These structures will be described in the remainder of the chapter, in the order in which they are listed in Table 3.2. (See *Table 3.2.*)

Details of Brain Development

Brain development begins with a thin tube and ends with a structure weighing approximately 1400 g (about 3 lb) and consisting of several hundreds of billions of cells. Where do these cells come from, and what controls their growth?

Let's consider the development of the cerebral cortex, about which most is known. The principles described here are similar to the ones that apply to development of other regions of the brain. (For details of this process, see Honda, Tabata, and

neural tube A hollow tube, closed at the rostral end, that forms from ectodermal tissue early in embryonic development; serves as the origin of the central nervous system.

FIGURE 3.5

Brain Development.   This schematic outline of brain development shows its relation to the ventricles. Views (a) and (c) show early development. Views (b) and (d) show later development. View (e) shows a lateral view of the left side of a semitransparent human brain with the brain stem "ghosted in." The colors of all figures denote corresponding regions.

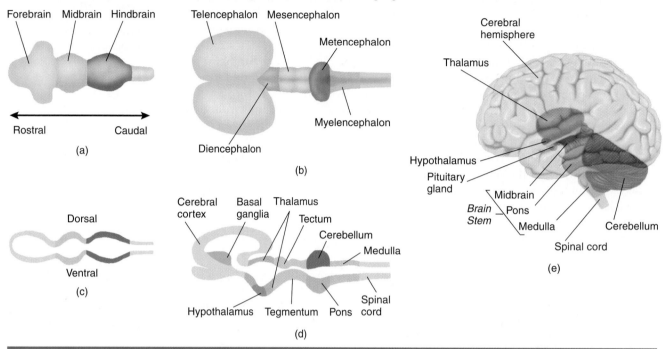

cerebral cortex The outermost layer of gray matter of the cerebral hemispheres.

ventricular zone A layer of cells that line the inside of the neural tube; contains progenitor cells that divide and give rise to cells of the central nervous system.

progenitor cells Cells of the ventricular zone that divide and give rise to cells of the central nervous system.

Nakajima, 2003; Ayala, Shu, and Tsai, 2007; and Cooper, 2008). *Cortex* means "bark," and the **cerebral cortex**, approximately 3 mm thick, surrounds the cerebral hemispheres like the bark of a tree. Corrected for body size, the cerebral cortex is larger in humans than in any other species. As we will see later in this book, circuits of neurons in the cerebral cortex play a vital role in cognition and control of movement.

The cells that line the inside of the neural tube—the **ventricular zone**—give rise to the cells of the central nervous system. The cerebral cortex develops from the inside out; that is, the first cells to be produced by the ventricular zone migrate a

TABLE 3.2   Anatomical Subdivisions of the Brain

Major Division	Ventricle	Subdivision	Principal Structures
Forebrain	Lateral	Telencephalon	Cerebral cortex
			Basal ganglia
			Limbic system
	Third	Diencephalon	Thalamus
			Hypothalamus
Midbrain	Cerebral aqueduct	Mesencephalon	Tectum Tegmentum
Hindbrain	Fourth	Metencephalon	Cerebellum
			Pons
		Myelencephalon	Medulla oblongata

short distance and establish the first—and deepest—layer. The next wave of newborn cells pass through the first layer and form the second one—and so on, until all six layers of the cerebral cortex are laid down. The last cells to be produced must pass through all the ones born before them.

The cells in the ventricular zone that give rise to the cells of the brain are known as **progenitor cells**. (A *progenitor* is a direct ancestor of a line of descendants.) During the first phase of development, progenitor cells divide, making new progenitor cells and increasing the size of the ventricular zone. This phase is referred to as **symmetrical division**, because the division of each progenitor cell produces two new progenitor cells. This form of division increases the size of the ventricular zone. Then, seven weeks after conception, progenitor cells receive a signal to begin a period of **asymmetrical division**. During this phase progenitor cells divide asymmetrically, producing another progenitor cell and a brain cell.

The first brain cells produced through asymmetrical division are **radial glia**. The cell bodies of radial glia remain in the ventricular zone, but they extend fibers radially outward from the ventricular zone, like spokes in a wheel. These fibers end in cuplike feet that attach to the pia mater, located at the outer surface of what becomes the cerebral cortex. As the cortex becomes thicker, the fibers of the radial glia grow longer and maintain their connections with the pia mater.

The next set of brain cells produced by asymmetrical division are special neurons known as **Cajal-Retzius (C-R) cells**. C-R cells establish themselves in a layer near the terminals of the radial glia, just inside the pia mater. A second set of neurons is produced that forms a layer just beneath the C-R cells. These neurons constitute the first, innermost of the six layers of the cerebral cortex. As *neurogenesis* (production of new neurons) continues, the cells leave the ventricular zone, pass the first layer of neurons, and establish themselves just inside the layer of C-R cells. Each successive wave of newborn neurons travels past the neurons that were born previously and establishes the next cortical layer. Newborn neurons are guided in their travel by the fibers of radial glial cells. Neurons crawl along radial fibers like amoebas, pushing their way through neurons that were born earlier and finally coming to rest against the layer of C-R cells. Chemicals secreted by the C-R cells causes the neurons to detach from the radial glia fibers and establish themselves in the outmost layer of the cortex. (See *Figure 3.6*.)

The period of asymmetrical division lasts about 3 months. Because the human cerebral cortex contains about 100 billion neurons, there are about one billion neurons migrating along radial glial fibers on a given day. The migration path of the earliest neurons is the shortest and takes about 1 day. The neurons that produce the last, outermost layer have to pass through five layers of neurons, and their migration takes about 2 weeks. The end of cortical development occurs when the progenitor cells receive a chemical signal that causes them to die—a phenomenon known as **apoptosis** (literally, a "falling away"). Molecules of the chemical that conveys this signal bind with receptors that activate killer genes within the cells. (All cells have these genes, but only certain cells possess the receptors that respond to the chemical signals that turn

symmetrical division Division of a progenitor cell that gives rise to two identical progenitor cells; increases the size of the ventricular zone and hence the brain that develops from it.

asymmetrical division Division of a progenitor cell that gives rise to another progenitor cell and a neuron, which migrates away from the ventricular zone toward its final resting place in the brain.

radial glia Special glia with fibers that grow radially outward from the ventricular zone to the surface of the cortex; provide guidance for neurons migrating outward during brain development.

Cajal-Retzius (C-R) cells Specialized neurons that establish themselves during cortical development in a layer near the terminals of the radial glia, just inside the pia mater; secrete a chemical that controls the establishment of migrating neurons in the layers of the cortex.

apoptosis (*ay pop **toe** is*) Death of a cell caused by a chemical signal that activates a genetic mechanism inside the cell.

FIGURE 3.6

Nervous System Development.   A portion of a cross section through the nervous system early in its development. Radially oriented glial cells help to guide the migration of newly formed neurons from the ventricular zone to their final resting place in the cerebral cortex. Each successive wave of neurons passes neurons that migrated earlier, so the most recently formed neurons occupy layers closer to the cortical surface.

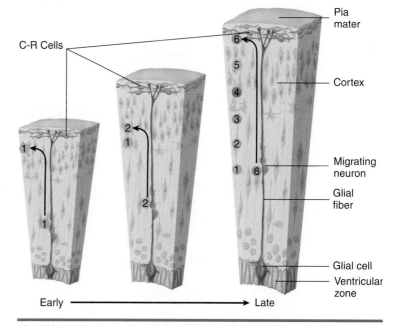

Adapted from Rakic, P. A small step for the cell, a giant leap for mankind: A hypothesis of neocortical expansion during evolution. *Trends in Neuroscience*, 1995, *18*, 383–388.

FIGURE 3.7

Effects of Learning on Neurogenesis.   This figure shows sections through a part of the hippocampus of rats that received training on a learning task or were exposed to a control condition that did not lead to learning. Arrows indicate newly formed cells.

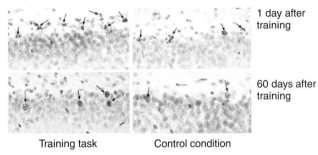

1 day after training

60 days after training

Training task   Control condition

From Leuner, B., Mendolia-Loffredo, S., Kozorovitskiy, Y., Samburg, D., Gould, E., and Shors, T. J. *Journal of Neuroscience*, 2004, *24*, 7477–7481.

them on.) At this time, some radial glia appear to undergo apoptosis, but many are transformed into astrocytes or neurons.

Once neurons have migrated to their final locations, they begin forming connections with other neurons. They grow dendrites, which receive the terminal buttons from the axons of other neurons, and they grow axons of their own. Some neurons extend their dendrites and axons laterally, connecting adjacent columns of neurons or even establishing connections with other neurons in distant regions of the brain.

During development, thousands of different pathways—groups of axons that connect one brain region with another—develop in the brain. Within many of these pathways the connections are orderly and systematic. For example, the axons of sensory neurons from the skin form orderly connections in the brain; axons from the little finger form synapses in one region, those of the ring finger form synapses in a neighboring region, and so on. In fact, the surface of the body is "mapped" on the surface of the brain. Similarly, the surface of the retina of the eye is "mapped" on another region of the surface of the brain.

For many years, researchers have believed that neurogenesis does not take place in the fully developed brain. However, more recent studies have shown this belief to be incorrect—the adult brain contains some stem cells (similar to the progenitor cells that give rise to the cells of the developing brain) that can divide and produce neurons. Detection of newly produced cells is done by administering a small amount of a radioactive form of one of the nucleotide bases that cells use to produce the DNA that is needed for neurogenesis. The next day, the animals' brains are removed and examined with methods described in Chapter 5. Such studies have found evidence for neurogenesis in just two parts of the adult brain: the hippocampus, primarily involved in learning, and the olfactory bulb, involved in the sense of smell (Doetsch and Hen, 2005). Evidence indicates that exposure to new odors can increase the survival rate of new neurons in the olfactory bulbs, and training on a learning task can enhance neurogenesis in the hippocampus. (See *Figure 3.7.*) In addition, as we will see in Chapter 15, depression or exposure to stress can suppress neurogenesis in the hippocampus, and drugs that reduce stress and depression can reinstate neurogenesis. Unfortunately, there is no evidence that growth of new neurons can repair the effects of brain damage, such as that caused by head injury or strokes.

Evolution of the Human Brain

The brains of the earliest vertebrates were smaller than those of later animals, and they were simpler as well. The evolutionary process brought about genetic changes that were responsible for the development of more complex brains, with more parts and more interconnections. The human brain is larger than that of any other large animal when corrected for body size. For example, our brain is more than three times larger than that of a chimpanzee, our closest relative. What types of genetic changes are required to produce a large brain?

Rakic (1988, 1995) suggests that the size differences between these two brains could be caused by a very simple process. We just saw that the size of the ventricular zone increases during symmetrical division of the progenitor cells located there. The ultimate size of the brain is determined by the size of the ventricular zone. As Rakic notes, each symmetrical division doubles the number of progenitor cells and thus doubles the size of the brain. The human brain is ten times larger than that of a rhesus macaque monkey. Thus, between three and four additional symmetrical divisions of progenitor cells would account for the difference in the size of these two brains. In fact, the stage of symmetrical division lasts about 2 days longer in humans, which provides enough time for three more divisions. The period of asymmetrical division is longer, too, which accounts for the fact that the human cortex is 15 percent thicker. Thus, delays in the termination of the symmetrical and asymmetrical periods of development could be responsible for the increased size of the human brain. A few simple mutations of the genes that control the timing of brain development could be responsible for these delays.

We do not yet know what genetic differences between humans and our primate relatives are responsible for our larger brains, but investigators are beginning to discover the factors that control brain size. For example, a protein called β-*catenin* is involved in regulation of cell division and tissue growth. Research indicates that this protein also plays a role in regulating the size of the cerebral cortex by controlling symmetrical cell division of progenitor cells. Chenn and Walsh (2002) employed a genetic engineering method that increased the production of β-catenin in neural progenitor cells in mouse fetuses. As a result, the number of progenitor cells increased dramatically, and the mice developed larger brains—and larger heads to accommodate these brains. The cerebral cortex grew so much that it developed convolutions normally seen only in larger, more complex brains. (See *Figure 3.8.*) A follow-up study (Woodhead et al., 2006) found that interfering with β-catenin signaling in the ventricular zone led to development of a smaller cerebral cortex. It is possible that mutations in the human genome have led to larger brains by affecting the production of β-catenin or some of the other chemicals with which this protein interacts.

FIGURE 3.8

Effect of β-Catenin on Development.   The photographs show (a) a normal mouse head and (b) the head of a genetically engineered mouse that produced excessive amounts of β-catenin, which causes development of a much larger head and brain and development of convolutions in the cerebral cortex that are normally seen only in the brains of larger mammals.

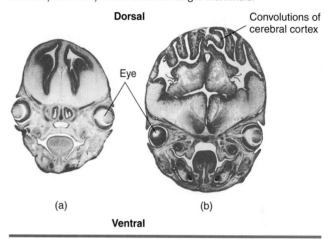

From Chenn, A., and Walsh, C. A. *Science*, 2002, *297*, 365–369. Copyright © 2002. Reprinted with permission from AAAS.

The Forebrain

As we saw, the **forebrain** surrounds the rostral end of the neural tube. Its two major components are the telencephalon and the diencephalon.

Telencephalon

The telencephalon includes most of the two symmetrical **cerebral hemispheres** that make up the cerebrum. The cerebral hemispheres are covered by the cerebral cortex and contain the limbic system and the basal ganglia. The latter two sets of structures are primarily in the **subcortical regions** of the brain—those located deep within it, beneath the cerebral cortex.

Cerebral Cortex   As we saw, *cortex* means "bark," and the cerebral cortex surrounds the cerebral hemispheres like the bark of a tree. In humans the cerebral cortex is greatly convoluted. These convolutions, consisting of **sulci** (small grooves), **fissures** (large grooves), and **gyri** (bulges between adjacent sulci or fissures), greatly enlarge the surface area of the cortex, compared with a smooth brain of the same size. In fact, two-thirds of the surface of the cortex is hidden in the grooves; thus, the presence of gyri and sulci triples the area of the cerebral cortex. The total surface area is approximately 2360 cm² (2.5 ft²), and the thickness is approximately 3 mm.

The cerebral cortex consists mostly of glia and the cell bodies, dendrites, and interconnecting axons of neurons. Because cells predominate, the cerebral cortex

forebrain The most rostral of the three major divisions of the brain; includes the telencephalon and diencephalon.

cerebral hemisphere (*sa ree brul*) One of the two major portions of the forebrain, covered by the cerebral cortex.

subcortical region The region located within the brain, beneath the cortical surface.

sulcus (plural: sulci) (*sul kus, sul sigh*) A groove in the surface of the cerebral hemisphere, smaller than a fissure.

fissure A major groove in the surface of the brain, larger than a sulcus.

gyrus (plural: gyri) (*jye russ, jye rye*) A convolution of the cortex of the cerebral hemispheres, separated by sulci or fissures.

FIGURE 3.9

Cross Section of the Human Brain.   The brain slice shows fissures and gyri and the layer of cerebral cortex that follows these convolutions.

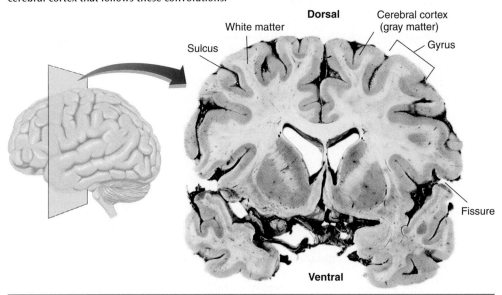

has a grayish brown appearance, and it is called *gray matter*. (See *Figure 3.9*.) Millions of axons run beneath the cerebral cortex and connect its neurons with those located elsewhere in the brain. The large concentration of myelin around these axons gives this tissue an opaque white appearance—hence the term *white matter*.

Different regions of the cerebral cortex perform different functions. Three regions receive information from the sensory organs. The **primary visual cortex**, which receives visual information, is located at the back of the brain, on the inner surfaces of the cerebral hemispheres—primarily on the upper and lower banks of the **calcarine fissure**. (*Calcarine* means "spur shaped." See *Figure 3.10*.) The **primary auditory cortex**, which receives auditory information, is located on the upper surface of a deep fissure in the side of the brain—the **lateral fissure**. (See inset, *Figure 3.10*.) The **primary somatosensory cortex**, a vertical strip of cortex just caudal to the **central sulcus**, receives information from the body senses. As Figure 3.10 shows, different regions of the primary somatosensory cortex receive information from different regions of the body. In addition, the base of the somatosensory cortex receives information concerning taste. (See *Figure 3.10*.)

With the exception of olfaction and gustation (taste), sensory information from the body or the environment is sent to primary sensory cortex of the contralateral hemisphere. Thus, the primary somatosensory cortex of the left hemisphere learns what the right hand is holding, the left primary visual cortex learns what is happening toward the person's right, and so on.

The region of the cerebral cortex that is most directly involved in the control of movement is the **primary motor cortex**, located just in front of the primary somatosensory cortex. Neurons in different parts of the primary motor cortex are connected to muscles in different parts of the body. The connections, like those of the sensory regions of the cerebral cortex, are contralateral; the left primary motor cortex controls the right side of the body and vice versa. Thus, if a surgeon places an electrode on the surface of the primary motor cortex and stimulates the neurons there with a weak electrical current, the result will be movement of a particular part of the body. Moving the electrode to a different spot will cause a different part of the body to move. (See *Figure 3.10*.) I like to think of the strip of primary motor cortex as the keyboard of a piano, with each key controlling a different movement. (We will see shortly who the "player" of this piano is.)

primary visual cortex The region of the posterior occipital lobe whose primary input is from the visual system.

calcarine fissure (*kal ka rine*) A fissure located in the occipital lobe on the medial surface of the brain; most of the primary visual cortex is located along its upper and lower banks.

primary auditory cortex The region of the superior temporal lobe whose primary input is from the auditory system.

lateral fissure The fissure that separates the temporal lobe from the overlying frontal and parietal lobes.

primary somatosensory cortex The region of the anterior parietal lobe whose primary input is from the somatosensory system.

central sulcus (*sul kus*) The sulcus that separates the frontal lobe from the parietal lobe.

primary motor cortex The region of the posterior frontal lobe that contains neurons that control movements of skeletal muscles.

FIGURE 3.10

The Primary Sensory Regions of the Brain.   The figure shows a lateral view of the left hemisphere of the brain and part of the inner surface of the right hemisphere. The inset shows a cutaway of part of the frontal lobe of the left hemisphere, permitting us to see the primary auditory cortex on the dorsal surface of the temporal lobe, which forms the ventral bank of the lateral fissure.

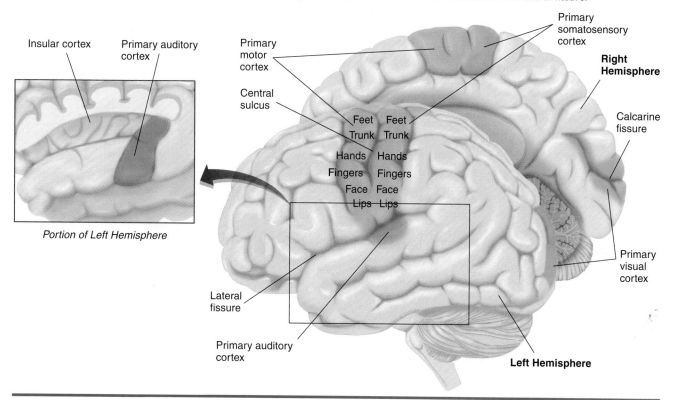

The regions of primary sensory and motor cortex occupy only a small part of the cerebral cortex. The rest of the cerebral cortex accomplishes what is done between sensation and action: perceiving, learning and remembering, planning, and acting. These processes take place in the *association areas* of the cerebral cortex. The central sulcus provides an important dividing line between the rostral and caudal regions of the cerebral cortex. (See *Figure 3.10*.) The rostral region is involved in movement-related activities, such as planning and executing behaviors. The caudal region is involved in perceiving and learning.

Discussing the various regions of the cerebral cortex is easier if we have names for them. In fact, the cerebral cortex is divided into four areas, or *lobes*, named for the bones of the skull that cover them: the frontal lobe, parietal lobe, temporal lobe, and occipital lobe. Of course, the brain contains two of each lobe, one in each hemisphere. The **frontal lobe** (the "front") includes everything in front of the central sulcus. The **parietal lobe** (the "wall") is located on the side of the cerebral hemisphere, just behind the central sulcus, caudal to the frontal lobe. The **temporal lobe** (the "temple") juts forward from the base of the brain, ventral to the frontal and parietal lobes. The **occipital lobe** (from the Latin *ob*, "in back of," and *caput*, "head") lies at the very back of the brain, caudal to the parietal and temporal lobes. Figure 3.11 shows these lobes in three views of the cerebral hemispheres: a ventral view (a view from the bottom), a midsagittal view (a view of the inner surface of the right hemisphere after the left hemisphere has been removed), and a lateral view. (See *Figure 3.11*.)

Each primary sensory area of the cerebral cortex sends information to adjacent regions, called the **sensory association cortex**. Circuits of neurons in the sensory association cortex analyze the information received from the primary sensory cortex;

frontal lobe   The anterior portion of the cerebral cortex, rostral to the parietal lobe and dorsal to the temporal lobe.

parietal lobe (*pa rye i tul*)   The region of the cerebral cortex caudal to the frontal lobe and dorsal to the temporal lobe.

temporal lobe (*tem por ul*)   The region of the cerebral cortex rostral to the occipital lobe and ventral to the parietal and frontal lobes.

occipital lobe (*ok sip i tul*)   The region of the cerebral cortex caudal to the parietal and temporal lobes.

sensory association cortex   Those regions of the cerebral cortex that receive information from the regions of primary sensory cortex.

The Four Lobes of the Cerebral Cortex.   This figure shows the location of the four lobes, the primary sensory and motor areas, and the association areas of the cerebral cortex: (a) ventral view, from the base of the brain; (b) midsagittal view, with the cerebellum and brain stem removed; and (c) lateral view.

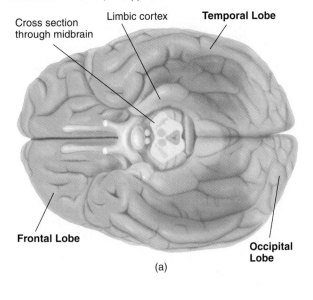

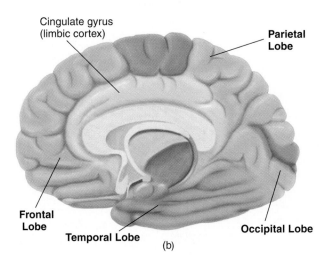

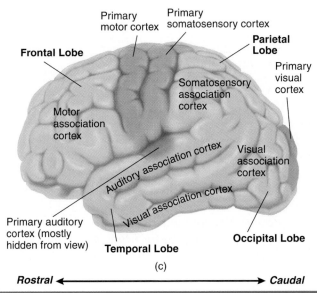

perception takes place there, and memories are stored there. The regions of the sensory association cortex located closest to the primary sensory areas receive information from only one sensory system. For example, the region closest to the primary visual cortex analyzes visual information and stores visual memories. Regions of the sensory association cortex located far from the primary sensory areas receive information from more than one sensory system; thus, they are involved in several kinds of perceptions and memories. These regions make it possible to integrate information from more than one sensory system. For example, we can learn the connection between the sight of a particular face and the sound of a particular voice. (See *Figure 3.11*.)

If people sustain damage to the somatosensory association cortex, their deficits are related to somatosensation and to the environment in general; for example, they may have difficulty perceiving the shapes of objects that they can touch but not see, they may be unable to name parts of their bodies (see the following case), or they may have trouble drawing maps or following them. Destruction of the primary visual cortex causes blindness. However, although people who sustain damage to the visual association cortex will not become blind, they may be unable to recognize objects by sight. People who sustain damage to the auditory association cortex may have difficulty perceiving speech or even producing meaningful speech of their own. People who sustain damage to regions of the association cortex at the junction of the three posterior lobes, where the somatosensory, visual, and auditory functions overlap, may have difficulty reading or writing.

Mr. M., a city bus driver, stopped to let a passenger climb aboard. The passenger asked him a question, and Mr. M. suddenly realized that he didn't understand what she was saying. He could hear her, but her words made no sense. He opened his mouth to reply. He made some sounds, but the look on the woman's face told him that she couldn't understand what he was trying to say. He turned off the engine and looked around at the passengers and tried to tell them to get some help. Although he was unable to say anything, they understood that something was wrong, and one of them called an ambulance.

An MRI scan showed that Mr. M. had sustained an intracerebral hemorrhage—a kind of stroke caused by rupture of blood vessels in the brain. The stroke had damaged his left parietal lobe. Mr. M. gradually regained the ability to talk and understand the speech of others, but some deficits remained. A colleague, Dr. D., and I studied Mr. M. several weeks after his stroke. The dialogue went something like this:

"Show me your hand."
"My hand . . . my hand." Looks at his arms, then touches his left forearm.
"Show me your chin."
"My chin." Looks at his arms, looks down, puts his hand on his abdomen.
"Show me your right elbow."
"My right . . ." (points to the right with his right thumb) "elbow." Looks up and down his right arm, finally touches his right shoulder.

As you can see, Mr. M. could understand that we were asking him to point out parts of his body and could repeat the names of the body parts when we spoke them, but he could not identify which body parts these names referred to. This strange deficit, which sometimes follows damage to the left parietal lobe, is called autotopagnosia, or "poor knowledge of one's own topography." (A better term would be autotopanomia, or "poor knowledge of the names of one's own topography," but, then, no one asked me to choose the term.) The parietal lobes are involved with space: the right primarily with external space, and the left with one's body and personal space. I'll say more about disorders such as this one in Chapter 13, which deals with brain mechanisms of language.

Just as regions of the sensory association cortex of the posterior part of the brain are involved in perceiving and remembering, the frontal association cortex is involved in the planning and execution of movements. The **motor association cortex** (also known as the *premotor cortex*) is located just rostral to the primary motor cortex. This region controls the primary motor cortex; thus, it directly controls behavior. If the primary motor cortex is the keyboard of the piano, then the motor association cortex is the piano player. The rest of the frontal lobe, rostral to the motor association cortex, is known as the **prefrontal cortex**. This region of the brain is less involved with the control of movement and more involved in formulating plans and strategies.

Although the two cerebral hemispheres cooperate with each other, they do not perform identical functions. Some functions are *lateralized*—located primarily on one side of the brain. In general, the left hemisphere participates in the *analysis* of information—the extraction of the elements that make up the whole of an experience. This ability makes the left hemisphere particularly good at recognizing *serial events*—events whose elements occur one after the other—and controlling

motor association cortex The region of the frontal lobe rostral to the primary motor cortex; also known as the premotor cortex.

prefrontal cortex The region of the frontal lobe rostral to the motor association cortex.

FIGURE 3.12

Bundles of Axons in the Corpus Callosum. This figure, obtained by means of diffusion tensor imaging, shows bundles of axons in the corpus callosum that serve different regions of the cerebral cortex that constitute the corpus callosum.

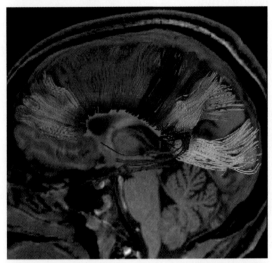

Reprinted from *NeuroImage, 32,* Hofer, S., and Frahm, J., Topography of the Human Corpus Callosum Revisited—Comprehensive Fiber Tractography Using Diffusion Tensor Magnetic Resonance Imaging, 989–994, Copyright 2006, with permission from Elsevier.

corpus callosum (*ka loh sum*) A large bundle of axons that interconnects corresponding regions of the association cortex on each side of the brain.

neocortex The phylogenetically newest cortex, including the primary sensory cortex, primary motor cortex, and association cortex.

limbic cortex Phylogenetically old cortex, located at the medial edge ("limbus") of the cerebral hemispheres; part of the limbic system.

cingulate gyrus (*sing yew lett*) A strip of limbic cortex lying along the lateral walls of the groove separating the cerebral hemispheres, just above the corpus callosum.

limbic system A group of brain regions including the anterior thalamic nuclei, amygdala, hippocampus, limbic cortex, and parts of the hypothalamus, as well as their interconnecting fiber bundles.

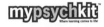

Animation 3.2
The Rotatable Brain

sequences of behavior. (In a few people the functions of the left and right hemispheres are reversed.) The serial functions that are performed by the left hemisphere include verbal activities, such as talking, understanding the speech of other people, reading, and writing. These abilities are disrupted by damage to the various regions of the left hemisphere. (I will say more about language and the brain in Chapter 13.)

In contrast, the right hemisphere is specialized for *synthesis*; it is particularly good at putting isolated elements together to perceive things as a whole. For example, our ability to draw sketches (especially of three-dimensional objects), read maps, and construct complex objects out of smaller elements depends heavily on circuits of neurons that are located in the right hemisphere. Damage to the right hemisphere disrupts these abilities.

We are not aware of the fact that each hemisphere perceives the world differently. Although the two cerebral hemispheres perform somewhat different functions, our perceptions and our memories are unified. This unity is accomplished by the **corpus callosum**, a large band of axons that connects corresponding parts of the association cortex of the left and right hemispheres: The left and right temporal lobes are connected, the left and right parietal lobes are connected, and so on. Because of the corpus callosum, each region of the association cortex knows what is happening in the corresponding region of the opposite side of the brain. The corpus callosum also makes a few asymmetrical connections that link different regions of the two hemispheres. *Figure 3.12* shows the bundles of axons that constitute the corpus callosum, obtained by means of *diffusion tensor imaging*, a special scanning method described in Chapter 5.

Figure 3.13 shows a midsagittal view of the brain. The brain (and part of the spinal cord) has been sliced down the middle, dividing it into its two symmetrical halves. The left half has been removed, so we see the inner surface of the right half. The cerebral cortex that covers most of the surface of the cerebral hemispheres (including the frontal, parietal, occipital, and temporal lobes) is called the **neocortex** ("new" cortex, because it is of relatively recent evolutionary origin). Another form of cerebral cortex, the **limbic cortex**, is located around the medial edge of the cerebral hemispheres (*limbus* means "border"). The **cingulate gyrus**, an important region of the limbic cortex, can be seen in this figure. (See *Figure 3.13*.) In addition, if you look back at Figures 3.11(a) and 3.11(b), you will see that the limbic cortex occupies the regions that have not been colored in. (Refer to *Figures 3.11a* and *3.11b*.)

Figure 3.13 also shows the corpus callosum. To slice the brain into its two symmetrical halves, one must slice through the middle of the corpus callosum. (Recall that I described the split-brain operation, in which the corpus callosum is severed, in Chapter 1.) (See *Figure 3.13*.)

As mentioned earlier, one of the animations I have prepared will permit you to view the brain from various angles and see the locations of the specialized regions of the cerebral cortex. (See *MyPsychKit 3.2, The Rotatable Brain.*)

Limbic System A neuroanatomist, Papez (1937), suggested that a set of interconnected brain structures formed a circuit whose primary function was motivation and emotion. This system included several regions of the limbic cortex (already described) and a set of interconnected structures surrounding the core of the forebrain. A physiologist, MacLean (1949), expanded the system to include other structures and coined the term **limbic system**. Besides the limbic cortex, the most important parts of the limbic system are the **hippocampus** ("sea horse") and the

FIGURE 3.13

A Midsagittal View of the Brain and Part of the Spinal Cord

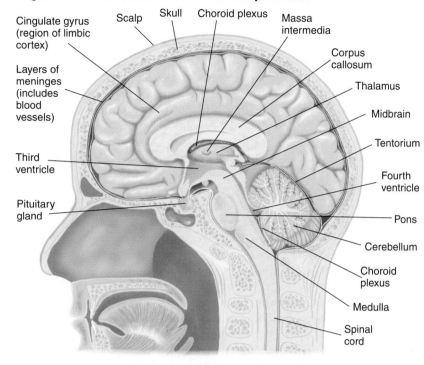

amygdala ("almond"), located next to the lateral ventricle in the temporal lobe. The **fornix** ("arch") is a bundle of axons that connects the hippocampus with other regions of the brain, including the **mammillary** ("breast-shaped") **bodies,** protrusions on the base of the brain that contain parts of the hypothalamus. (See *Figure 3.14.*)

MacLean noted that the evolution of this system, which includes the first and simplest form of cerebral cortex, appears to have coincided with the development of emotional responses. As you will see in Chapter 12, we now know that parts of the limbic system (notably, the hippocampal formation and the region of limbic cortex that surrounds it) are involved in learning and memory. The amygdala and some regions of limbic cortex are specifically involved in emotions: feelings and expressions of emotions, emotional memories, and recognition of the signs of emotions in other people.

Basal Ganglia The **basal ganglia** are a collection of subcortical nuclei in the forebrain, which lie beneath the anterior portion of the lateral ventricles. **Nuclei** are groups of neurons of similar shape. (The word *nucleus*, from the Greek word for "nut," can refer to the inner portion of an atom, to the structure of a cell that contains the chromosomes, and—as in this case—to a collection of neurons located within the brain.) The major parts of the basal ganglia are the *caudate nucleus*, the *putamen*, and the *globus pallidus* (the "nucleus with a tail," the "shell," and the "pale globe"). (See *Figure 3.15.*) The basal ganglia are involved in the control of movement. For example,

hippocampus A forebrain structure of the temporal lobe, constituting an important part of the limbic system; includes the hippocampus proper (Ammon's horn), dentate gyrus, and subiculum.

amygdala (*a mig da la*) A structure in the interior of the rostral temporal lobe, containing a set of nuclei; part of the limbic system.

fornix A fiber bundle that connects the hippocampus with other parts of the brain, including the mammillary bodies of the hypothalamus; part of the limbic system.

mammillary bodies (*mam i lair ee*) A protrusion of the bottom of the brain at the posterior end of the hypothalamus, containing some hypothalamic nuclei; part of the limbic system.

basal ganglia A group of subcortical nuclei in the telencephalon, the caudate nucleus, the globus pallidus, and the putamen; important parts of the motor system.

nucleus (plural: nuclei) An identifiable group of neural cell bodies in the central nervous system.

FIGURE 3.14

The Major Components of the Limbic System. All of the left hemisphere except for the limbic system has been removed.

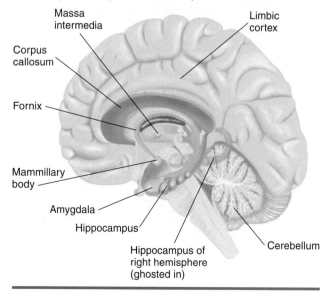

Parkinson's disease is caused by degeneration of certain neurons located in the mid-brain that send axons to the caudate nucleus and the putamen. The symptoms of this disease are of weakness, tremors, rigidity of the limbs, poor balance, and difficulty in initiating movements.

Diencephalon

The second major division of the forebrain, the **diencephalon**, is situated between the telencephalon and the mesencephalon; it surrounds the third ventricle. Its two most important structures are the thalamus and the hypothalamus. (See *Figure 3.15*.)

Thalamus   The **thalamus** (from the Greek *thalamos*, "inner chamber") makes up the dorsal part of the diencephalon. It is situated near the middle of the cerebral hemispheres, immediately medial and caudal to the basal ganglia. The thalamus has two lobes, connected by a bridge of gray matter called the *massa intermedia*, which pierces the middle of the third ventricle. (See *Figure 3.15*.) The massa intermedia is probably not an important structure, because it is absent in the brains of many people. However, it serves as a useful reference point in looking at diagrams of the brain; it appears in Figures 3.4, 3.13, 3.14, and 3.16.

Most neural input to the cerebral cortex is received from the thalamus; indeed, much of the cortical surface can be divided into regions that receive projections from specific parts of the thalamus. **Projection fibers** are sets of axons that arise from cell bodies located in one region of the brain and synapse on neurons located within another region (that is, they *project to* these regions).

The thalamus is divided into several nuclei. Some thalamic nuclei receive sensory information from the sensory systems. The neurons in these nuclei then relay the sensory information to specific sensory projection areas of the cerebral cortex. For example, the **lateral geniculate nucleus** receives information from the eye and sends axons to the primary visual cortex, and the **medial geniculate nucleus** receives information from the inner ear and sends axons to the primary auditory cortex. Other thalamic nuclei project to specific regions of the cerebral cortex, but they do not relay sensory information. For example, the **ventrolateral nucleus** receives information from the cerebellum and projects it to the primary motor cortex. As we will see in Chapter 8, several nuclei are involved in controlling the general excitability of the cerebral cortex. To accomplish this task, these nuclei have widespread projections to the cerebral cortex.

Hypothalamus   As its name implies, the **hypothalamus** lies at the base of the brain, under the thalamus. Although the hypothalamus is a relatively small structure, it is an important one. It controls the autonomic nervous system and the endocrine system and organizes behaviors related to survival of the species—the so-called four F's: fighting, feeding, fleeing, and mating.

The hypothalamus is situated on both sides of the ventral portion of the third ventricle. The hypothalamus is a complex structure, containing many nuclei and fiber tracts. Figure 3.16 indicates its location and size. Note that the pituitary gland is attached to the base of the hypothalamus via the pituitary stalk. Just in front of the pituitary stalk is the **optic chiasm**, where half of the axons in the optic nerves (from the eyes) cross from one side of the brain to the other. (See *Figure 3.16*.) The role of the hypo-

---

diencephalon (*dy en **seff** a lahn*) A region of the forebrain surrounding the third ventricle; includes the thalamus and the hypothalamus.

thalamus The largest portion of the diencephalon, located above the hypothalamus; contains nuclei that project information to specific regions of the cerebral cortex and receive information from it.

projection fiber An axon of a neuron in one region of the brain whose terminals form synapses with neurons in another region.

lateral geniculate nucleus A group of cell bodies within the lateral geniculate body of the thalamus that receives fibers from the retina and projects fibers to the primary visual cortex.

medial geniculate nucleus A group of cell bodies within the medial geniculate body of the thalamus; receives fibers from the auditory system and projects fibers to the primary auditory cortex.

ventrolateral nucleus A nucleus of the thalamus that receives inputs from the cerebellum and sends axons to the primary motor cortex.

FIGURE 3.15

The Basal Ganglia and Diencephalon.   The basal ganglia and diencephalon (thalamus and hypothalamus) are ghosted in to a semitransparent brain.

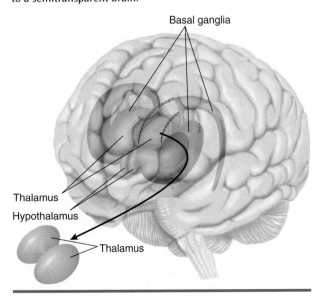

Basal ganglia

Thalamus

Hypothalamus

Thalamus

FIGURE 3.16

A Midsagittal View of Part of the Brain.   This view shows some of the nuclei of the hypothalamus. The nuclei are situated on the far side of the wall of the third ventricle, inside the right hemisphere.

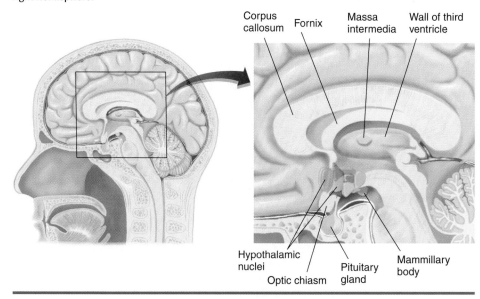

Corpus callosum   Fornix   Massa intermedia   Wall of third ventricle

Hypothalamic nuclei   Optic chiasm   Pituitary gland   Mammillary body

hypothalamus The group of nuclei of the diencephalon situated beneath the thalamus; involved in regulation of the autonomic nervous system, control of the anterior and posterior pituitary glands, and integration of species-typical behaviors.

optic chiasm (*kye az'm*) An X-shaped connection between the optic nerves, located below the base of the brain, just anterior to the pituitary gland.

anterior pituitary gland The anterior part of the pituitary gland; an endocrine gland whose secretions are controlled by the hypothalamic hormones.

neurosecretory cell A neuron that secretes a hormone or hormonelike substance.

posterior pituitary gland The posterior part of the pituitary gland; an endocrine gland that contains hormone-secreting terminal buttons of axons whose cell bodies lie within the hypothalamus.

thalamus in the control of the four F's (and other behaviors, such as drinking and sleeping) will be considered in several chapters later in this book.

Much of the endocrine system is controlled by hormones produced by cells in the hypothalamus. A special system of blood vessels directly connects the hypothalamus with the **anterior pituitary gland**. (See *Figure 3.17*.) The hypothalamic hormones are secreted by specialized neurons called **neurosecretory cells**, located near the base of the pituitary stalk. These hormones stimulate the anterior pituitary gland to secrete its hormones. For example, *gonadotropin-releasing hormone* causes the anterior pituitary gland to secrete the *gonadotropic hormones*, which play a role in reproductive physiology and behavior.

Most of the hormones secreted by the anterior pituitary gland control other endocrine glands. Because of this function, the anterior pituitary gland has been called the body's "master gland." For example, the gonadotropic hormones stimulate the gonads (ovaries and testes) to release male or female sex hormones. These hormones affect cells throughout the body, including some in the brain. Two other anterior pituitary hormones—prolactin and somatotropic hormone (growth hormone)—do not control other glands but act as the final messenger. The behavioral effects of many of the anterior pituitary hormones are discussed in later chapters.

The **posterior pituitary gland** is in many ways an extension of the hypothalamus. The hypothalamus produces the posterior pituitary hormones and directly controls their secretion. These hormones include oxytocin, which stimulates ejection of milk and uterine contractions at the time of childbirth, and vasopressin, which regulates urine output by the kidneys. They are produced by two different sets of neurons in the hypothalamus whose axons travel down the pituitary stalk and terminate in the posterior pituitary gland. The hormones are carried in vesicles through the axoplasm of these neurons and collect in the terminal buttons in

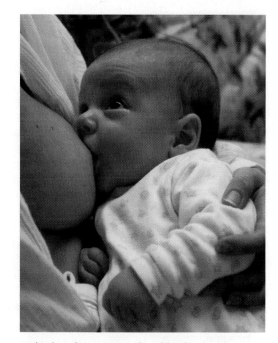

Prolactin, a hormone produced by the anterior pituitary gland, stimulates milk production in a nursing mother. Oxytocin, a hormone released by the posterior pituitary gland, stimulates the ejection of milk when the baby sucks on a nipple.

FIGURE 3.17

The Pituitary Gland.   Hormones released by the neurosecretory cells in the hypothalamus enter capillaries and are conveyed to the anterior pituitary gland, where they control its secretion of hormones. The hormones of the posterior pituitary gland are produced in the hypothalamus and carried there in vesicles by means of axoplasmic transport.

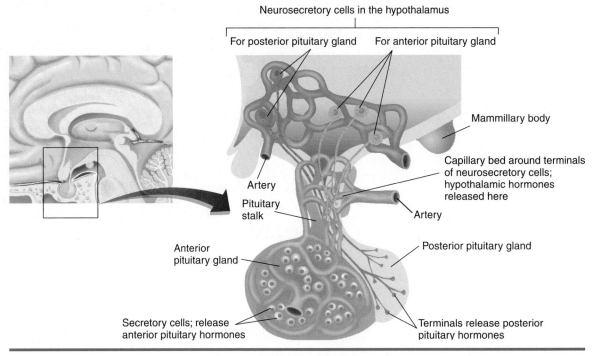

the posterior pituitary gland. When these axons fire, the hormone contained within their terminal buttons is liberated and enters the circulatory system.

The Midbrain

The **midbrain** (also called the **mesencephalon**) surrounds the cerebral aqueduct and consists of two major parts: the tectum and the tegmentum.

Tectum

The **tectum** ("roof") is located in the dorsal portion of the mesencephalon. Its principal structures are the **superior colliculi** and the **inferior colliculi**, which appear as four bumps on the dorsal surface of the **brain stem**. The brain stem includes the diencephalon, midbrain, and hindbrain; it is so called because it looks just like that—a stem. Figure 3.18 shows several views of the brain stem: lateral and posterior views of the brain stem inside a semitransparent brain, an enlarged view of the brain stem with part of the cerebellum cut away to reveal the inside of the fourth ventricle, and a cross section through the midbrain. (See *Figure 3.18.*) The inferior colliculi are a part of the auditory system. The superior colliculi are part of the visual system. In mammals they are primarily involved in visual reflexes and reactions to moving stimuli.

Tegmentum

The **tegmentum** ("covering") consists of the portion of the mesencephalon beneath the tectum. It includes the rostral end of the reticular formation, several nuclei controlling eye movements, the periaqueductal gray matter, the red nucleus, the substantia nigra, and the ventral tegmental area. (See *Figure 3.18d.*)

The **reticular formation** is a large structure consisting of many nuclei (over ninety in all). It is also characterized by a diffuse, interconnected network of neurons with complex dendritic and axonal processes. (Indeed, *reticulum* means "little net";

midbrain The mesencephalon; the central of the three major divisions of the brain.

mesencephalon (*mezz en seff a lahn*) The midbrain; a region of the brain that surrounds the cerebral aqueduct; includes the tectum and the tegmentum.

tectum The dorsal part of the midbrain; includes the superior and inferior colliculi.

superior colliculi (*ka lik yew lee*) Protrusions on top of the midbrain; part of the visual system.

inferior colliculi Protrusions on top of the midbrain; part of the auditory system.

brain stem The "stem" of the brain, from the medulla to the diencephalon, excluding the cerebellum.

tegmentum The ventral part of the midbrain; includes the periaqueductal gray matter, reticular formation, red nucleus, and substantia nigra.

FIGURE 3.18

The Cerebellum and Brain Stem.   The figure shows (a) a lateral view of a semitransparent brain, showing the cerebellum and brain stem ghosted in, (b) a view from the back of the brain, and (c) a dorsal view of the brain stem. The left hemisphere of the cerebellum and part of the right hemisphere have been removed to show the inside of the fourth ventricle and the cerebellar peduncles. Part (d) shows a cross section of the midbrain.

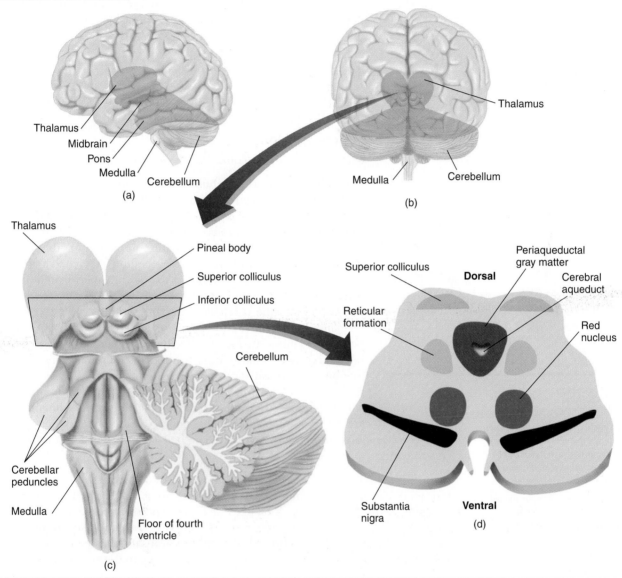

early anatomists were struck by the netlike appearance of the reticular formation.) The reticular formation occupies the core of the brain stem, from the lower border of the medulla to the upper border of the midbrain. (See *Figure 3.18d.*) The reticular formation receives sensory information by means of various pathways and projects axons to the cerebral cortex, thalamus, and spinal cord. It plays a role in sleep and arousal, attention, muscle tonus, movement, and various vital reflexes. Its functions will be described more fully in later chapters.

The **periaqueductal gray matter** is so called because it consists mostly of cell bodies of neurons ("gray matter," as contrasted with the "white matter" of axon bundles) that surround the cerebral aqueduct as it travels from the third to the fourth ventricle. The periaqueductal gray matter contains neural circuits that control sequences of movements that constitute species-typical behaviors, such as fighting and mating. As we will see in Chapter 7, opiates such as morphine decrease an organism's sensitivity to pain by stimulating receptors on neurons located in this region.

reticular formation A large network of neural tissue located in the central region of the brain stem, from the medulla to the diencephalon.

periaqueductal gray matter The region of the midbrain surrounding the cerebral aqueduct; contains neural circuits involved in species-typical behaviors.

FIGURE 3.19

Ventral View of the Spinal Column. Details show the anatomy of the bony vertebrae.

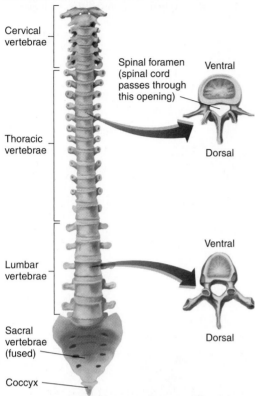

Cervical vertebrae

Spinal foramen (spinal cord passes through this opening)

Ventral

Dorsal

Thoracic vertebrae

Ventral

Lumbar vertebrae

Dorsal

Sacral vertebrae (fused)

Coccyx

red nucleus A large nucleus of the midbrain that receives inputs from the cerebellum and motor cortex and sends axons to motor neurons in the spinal cord.

substantia nigra A darkly stained region of the tegmentum that contains neurons that communicate with the caudate nucleus and putamen in the basal ganglia.

hindbrain The most caudal of the three major divisions of the brain; includes the metencephalon and myelencephalon.

cerebellum (*sair a bel lum*) A major part of the brain located dorsal to the pons, containing the two cerebellar hemispheres, covered with the cerebellar cortex; an important component of the motor system.

cerebellar cortex The cortex that covers the surface of the cerebellum.

deep cerebellar nuclei Nuclei located within the cerebellar hemispheres; receive projections from the cerebellar cortex and send projections out of the cerebellum to other parts of the brain.

The **red nucleus** and **substantia nigra** ("black substance") are important components of the motor system. A bundle of axons that arises from the red nucleus constitutes one of the two major fiber systems that bring motor information from the cerebral cortex and cerebellum to the spinal cord. The substantia nigra contains neurons whose axons project to the caudate nucleus and putamen, parts of the basal ganglia. As we will see in Chapter 4, degeneration of these neurons causes Parkinson's disease.

The Hindbrain

The **hindbrain**, which surrounds the fourth ventricle, consists of two major divisions: the metencephalon and the myelencephalon.

Metencephalon

The metencephalon consists of the cerebellum and the pons.

Cerebellum The **cerebellum** ("little brain"), with its two hemispheres, resembles a miniature version of the cerebrum. It is covered by the **cerebellar cortex** and has a set of **deep cerebellar nuclei**. These nuclei receive projections from the cerebellar cortex and themselves send projections out of the cerebellum to other parts of the brain. Each hemisphere of the cerebellum is attached to the dorsal surface of the pons by bundles of axons: the superior, middle, and inferior **cerebellar peduncles** ("little feet"). (See *Figure 3.18c.*)

Damage to the cerebellum impairs standing, walking, or performance of coordinated movements. (A virtuoso pianist or other performing musician owes much to his or her cerebellum.) The cerebellum receives visual, auditory, vestibular, and somatosensory information, and it also receives information about individual muscle movements being directed by the brain. The cerebellum integrates this information and modifies the motor outflow, exerting a coordinating and smoothing effect on the movements. Cerebellar damage results in jerky, poorly coordinated, exaggerated movements; extensive cerebellar damage makes it impossible even to stand.

Pons The **pons**, a large bulge in the brain stem, lies between the mesencephalon and medulla oblongata, immediately ventral to the cerebellum. *Pons* means "bridge," but it does not really look like one. (Refer to *Figures 3.13* and *3.18a.*) The pons contains, in its core, a portion of the reticular formation, including some nuclei that appear to be important in sleep and arousal. It also contains a large nucleus that relays information from the cerebral cortex to the cerebellum.

Myelencephalon

The myelencephalon contains one major structure, the **medulla oblongata** (literally, "oblong marrow"), usually just called the *medulla.* This structure is the most caudal portion of the brain stem; its lower border is the rostral end of the spinal cord. (Refer to *Figures 3.13* and *3.18a.*) The medulla contains part of the reticular formation, including nuclei that control vital functions such as regulation of the cardiovascular system, respiration, and skeletal muscle tonus.

The Spinal Cord

The **spinal cord** is a long, conical structure, approximately as thick as an adult's little finger. The principal function of the spinal cord is to distribute motor fibers to the effector organs of the body (glands and muscles) and to collect somatosensory information to be passed on to the brain. The spinal cord also has a certain degree of autonomy from the brain; various reflexive control circuits are located there.

The spinal cord is protected by the vertebral column, which is composed of twenty-four individual vertebrae of the *cervical* (neck), *thoracic* (chest), and *lumbar* (lower back) regions and the fused vertebrae making up the *sacral* and *coccygeal* portions of the column (located in the pelvic region). The spinal cord passes through a hole in each of the vertebrae (the *spinal foramens*). Figure 3.19 illustrates the divisions and structures of the spinal cord and vertebral column. (See *Figure 3.19.*) Note that the spinal cord is only about two-thirds as long as the vertebral column; the rest of the space is filled by a mass of **spinal roots** composing the **cauda equine** ("horse's tail"). (Refer to *Figure 3.3c.*)

Early in embryological development the vertebral column and spinal cord are the same length. As development progresses, the vertebral column grows faster than the spinal cord. This differential growth rate causes the spinal roots to be displaced downward; the most caudal roots travel the farthest before they emerge through openings between the vertebrae and thus compose the cauda equina. To produce the **caudal block** that is sometimes used in pelvic surgery or childbirth, a local anesthetic can be injected into the CSF contained within the sac of dura mater surrounding the cauda equina. The drug blocks conduction in the axons of the cauda equina.

Figure 3.20(a) shows a portion of the spinal cord, with the layers of the meninges that wrap it. Small bundles of fibers emerge from each side of the spinal cord in two straight lines along its dorsolateral and ventrolateral surfaces. Groups of these bundles fuse together and become the thirty-one paired sets of **dorsal roots**

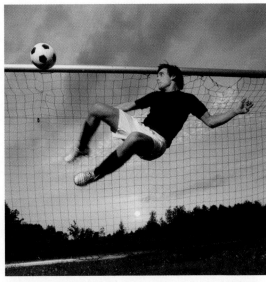

The cerebellum plays an important role in coordinating skilled movements.

FIGURE 3.20

Ventral View of the Spinal Cord. The figure shows (a) a portion of the spinal cord, showing the layers of the meninges and the relation of the spinal cord to the vertebral column, and (b) a cross section through the spinal cord. Ascending tracts are shown in blue; descending tracts are shown in red.

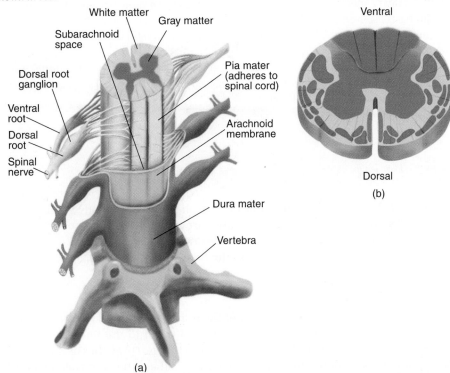

(a)

(b)

cerebellar peduncle (*pee dun kul*) One of three bundles of axons that attach each cerebellar hemisphere to the dorsal pons.

pons The region of the metencephalon rostral to the medulla, caudal to the midbrain, and ventral to the cerebellum.

medulla oblongata (*me doo la*) The most caudal portion of the brain; located in the myelencephalon, immediately rostral to the spinal cord.

spinal cord The cord of nervous tissue that extends caudally from the medulla.

spinal root A bundle of axons surrounded by connective tissue that occurs in pairs, which fuse and form a spinal nerve.

cauda equina (*ee kwye na*) A bundle of spinal roots located caudal to the end of the spinal cord.

caudal block The anesthesia and paralysis of the lower part of the body produced by injection of a local anesthetic into the cerebrospinal fluid surrounding the cauda equina.

dorsal root The spinal root that contains incoming (afferent) sensory fibers.

and **ventral roots**. The dorsal and ventral roots join together as they pass through the intervertebral foramens and become spinal nerves. (See *Figure 3.20a*.)

Figure 3.20(b) shows a cross section of the spinal cord. Like the brain, the spinal cord consists of white matter and gray matter. Unlike the white matter of the brain, the white matter of the spinal cord (consisting of ascending and descending bundles of myelinated axons) is on the outside; the gray matter (mostly neural cell bodies and short, unmyelinated axons) is on the inside. In Figure 3.20(b), ascending tracts are indicated in blue; descending tracts are indicated in red. (See *Figure 3.20b*.)

InterimSummary

The Central Nervous System

The brain consists of three major divisions, organized around the three chambers of the tube that develop early in embryonic life: the forebrain, the midbrain, and the hindbrain. The development of the neural tube into the mature central nervous system is illustrated in Figure 3.5; Table 3.2 outlines the major divisions and subdivisions of the brain.

During the first phase of brain development, symmetrical division of the progenitor cells of the ventricular zone, which lines the neural tube, increases its size. During the second phase, asymmetrical division of these cells gives rise to neurons, which migrate up the fibers of radial glial cells to their final resting places. There, neurons develop dendrites and axons and establish synaptic connections with other neurons. Later, neurons that fail to develop a sufficient number of synaptic connections are killed through apoptosis. The large size of the human brain, relative to the brains of other primates, appears to be accomplished primarily by lengthening the first and second periods of brain development.

The forebrain, which surrounds the lateral and third ventricles, consists of the telencephalon and diencephalon. The telencephalon contains the cerebral cortex, the limbic system, and the basal ganglia. The cerebral cortex is organized into the frontal, parietal, temporal, and occipital lobes. The central sulcus divides the frontal lobe, which deals specifically with movement and the planning of movement, from the other three lobes, which deal primarily with perceiving and

learning. The limbic system, which includes the limbic cortex, the hippocampus, and the amygdala, is involved in emotion, motivation, and learning. The basal ganglia participate in the control of movement. The diencephalon consists of the thalamus, which directs information to and from the cerebral cortex, and the hypothalamus, which controls the endocrine system and modulates species-typical behaviors.

The midbrain, which surrounds the cerebral aqueduct, consists of the tectum and tegmentum. The tectum is involved in audition and the control of visual reflexes and reactions to moving stimuli. The tegmentum contains the reticular formation, which is important in sleep, arousal, and movement; the periaqueductal gray matter, which controls various species-typical behaviors; and the red nucleus and the substantia nigra, both of which are parts of the motor system. The hindbrain, which surrounds the fourth ventricle, contains the cerebellum, the pons, and the medulla. The cerebellum plays an important role in integrating and coordinating movements. The pons contains some nuclei that are important in sleep and arousal. The medulla oblongata, too, is involved in sleep and arousal, but it also plays a role in control of movement and in control of vital functions such as heart rate, breathing, and blood pressure.

The outer part of the spinal cord consists of white matter: axons conveying information up or down. The central gray matter contains cell bodies.

The Peripheral Nervous System

The brain and spinal cord communicate with the rest of the body via the cranial nerves and spinal nerves. These nerves are part of the peripheral nervous system, which conveys sensory information to the central nervous system and conveys messages from the central nervous system to the body's muscles and glands.

Spinal Nerves

ventral root The spinal root that contains outgoing (efferent) motor fibers.

spinal nerve A peripheral nerve attached to the spinal cord.

The **spinal nerves** begin at the junction of the dorsal and ventral roots of the spinal cord. The nerves leave the vertebral column and travel to the muscles or sensory receptors they innervate, branching repeatedly as they go. Branches of spinal nerves often follow blood vessels, especially those branches that innervate skeletal muscles. (Refer to *Figure 3.3*.)

Now let us consider the pathways by which sensory information enters the spinal cord and motor information leaves it. The cell bodies of all axons that bring sensory information into the brain and spinal cord are located outside the CNS. (The sole exception is the visual system; the retina of the eye is actually a part of the brain.) These incoming axons are referred to as **afferent axons** because they "bear toward" the CNS. The cell bodies that give rise to the axons that bring somatosensory information to the spinal cord reside in the **dorsal root ganglia**, rounded swellings of the dorsal root. (See *Figure 3.21*.) These neurons are of the unipolar type (described in Chapter 2). The axonal stalk divides close to the cell body, sending one limb into the spinal cord and the other limb out to the sensory organ. Note that all of the axons in the dorsal root convey somatosensory information.

Cell bodies that give rise to the ventral root are located within the gray matter of the spinal cord. The axons of these multipolar neurons leave the spinal cord via a ventral root, which joins a dorsal root to make a spinal nerve. The axons that leave the spinal cord through the ventral roots control muscles and glands. They are referred to as **efferent axons** because they "bear away from" the CNS. (See *Figure 3.21*.)

Cranial Nerves

Twelve pairs of **cranial nerves** are attached to the ventral surface of the brain. Most of these nerves serve sensory and motor functions of the head and neck region. One of them, the *tenth*, or **vagus nerve**, regulates the functions of organs in the thoracic and abdominal cavities. It is called the *vagus* ("wandering") nerve because its branches wander throughout the thoracic and abdominal cavities. (The word *vagabond* has the same root.) Figure 3.22 presents a view of the base of the brain and illustrates the cranial nerves and the structures they serve. Note that efferent (motor) fibers are drawn in red and that afferent (sensory) fibers are drawn in blue. (See *Figure 3.22*.)

afferent axon An axon directed toward the central nervous system, conveying sensory information.

dorsal root ganglion A nodule on a dorsal root that contains cell bodies of afferent spinal nerve neurons.

efferent axon (*eff ur ent*) An axon directed away from the central nervous system, conveying motor commands to muscles and glands.

cranial nerve A peripheral nerve attached directly to the brain.

vagus nerve The largest of the cranial nerves, conveying efferent fibers of the parasympathetic division of the autonomic nervous system to organs of the thoracic and abdominal cavities.

FIGURE 3.21

A Cross Section of the Spinal Cord.   The figure shows the routes taken by afferent and efferent axons through the dorsal and ventral roots.

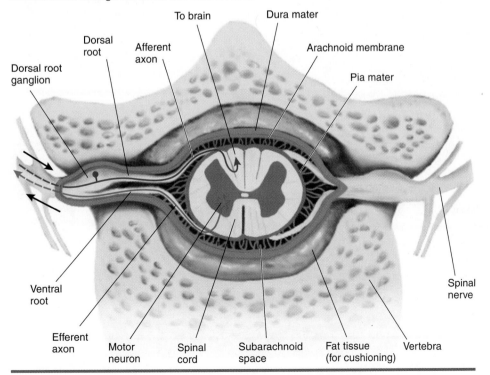

As mentioned in the previous section, cell bodies of sensory nerve fibers that enter the brain and spinal cord (except for the visual system) are located outside the central nervous system. Somatosensory information (and the sense of taste) is received, via the cranial nerves, from unipolar neurons. Auditory, vestibular, and visual information is received via fibers of bipolar neurons (described in Chapter 2). Olfactory information is received via the **olfactory bulbs**, which receive information from the olfactory receptors in the nose. The olfactory bulbs are complex structures containing a considerable amount of neural circuitry; actually, they are part of the brain. Sensory mechanisms are described in greater detail in Chapters 6 and 7.

olfactory bulb The protrusion at the end of the olfactory nerve; receives input from the olfactory receptors.

FIGURE 3.22

The Cranial Nerves.   The figure shows the twelve pairs of cranial nerves and the regions and functions they serve. Red lines denote axons that control muscles or glands; blue lines denote sensory axons.

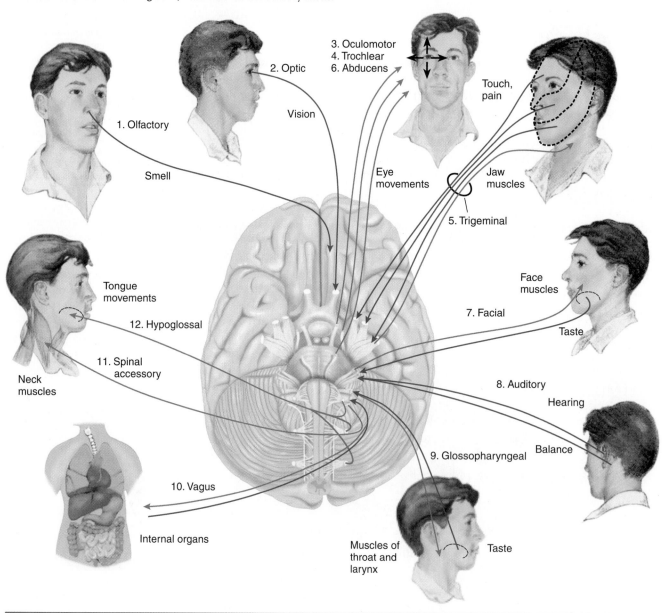

3. Oculomotor
4. Trochlear
6. Abducens

2. Optic

Vision

Touch, pain

1. Olfactory

Smell

Eye movements

Jaw muscles

5. Trigeminal

Tongue movements

Face muscles

12. Hypoglossal

7. Facial

Taste

11. Spinal accessory

8. Auditory

Neck muscles

Hearing

Balance

9. Glossopharyngeal

10. Vagus

Internal organs

Muscles of throat and larynx

Taste

The Autonomic Nervous System

The part of the peripheral nervous system discussed so far—which receives sensory information from the sensory organs and that controls movements of the skeletal muscles—is called the **somatic nervous system**. The other branch of the peripheral nervous system—the **autonomic nervous system (ANS)**—is concerned with regulation of smooth muscle, cardiac muscle, and glands. (*Autonomic* means "self-governing.") Smooth muscle is found in the skin (associated with hair follicles), in blood vessels, in the eyes (controlling pupil size and accommodation of the lens), and in the walls and sphincters of the gut, gallbladder, and urinary bladder. Merely describing the organs that are innervated by the autonomic nervous system suggests the function of this system: regulation of "vegetative processes" in the body.

The ANS consists of two anatomically separate systems: the *sympathetic division* and the *parasympathetic division*. With few exceptions, organs of the body are innervated by both of these subdivisions, and each has a different effect. For example, the sympathetic division speeds the heart rate, whereas the parasympathetic division slows it.

Sympathetic Division of the ANS

The **sympathetic division** is most involved in activities associated with expenditure of energy from reserves that are stored in the body. For example, when an organism is excited, the sympathetic nervous system increases blood flow to skeletal muscles, stimulates the secretion of epinephrine (resulting in increased heart rate and a rise in blood sugar level), and causes piloerection (erection of fur in mammals that have it and production of "goose bumps" in humans).

The cell bodies of sympathetic motor neurons are located in the gray matter of the thoracic and lumbar regions of the spinal cord (hence the sympathetic nervous system is also known as the *thoracolumbar system*). The fibers of these neurons exit via the ventral roots. After joining the spinal nerves, the fibers branch off and pass into **sympathetic ganglia** (not to be confused with the dorsal root ganglia). Figure 3.23 shows the relation of these ganglia to the spinal cord. Note that individual sympathetic ganglia are connected to the neighboring ganglia above and below, thus forming the **sympathetic ganglion chain**. (See *Figure 3.23.*)

The axons that leave the spinal cord through the ventral root belong to the **preganglionic neurons**. With one exception, all sympathetic preganglionic axons enter the ganglia of the sympathetic chain, but not all of them form synapses there. (The exception is the medulla of the adrenal gland, described in Chapter 10.) Some axons leave and travel to one of the other sympathetic ganglia, located among the internal organs. All sympathetic preganglionic axons form synapses with neurons located in one of the ganglia. The neurons with which they form synapses are called **postganglionic neurons**. In turn, the postganglionic neurons send axons to the target organs, such as the intestines, stomach, kidneys, or sweat glands. (See *Figure 3.23.*)

Parasympathetic Division of the ANS

The **parasympathetic division** of the autonomic nervous system supports activities that are involved with increases in the body's supply of stored energy. These activities include salivation, gastric and intestinal motility, secretion of digestive juices, and increased blood flow to the gastrointestinal system.

Cell bodies that give rise to preganglionic axons in the parasympathetic nervous system are located in two regions: the nuclei of some of the cranial nerves (especially the vagus nerve) and the intermediate horn of the gray matter in the sacral region of the spinal cord. Thus, the parasympathetic division of the ANS has often been

somatic nervous system The part of the peripheral nervous system that controls the movement of skeletal muscles or transmits somatosensory information to the central nervous system.

autonomic nervous system (ANS) The portion of the peripheral nervous system that controls the body's vegetative functions.

sympathetic division The portion of the autonomic nervous system that controls functions that accompany arousal and expenditure of energy.

sympathetic ganglia Nodules that contain synapses between preganglionic and postganglionic neurons of the sympathetic nervous system.

sympathetic ganglion chain One of a pair of groups of sympathetic ganglia that lie ventrolateral to the vertebral column.

preganglionic neuron The efferent neuron of the autonomic nervous system whose cell body is located in a cranial nerve nucleus or in the intermediate horn of the spinal gray matter and whose terminal buttons synapse upon postganglionic neurons in the autonomic ganglia.

postganglionic neuron Neurons of the autonomic nervous system that form synapses directly with their target organ.

parasympathetic division The portion of the autonomic nervous system that controls functions that occur during a relaxed state.

FIGURE 3.23

The Autonomic Nervous System.   The schematic figure shows the target organs and functions served by the sympathetic and parasympathetic branches of the autonomic nervous system.

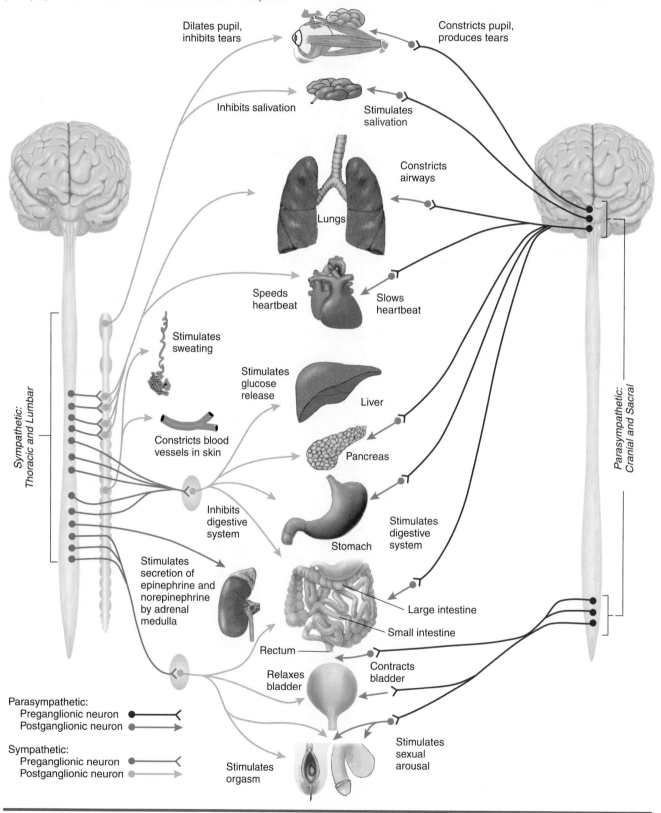

TABLE 3.3 The Major Divisions of the Peripheral Nervous System

Somatic Nervous System	Autonomic Nervous System (ANS)
Spinal Nerves	**Sympathetic Branch**
Afferents from sense organs	Spinal nerves (from thoracic and lumbar regions)
Efferents to muscles	Sympathetic ganglia
Cranial Nerves	**Parasympathetic Branch**
Afferents from sense organs	Cranial nerves (3rd, 7th, 9th, and 10th)
Efferents to muscles	Spinal nerves (from sacral region)
	Parasympathetic ganglia (adjacent to target organs)

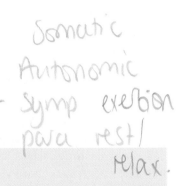

referred to as the *craniosacral system*. Parasympathetic ganglia are located in the immediate vicinity of the target organs; the postganglionic fibers are therefore relatively short. The terminal buttons of both preganglionic and postganglionic neurons in the parasympathetic nervous system secrete acetylcholine.

Table 3.3 summarizes the major divisions of the peripheral nervous system.

InterimSummary

The Peripheral Nervous System

The spinal nerves and the cranial nerves convey sensory axons into the central nervous system and motor axons out from it. Spinal nerves are formed by the junctions of the dorsal roots, which contain incoming (afferent) axons, and the ventral roots, which contain outgoing (efferent) axons. The autonomic nervous system consists of two divisions: the sympathetic division, which controls activities that occur during excitement or exertion, such as increased heart rate; and the parasympathetic division, which controls activities that occur during relaxation, such as decreased heart rate and increased activity of the digestive system. The pathways of the autonomic nervous system contain preganglionic axons, from the brain or spinal cord to the sympathetic or parasympathetic ganglia, and postganglionic axons, from the ganglia to the target organ.

⋮ EPILOGUE   Unilateral Neglect

When we see people like Miss S., the woman with unilateral neglect described in the prologue to this chapter, we realize that perception and attention are somewhat independent. The perceptual mechanisms of our brain provide the information, and the mechanisms involved in attention determine whether we become conscious of this information.

Unilateral ("one-sided") neglect occurs when the right parietal lobe is damaged. The parietal lobe contains the primary somatosensory cortex. It receives information from the skin, the muscles, the joints, the internal organs, and the part of the inner ear that is concerned with balance. Thus, it is concerned with the body and its position—but that is not all; the association cortex of the parietal lobe also receives auditory and visual information from the association cortex of the occipital and temporal lobes. Its

most important function seems to be to put together information about the movements and location of the parts of the body with the locations of objects in space around us.

If unilateral neglect simply consisted of blindness in the left side of the visual field and anesthesia of the left side of the body, it would not be nearly as interesting, but individuals with unilateral neglect are neither half blind nor half numb. Under the proper circumstances, they *can* see things located to their left, and they *can* tell when someone touches the left side of their bodies. However, they normally ignore such stimuli and act as if the left side of the world and of their bodies did not exist.

Volpe, LeDoux, and Gazzaniga (1979) presented pairs of visual stimuli to people with unilateral neglect—one stimulus in the left visual field and one stimulus in the right. Invariably, the people reported seeing only the right-hand stimulus. But when the investigators asked the people to say whether or not the two stimuli were identical, they answered correctly *even though they said that they were unaware of the left-hand stimulus*.

If you think about the story that the chief of neurology told about the man who ate only the right half of a pancake, you will realize that people with unilateral neglect *must* be able to perceive more than the right visual field. Remember that people with unilateral neglect fail to notice not only things to their left but also the *left halves* of things. But to distinguish between the left and right halves of an object, you first have to perceive the entire object—otherwise, how would you know where the middle was?

People with unilateral neglect also demonstrate their unawareness of the left half of things when they draw pictures. For example, when asked to draw a clock, they almost always successfully draw a circle, but then when they fill in the numbers, they scrunch them all in on the right side. Sometimes they simply stop after reaching 6 or 7, and sometimes they write the rest of the numbers underneath the circle. When asked to draw a daisy, they begin with a stem and a leaf or two and then draw all the petals to the right. (See *Figure 3.24*.)

Bisiach and Luzzatti (1978) demonstrated a similar phenomenon, which suggests that unilateral neglect extends even to a person's own visual imagery. The investigators asked two patients with unilateral neglect to describe the Piazza del Duomo, a well-known landmark in Milan, the city in which they and the patients lived. They asked the patients to imagine that they were standing at the north end of the piazza and to tell them what they saw. The patients duly named the buildings, but only those on the west, to their right. Then the investigators asked the patients to imagine themselves at the south end of the piazza. This time, they named the buildings on the east—again, to their right. Obviously, they knew about *all* of the buildings and their locations, but they visualized them only when the buildings were located in the right side of their (imaginary) visual field.

Although neglect of the left side of one's own body can be studied only in people with brain abnormalities, an interesting phenomenon seen in people with undamaged brains confirms the importance of the parietal lobe (and another region of the brain) in feelings of body ownership. Ehrsson, Spence, and Passingham (2004) studied the *rubber hand illusion*. Normal subjects were positioned with their left hand hidden out of sight. They saw a lifelike rubber left hand in front of them. The experimenters stroked both the subject's hidden left hand and the visible rubber hand with a small paintbrush. If the two hands were stroked synchronously and in the same direction, the subjects began to experience the rubber hand as their own. In fact, if they were then asked to use their right hand to point to their left hand, they tended to point toward the rubber hand. However, if the real and artificial hands were stroked in different directions or at different

FIGURE 3.24

Unilateral Neglect.   When people with unilateral neglect attempt to draw simple objects, they demonstrate their unawareness of the left half of things by drawing only those features that appear on the right.

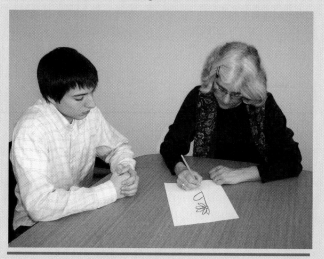

times, the subjects did *not* experience the rubber hand as their own. (See *Figure 3.25*.)

While the subjects were participating in the experiment, the experimenters recorded the activity of their brains with a functional MRI scanner. (Brain scanning is described in Chapter 5.) The

FIGURE 3.25

The Rubber Hand Illusion.   If the subject's hidden left hand and the visible rubber hand are stroked synchronously in the same direction, the subject will come to experience the artificial hand as his or her own. If the hands are stroked asynchronously or in different directions, this illusion will not occur.

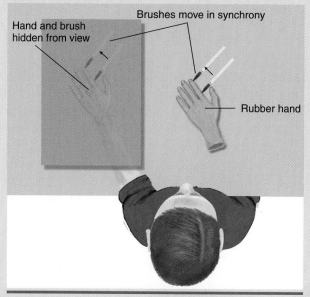

Adapted from Botwinick, M. *Science*, 2004, *305*, 782–783.

scans showed increased activity in the parietal lobe, and then, as the subjects began to experience the rubber hand as belonging to their body, in the *premotor cortex*, a region of the brain involved in planning movements. When the stroking of the real and artificial hands was uncoordinated and the subjects did not experience the rubber hand as their own, the premotor cortex did not become activated. The experimenters concluded that the parietal cortex analyzed the sight and the feeling of brush strokes. When the parietal cortex detected that they were congruent, this information was transmitted to the premotor cortex, which gave rise to the feeling of ownership of the rubber hand.

A second study from the same laboratory provided a particularly convincing demonstration that people experience a genuine feeling of ownership of the rubber hand (Ehrsson et al., 2007). The investigators used the procedure just described to establish a feeling of ownership and then threatened the rubber hand by making a stabbing movement toward the hand with a needle. (They did not actually touch the hand with the needle.) Brain scans showed increased activity in a region of the brain (the anterior cingulate cortex) that is normally activated when a person anticipates pain, and also in a region (the supplementary motor area) this is normally activated when a person feels the urge to move his or her arm (Fried et al., 1991; Peyron, Laurent, and Garcia-Larrea, 2000). So the impression that the rubber hand was about to receive a painful stab from a needle made people react as they would if their own hand were the target of the threat.

Key Concepts

BASIC FEATURES OF THE NERVOUS SYSTEM

1. The central nervous system consists of the brain and spinal cord; it is covered with the meninges and floats in cerebrospinal fluid.

THE CENTRAL NERVOUS SYSTEM

2. The nervous system develops first as a tube, which thickens and forms pockets and folds as cells are produced. The tube becomes the ventricular system.
3. The primary cause of the difference between the human brain and that of other primates is a slightly extended period of symmetrical and asymmetrical division of progenitor cells located in the ventricular zone.

4. The forebrain, surrounding the lateral and third ventricles, consists of the telencephalon (cerebral cortex, limbic system, and basal ganglia) and diencephalon (thalamus and hypothalamus).
5. The midbrain, which surrounds the cerebral aqueduct, consists of the tectum and tegmentum.
6. The hindbrain, which surrounds the fourth ventricle, contains the cerebellum, the pons, and the medulla.

THE PERIPHERAL NERVOUS SYSTEM

7. The spinal and cranial nerves connect the central nervous system with the rest of the body. The autonomic nervous system consists of two divisions: sympathetic and parasympathetic.

Suggested Readings

Diamond, M. C., Scheibel, A. B., and Elson, L. M. *The Human Brain Coloring Book.* New York: Barnes & Noble, 1985.

Gluhbegovic, N., and Williams, T. H. *The Human Brain: A Photographic Guide.* New York: Harper & Row, 1980.

Heimer, L. *The Human Brain and Spinal Cord: Functional Neuroanatomy and Dissection Guide,* 2nd ed. New York: Springer-Verlag, 1995.

Nauta, W. J. H., and Feirtag, M. *Fundamental Neuroanatomy.* New York: W. H. Freeman, 1986.

Netter, F. H. *The CIBA Collection of Medical Illustrations. Vol. 1: Nervous System. Part 1: Anatomy and Physiology.* Summit, NJ: CIBA Pharmaceutical Products Co., 1991.

Woolsey, T. A., Hanaway, J., and Gado, M. H. *The Brain Atlas: A Guide to the Human Central Nervous System,* 2nd. ed. Hoboken, NJ: John Wiley & Sons, 2003.

Additional Resources

Visit www.mypsychkit.com for additional review and practice of the material covered in this chapter. Within MyPsychKit, you can take practice tests and receive a customized study plan to help you review. Dozens of animations, tutorials, and Web links are also available. You can even review using the interactive electronic version of this textbook. You will need to register for MyPsychKit. See www.mypsychkit.com for complete details.

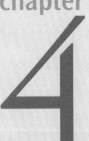

chapter

4

Psychopharmacology

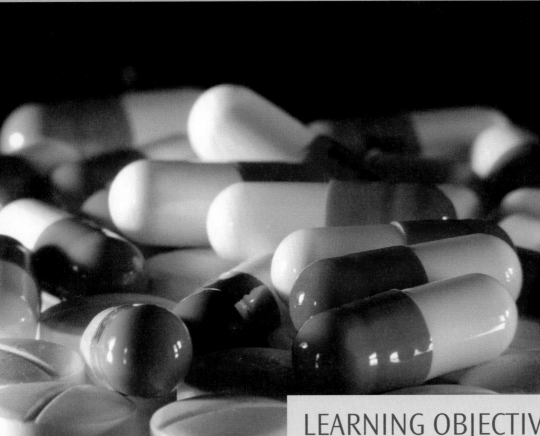

LEARNING OBJECTIVES

1. Describe the routes of administration of drugs and their subsequent distribution within the body.

2. Describe drug effectiveness, the effects of repeated administration of drugs, and the placebo effect.

3. Describe the effects of drugs on synaptic activity.

4. Review the general role of neurotransmitters and neuromodulators, and describe the acetylcholinergic pathways in the brain and the drugs that affect these neurons.

5. Describe the monoaminergic pathways in the brain and the drugs that affect these neurons.

6. Review the role of neurons that release amino acid neurotransmitters and describe drugs that affect these neurons.

7. Describe the effects of peptides, lipids, nucleosides, and soluble gases released by neurons.

PROLOGUE   A Contaminated Drug

In July 1982, some people in northern California began showing up at neurology clinics displaying dramatic, severe symptoms (Langston, Ballard, Tetrud, and Irwin, 1983). The most severely affected patients were almost totally paralyzed. They were unable to speak intelligibly, they drooled constantly, and their eyes were open with a fixed stare. Others, less severely affected, walked with a slow, shuffling gait and moved slowly and with great difficulty. The symptoms looked like those of Parkinson's disease, but that disorder has a very gradual onset. In addition, it rarely strikes people before late middle age, and the patients were all in their twenties or early thirties.

The common factor linking these patients was intravenous drug use; all of them had been taking a "new heroin," a synthetic opiate related to meperidine (Demerol). Because the symptoms looked like those of Parkinson's disease, the patients were given L-DOPA, the drug used to treat this disease, and they all showed significant improvement in their symptoms, however, even with this treatment, the symptoms were debilitating. In normal cases of Parkinson's disease L-DOPA therapy works for a time, but as the degeneration of dopamine-secreting neurons continues, the drug loses its effectiveness. This pattern of response also appears to have occurred in the young patients (Langston and Ballard, 1984).

Some detective work revealed that the chemical that caused the neurological symptoms was not the synthetic opiate itself but another chemical with which it was contaminated. According to researcher William Langston, the mini-epidemic appears to have started "when a young man in Silicon Valley was sloppy in his synthesis of synthetic heroin. That sloppiness led to the presence of MPTP, which by an extraordinary trick of fate is highly toxic to the very same neurons that are lost in Parkinson's disease" (Lewin, 1989, p. 467). Because of the research that followed up on that "trick of fate," patients with Parkinson's disease are now receiving a drug that appears to slow the rate of degeneration of their dopamine-secreting neurons. There is hope that new drugs may even halt the degeneration, giving patients many more years of useful, productive lives and preventing others from ever developing the disease.

Chapter 2 introduced you to the cells of the nervous system, and Chapter 3 described its basic structure. Now it is time to build on this information by introducing the field of **psychopharmacology**, which is the study of the effects of drugs on the nervous system and on behavior. (*Pharmakon* is the Greek word for "drug.")

As we will see in this chapter, drugs have *effects* and *sites of action*. **Drug effects** are the changes we can observe in an animal's physiological processes and behavior. For example, the effects of morphine, heroin, and other opiates include decreased sensitivity to pain, slowing of the digestive system, sedation, muscular relaxation, constriction of the pupils, and euphoria. The **sites of action** of drugs are the points at which molecules of drugs interact with molecules located on or in cells of the body, thus affecting some biochemical processes of these cells. For example, the sites of action of the opiates are specialized receptors situated in the membrane of certain neurons. When molecules of opiates attach to and activate these receptors, the drugs alter the activity of these neurons and produce their effects. This chapter considers both the effects of drugs and their sites of action.

Psychopharmacology is an important field of neuroscience. It has been responsible for the development of psychotherapeutic drugs, which are used to treat psychological and behavioral disorders. It has also provided tools that have enabled other investigators to study the functions of cells of the nervous system and the behaviors controlled by particular neural circuits.

Principles of Psychopharmacology

This chapter begins with a description of the basic principles of psychopharmacology: the routes of administration of drugs and their fate in the body. The second section discusses the sites of drug actions. The final section discusses specific neurotransmitters and neuromodulators and the physiological and behavioral effects of specific drugs that interact with them.

psychopharmacology The study of the effects of drugs on the nervous system and on behavior.

drug effect The changes a drug produces in an animal's physiological processes and behavior.

site of action A location at which molecules of drugs interact with molecules located on or in cells of the body, thus affecting some biochemical processes of these cells.

Pharmacokinetics

To be effective, a drug must reach its sites of action. To do so, molecules of the drug must enter the body and then enter the bloodstream so that they can be carried to the organ (or organs) they act on. Once there, they must leave the bloodstream and come into contact with the molecules with which they interact. For almost all of the drugs we are interested in, this means that the molecules of the drug must enter the central nervous system. Some behaviorally active drugs exert their effects on the peripheral nervous system, but these drugs are less important to neuroscientists than those that affect cells of the CNS.

Molecules of drugs must cross several barriers to enter the body and find their way to their sites of action. Some molecules pass through these barriers easily and quickly; others do so very slowly. Once molecules of drugs enter the body, they begin to be metabolized—broken down by enzymes—or excreted in the urine (or both). In time, the molecules either disappear or are transformed into inactive fragments. The process by which drugs are absorbed, distributed within the body, metabolized, and excreted is referred to as **pharmacokinetics** ("movements of drugs").

Routes of Administration

First, let's consider the routes by which drugs can be administered. For laboratory animals the most common route is injection. The drug is dissolved in a liquid (or, in some cases, suspended in a liquid in the form of fine particles) and injected through a hypodermic needle. The fastest route is **intravenous (IV) injection**—injection into a vein. The drug immediately enters the bloodstream, and it reaches the brain within a few seconds. The disadvantages of IV injections are the increased care and skill they require in comparison to most other forms of injection and the fact that the entire dose reaches the bloodstream at once. If an animal is especially sensitive to the drug, there may be little time to administer another drug to counteract its effects.

An **intraperitoneal (IP) injection** is rapid, but not as rapid as an IV injection. The drug is injected through the abdominal wall into the *peritoneal cavity*—the space that surrounds the stomach, intestines, liver, and other abdominal organs. IP injections are the most common route for administering drugs to small laboratory animals. An **intramuscular (IM) injection** is made directly into a large muscle, such as those found in the upper arm, thigh, or buttocks. The drug is absorbed into the bloodstream through the capillaries that supply the muscle. If very slow absorption is desirable, the drug can be mixed with another drug (such as ephedrine) that constricts blood vessels and retards the flow of blood through the muscle.

A drug can also be injected into the space beneath the skin, by means of a **subcutaneous (SC) injection**. A subcutaneous injection is useful only if small amounts of drug need to be administered, because large amounts would be painful. Some fat-soluble drugs can be dissolved in vegetable oil and administered subcutaneously. In this case, molecules of the drug will slowly leave the deposit of oil over a period of several days. If *very* slow and prolonged absorption of a drug is desired, the drug can be formed into a dry pellet or placed in a sealed silicone rubber capsule and implanted beneath the skin.

Oral administration is the most common form of administering medicinal drugs to humans. Because of the difficulty of getting laboratory animals to eat something that does not taste good to them, researchers seldom use this route. Some chemicals cannot be administered orally because they will be destroyed by stomach acid or digestive enzymes or because they are not absorbed from the digestive system into the bloodstream. For example, insulin, a peptide hormone, must be injected. **Sublingual administration** of certain drugs can be accomplished by placing them beneath the tongue. The drug is absorbed into the bloodstream by the capillaries that supply the mucous membrane that lines the mouth. (Obviously, this method works only with humans, who can cooperate and leave the capsule beneath

pharmacokinetics The process by which drugs are absorbed, distributed within the body, metabolized, and excreted.

intravenous (IV) injection Injection of a substance directly into a vein.

intraperitoneal (IP) injection (*in tra pair i toe nee ul*) Injection of a substance into the *peritoneal cavity*—the space that surrounds the stomach, intestines, liver, and other abdominal organs.

intramuscular (IM) injection Injection of a substance into a muscle.

subcutaneous (SC) injection Injection of a substance into the space beneath the skin.

oral administration Administration of a substance into the mouth, so that it is swallowed.

sublingual administration (*sub ling wul*) Administration of a substance by placing it beneath the tongue.

their tongue.) Nitroglycerine, a drug that causes blood vessels to dilate, is taken sublingually by people who suffer the pains of angina pectoris, caused by obstructions in the coronary arteries.

Drugs can also be administered at the opposite end of the digestive tract, in the form of suppositories. **Intrarectal administration** is rarely used to give drugs to experimental animals. For obvious reasons this process would be difficult with a small animal. In addition, when agitated, small animals such as rats tend to defecate, which would mean that the drug would not remain in place long enough to be absorbed (and I'm not sure I would want to try to administer a rectal suppository to a large animal). Rectal suppositories are most commonly used to administer drugs that might upset a person's stomach.

The lungs provide another route for drug administration: **inhalation**. Nicotine, freebase cocaine, and marijuana are usually smoked. In addition, drugs used to treat lung disorders are often inhaled in the form of a vapor or fine mist, and many general anesthetics are gasses that are administered through inhalation The route from the lungs to the brain is very short, and drugs administered this way have very rapid effects.

Some drugs can be absorbed directly through the skin, so they can be given by means of **topical administration**, usually in the form of creams, ointments, or patches. Natural or artificial steroid hormones can be administered this way, as can nicotine (as a treatment to make it easier for a person to stop smoking). The mucous membrane lining the nasal passages also provides a route for topical administration. Commonly abused drugs such as cocaine hydrochloride are often sniffed so that they come into contact with the nasal mucosa. This route delivers the drug to the brain very rapidly. (The technical, rarely used name for this route is *insufflation*. And note that sniffing is not the same as inhalation; when powdered cocaine is sniffed, it ends up in the mucous membrane of the nasal passages, not in the lungs.)

Finally, drugs can be administered directly into the brain. As we saw in Chapter 2, the blood–brain barrier prevents certain chemicals from leaving capillaries and entering the brain. Some drugs cannot cross the blood–brain barrier. If these drugs are to reach the brain, they must be injected directly into the brain or into the cerebrospinal fluid in the brain's ventricular system. To study the effects of a drug in a specific region of the brain (for example, in a particular nucleus of the hypothalamus), a researcher will inject a very small amount of the drug directly into the brain. This procedure, known as **intracerebral administration**, is described in greater detail in Chapter 5. To achieve a widespread distribution of a drug in the brain, a researcher will get past the blood–brain barrier by injecting the drug into a cerebral ventricle. The drug is then absorbed into the brain tissue, where it can exert its effects. This route, **intracerebroventricular (ICV) administration**, is used very rarely in humans—primarily to deliver antibiotics directly to the brain to treat certain types of infections.

Figure 4.1 shows the time course of blood levels of a commonly abused drug, cocaine, after intravenous injection, inhalation, sniffing, and oral administration. The amounts received were not identical, but the graph illustrates the relative rapidity with which the drug reaches the blood. (See *Figure 4.1.*)

Distribution of Drugs Within the Body

As we saw, drugs exert their effects only when they reach their sites of action. In the case of drugs that affect behavior, most of these sites are located on or in particular cells in the CNS. The previous section described the routes by which drugs can be introduced into the body. With the exception of intracerebral or intracerebroventricular administration, the differences in the routes of drug administration vary only in the rate at which a drug reaches the blood plasma (that is, the liquid part of the blood). But what happens next? All the sites of action of drugs that are of interest to psychopharmacologists lie outside the blood vessels.

intrarectal administration Administration of a substance into the rectum.

inhalation Administration of a vaporous substance into the lungs.

topical administration Administration of a substance directly onto the skin or mucous membrane.

intracerebral administration Administration of a substance directly into the brain.

intracerebroventricular (ICV) administration Administration of a substance into one of the cerebral ventricles.

FIGURE 4.1

Cocaine in Blood Plasma. The graph shows the concentration of cocaine in blood plasma after intravenous injection, inhalation, sniffing, and oral administration.

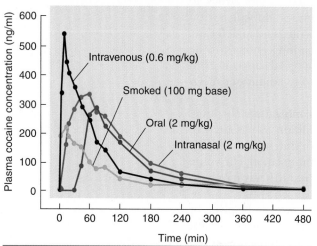

Adapted from Feldman, R. S., Meyer, J. S., and Quenzer, L. F. *Principles of Neuropsychopharmacology.* Sunderland, MA: Sinauer Associates, 1997; after Jones, R. T. *NIDA Research Monographs,* 1990, *99,* 30–41.

Several factors determine the rate at which a drug in the bloodstream reaches sites of action within the brain. The most important is lipid solubility. The blood–brain barrier is a barrier only for water-soluble molecules. Molecules that are soluble in lipids pass through the cells that line the capillaries in the central nervous system, and they rapidly distribute themselves throughout the brain. For example, diacetylmorphine (more commonly known as heroin) is more lipid soluble than morphine is. Thus, an intravenous injection of heroin produces more rapid effects than does one of morphine. Even though the molecules of the two drugs are equally effective when they reach their sites of action in the brain, the fact that heroin molecules get there faster means that they produce a more intense "rush" and thus explains why drug addicts prefer heroin to morphine.

Inactivation and Excretion

Drugs do not remain in the body indefinitely. Many are deactivated by enzymes, and all are eventually excreted, primarily by the kidneys. The liver plays an especially active role in enzymatic deactivation of drugs, but some deactivating enzymes are also found in the blood. The brain also contains enzymes that destroy some drugs. In some cases enzymes transform molecules of a drug into other forms that themselves are biologically active. Occasionally, the transformed molecule is *even more* active than the one that is administered. In such cases the effects of a drug can have a very long duration.

Drug Effectiveness

Drugs vary widely in their effectiveness. The effects of a small dose of a relatively effective drug can equal or exceed the effects of larger amounts of a relatively ineffective drug. The best way to measure the effectiveness of a drug is to plot a **dose-response curve**. To do this, subjects are given various doses of a drug, usually defined as milligrams of drug per kilogram of a subject's body weight, and the effects of the drug are plotted. Because the molecules of most drugs distribute themselves throughout the blood and then throughout the rest of the body, a heavier subject (human or laboratory animal) will require a larger quantity of a drug to achieve the same concentration as that in a smaller subject. As Figure 4.2 shows, increasingly stronger doses of a drug cause increasingly larger effects, until the point of maximum effect is reached. At this point, increasing the dose of the drug does not produce any more effect. (See *Figure 4.2.*)

Most drugs have more than one effect. Opiates such as morphine and codeine produce analgesia (reduced sensitivity to pain), but they also depress the activity of neurons in the medulla that control heart rate and respiration. A physician who prescribes an opiate to relieve a patient's pain wants to administer a dose that is large enough to produce analgesia but not enough to depress heart rate and respiration—effects that could be fatal. Figure 4.3 shows two dose-response curves, one for the analgesic effects of a painkiller and one for the drug's depressant effects on respiration. The difference between these curves indicates the drug's margin of safety. Obviously, the most desirable drugs have a large margin of safety. (See *Figure 4.3.*)

One measure of a drug's margin of safety is its **therapeutic index**. This measure is obtained by administering varying doses of the drug to a group of laboratory animals such as mice. Two numbers are obtained: the dose that produces the desired effects in 50 percent of the animals and the dose that produces toxic effects in 50

dose-response curve A graph of the magnitude of an effect of a drug as a function of the amount of drug administered.

therapeutic index The ratio between the dose that produces the desired effect in 50 percent of the animals and the dose that produces toxic effects in 50 percent of the animals.

affinity The readiness with which two molecules join together.

tolerance A decrease in the effectiveness of a drug that is administered repeatedly.

sensitization An increase in the effectiveness of a drug that is administered repeatedly.

withdrawal symptom The appearance of symptoms opposite to those produced by a drug when the drug is administered repeatedly and then suddenly no longer taken.

percent of the animals. The therapeutic index is the ratio of these two numbers. For example, if the toxic dose is five times higher than the effective dose, then the therapeutic index is 5.0. The lower the therapeutic index, the more care must be taken in prescribing the drug. For example, barbiturates have relatively low therapeutic indexes—as low as 2 or 3. In contrast, tranquilizers such as Valium have therapeutic indexes of well over 100. As a consequence, an accidental overdose of a barbiturate is much more likely to have tragic effects than a similar overdose of Valium.

Why do drugs vary in their effectiveness? There are two reasons. First, different drugs—even those with the same behavioral effects—may have different sites of action. For example, both morphine and aspirin have analgesic effects, but morphine suppresses the activity of neurons in the spinal cord and brain that are involved in pain perception, whereas aspirin reduces the production of a chemical involved in transmitting information from damaged tissue to pain-sensitive neurons. Because the drugs act very differently, a given dose of morphine (expressed in terms of milligrams of drug per kilogram of body weight) produces much more pain reduction than does the same dose of aspirin.

The second reason that drugs vary in their effectiveness has to do with the affinity of the drug with its site of action. As we will see in the next major section of this chapter, most drugs of interest to psychopharmacologists exert their effects by binding with other molecules located in the central nervous system—with presynaptic or postsynaptic receptors, with transporter molecules, or with enzymes involved in the production or deactivation of neurotransmitters. Drugs vary widely in their **affinity** for the molecules to which they attach—the readiness with which the two molecules join together. A drug with a high affinity will produce effects at a relatively low concentration, whereas one with a low affinity must be administered in relatively high doses. Thus, even two drugs with identical sites of action can vary widely in their effectiveness if they have different affinities for their binding sites. In addition, because most drugs have multiple effects, a drug can have high affinities for some of its sites of action and low affinities for others. The most desirable drug has a high affinity for sites of action that produce therapeutic effects and a low affinity for sites of action that produce toxic side effects. One of the goals of research by drug companies is to find chemicals with just this pattern of effects.

Effects of Repeated Administration

Often, when a drug is administered repeatedly, its effects will not remain constant. In most cases its effects will diminish—a phenomenon known as **tolerance**. In other cases a drug becomes more and more effective—a phenomenon known as **sensitization**.

Let's consider tolerance first. Tolerance is seen in many drugs that are commonly abused. For example, a regular user of heroin must take larger and larger amounts of the drug for it to be effective—and once a person has taken an opiate regularly enough to develop tolerance, that individual will suffer **withdrawal symptoms** if he or she suddenly stops taking the drug. Withdrawal symptoms are primarily the opposite of the effects of the drug itself. For example, heroin produces euphoria; withdrawal from it produces *dysphoria*—a feeling of anxious misery. (*Euphoria* and *dysphoria* mean "easy to bear" and "hard to bear," respectively.) Heroin

FIGURE 4.2

A Dose-Response Curve.   Increasingly stronger doses of the drug produce increasingly larger effects until the maximum effect is reached. After that point, increments in the dose do not produce any increments in the drug's effect. However, the risk of adverse side effects increases.

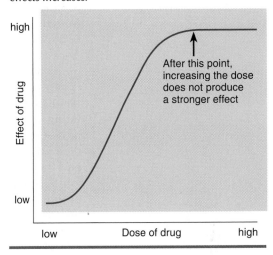

FIGURE 4.3

Dose-Response Curves for Morphine.   The dose-response curve on the left shows the analgesic effect of morphine, and the curve on the right shows one of the drug's adverse side effects: its depressant effect on respiration. A drug's margin of safety is reflected by the difference between the dose-response curve for its therapeutic effects and that for its adverse side effects.

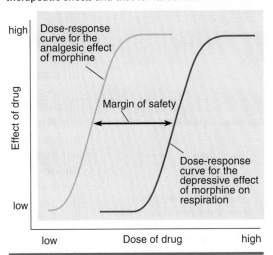

produces constipation; withdrawal from heroin produces nausea and cramping. Heroin produces relaxation; withdrawal from it produces agitation.

Withdrawal symptoms are caused by the same mechanisms that are responsible for tolerance. Tolerance is the result of the body's attempt to compensate for the effects of the drug. That is, most systems of the body, including those controlled by the brain, are regulated so that they stay at an optimal value. When the effects of a drug alter these systems for a prolonged time, compensatory mechanisms begin to produce the opposite reaction, at least partially compensating for the disturbance from the optimal value. These mechanisms account for the fact that more and more of the drug must be taken to achieve a given level of effects. Then, when the person stops taking the drug, the compensatory mechanisms make themselves felt, unopposed by the action of the drug.

Research suggests that there are several types of compensatory mechanisms. As we will see, many drugs that affect the brain do so by binding with receptors and activating them. The first compensatory mechanism involves a decrease in the effectiveness of such binding. Either the receptors become less sensitive to the drug (that is, their affinity for the drug decreases) or the receptors decrease in number. The second compensatory mechanism involves the process that couples the receptors to ion channels in the membrane or to the production of second messengers. After prolonged stimulation of the receptors, one or more steps in the coupling process become less effective. (Of course, *both* effects can occur.) The details of these compensatory mechanisms are described in Chapter 16, which discusses the causes and effects of drug abuse.

As we have just seen, many drugs have several different sites of action and thus produce several different effects. This means that some of the effects of a drug may show tolerance but others may not. For example, barbiturates cause sedation and also depress neurons that control respiration. The sedative effects show tolerance, but the respiratory depression does not. This means that if larger and larger doses of a barbiturate are taken to achieve the same level of sedation, the person begins to run the risk of taking a dangerously large dose of the drug.

Sensitization is, of course, the exact opposite of tolerance: Repeated doses of a drug produce larger and larger effects. Because compensatory mechanisms tend to correct for deviations away from the optimal values of physiological processes, sensitization is less common than tolerance—and some of the effects of a drug may show sensitization while others show tolerance. For example, repeated injections of cocaine become more and more likely to produce movement disorders and convulsions, whereas the euphoric effects of the drug do not show sensitization—and may even show tolerance.

Placebo Effects

A **placebo** is an innocuous substance that has no specific physiological effect. The word comes from the Latin *placere*, "to please." A physician may sometimes give a placebo to anxious patients to placate them. (You can see that the word *placate* also has the same root.) However, although placebos have no *specific* physiological effect, it is incorrect to say that they have *no* effect. If a person thinks that a placebo has a physiological effect, then administration of the placebo may actually produce that effect.

When experimenters want to investigate the behavioral effects of drugs in humans, they must use control groups whose members receive placebos, or they cannot be sure that the behavioral effects they observe were caused by specific effects of the drug. Studies with laboratory animals must also use placebos, even though we need not worry about the animals' "beliefs" about the effects of the drugs we give them. Consider what you must do to give a rat an intraperitoneal injection of a drug: You reach into the animal's cage, pick the animal up, hold it in such a way that its abdomen is exposed and its head is positioned to prevent it from biting you, insert a hypodermic needle through its abdominal wall, press the plunger of the syringe, and replace the animal in its cage, being sure to let go of it quickly so that it cannot turn

placebo (*pla see boh*) An inert substance that is given to an organism in lieu of a physiologically active drug; used experimentally to control for the effects of mere administration of a drug.

and bite you. Even if the substance you inject is innocuous, the experience of receiving the injection would activate the animal's autonomic nervous system, cause the secretion of stress hormones, and have other physiological effects. If we want to know what the behavioral effects of a drug are, we must compare the drug-treated animals with other animals who receive a placebo, administered in exactly the same way as the drug. (By the way, a skilled and experienced researcher can handle a rat so gently that it shows very little reaction to a hypodermic injection.)

Interim Summary

Principles of Psychopharmacology

Psychopharmacology is the study of the effects of drugs on the nervous system and behavior. Drugs are exogenous chemicals that are not necessary for normal cellular functioning that significantly alter the functions of certain cells of the body when taken in relatively low doses. Drugs have *effects*, physiological and behavioral, and they have *sites of action*—molecules with which they interact to produce these effects.

Pharmacokinetics is the fate of a drug as it is absorbed into the body, circulates throughout the body, and reaches its sites of action. Drugs may be administered by intravenous, intraperitoneal, intramuscular, and subcutaneous injection; they may be administered orally, sublingually, intrarectally, by inhalation, and topically (on skin or mucous membrane); and they may be injected intracerebrally or intracerebroventricularly. Lipid-soluble drugs easily pass through the blood–brain barrier, whereas others pass this barrier slowly or not at all.

The dose-response curve represents a drug's effectiveness; it relates the amount administered (usually in milligrams per kilogram of the subject's body weight) to the resulting effect. Most drugs have more than one site of action and therefore more than one effect. The safety of a drug is measured by the difference between doses that produce desirable effects and those that produce toxic side effects. Drugs vary in their effectiveness because of the nature of their sites of actions and the affinity between molecules of the drug and these sites of action.

Repeated administration of a drug can cause either tolerance, often resulting in withdrawal symptoms, or sensitization. Tolerance can be caused by decreased affinity of a drug with its receptors, by decreased numbers of receptors, or by decreased coupling of receptors with the biochemical steps it controls. Some of the effects of a drug may show tolerance, while others may not—or may even show sensitization.

Sites of Drug Action

Throughout the history of our species, people have discovered that plants—and a few animals—produce chemicals that act on synapses. (Of course, the people who discovered these chemicals knew nothing about neurons and synapses.) Some of these chemicals have been used for their pleasurable effects; others have been used to treat illness, reduce pain, or poison other animals (or enemies). More recently, scientists have learned to produce completely artificial drugs, some with potencies far greater than those of the naturally occurring ones. The traditional uses of drugs remain, but in addition, they can be used in research laboratories to investigate the operations of the nervous system. Most drugs that affect behavior do so by affecting synaptic transmission. Drugs that affect synaptic transmission are classified into two general categories. Those that block or inhibit the postsynaptic effects are called **antagonists**. Those that facilitate them are called **agonists**. (The Greek word *agon* means "contest." Thus, an *agonist* is one who takes part in the contest.)

This section will describe the basic effects of drugs on synaptic activity. The sequence of synaptic activity goes like this: Neurotransmitters are synthesized and stored in synaptic vesicles. The synaptic vesicles travel to the presynaptic membrane. When an axon fires, voltage-dependent calcium channels in the presynaptic membrane open, permitting the entry of calcium ions. The calcium ions interact with proteins in the synaptic vesicles and presynaptic membrane and initiate the release of

antagonist A drug that opposes or inhibits the effects of a particular neurotransmitter on the postsynaptic cell.

agonist A drug that facilitates the effects of a particular neurotransmitter on the postsynaptic cell.

the neurotransmitters into the synaptic cleft. Molecules of the neurotransmitter bind with postsynaptic receptors, causing particular ion channels to open, which produces excitatory or inhibitory postsynaptic potentials. The effects of the neurotransmitter are kept relatively brief by their reuptake by transporter molecules in the presynaptic membrane or by their destruction by enzymes. In addition, the stimulation of presynaptic autoreceptors regulates the synthesis and release of the neurotransmitter. The discussion of the effects of drugs in this section follows the same basic sequence. All of the effects I will describe are summarized in Figure 4.4, with some details shown in additional figures. I should warn you that some of the effects are complex, so the discussion that follows bears careful reading. I recommend that you study *MyPsychKit 4.1, Actions of Drugs*, which reviews this material.

Animation 4.1
Actions of Drugs

Effects on Production of Neurotransmitters

The first step is the synthesis of the neurotransmitter from its precursors. In some cases the rate of synthesis and release of a neurotransmitter is increased when a precursor is administered; in these cases the precursor itself serves as an agonist. (See step 1 in *Figure 4.4.*)

The steps in the synthesis of neurotransmitters are controlled by enzymes. Therefore, if a drug inactivates one of these enzymes, it will prevent the neurotransmitter from being produced. Such a drug serves as an antagonist. (See step 2 in *Figure 4.4.*)

FIGURE 4.4

Drug Effects on Synaptic Transmission.   The figure summarizes the ways in which drugs can affect the synaptic transmission (AGO = agonist; ANT = antagonist; NT = neurotransmitter). Drugs that act as agonists are marked in blue; drugs that act as antagonists are marked in red.

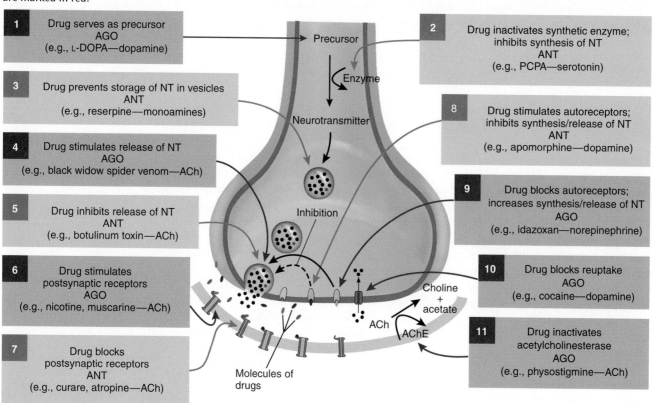

1 Drug serves as precursor
AGO
(e.g., L-DOPA—dopamine)

2 Drug inactivates synthetic enzyme; inhibits synthesis of NT
ANT
(e.g., PCPA—serotonin)

3 Drug prevents storage of NT in vesicles
ANT
(e.g., reserpine—monoamines)

8 Drug stimulates autoreceptors; inhibits synthesis/release of NT
ANT
(e.g., apomorphine—dopamine)

4 Drug stimulates release of NT
AGO
(e.g., black widow spider venom—ACh)

9 Drug blocks autoreceptors; increases synthesis/release of NT
AGO
(e.g., idazoxan—norepinephrine)

5 Drug inhibits release of NT
ANT
(e.g., botulinum toxin—ACh)

6 Drug stimulates postsynaptic receptors
AGO
(e.g., nicotine, muscarine—ACh)

10 Drug blocks reuptake
AGO
(e.g., cocaine—dopamine)

7 Drug blocks postsynaptic receptors
ANT
(e.g., curare, atropine—ACh)

11 Drug inactivates acetylcholinesterase
AGO
(e.g., physostigmine—ACh)

Precursor
Enzyme
Neurotransmitter
Inhibition
Molecules of drugs
Choline + acetate
ACh
AChE

Effects on Storage and Release of Neurotransmitters

Neurotransmitters are stored in synaptic vesicles, which are transported to the presynaptic membrane, where the chemicals are released. The storage of neurotransmitters in vesicles is accomplished by the same kind of transporter molecules that are responsible for reuptake of a neurotransmitter into a terminal button. The transporter molecules are located in the membrane of synaptic vesicles, and their action is to pump molecules of the neurotransmitter across the membrane, filling the vesicles. Some of the transporter molecules that fill synaptic vesicles are capable of being blocked by a drug. Molecules of the drug bind with a particular site on the transporter and inactivate it. Because the synaptic vesicles remain empty, nothing is released when the vesicles eventually rupture against the presynaptic membrane. The drug serves as an antagonist. (See step 3 in *Figure 4.4*.)

Some drugs act as antagonists by preventing the release of neurotransmitters from the terminal button. They do so by deactivating the proteins that cause synaptic vesicles to fuse with the presynaptic membrane and expel their contents into the synaptic cleft. Other drugs have just the opposite effect: They act as agonists by binding with these proteins and directly triggering release of the neurotransmitter. (See steps 4 and 5 in *Figure 4.4*.)

Effects on Receptors

The most important—and most complex—site of action of drugs in the nervous system is on receptors, both presynaptic and postsynaptic. Let's consider postsynaptic receptors first. (Here is where the careful reading should begin.) Once a neurotransmitter has been released, it must stimulate the postsynaptic receptors. Some drugs bind with these receptors, just as the neurotransmitter does. Once a drug has bound with the receptor, it can serve as either an agonist or an antagonist.

A drug that mimics the effects of a neurotransmitter acts as a **direct agonist**. Molecules of the drug attach to the binding site to which the neurotransmitter normally attaches. This binding causes ion channels controlled by the receptor to open, just as they do when the neurotransmitter is present. Ions then pass through these channels and produce postsynaptic potentials. (See step 6 in *Figure 4.4*.)

Drugs that bind with postsynaptic receptors can also serve as antagonists. Molecules of such drugs bind with the receptors but do not open the ion channel. Because they occupy the receptor's binding site, they prevent the neurotransmitter from opening the ion channel. These drugs are called **receptor blockers** or **direct antagonists**. (See step 7 in *Figure 4.4*.)

Some receptors have multiple binding sites, to which different ligands can attach. Molecules of the neurotransmitter bind with one site, and other substances (such as neuromodulators and various drugs) bind with the others. Binding of a molecule with one of these alternative sites is referred to as **noncompetitive binding**, because the molecule does not compete with molecules of the neurotransmitter for the same binding site. If a drug attaches to one of these alternative sites and prevents the ion channel from opening, the drug is said to be an **indirect antagonist**. The ultimate *effect* of an indirect antagonist is similar to that of a direct antagonist, but its site of action is different. If a drug attaches to one of the alternative sites and *facilitates* the opening of the ion channel, it is said to be an **indirect agonist**. (See *Figure 4.5*.)

As we saw in Chapter 2, the presynaptic membranes of some neurons contain autoreceptors that regulate the amount of neurotransmitter that is released. Because stimulation of these receptors causes less neurotransmitter to be released, drugs that selectively activate presynaptic receptors act as antagonists. Drugs that *block* presynaptic autoreceptors have the opposite effect: They *increase* the release of the neurotransmitter, acting as agonists. (Refer to steps 8 and 9 in *Figure 4.4*.)

direct agonist A drug that binds with and activates a receptor.

receptor blocker or **direct antagonists** A drug that binds with a receptor but does not activate it; prevents the natural ligand from binding with the receptor.

noncompetitive binding Binding of a drug to a site on a receptor; does not interfere with the binding site for the principal ligand.

indirect antagonist A drug that attaches to a binding site on a receptor and interferes with the action of the receptor; does not interfere with the binding site for the principal ligand.

indirect agonist A drug that attaches to a binding site on a receptor and facilitates the action of the receptor; does not interfere with the binding site for the principal ligand.

FIGURE 4.5

Drug Actions as Binding Sites.   This figure shows (a) competitive binding (direct agonists and antagonists act directly on the neurotransmitter binding site) and (b) noncompetitive binding (indirect agonists and antagonists act on an alternative binding site and modify the effects of the neurotransmitter on opening of the ion channel).

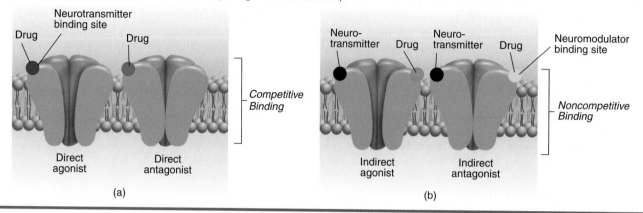

(a)   (b)

Effects on Reuptake or Destruction of Neurotransmitters

The next step after stimulation of the postsynaptic receptor is termination of the postsynaptic potential. Two processes accomplish that task: Molecules of the neurotransmitter are taken back into the terminal button through the process of reuptake, or they are destroyed by an enzyme. Drugs can interfere with either of these processes. In the first case molecules of the drug attach to the transporter molecules that are responsible for reuptake and inactivate them, thus blocking reuptake. In the second case molecules of the drug bind with the enzyme that normally destroys the neurotransmitter and prevents the enzymes from working. The most important example of such an enzyme is acetylcholinesterase, which destroys acetylcholine. Because both types of drugs prolong the presence of the neurotransmitter in the synaptic cleft (and hence in a location where they can stimulate postsynaptic receptors), they serve as *agonists*. (Refer to steps 10 and 11 in *Figure 4.4.*)

InterimSummary

Sites of Drug Action

The process of synaptic transmission entails the synthesis of the neurotransmitter, its storage in synaptic vesicles, its release into the synaptic cleft, its interaction with postsynaptic receptors, and the consequent opening of ion channels in the postsynaptic membrane. The effects of the neurotransmitter are then terminated by reuptake into the terminal button or by enzymatic deactivation.

Each of the steps necessary for synaptic transmission can be interfered with by drugs that serve as *antagonists*, and a few of these steps can be stimulated by drugs that serve as *agonists*. In particular, drugs can increase the pool of available precursor, block a biosyn-thetic enzyme, prevent the storage of neurotransmitter in the synaptic vesicles, stimulate or block the release of the neurotransmitter, stimulate or block presynaptic or postsynaptic receptors, retard reuptake, or deactivate enzymes that destroy the neurotransmitter postsynaptically or presynaptically. A drug that activates postsynaptic receptors serves as an agonist, whereas one that activates presynaptic autoreceptors serves as an antagonist. A drug that blocks postsynaptic receptors serves as an antagonist, whereas one that blocks autoreceptors serves as an agonist.

Neurotransmitters and Neuromodulators

Because neurotransmitters have two general effects on postsynaptic membranes—depolarization (EPSP) or hyperpolarization (IPSP)—one might expect that there would be two kinds of neurotransmitters: excitatory and inhibitory. Instead, there are many different kinds—several dozen, at least. In the brain most synaptic communication is accomplished by two neurotransmitters: one with excitatory effects (glutamate) and one with inhibitory effects (GABA). (Another inhibitory neurotransmitter, glycine, is found in the spinal cord and lower brain stem.) Most of the activity of local circuits of neurons involves balances between the excitatory and inhibitory effects of these chemicals, which are responsible for most of the information transmitted from place to place within the brain. In fact, there are probably no neurons in the brain that do not receive excitatory input from glutamate-secreting terminal buttons and inhibitory input from neurons that secrete either GABA or glycine—and with the exception of neurons that detect painful stimuli, all sensory organs transmit information to the brain through axons whose terminals release glutamate. (Pain-detecting neurons secrete a peptide.)

What do all the other neurotransmitters do? In general, they have modulating effects rather than information-transmitting effects. That is, the release of neurotransmitters other than glutamate and GABA tends to activate or inhibit entire circuits of neurons that are involved in particular brain functions. For example, secretion of acetylcholine activates the cerebral cortex and facilitates learning, but the information that is learned and remembered is transmitted by neurons that secrete glutamate and GABA. Secretion of norepinephrine increases vigilance and enhances readiness to act when a signal is detected. Secretion of serotonin suppresses certain categories of species-typical behaviors and reduces the likelihood that the animal acts impulsively. Secretion of dopamine in some regions of the brain generally activates voluntary movements but does not specify which movements will occur. In other regions secretion of dopamine reinforces ongoing behaviors and makes them more likely to occur at a later time. Because particular drugs can selectively affect neurons that secrete particular neurotransmitters, they can have specific effects on behavior.

This section introduces the most important neurotransmitters, discusses some of their behavioral functions, and describes the drugs that interact with them. As we saw in the previous section of this chapter, drugs have many different sites of action. Fortunately for your information-processing capacity (and perhaps your sanity), not all types of neurons are affected by all types of drugs. As you will see, that still leaves a good number of drugs to be mentioned by name. Obviously, some are more important than others. Those whose effects I describe in some detail are more important than those I mention in passing. If you want to learn more details about these drugs (and many others), you should consult one of the psychopharmacology texts listed in the suggested readings at the end of this chapter.

Acetylcholine

Acetylcholine is the primary neurotransmitter secreted by efferent axons of the central nervous system. All muscular movement is accomplished by the release of acetylcholine, and ACh is also found in the ganglia of the autonomic nervous system and at the target organs of the parasympathetic branch of the ANS. Because ACh is found outside the central nervous system in locations that are easy to study, this neurotransmitter was the first to be discovered, and it has received much attention from neuroscientists. Some terminology: These synapses are said to be *acetylcholinergic. Ergon* is the Greek word for "work." Thus, *dopaminergic* synapses release dopamine, *serotonergic* synapses release serotonin, and so on. (The suffix *-ergic* is pronounced "*ur jik.*")

FIGURE 4.6

Biosynthesis of Acetylcholine

Acetyl coenzyme A
(acetyl-CoA)

Coenzyme A
(CoA)

Acetylcholine (ACh)

Choline

ChAT transfers
acetate ion from
acetyl-CoA to
choline

Choline
acetyltransferase
(ChAT)

acetyl-CoA (*a see tul*) A cofactor that supplies acetate for the synthesis of acetylcholine.

choline acetyltransferase (ChAT) (**koh** *leen a see tul* **trans** *fer ace*) The enzyme that transfers the acetate ion from acetyl coenzyme A to choline, producing the neurotransmitter acetylcholine.

botulinum toxin (*bot you* **lin** *um*) An acetylcholine antagonist; prevents release of ACh by terminal buttons.

black widow spider venom A poison produced by the black widow spider that triggers the release of acetylcholine.

neostigmine (*nee o* **stig** *meen*) A drug that inhibits the activity of acetylcholinesterase.

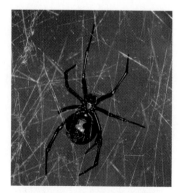

The venom of the black widow spider is much less toxic than botulinum toxin, but both toxins affect the release of acetylcholine.

The axons and terminal buttons of acetylcholinergic neurons are distributed widely throughout the brain. Three systems have received the most attention from neuroscientists: those originating in the dorsolateral pons, the basal forebrain, and the medial septum. The effects of ACh release in the brain are generally facilitatory. The acetylcholinergic neurons located in the dorsolateral pons play a role in REM sleep (the phase of sleep during which dreaming occurs). Those located in the basal forebrain are involved in activating the cerebral cortex and facilitating learning, especially perceptual learning. Those located in the medial septum control the electrical rhythms of the hippocampus and modulate its functions, which include the formation of particular kinds of memories.

Acetylcholine is composed of two components: *choline*, a substance derived from the breakdown of lipids, and *acetate*, the anion found in vinegar, also called acetic acid. Acetate cannot be attached directly to choline; instead, it is transferred from a molecule of *acetyl-CoA*. CoA (coenzyme A) is a complex molecule, consisting in part of the vitamin pantothenic acid (one of the B vitamins). CoA is produced by the mitochondria, and it takes part in many reactions in the body. **Acetyl-CoA** is simply CoA with an acetate ion attached to it. ACh is produced by the following reaction: In the presence of the enzyme **choline acetyltransferase (ChAT)**, the acetate ion is transferred from the acetyl-CoA molecule to the choline molecule, yielding a molecule of ACh and one of ordinary CoA. (See *Figure 4.6*.)

A simple analogy will illustrate the role of coenzymes in chemical reactions. Think of acetate as a hot dog and choline as a bun. The task of the person (enzyme) who operates the hot dog vending stand is to put a hot dog into the bun (make acetylcholine). To do so, the vendor needs a fork (coenzyme) to remove the hot dog from the boiling water. The vendor inserts the fork into the hot dog (attaches acetate to CoA) and transfers the hot dog from fork to bun.

Two drugs, botulinum toxin and the venom of the black widow spider, affect the release of acetylcholine. **Botulinum toxin** is produced by *clostridium botulinum*, a bacterium that can grow in improperly canned food. This drug prevents the release of ACh (step 5 of Figure 4.4). The drug is an extremely potent poison; someone once calculated that a teaspoonful of pure botulinum toxin could kill the world's entire human population. You undoubtedly know that *botox* treatment has become fashionable. A very dilute (obviously!) solution of botulinum toxin is injected into people's facial muscles to stop muscular contractions that are causing wrinkles in the skin. In contrast, **black widow spider venom** has the opposite effect: It stimulates the release of ACh (step 4 of Figure 4.4). Although the effects of black widow spider venom can also be fatal, the venom is much less toxic than botulinum toxin. In fact, most healthy adults would have to receive several bites, but infants or frail, elderly people would be more susceptible.

You will recall from Chapter 2 that after being released by the terminal button, ACh is deactivated by the enzyme acetylcholinesterase (AChE), which is present in the postsynaptic membrane. (See *Figure 4.7*.)

Drugs that deactivate AChE (step 11 of Figure 4.4) are used for several purposes. Some are used as insecticides. These drugs readily kill insects but not humans and other mammals, because our blood contains enzymes that destroy them. (Insects lack the enzyme.) Other AChE inhibitors are used medically. For example, a hereditary disorder called *myasthenia gravis* is caused by an attack of a person's immune system against acetylcholine receptors located on skeletal muscles. The person becomes weaker and weaker as the muscles become less responsive to the neurotransmitter. If the person is given an AChE inhibitor such as **neostigmine**, the person will regain some strength, because the acetylcholine that is released has a more prolonged effect on the remaining receptors. (Fortunately, neostigmine cannot cross the blood–brain barrier, so it does not affect the AChE found in the central nervous system.)

There are two types of ACh receptors: one ionotropic and one metabotropic. These receptors were identified when investigators discovered that different drugs activated them (step 6 of Figure 4.4). The ionotropic ACh receptor is stimulated by nicotine, a drug found in tobacco leaves. (The Latin name of the plant is *Nicotiniana tabacum*.) The metabotropic ACh receptor is stimulated by muscarine, a drug found in the poison mushroom *Amanita muscaria*. Consequently, these two ACh receptors are referred to as **nicotinic receptors** and **muscarinic receptors**, respectively. Because muscle fibers must be able to contract rapidly, they contain the rapid, ionotropic nicotinic receptors. Because muscarinic receptors are metabotropic in nature and thus control ion channels through the production of second messengers, their actions are slower and more prolonged than those of nicotinic receptors. The central nervous system contains both kinds of ACh receptors, but muscarinic receptors predominate. Some nicotinic receptors are found at axoaxonic synapses in the brain, where they produce presynaptic facilitation. Activation of these receptors is responsible for the addictive effect of the nicotine found in tobacco smoke.

Just as two different drugs stimulate the two classes of acetylcholine receptors, two different drugs *block* them (step 7 of Figure 4.4). Both drugs were discovered in nature long ago, and both are still used by modern medicine. The first, **atropine**, blocks muscarinic receptors. The drug is named after Atropos, the Greek fate who cut the thread of life (which a sufficient dose of atropine will certainly do). Atropine is one of several *belladonna alkaloids* extracted from a plant called the deadly nightshade, and therein lies a tale. Many years ago, women who wanted to increase their attractiveness to men put drops containing belladonna alkaloids into their eyes. In fact, *belladonna* means "pretty lady." Why was the drug used this way? One of the unconscious responses that occurs when we are interested in something is dilation of our pupils. By blocking the effects of acetylcholine on the pupil, belladonna alkaloids such as atropine make the pupils dilate. This change makes a woman appear more interested in a man when she looks at him, and, of course, this apparent sign of interest makes him regard her as more attractive.

Another drug, **curare**, blocks nicotinic receptors. Because these receptors are the ones found on muscles, curare, like botulinum toxin, causes paralysis. However, the effects of curare are much faster. The drug is extracted from several different species of plants found in South America, where it was discovered long ago by people who used it to coat the tips of arrows and darts. Within minutes of being struck by one of these points, an animal collapses, ceases breathing, and dies. Nowadays, curare (and other drugs with the same site of action) are used to paralyze patients who are to undergo surgery so that their muscles will relax completely and not contract when they are cut with a scalpel. An anesthetic must also be used, because a person who receives only curare will remain perfectly conscious and sensitive to pain, even though paralyzed—and, of course, a respirator must be used to supply air to the lungs.

The Monoamines

Dopamine, norepinephrine, epinephrine, and serotonin are four chemicals that belong to a family of compounds called **monoamines**. Because the molecular structures of these substances are similar, some drugs affect the activity of all of them to some degree. The first three—dopamine, norepinephrine, and epinephrine—

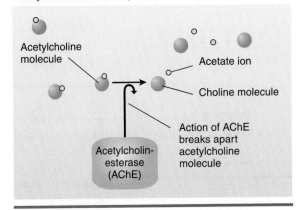

nicotinic receptor An ionotropic acetylcholine receptor that is stimulated by nicotine and blocked by curare.

muscarinic receptor (*muss ka **rin** ic*) A metabotropic acetylcholine receptor that is stimulated by muscarine and blocked by atropine.

atropine (*a tro peen*) A drug that blocks muscarinic acetylcholine receptors.

curare (*kew **rahr** ee*) A drug that blocks nicotinic acetylcholine receptors.

monoamine (*mahn o a meen*) A class of amines that includes indolamines such as serotonin and catecholamines such as dopamine, norepinephrine, and epinephrine.

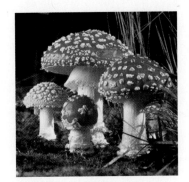

Amanita muscaria, a colorful mushroom, is the source of muscarine, a drug that stimulates muscarinic actylcholine receptors.

FIGURE 4.8

Biosynthesis of the Catecholamines

Tyrosine

⬇ ❰ *Enzyme*

L-DOPA

⬇ ❰ *Enzyme*

Dopamine

⬇ ❰ *Enzyme*

Norepinephrine

---

catecholamine (*cat a **kohl** a meen*) A class of amines that includes the neurotransmitters dopamine, norepinephrine, and epinephrine.

dopamine (DA) (*dope a meen*) A neurotransmitter; one of the catecholamines.

L-DOPA (*ell dope a*) The levorotatory form of DOPA; the precursor of the catecholamines; often used to treat Parkinson's disease because of its effect as a dopamine agonist.

nigrostriatal system (*nigh grow stry ay tul*) A system of neurons originating in the substantia nigra and terminating in the neostriatum (caudate nucleus and putamen).

mesolimbic system (*mee zo lim bik*) A system of dopaminergic neurons originating in the ventral tegmental area and terminating in the nucleus accumbens, amygdala, and hippocampus.

mesocortical system (*mee zo kor ti kul*) A system of dopaminergic neurons originating in the ventral tegmental area and terminating in the prefrontal cortex.

Parkinson's disease A neurological disease characterized by tremors, rigidity of the limbs, poor balance, and difficulty in initiating movements; caused by degeneration of the nigrostriatal system.

TABLE 4.1   Classification of the Monoamine Transmitter Substances

Catecholamines	Indolamines
Dopamine	Serotonin
Norepinephrine	
Epinephrine	

---

belong to a subclass of monoamines called **catecholamines**. It is worthwhile learning the terms in Table 4.1, because they will be used many times throughout the rest of this book. (See *Table 4.1*.)

The monoamines are produced by several systems of neurons in the brain. Most of these systems consist of a relatively small number of cell bodies located in the brain stem, whose axons branch repeatedly and give rise to an enormous number of terminal buttons distributed throughout many regions of the brain. Monoaminergic neurons thus serve to modulate the function of widespread regions of the brain, increasing or decreasing the activities of particular brain functions.

Dopamine

The first catecholamine in Table 4.1, **dopamine (DA)**, produces both excitatory and inhibitory postsynaptic potentials, depending on the postsynaptic receptor. Dopamine is one of the more interesting neurotransmitters because it has been implicated in several important functions, including movement, attention, learning, and the reinforcing effects of drugs that people tend to abuse.

The synthesis of the catecholamines is somewhat more complicated than that of ACh, but each step is a simple one. The precursor molecule is modified slightly, step by step, until it achieves its final shape. Each step is controlled by a different enzyme, which causes a small part to be added or taken off. The precursor for the two major catecholamine neurotransmitters (dopamine and norepinephrine) is *tyrosine*, an essential amino acid that we must obtain from our diet. An enzyme converts tyrosine into **L-DOPA**. Another enzyme converts L-DOPA into dopamine. In dopaminergic neurons that conversion is the last step, but in noradrenergic neurons, dopamine is converted into norepinephrine. These reactions are shown in *Figure 4.8*.

The brain contains several systems of dopaminergic neurons. The three most important of these originate in the midbrain. The cell bodies of neurons of the **nigrostriatal system** are located in the substantia nigra and project their axons to the neostriatum: the caudate nucleus and the putamen. The neostriatum is an important part of the basal ganglia, involved in the control of movement. The cell bodies of neurons of the **mesolimbic system** are located in the ventral tegmental area and project their axons to several parts of the limbic system, including the nucleus accumbens, amygdala, and hippocampus. (The term *meso-* refers to the midbrain, or mesencephalon.) The nucleus accumbens plays an important role in the reinforcing (rewarding) effects of certain categories of stimuli, including those of drugs that people abuse. The cell bodies of neurons of the **mesocortical system** are also located in the ventral tegmental area. Their axons project to the prefrontal cortex. These neurons have an excitatory effect on the frontal cortex and thus affect such functions as formation of short-term memories, planning, and strategy preparation for problem solving. (See *Table 4.2*.)

Degeneration of dopaminergic neurons that connect the substantia nigra with the caudate nucleus causes **Parkinson's disease**, a movement disorder characterized by tremors, rigidity of the limbs, poor balance, and difficulty in initiating movements. The cell bodies of these neurons are located in a region of the brain called

TABLE 4.2	The Three Major Dopaminergic Pathways		
Name	**Origin (Location of Cell Bodies)**	**Location of Terminal Buttons**	**Behavioral Effects**
Nigrostriatal system	Substantia nigra	Neostriatum (caudate nucleus and putamen)	Control of movement
Mesolimbic system	Ventral tegmental area	Nucleus accumbens and amygdala	Reinforcement, effects of addictive drugs
Mesocortical system	Ventral tegmental area	Prefrontal cortex	Short-term memories, planning, strategies for problem solving

the *substantia nigra* ("black substance"). This region is normally stained black with melanin, the substance that gives color to skin. This compound is produced by the breakdown of dopamine. (The brain damage that causes Parkinson's disease was discovered by pathologists who observed that the substantia nigra of a deceased person who had had this disorder was pale rather than black.) People with Parkinson's disease are given L-DOPA, the precursor to dopamine. Although dopamine cannot cross the blood–brain barrier, L-DOPA can. Once L-DOPA reaches the brain, it is taken up by dopaminergic neurons and is converted to dopamine (step 1 of Figure 4.4). The increased synthesis of dopamine causes more dopamine to be released by the surviving dopaminergic neurons in patients with Parkinson's disease. As a consequence, the patients' symptoms are alleviated.

Another drug, **AMPT** (or α-methyl-*p*-tyrosine), inactivates tyrosine hydroxylase, the enzyme that converts tyrosine to L-DOPA (step 2 of Figure 4.4). Because this drug interferes with the synthesis of dopamine (and of norepinephrine, as well), it serves as a catecholamine antagonist. The drug is not normally used medically, but it has been used as a research tool in laboratory animals.

The drug **reserpine** prevents the storage of monoamines in synaptic vesicles by blocking the transporters in the membrane of vesicles in the terminals of monoaminergic neurons (step 3 of Figure 4.4). Because the synaptic vesicles remain empty, no neurotransmitter is released when an action potential reaches the terminal button. Reserpine, then, is a monoamine antagonist. The drug, which comes from the root of a shrub, was discovered over three thousand years ago in India, where it was found to be useful in treating snakebite and seemed to have a calming effect. Pieces of the root are still sold in markets in rural areas of India. In Western medicine reserpine was previously used to treat high blood pressure, but it has been replaced by drugs that have fewer side effects.

Several different types of dopamine receptors have been identified, all metabotropic. Of these, two are the most common: D_1 *dopamine receptors* and D_2 *dopamine receptors*. It appears that D_1 receptors are exclusively postsynaptic, whereas D_2 receptors are found both presynaptically and postsynaptically in the brain. Several drugs stimulate or block specific types of dopamine receptors.

Several drugs inhibit the reuptake of dopamine, thus serving as potent dopamine agonists (step 10 of Figure 4.4). The best known of these drugs are amphetamine, cocaine, and methylphenidate. Amphetamine has an interesting effect: It causes the release of both dopamine and norepinephrine by causing the transporters for these neurotransmitters to run in reverse, propelling DA and NE into the synaptic cleft. Of course, this action also blocks reuptake of these neurotransmitters. Cocaine and **methylphenidate** simply block dopamine reuptake. Because cocaine also blocks voltage-dependent sodium channels, it is sometimes used as a topical anesthetic, especially in the form of eye drops for eye surgery. Methylphenidate (Ritalin) is used to treat children with attention deficit disorder.

AMPT A drug that blocks the activity of tyrosine hydroxylase and thus interferes with the synthesis of the catecholamines.

reserpine (*ree sur peen*) A drug that interferes with the storage of monoamines in synaptic vesicles.

methylphenidate (*meth ul fen i date*) A drug that inhibits the reuptake of dopamine.

FIGURE 4.9

Role of Monoamine Oxidase (MAO). This schematic illustration shows the role of monoamine oxidase in dopaminergic terminal buttons and the action of deprenyl.

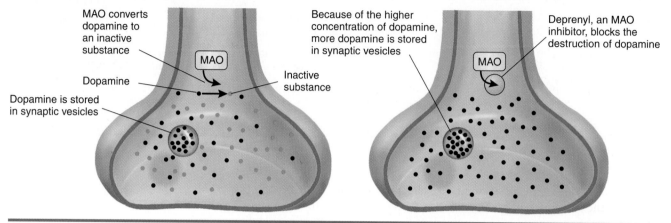

The production of the catecholamines is regulated by an enzyme called **monoamine oxidase (MAO)**. This enzyme is found within monoaminergic terminal buttons, where it destroys excessive amounts of neurotransmitter. A drug called **deprenyl** destroys the particular form of monoamine oxidase (MAO-B) that is found in dopaminergic terminal buttons. Because deprenyl prevents the destruction of dopamine, more dopamine is released when an action potential reaches the terminal button. Thus, deprenyl serves as a dopamine agonist. (See *Figure 4.9*.)

MAO is also found in the blood, where it deactivates amines that are present in foods such as chocolate and cheese; without such deactivation these amines could cause dangerous increases in blood pressure.

Dopamine has been implicated as a neurotransmitter that might be involved in schizophrenia, a serious mental disorder whose symptoms include hallucinations, delusions, and disruption of normal, logical thought processes. Drugs such as **chlorpromazine**, which block D_2 receptors, alleviate these symptoms (step 7 of Figure 4.4). Hence, investigators have speculated that schizophrenia is produced by overactivity of dopaminergic neurons. More recently discovered drugs—the so-called *atypical antipsychotics*—have more complicated actions, which are discussed in Chapter 15.

Norepinephrine

Because **norepinephrine (NE)**, like ACh, is found in neurons in the autonomic nervous system, this neurotransmitter has received much experimental attention. I should note that the terms *Adrenalin* and *epinephrine* are synonymous, as are *noradrenalin* and *norepinephrine*. Let me explain why. **Epinephrine** is a hormone produced by the adrenal medulla, the central core of the adrenal glands, located just above the kidneys. Epinephrine also serves as a neurotransmitter in the brain, but it is of minor importance compared with norepinephrine. *Ad renal* is Latin for "toward kidney." In Greek, one would say *epi nephron* ("upon the kidney"), hence the term *epinephrine*. The latter term has been adopted by pharmacologists, probably because the word *Adrenalin* was appropriated by a drug company as a proprietary name; therefore, to be consistent with general usage, I will refer to the neurotransmitter as *norepinephrine*. The accepted adjectival form is *noradrenergic*; I suppose that *norepinephrinergic* never caught on because it takes so long to pronounce.

We have already seen the biosynthetic pathway for norepinephrine in Figure 4.8. The drug **fusaric acid**, which prevents the conversion of dopamine to norepinephrine, blocks the production of NE.

Almost every region of the brain receives input from noradrenergic neurons. The cell bodies of most of these neurons are located in seven regions of the pons and

monoamine oxidase (MAO) (*mahn o a meen*) A class of enzymes that destroy the monoamines: dopamine, norepinephrine, and serotonin.

deprenyl (*dep ra nil*) A drug that blocks the activity of MAO-B; acts as a dopamine agonist.

chlorpromazine (*klor proh ma zeen*) A drug that reduces the symptoms of schizophrenia by blocking dopamine D_2 receptors.

norepinephrine (NE) (*nor epp i neff rin*) One of the catecholamines; a neurotransmitter found in the brain and in the sympathetic division of the autonomic nervous system.

epinephrine (*epp i neff rin*) One of the catecholamines; a hormone secreted by the adrenal medulla; serves also as a neurotransmitter in the brain.

fusaric acid (*few sahr ik*) A drug that inhibits the activity of the enzyme dopamine-β-hydroxylase and thus blocks the production of norepinephrine.

medulla and one region of the thalamus. The cell bodies of the most important noradrenergic system begin in the **locus coeruleus**, a nucleus located in the dorsal pons. The axons of these neurons project to widespread regions of the brain. As we will see in Chapter 8, one effect of activation of these neurons is an increase in vigilance—attentiveness to events in the environment.

There are several types of noradrenergic receptors, identified by their differing sensitivities to various drugs. Actually, these receptors are usually called *adrenergic* receptors rather than *noradrenergic* receptors, because they are sensitive to epinephrine (Adrenalin) as well as norepinephrine. Neurons in the central nervous system contain β_1- and β_2-*adrenergic receptors* and α_1- and α_2-*adrenergic receptors*. All four kinds of receptors are also found in various organs of the body besides the brain and are responsible for the effects of the catecholamines when they act as hormones outside the central nervous system. In the brain, all autoreceptors appear to be of the α_2 type. The drug **idazoxan** blocks α_2 autoreceptors and hence acts as an agonist. All adrenergic receptors are metabotropic, coupled to G proteins that control the production of second messengers.

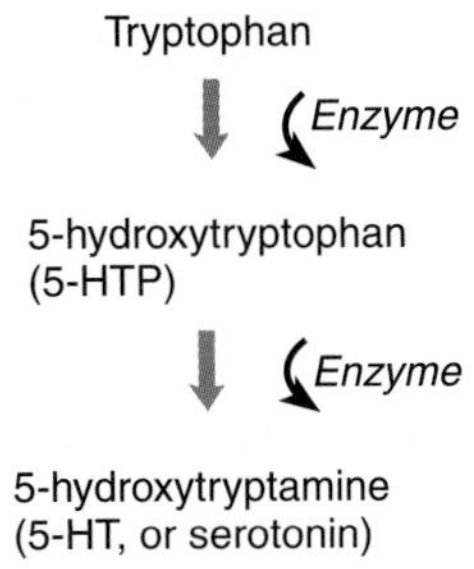

Serotonin

The third monoamine neurotransmitter, **serotonin** (also called **5-HT**, or 5-hydroxytryptamine), has also received much experimental attention. Its behavioral effects are complex. Serotonin plays a role in the regulation of mood; in the control of eating, sleep, and arousal; and in the regulation of pain. Serotonergic neurons are involved somehow in the control of dreaming.

The precursor for serotonin is the amino acid *tryptophan.* An enzyme converts tryptophan to *5-HTP* (5-hydroxytryptophan). Another enzyme converts 5-HTP to 5-HT (serotonin). (See *Figure 4.10.*) The drug **PCPA** (*p*-chlorophenylalanine) blocks the conversion of tryptophan to 5-HTP and thus serves as a serotonergic antagonist.

The cell bodies of serotonergic neurons are found in nine clusters, most of which are located in the raphe nuclei of the midbrain, pons, and medulla. The two most important clusters are found in the dorsal and medial raphe nuclei, and I will restrict my discussion to these clusters. The word *raphe* means "seam" or "crease" and refers to the fact that most of the raphe nuclei are found at or near the midline of the brain stem. Both the dorsal and median raphe nuclei project axons to the cerebral cortex. In addition, neurons in the dorsal raphe innervate the basal ganglia, and those in the median raphe innervate the dentate gyrus, a part of the hippocampal formation.

Investigators have identified at least nine different types of serotonin receptors, and pharmacologists have discovered drugs that serve as agonists or antagonists for many of the types of 5-HT receptors.

Drugs that inhibit the reuptake of serotonin have found a very important place in the treatment of mental disorders. The best known of these, **fluoxetine** (Prozac), is used to treat depression, some forms of anxiety disorders, and obsessive-compulsive disorder. These disorders—and their treatment—are discussed in Chapter 15. Another drug, **fenfluramine**, which causes the release of serotonin as well as inhibits its reuptake, has been used as an appetite suppressant in the treatment of obesity. Chapter 11 discusses the topic of obesity and its control by means of drugs.

Several hallucinogenic drugs produce their effects by interacting with serotonergic transmission. **LSD** (lysergic acid diethylamide) produces distortions of visual perceptions that some people find awesome and fascinating but that simply frighten other people. This drug, which is effective in extremely small doses, is a direct agonist for postsynaptic 5-HT$_{2A}$ receptors in the forebrain. Another drug, **MDMA** (methylenedioxymethamphetamine), is both a noradrenergic and serotonergic agonist and has both excitatory and hallucinogenic effects. Like its relative amphetamine, MDMA (popularly called "ecstasy") causes noradrenergic transporters to run backwards, thus causing the release of NE and inhibiting its reuptake. This site of action is apparently responsible for the drug's excitatory effect. MDMA also causes serotonergic transporters to run backwards, and this site of action is

FIGURE 4.10

Biosynthesis of Serotonin (5-hydroxytryptamine, or 5-HT)

Tryptophan

Enzyme

5-hydroxytryptophan
(5-HTP)

Enzyme

5-hydroxytryptamine
(5-HT, or serotonin)

locus coeruleus (*sur oo lee us*) A dark-colored group of noradrenergic cell bodies located in the pons near the rostral end of the floor of the fourth ventricle.

idazoxan A drug that blocks presynaptic noradrenergic α_2 receptors and hence acts as an agonist, stimulating the synthesis and release of NE.

serotonin (5-HT) (*sair a toe nin*) An indolamine neurotransmitter; also called 5-hydroxytryptamine.

PCPA A drug that inhibits the activity of tryptophan hydroxylase and thus interferes with the synthesis of 5-HT.

fluoxetine (*floo ox i teen*) A drug that inhibits the reuptake of 5-HT.

fenfluramine (*fen fluor i meen*) A drug that stimulates the release of 5-HT.

LSD A drug that stimulates 5-HT$_{2A}$ receptors.

MDMA A drug that serves as a noradrenergic and serotonergic agonist, also known as "ecstasy"; has excitatory and hallucinogenic effects.

apparently responsible for the drug's hallucinogenic effects. Unfortunately, research indicates that MDMA can damage serotonergic neurons and cause cognitive deficits.

Amino Acids

So far, all of the neurotransmitters I have described are synthesized within neurons: acetylcholine from choline, the catecholamines from the amino acid tyrosine, and serotonin from the amino acid tryptophan. Some neurons secrete simple amino acids as neurotransmitters. Because amino acids are used for protein synthesis by all cells of the brain, it is difficult to prove that a particular amino acid is a neurotransmitter. However, investigators suspect that at least eight amino acids may serve as neurotransmitters in the mammalian central nervous system. As we saw in the introduction to this section, three of them are especially important because they are the most common neurotransmitters in the CNS: glutamate, gamma-aminobutyric acid (GABA), and glycine.

Glutamate

Because **glutamate** (also called *glutamic acid*) and GABA are found in very simple organisms, many investigators believe that these neurotransmitters are the first to have evolved. Besides producing postsynaptic potentials by activating postsynaptic receptors, they also have direct excitatory effects (glutamic acid) and inhibitory effects (GABA) on axons; they raise or lower the threshold of excitation, thus affecting the rate at which action potentials occur. These direct effects suggest that these substances had a general modulating role even before the evolutionary development of specific receptor molecules.

Glutamate is the principal excitatory neurotransmitter in the brain and spinal cord. It is produced in abundance by the cells' metabolic processes. There is no effective way to prevent its synthesis without disrupting other activities of the cell.

Investigators have discovered four major types of glutamate receptors. Three of these receptors are ionotropic and are named after the artificial ligands that stimulate them: the **NMDA receptor**, the **AMPA receptor**, and the **kainate receptor**. The other glutamate receptor—the **metabotropic glutamate receptor**—is (obviously!) metabotropic. Actually, there appear to be at least seven subtypes of metabotropic glutamate receptors, but little is known about their functions except that some of them serve as presynaptic autoreceptors. The AMPA receptor is the most common glutamate receptor. It controls a sodium channel, so when glutamate attaches to the binding site, it produces EPSPs. The kainate receptor, which is stimulated by the drug kainic acid, has similar effects.

The NMDA receptor has some special—and very important—characteristics. It contains at least six different binding sites: four located on the exterior of the receptor and two located deep within the ion channel. When it is open, the ion channel controlled by the NMDA receptor permits both sodium and calcium ions to enter the cell. The influx of both of these ions causes a depolarization, of course, but the entry of calcium (Ca^{2+}) is especially important. Calcium serves as a second messenger, binding with—and activating—various enzymes within the cell. These enzymes have profound effects on the biochemical and structural properties of the cell. As we shall see, one important result is alteration in the characteristics of the synapse that provide one of the building blocks of a newly formed memory. These effects of NMDA receptors will be discussed in much greater detail in Chapter 12. The drug **AP5** (2-amino-5-phosphonopentanoate) blocks the glutamate-binding site on the NMDA receptor and impairs synaptic plasticity and certain forms of learning.

Figure 4.11 presents a schematic diagram of an NMDA receptor and its binding sites. Obviously, glutamate binds with one of these sites, or we would not call it a glutamate receptor. However, glutamate by itself cannot open the calcium channel. For that to happen, a molecule of glycine must be attached to the glycine-binding site,

glutamate An amino acid; the most important excitatory neurotransmitter in the brain.

NMDA receptor A specialized ionotropic glutamate receptor that controls a calcium channel that is normally blocked by Mg^{2+} ions; has several other binding sites.

AMPA receptor An ionotropic glutamate receptor that controls a sodium channel; stimulated by AMPA.

kainate receptor (*kay i nate*) An ionotropic glutamate receptor that controls a sodium channel; stimulated by kainic acid.

metabotropic glutamate receptor (*meh tab a troh pik*) A category of metabotropic receptors that are sensitive to glutamate.

AP5 (2-amino-5-phosphonopentanoate) A drug that blocks the glutamate-binding site on NMDA receptors.

located on the outside of the receptor. (We do not yet understand why glycine—which also serves as an inhibitory neurotransmitter in some parts of the central nervous system—is required for this ion channel to open.) (See *Figure 4.11.*)

One of the six binding sites on the NMDA receptor is sensitive to alcohol. In fact, as we will see in Chapter 14, researchers believe that this binding site is responsible for the dangerous convulsions that can be caused by sudden withdrawal from heavy, long-term alcohol abuse. Another binding site is sensitive to a hallucinogenic drug, **PCP** (phencyclidine, also known as "angel dust"). PCP serves as an indirect antagonist; when it attaches to its binding site, calcium ions cannot pass through the ion channel. PCP is a synthetic drug and is not produced by the brain. Thus, it is not the natural ligand of the PCP-binding site. What that ligand is and what useful functions it serves are not yet known.

Several drugs affect glutamatergic synapses. As you already know, NMDA, AMPA, and kainate (more precisely, *kainic acid*) serve as direct agonists at the receptors named after them.

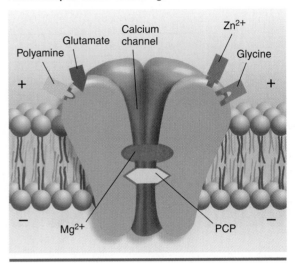

FIGURE 4.11

NMDA Receptor. This schematic illustration of an NMDA receptor shows its binding sites.

GABA

GABA (gamma-aminobutyric acid) is produced from glutamic acid by the action of an enzyme (glutamic acid decarboxylase, or GAD) that removes a carboxyl group. The drug **allylglycine** inactivates GAD and thus prevents the synthesis of GABA (step 2 of Figure 4.4). GABA is an inhibitory neurotransmitter, and it appears to have a widespread distribution throughout the brain and spinal cord. Two GABA receptors have been identified: GABA$_A$ and GABA$_B$. The GABA$_A$ receptor is ionotropic and controls a chloride channel; the GABA$_B$ receptor is metabotropic and controls a potassium channel.

As you know, neurons in the brain are greatly interconnected. Without the activity of inhibitory synapses, these interconnections would make the brain unstable. That is, through excitatory synapses neurons would excite their neighbors, which would then excite *their* neighbors, which would then excite the originally active neurons, and so on, until most of the neurons in the brain would be firing uncontrollably. In fact, this event does sometimes occur, and we refer to it as a *seizure.* (*Epilepsy* is a neurological disorder characterized by the presence of seizures.) Normally, an inhibitory influence is supplied by GABA-secreting neurons, which are present in large numbers in the brain. Some investigators believe that one of the causes of epilepsy is an abnormality in the biochemistry of GABA-secreting neurons or in GABA receptors.

Like NMDA receptors, GABA$_A$ receptors are complex; they contain at least five different binding sites. The primary binding site is, of course, for GABA. The drug **muscimol** (derived from the ACh agonist, muscarine) serves as a direct agonist for this site (step 6 of Figure 4.4). Another drug, **bicuculline**, blocks this GABA-binding site, serving as a direct antagonist (step 7 of Figure 4.4). A second site on the GABA$_A$ receptor binds with a class of tranquilizing drugs called the **benzodiazepines**. These drugs include diazepam (Valium) and chlordiazepoxide (Librium), which are used to reduce anxiety, promote sleep, reduce seizure activity, and produce muscle relaxation. The third site binds with barbiturates. The fourth site binds with various steroids, including some steroids used to produce general anesthesia. The fifth site binds with picrotoxin, a poison found in an East Indian shrub. In addition, alcohol binds with one of these sites—probably the benzodiazepine-binding site. (See *Figure 4.12.*)

Barbiturates, drugs that bind to the steroid site, and benzodiazepines all promote the activity of the GABA$_A$ receptor; thus, all these drugs serve as indirect agonists. The benzodiazepines are very effective **anxiolytics**, or "anxiety-dissolving"

PCP Phencyclidine; a drug that binds with the PCP-binding site of the NMDA receptor and serves as an indirect antagonist.

GABA An amino acid; the most important inhibitory neurotransmitter in the brain.

allylglycine A drug that inhibits the activity of GAD and thus blocks the synthesis of GABA.

muscimol (*musk i mawl*) A direct agonist for the GABA-binding site on the GABA$_A$ receptor.

bicuculline (*by kew kew leen*) A direct antagonist for the GABA-binding site on the GABA$_A$ receptor.

benzodiazepine (*ben zo di az a peen*) A category of anxiolytic drugs; an indirect agonist for the GABA$_A$ receptor.

anxiolytic (*ang zee oh lit ik*) An anxiety-reducing effect.

FIGURE 4.12

GABA$_A$ Receptor. This schematic illustration of a GABA$_A$ receptor, with its binding sites.

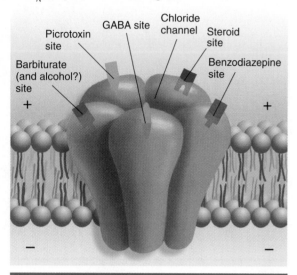

drugs. They are often used to treat people with anxiety disorders. In addition, some benzodiazepines serve as effective sleep medications, and others are used to treat some types of seizure disorder.

In low doses barbiturates have a calming effect. In progressively higher doses, they produce difficulty in walking and talking, unconsciousness, coma, and death. Although veterinarians sometimes use barbiturates to produce anesthesia for surgery, the therapeutic index—the ratio between a dose that produces anesthesia and one that causes fatal depression of the respiratory centers of the brain—is small. As a consequence, these drugs are rarely used by themselves to produce surgical anesthesia in humans.

Picrotoxin has effects opposite to those of benzodiazepines and barbiturates: It *inhibits* the activity of the GABA$_A$ receptor, thus serving as an indirect antagonist. In high enough doses, this drug causes convulsions.

Various steroid hormones are normally produced in the body, and some hormones related to progesterone (the principal pregnancy hormone) act on the steroid-binding site of the GABA$_A$ receptor, producing a relaxing, anxiolytic effect. However, the brain does not produce Valium, barbiturates, or picrotoxin. What are the natural ligands for these binding sites? So far, most research has concentrated on the benzodiazepine-binding site. These binding sites are more complex than the others. They can be activated by drugs such as the benzodiazepines, which promote the activity of the receptor and thus serve as indirect agonists. They can also be activated by other drugs that have the opposite effect—that inhibit the activity of the receptor, thus serving as indirect antagonists. Presumably, the brain produces natural ligands that act as indirect agonists or antagonists at the benzodiazepine-binding site, but so far, such a chemical has not been identified.

What about the GABA$_B$ receptor? This metabotropic receptor, coupled to a G protein, serves as both a postsynaptic receptor and a presynaptic autoreceptor. A GABA$_B$ agonist, baclofen, serves as a muscle relaxant. Another drug, CGP 335348, serves as an antagonist. The activation of GABA$_B$ receptors opens potassium channels, producing hyperpolarizing inhibitory postsynaptic potentials.

Glycine

The amino acid **glycine** appears to be the inhibitory neurotransmitter in the spinal cord and lower portions of the brain. Little is known about its biosynthetic pathway; there are several possible routes, but not enough is known to decide how neurons produce glycine. The bacteria that cause tetanus (lockjaw) release a chemical that prevents the release of glycine (and GABA as well); the removal of the inhibitory effect of these synapses causes muscles to contract continuously.

The glycine receptor is ionotropic, and it controls a chloride channel. Thus, when it is active, it produces inhibitory postsynaptic potentials. The drug **strychnine**, an alkaloid found in the seeds of the *Strychnos nux vomica*, a tree found in India, serves as a glycine antagonist. Strychnine is very toxic, and even relatively small doses cause convulsions and death. No drugs have yet been found that serve as specific glycine agonists.

Peptides

Recent studies have discovered that the neurons of the central nervous system release a large variety of peptides. Peptides consist of two or more amino acids

glycine (*gly seen*) An amino acid; an important inhibitory neurotransmitter in the lower brain stem and spinal cord.

strychnine (*strik neen*) A direct antagonist for the glycine receptor.

linked together by peptide bonds. All the peptides that have been studied so far are produced from precursor molecules. These precursors are large polypeptides that are broken into pieces by special enzymes. Neurons manufacture both the polypeptides and the enzymes needed to break them apart in the right places. The appropriate sections of the polypeptides are retained, and the rest are destroyed. Because the synthesis of peptides takes place in the soma, vesicles containing these chemicals must be delivered to the terminal buttons by axoplasmic transport.

Peptides are released from all parts of the terminal button, not just from the presynaptic membrane; thus, only a portion of the molecules are released into the synaptic cleft. The rest presumably act on receptors belonging to other cells in the vicinity. Once released, peptides are destroyed by enzymes. There is no mechanism for reuptake and recycling of peptides.

Several different peptides are released by neurons. Although most peptides appear to serve as neuromodulators, some act as neurotransmitters. One of the best-known families of peptides is the **endogenous opioids**. (*Endogenous* means "produced from within"; *opioid* means "like opium.") Several years ago it became clear that opiates (drugs such as opium, morphine, and heroin) reduce pain because they have direct effects on the brain. (Please note that the term *opioid* refers to endogenous chemicals, and *opiate* refers to drugs.) Pert, Snowman, and Snyder (1974) discovered that neurons in a localized region of the brain contain specialized receptors that respond to opiates. Then, soon after the discovery of the opiate receptor, other neuroscientists discovered the natural ligands for these receptors (Terenius and Wahlström, 1975; Hughes et al., 1975), which they called **enkephalins** (from the Greek word *enkephalos*, "in the head"). We now know that the enkephalins are only two members of a family of endogenous opioids, all of which are synthesized from one of three large peptides that serve as precursors. In addition, we know that there are at least three different types of opiate receptors: μ (mu), δ (delta), and κ (kappa).

Several different neural systems are activated when opiate receptors are stimulated. One type produces analgesia, another inhibits species-typical defensive responses such as fleeing and hiding, and another stimulates a system of neurons involved in reinforcement ("reward"). The last effect explains why opiates are often abused. The situations that cause neurons to secrete endogenous opioids are discussed in Chapter 7, and the brain mechanisms of opiate addiction are discussed in Chapter 16.

So far, pharmacologists have developed only two types of drugs that affect neural communication by means of opioids: direct agonists and antagonists. Many synthetic opiates, including heroin (dihydromorphine) and Percodan (levorphanol), have been developed and some are used clinically as analgesics (step 6 of Figure 4.4). Several opiate receptor blockers have also been developed (step 7 of Figure 4.4). One of them, **naloxone**, is used clinically to reverse opiate intoxication. This drug has saved the lives of many drug abusers who would otherwise have died of an overdose of heroin.

Several peptide hormones released by endocrine glands are also produced in the brain, where they serve as neuromodulators. In some cases the peripheral and central peptides perform related functions. For example, outside the nervous system the hormone angiotensin acts directly on the kidneys and blood vessels to produce effects that help the body cope with the loss of fluid, and inside the nervous system circuits of neurons that use angiotensin as a neurotransmitter perform complementary functions, including the activation of neural circuits that produce thirst. The existence of the blood–brain barrier keeps most peptide hormones in the general circulation separate from the extracellular fluid in the brain, which means that the same peptide molecule can have different effects in these two regions.

Many peptides produced in the brain have interesting behavioral effects, which will be discussed in subsequent chapters.

endogenous opioid (*en dodge en us oh pee oyd*) A class of peptides secreted by the brain that act as opiates.

enkephalin (*en keff a lin*) One of the endogenous opioids.

naloxone (*na lox own*) A drug that blocks opiate receptors.

FIGURE 4.13

Cannabinoid Receptors in a Rat Brain. To produce this autoradiogram, the brain was incubated in a solution containing a radioactive ligand for THC receptors. The receptors are indicated by dark areas. (Autoradiography is described in Chapter 5.) (Br St = brain stem, Cer = cerebellum, CP = caudate nucleus/putamen, Cx = cortex, EP = entopeduncular nucleus, GP = globus pallidus, Hipp = hippocampus, SNr = substantia nigra.)

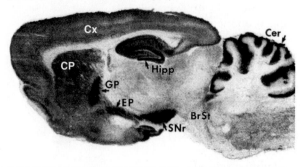

Courtesy of Miles Herkenham, National Institute of Mental Health, Bethesda, MD.

Lipids

Various substances derived from lipids can serve to transmit messages within or between cells. The best known, and probably the most important, are the two **endocannabinoids** ("endogenous cannabis-like substances")—natural ligands for the receptors that are responsible for the physiological effects of the active ingredient in marijuana. Matsuda et al. (1990) discovered that THC (tetrahydrocannibinal, the active ingredient of marijuana) stimulates cannabinoid receptors located in specific regions of the brain. (See *Figure 4.13*.) Two types of cannabinoid receptors, CB_1 and CB_2, both metabotropic, have since been discovered. Devane et al. (1992) discovered the first endocannabinoid: a lipidlike substance that they named **anandamide**, from the Sanskrit word *ananda*, or "bliss." Anandamide seems to be synthesized on demand; that is, it is produced and released as it is needed and is not stored in synaptic vesicles. CB_1 receptors are found in the brain, especially in the frontal cortex, anterior cingulate cortex, basal ganglia, cerebellum, hypothalamus, and hippocampus. They are located on terminal buttons of glutamatergic, GABAergic, acetylcholinergic, noradrenergic, dopaminergic, and serotonergic neurons, where they serve to regulate neurotransmitter release (Iversen, 2003). Very low levels of CB_1 receptors are found in the brain stem, which accounts for the low toxicity of THC. CB_1 receptors are blocked by the drug **rimonabant**. CB_2 receptors are found outside the brain, especially in cells of the immune system.

THC produces analgesia and sedation, stimulates appetite, reduces nausea caused by drugs used to treat cancer, relieves asthma attacks, decreases pressure within the eyes in patients with glaucoma, and reduces the symptoms of certain motor disorders. On the other hand, THC interferes with concentration and memory, alters visual and auditory perception, and distorts perceptions of the passage of time (Iversen, 2003). The short-term memory impairment that accompanies marijuana use appears to be caused by the action of THC on CB_1 receptors in the hippocampus. Endocannabinoids appear to play an essential role in the reinforcing effects of opiates: A targeted mutation that prevents the production of CB_1 receptors abolishes the reinforcing effects of morphine but not of cocaine, amphetamine, or nicotine (Cossu et al., 2001). These effects of cannabinoids are discussed further in Chapter 16.

I just mentioned that THC (and, of course, the endocannabinoids) has an analgesic effect. Agarwal et al. (2007) found that THC exerts its analgesic effects by stimulating CB_1 receptors in the peripheral nervous system. In addition, a commonly used over-the-counter analgesic, *acetaminophen* (known as *paracetamol* in many countries), also acts on these receptors. Once it enters the blood, acetaminophen is converted into another compound that then joins with arachidonic acid, the precursor of anandamide. This compound binds with peripheral CB_1 receptors and activates them, reducing pain sensation. Administration of a CB_1 antagonist completely blocks the analgesic effect of acetaminophen (Bertolini et al., 2006).

Nucleosides

A nucleoside is a compound that consists of a sugar molecule bound with a purine or pyrimidine base. One of these compounds, **adenosine** (a combination of ribose and adenine), serves as a neuromodulator in the brain.

endocannabinoid (*can* **nob** *i noid*) A lipid; an endogenous ligand for receptors that bind with THC, the active ingredient of marijuana.

anandamide (*a* **nan** *da mide*) The first cannabinoid to be discovered and probably the most important one.

rimonabant A drug that blocks cannabinoid CB_1 receptors.

adenosine (*a* **den** *oh seen*) A nucleoside; a combination of ribose and adenine; serves as a neuromodulator in the brain.

Adenosine is known to be released, apparently by glial cells as well as neurons, when cells are short of fuel or oxygen. The release of adenosine activates receptors on nearby blood vessels and causes them to dilate, increasing the flow of blood and helping bring more of the needed substances to the region. Adenosine also acts as a neuromodulator, through its action on at least three different types of adenosine receptors. Adenosine receptors are coupled to G proteins, and their effect is to open potassium channels, producing inhibitory postsynaptic potentials. Because adenosine is present in all cells, investigators have not yet succeeded in distinguishing neurons that release this chemical as a neuromodulator. Thus, circuits of adenosinergic neurons have not yet been identified.

Because adenosine receptors suppress neural activity, adenosine and other adenosine receptor agonists have generally inhibitory effects on behavior. In fact, as we will see in Chapter 8, investigators believe that adenosine receptors play an important role in the control of sleep. For example, the amount of adenosine in the brain increases during wakefulness and decreases during sleep. In fact, the accumulation of adenosine after prolonged wakefulness may be the most important cause of the sleepiness that ensues. A very common drug, **caffeine**, blocks adenosine receptors (step 7 of Figure 4.4) and hence produces excitatory effects. Caffeine is a bitter-tasting alkaloid found in coffee, tea, cocoa beans, and other plants. In much of the world, a majority of the adult population ingests caffeine every day—fortunately, without apparent harm.

Soluble Gases

Recently, investigators have discovered that neurons use at least two simple, soluble gases—nitric oxide and carbon monoxide—to communicate with one another. One of these, **nitric oxide (NO)**, has received the most attention. Nitric oxide (not to be confused with nitrous oxide, or laughing gas) is a soluble gas that is produced by the activity of an enzyme found in certain neurons. Researchers have found that NO is used as a messenger in many parts of the body; for example, it is involved in the control of the muscles in the wall of the intestines, it dilates blood vessels in regions of the brain that become metabolically active, and it stimulates the changes in blood vessels that produce penile erections (Culotta and Koshland, 1992). As we will see in Chapter 12, it may also play a role in the establishment of neural changes that are produced by learning.

All of the neurotransmitters and neuromodulators discussed so far (with the exception of anandamide and perhaps adenosine) are stored in synaptic vesicles and released by terminal buttons. Nitric oxide is produced in several regions of a nerve cell—including dendrites—and is released as soon as it is produced. More accurately, it diffuses out of the cell as soon as it is produced. It does not activate membrane-bound receptors but enters neighboring cells, where it activates an enzyme responsible for the production of a second messenger, cyclic GMP. Within a few seconds of being produced, nitric oxide is converted into biologically inactive compounds.

Nitric oxide is produced from arginine, an amino acid, by the activation of an enzyme known as **nitric oxide synthase**. This enzyme can be inactivated (step 2 of Figure 4.4) by a drug called L-NAME (nitro-L-arginine methyl ester).

You have undoubtedly heard of a drug called *sildenafil* (more commonly known as Viagra), which is used to treat men with erectile dysfunction—difficulty maintaining a penile erection. As we just saw, nitric oxide produces its physiological effects by stimulating the production of cyclic GMP. Although nitric oxide lasts only for a few seconds, cyclic GMP lasts somewhat longer but is ultimately destroyed by an enzyme. Molecules of sildenafil bind with this enzyme and thus cause cyclic GMP to be destroyed at a much slower rate. As a consequence, an erection is maintained for a longer time. (By the way, sildenafil has effects on other parts of the body and is used to treat altitude sickness and other vascular disorders.)

caffeine A drug that blocks adenosine receptors.

nitric oxide (NO) A gas produced by cells in the nervous system; used as a means of communication between cells.

nitric oxide synthase The enzyme responsible for the production of nitric oxide.

TABLE 4.3   Drugs Mentioned in This Chapter

Neurotransmitter	Name of Drug	Effect of Drug	Effect on Synaptic Transmission
Acetylcholine (ACh)	botulinum toxin	blocks release of ACh	antagonist
	black widow spider venom	stimulates release of ACh	agonist
	nicotine	stimulates nicotinic receptors	agonist
	curare	blocks nicotinic receptors	antagonist
	muscarine	stimulates muscarinic receptors	agonist
	atropine	blocks muscarinic receptors	antagonist
	neostigmine	inhibits acetylcholinesterase	agonist
Dopamine (DA)	L-DOPA	facilitates synthesis of DA	agonist
	AMPT	inhibits synthesis of DA	antagonist
	reserpine	inhibits storage of DA in synaptic vesicles	antagonist
	chlorpromazine	blocks D_2 receptors	antagonist
	cocaine, methylphenidate	blocks DA reuptake	agonist
	amphetamine	stimulates release of DA	agonist
	deprenyl	blocks MAO-B	agonist
Norepinephrine (NE)	fusaric acid	inhibits synthesis of NE	antagonist
	reserpine	inhibits storage of NE in synaptic vesicles	antagonist
	idazoxan	blocks α_2 autoreceptors	agonist
	MDMA, amphetamine	stimulates release of NE	agonist
Serotonin (5-HT)	PCPA	inhibits synthesis of 5-HT	antagonist
	reserpine	inhibits storage of 5-HT in synaptic vesicles	antagonist
	fenfluramine	stimulates release of 5-HT	agonist
	fluoxetine	inhibits reuptake of 5-HT	agonist
	LSD	stimulates 5-HT_{2A} receptors	agonist
	MDMA	stimulates release of 5-HT	agonist
Glutamate	AMPA	stimulates AMPA receptor	agonist
	kainic acid	stimulates kainate receptor	agonist
	NMDA	stimulates NMDA receptor	agonist
	AP5	blocks NMDA receptor	antagonist
GABA	allylglycine	inhibits synthesis of GABA	antagonist
	muscimol	stimulates GABA receptors	agonist
	bicuculline	blocks GABA receptors	antagonist
	benzodiazepines	serve as indirect GABA agonists	agonist
Glycine	strychnine	blocks glycine receptors	antagonist
Opioids	opiates (morphine, heroin, etc.)	stimulates opiate receptors	agonist
	naloxone	blocks opiate receptors	antagonist
Anandamide	rimonabant	blocks cannabinoid CB_1 receptors	antagonist
	THC	stimulates cannabinoid CB_1 receptors	agonist
Adenosine	caffeine	blocks adenosine receptors	antagonist
Nitric oxide (NO)	L-NAME	inhibits synthesis of NO	antagonist

InterimSummary

Neurotransmitters and Neuromodulators

The nervous system contains a variety of neurotransmitters, each of which interacts with a specialized receptor. Those that have received the most study are acetylcholine and the monoamines: dopamine, norepinephrine, and 5-hydroxytryptamine (serotonin). The synthesis of these neurotransmitters is controlled by a series of enzymes. Several amino acids also serve as neurotransmitters, the most important of which are glutamate (glutamic acid), GABA, and glycine. Glutamate serves as an excitatory neurotransmitter; the others serve as inhibitory neurotransmitters.

Peptide neurotransmitters consist of chains of amino acids. Like proteins, peptides are synthesized at the ribosomes according to sequences coded for by the chromosomes. The best-known class of peptides in the nervous system includes the endogenous opioids, whose effects are mimicked by drugs such as opium and heroin. One lipid appears to serve as a chemical messenger: anandamide, the endogenous ligand for the CB_1 cannabinoid receptor. Adenosine, a nucleoside that has inhibitory effects on synaptic transmission, is released by neurons and glial cells in the brain. In addition, two soluble gases—nitric oxide and carbon monoxide—can diffuse out of the cell in which they are produced and trigger the production of a second messenger in adjacent cells.

This chapter has mentioned many drugs and their effects. They are summarized for your convenience in **Table 4.3.**

EPILOGUE   Helpful Hints from a Tragedy

The discovery that MPTP damages the brain and causes the symptoms of Parkinson's disease galvanized researchers interested in the disease. (I recently checked PubMed, a web site maintained by the U.S. National Institutes of Health, and found that 3780 scientific publications referred to MPTP.) The first step was to find out whether the drug would have the same effect in laboratory animals so that the details of the process could be studied. It did; Langston and Ballard (1984) found that injections of MPTP produced parkinsonian symptoms in squirrel monkeys and that these symptoms could be reduced by L-DOPA therapy—and just as the investigators had hoped, examination of the animals' brains showed a selective loss of dopamine-secreting neurons in the substantia nigra.

It turns out that MPTP itself does not cause neural damage; instead, the drug is converted by an enzyme present in glial cells into another substance, MPP⁺. *That* chemical is taken up by dopamine-secreting neurons, by means of the reuptake mechanism that normally retrieves dopamine that is released by terminal buttons. MPP⁺ accumulates in mitochondria in these cells and blocks their ability to metabolize nutrients, thus killing the cells (Maret et al., 1990). The enzyme that converts MPTP into MPP⁺ is none other than monoamine oxidase (MAO), which, as you now know, is responsible for deactivating excess amounts of monoamines present in terminal buttons. Because pharmacolo-gists had already developed MAO inhibitors, Langston and his colleagues decided to find out whether one of these drugs (pargyline) would protect squirrel monkeys from the toxic effects of MPTP by preventing its conversion into MPP⁺ (Langston and Ballard, 1984). It worked; when MAO was inhibited by pargyline, MPTP injections had no effects.

These results made researchers wonder whether MAO inhibitors might possibly protect against the degeneration of dopamine-secreting neurons in patients with Parkinson's disease. No one thought that Parkinson's disease was caused by MPP⁺, but perhaps some other toxins were involved. Epidemiologists have found that Parkinson's disease is more common in highly industrialized countries, which suggests that environmental toxins produced in these societies may be responsible for the brain damage (Tanner, 1989; Veldman et al., 1998). Fortunately, several MAO inhibitors have been tested and approved for use in humans. One of them, deprenyl, was tested and appeared to slow down the progression of neurological symptoms (Tetrud and Langston, 1989).

As a result of this study, many neurologists are now treating their Parkinson's patients with deprenyl, especially during the early stages of the disease. More recent studies found that deprenyl does not protect dopaminergic neurons indefinitely (Shoulson et al., 2002), but researchers are trying to develop other drugs with more sustained neuroprotective effects.

Key Concepts

PRINCIPLES OF PSYCHOPHARMACOLOGY

1. Pharmacokinetics is the process by which drugs are absorbed, distributed within the body, metabolized, and excreted.
2. Drugs can act at several different sites and have several different effects. The effectiveness of a drug is the magnitude of the effects of a given quantity of the drug.
3. A drug's therapeutic index is its margin of safety: the difference between an effective dose and a dose that produces toxic side effects.
4. When a drug is administered repeatedly, it often produces tolerance, and withdrawal effects often occur when the drug is discontinued. Sometimes, repeated administration of a drug causes sensitization.
5. Researchers must control for placebo effects in both humans and laboratory animals.

SITES OF DRUG ACTION

6. Each of the steps involved in synaptic transmission can be interfered with by drugs, and some can be facilitated. These steps include synthesis of the neurotransmitter, storage in synaptic vesicles, release, activation of postsynaptic and presynaptic receptors, and termination of postsynaptic potentials through reuptake or enzymatic deactivation.

NEUROTRANSMITTERS AND NEUROMODULATORS

7. Neurons use a variety of chemicals as neurotransmitters, including acetylcholine, the monoamines (dopamine, norepinephrine, and 5-HT), the amino acids (glutamic acid, GABA, and glycine), various peptides, lipids, nucleosides, and soluble gases.

Suggested Readings

Cooper, J. R., Bloom, F. E., and Roth, R. H. *The Biochemical Basis of Neuropharmacology*, 8th ed. New York: Oxford University Press, 2002.

Grilly, D. M. *Drugs and Human Behavior*, 5th ed. Boston: Allyn and Bacon, 2005.

Meyer, J. S., and Quenzer, L. F. *Psychopharmacology: Drugs, the Brain, and Behavior*. Sunderland, MA: Sinauer Associates, 2005.

Additional Resources

Visit www.mypsychkit.com for additional review and practice of the material covered in this chapter. Within MyPsychKit, you can take practice tests and receive a customized study plan to help you review. Dozens of animations, tutorials, and Web links are also available. You can even review using the interactive electronic version of this textbook. You will need to register for MyPsychKit. See www.mypsychkit.com for complete details.

chapter 5

Methods and Strategies of Research

LEARNING OBJECTIVES

1. Discuss the research method of experimental ablation: the rationale for this procedure, the distinction between brain function and behavior, and the production of brain lesions.

2. Describe stereotaxic surgery and its uses.

3. Describe research methods for preserving, sectioning, and staining the brain and for studying its parts.

4. Describe research methods for tracing efferent and afferent axons and for studying the structure of the living human brain.

5. Describe how the neural and metabolic activity of the brain is recorded.

6. Describe how neural activity in the brain is stimulated, both electrically and chemically.

7. Describe research methods for locating particular neurochemicals, the neurons that produce them, and the receptors that respond to them.

8. Describe research techniques to identify genetic factors that may affect the development of the nervous system and influence behavior.

9. Describe the use of targeted mutations and the administration of antisense oligonucleotides in the study of functions of particular sets of neurons in the brain.

⋮ PROLOGUE   Heart Repaired, Brain Damaged

All her life, Mrs. H. had been active. She had never been particularly athletic, but she and her husband often went hiking and camping with their children when they were young, and they continued to hike and go for bicycle rides after their children left home. Her husband died when she was 60, and even though she no longer rode her bicycle, she enjoyed gardening and walking around the neighborhood with her friends.

A few years later, Mrs. H. was digging in her garden when a sudden pain gripped her chest. She felt as if a hand were squeezing her heart. She gasped and dropped her spade. The pain crept toward her left shoulder and then traveled down her left arm. The sensation was terrifying; she was sure that she was having a heart attack and was going to die. However, after a few minutes the pain melted away, and she walked slowly back to her house.

Her physician examined her and performed some tests and later told her that she had not had a heart attack. Her pain was that of angina pectoris, caused by insufficient flow of blood to the heart. Some of her coronary arteries had become partially obstructed with atherosclerotic plaque—cholesterol-containing deposits on the walls of the blood vessels. Her efforts in her garden had increased her heart rate, and as a consequence, the metabolic activity of her heart muscle had also increased. Her clogged coronary arteries simply could not keep up with the demand, and the accumulation of metabolic by-products caused intense pain. Her physician cautioned her to avoid unnecessary exertion and prescribed nitroglycerine tablets to place under her tongue if another attack occurred.

Mrs. H. stopped working in her garden but continued to walk around the neighborhood with her friends. Then one evening, while climbing the stairs to get ready for bed, she felt another attack grip her heart. With difficulty, she made her way to her bathroom cabinet, where she found her nitroglycerine tablets.

Fumbling with the childproof cap, she extracted a tablet and placed it under her tongue. As the tablet dissolved and the nitroglycerine entered her bloodstream, she felt the tightness in her chest loosen, and she stumbled to her bed.

Over the next year the frequency and intensity of Mrs. H.'s attacks increased. Finally, the specialist to whom her physician had referred her recommended that she consider having a coronary artery bypass performed. She readily agreed. The surgeon, Dr. G., replaced two of her coronary arteries with sections of vein that he had removed from her leg. During the procedure, an artificial heart took over the pumping of her blood so that the surgeon could cut out the diseased section of the arteries and delicately sew in the replacements.

Several days later, Dr. G. visited Mrs. H. in her hospital room. "How are you feeling, Mrs. H?"

"I'm feeling fine," she said, "but I'm having trouble with my vision. Everything looks so confusing, and I feel disoriented. I can't. . . ."

"Don't worry," he cut in. "It's normal to feel confused after such serious surgery. Your tests look fine, and we don't expect a recurrence of your angina. You should be good for many years!" He flashed a broad smile at her and left the room.

But Mrs. H.'s visual problems and her confusion did not get better. Although the surgeon's notes indicated a successful outcome, her family physician saw that something was wrong and asked Dr. J., a neuropsychologist, to evaluate her. Dr. J.'s report confirmed the physician's fears: Mrs. H. had Balint's syndrome. She could still see, but she could not control her eye movements. The world confused her because she saw only fleeting, fragmentary images. She could no longer read, and she could no longer locate and grasp objects in front of her. In short, her vision was almost useless. Her heart was fine, but she would henceforth have to live in a nursing home, where others could care for her.

Study of the physiology of behavior involves the efforts of scientists in many disciplines, including physiology, neuroanatomy, biochemistry, psychology, endocrinology, and histology. Pursuing a research project in behavioral neuroscience requires competence in many experimental techniques. Because different procedures often produce contradictory results, investigators must be familiar with the advantages and limitations of the methods they employ. Scientific investigation entails a process of asking questions of nature. The method that is used frames the question. Often we receive a puzzling answer, only to realize later that we were not asking the question we thought we were. As we will see, the best conclusions about the physiology of behavior are made not by any single experiment, but by a program of research that enables us to compare the results of studies that approach the problem with different methods.

An enormous—and bewildering—array of research methods is available to the investigator. If I merely presented a catalog of them, it would not be surprising if you got lost—or simply lost interest. Instead, I will present only the most important and commonly used procedures, organized around a few problems that researchers have studied. This way, it should be easier to see the types of information provided by various research methods and to understand their advantages and disadvantages. It will also permit me to describe the strategies that researchers employ as they follow up the results of one experiment by designing and executing another one.

Experimental Ablation

One of the most important research methods used to investigate brain functions involves destroying part of the brain and evaluating the animal's subsequent behavior. This method is called **experimental ablation** (from the Latin word *ablatus*, a "carrying away"). In most cases experimental ablation does not involve the removal of brain tissue; instead, the researcher destroys some tissue and leaves it in place. Experimental ablation is the oldest method used in neuroscience, and it remains in common use today.

Evaluating the Behavioral Effects of Brain Damage

A *lesion* is a wound or injury, and a researcher who destroys part of the brain usually refers to the damage as a *brain lesion*. Experiments in which part of the brain is damaged and the animal's behavior is subsequently observed are called **lesion studies**. The rationale for lesion studies is that the function of an area of the brain can be inferred from the behaviors that the animal can no longer perform after the area has been damaged. For example, if, after part of the brain is destroyed, an animal can no longer perform tasks that require vision, we can conclude that the animal is blind—and that the damaged area plays some role in vision.

Just what can we learn from lesion studies? Our goal is to discover what functions are performed by different regions of the brain and then to understand how these functions are combined to accomplish particular behaviors. The distinction between *brain function* and *behavior* is an important one. Circuits within the brain perform functions, not behaviors. No one brain region or neural circuit is solely responsible for a behavior; each region performs a function (or set of functions) that contributes to performance of the behavior. For example, the act of reading involves functions required for controlling eye movements, focusing the lens of the eye, perceiving and recognizing words and letters, comprehending the meaning of the words, and so on. Some of these functions also participate in other behaviors; for example, controlling eye movement and focusing are required for any task that involves looking, and brain mechanisms used for comprehending the meanings of words also participate in comprehending speech. The researcher's task is to understand the functions that are required for performing a particular behavior and to determine what circuits of neurons in the brain are responsible for each of these functions.

Producing Brain Lesions

How do we produce brain lesions? It is easy to destroy parts of the brain immediately beneath the skull; we anesthetize the animal, cut open its scalp, remove part of its skull, and cut through the dura mater, bringing the cortex into view. Then we can use a suction device to aspirate the brain tissue. To accomplish this tissue removal, we place a glass pipette on the surface of the brain and suck away brain tissue with a vacuum pump attached to the pipette.

More often, we want to destroy regions that are hidden away in the depths of the brain. Brain lesions of subcortical regions (regions located beneath the cortex) are

experimental ablation The removal or destruction of a portion of the brain of a laboratory animal; presumably, the functions that can no longer be performed are the ones the region previously controlled.

lesion study A synonym for experimental ablation.

FIGURE 5.1

Radio Frequency Lesion. The arrows point to very small lesions produced by passing radio frequency current through the tips of stainless steel electrodes placed in the medial preoptic nucleus of a rat brain. The oblong hole in the middle of the photograph is the third ventricle. (Frontal section, cell-body stain.)

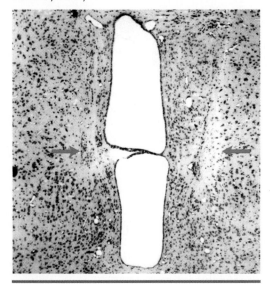

From Turkenburg, J. L., Swaab, D. F., Endert, E., et al. *Brain Research Bulletin*, 1988, *21*, 215–224. Reprinted with permission.

excitotoxic lesion (ek sigh tow **tok** sik) A brain lesion produced by intracerebral injection of an excitatory amino acid, such as kainic acid.

usually produced by passing electrical current through a stainless steel wire that is coated with an insulating varnish except for the very tip. We guide the wire stereotaxically so that its end reaches the appropriate location. (Stereotaxic surgery is described in the next subsection.) Then we turn on a lesion-making device, which produces radio frequency (RF) current—alternating current of a very high frequency. The passage of the current through the brain tissue produces heat that kills cells in the region surrounding the tip of the electrode. (See *Figure 5.1*.)

Lesions produced by these means destroy everything in the vicinity of the electrode tip, including neural cell bodies and the axons of neurons that pass through the region. A more selective method of producing brain lesions employs an excitatory amino acid such as *kainic acid*, which kills neurons by stimulating them to death. (As we saw in Chapter 4, kainic acid stimulates glutamate receptors.) Lesions produced this way are referred to as **excitotoxic lesions**. When an excitatory amino acid is injected through a cannula into a region of the brain, the chemical destroys neural cell bodies in the vicinity but spares axons that belong to different neurons that happen to pass nearby. (See *Figure 5.2*.) This selectivity permits the investigator to determine whether the behavioral effects of destroying a particular brain structure are caused by the death of neurons located there or by the destruction of axons that pass nearby.

Even more specific methods of targeting and killing particular types of neurons are available. For example, molecular biologists have devised ways to attach toxic chemicals to antibodies that will bind with particular proteins found only on certain types of neurons in the brain. The antibodies target these proteins, and the toxic chemicals kill the cells to which the proteins are attached.

Note that when we produce subcortical lesions by passing RF current through an electrode or infusing a chemical through a cannula, we always cause additional damage to the brain. When we pass an electrode or a cannula through the brain to get to our target, we inevitably cause a small amount of damage even before turning on the lesion maker or starting the infusion. Therefore, we cannot simply compare the behavior of brain-lesioned animals with that of unoperated control animals; the incidental damage to the brain regions above the lesion may actually be responsible

FIGURE 5.2

Excitotoxic Lesion. This figure shows slices through the hippocampus of a rat brain: (a) depicts a normal hippocampus, while (b) shows a hippocampus with a lesion produced by an infusion of an excitatory amino acid. The arrowheads mark the ends of the region in which neurons have been destroyed.

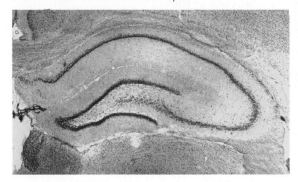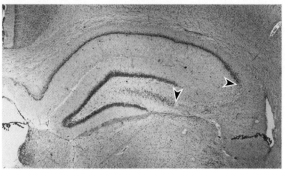

(a)   (b)

Courtesy of Benno Roozendaal, University of California, Irvine.

for some of the behavioral deficits we see. What we do is operate on a group of animals and produce **sham lesions**. To do so, we anesthetize each animal, put it in the stereotaxic apparatus (described later), cut open the scalp, drill the holes, insert the electrode or cannula, and lower it to the proper depth. In other words, we do everything we would do to produce the lesion except turn on the lesion maker or start the infusion. This group of animals serves as a control group; if the behavior of the animals with brain lesions is different from that of the sham-operated control animals, we can conclude that the lesions caused the behavioral deficits. (As you can see, a sham lesion serves the same purpose as a placebo does in a pharmacology study.)

Most of the time, investigators produce permanent brain lesions, but sometimes it is advantageous to disrupt the activity of a particular region of the brain temporarily. The easiest way to do so is to inject a local anesthetic or a drug called *muscimol* into the appropriate part of the brain. The anesthetic blocks action potentials in axons from entering or leaving that region, thus effectively producing a temporary lesion (usually called a *reversible* brain lesion). Muscimol, a drug that stimulates GABA receptors, inactivates a region of the brain by inhibiting the neurons located there. (You will recall that GABA is the most important inhibitory neurotransmitter in the brain.)

sham lesion A "placebo" procedure that duplicates all the steps of producing a brain lesion except for the one that actually causes the brain damage.

stereotaxic surgery (*stair ee oh* **tak** *sik*) Brain surgery using a stereotaxic apparatus to position an electrode or cannula in a specified position of the brain.

bregma The junction of the sagittal and coronal sutures of the skull; often used as a reference point for stereotaxic brain surgery.

stereotaxic atlas A collection of drawings of sections of the brain of a particular animal with measurements that provide coordinates for stereotaxic surgery.

Stereotaxic Surgery

So how do we get the tip of an electrode or cannula to a precise location in the depths of an animal's brain? The answer is **stereotaxic surgery**. *Stereotaxis* literally means "solid arrangement"; more specifically, it refers to the ability to locate objects in space. A *stereotaxic apparatus* contains a holder that fixes the animal's head in a standard position and a carrier that moves an electrode or a cannula through measured distances in all three axes of space. However, to perform stereotaxic surgery, one must first study a *stereotaxic atlas*.

The Stereotaxic Atlas

No two brains of animals of a given species are completely identical, but there is enough similarity among individuals to predict the location of particular brain structures relative to external features of the head. For instance, a subcortical nucleus of a rat might be so many millimeters ventral, anterior, and lateral to a point formed by the junction of several bones of the skull. Figure 5.3 shows two views of a rat skull: a drawing of the dorsal surface and, beneath it, a midsagittal view. (See *Figure 5.3*.) The skull is composed of several bones that grow together and form *sutures* (seams). The heads of newborn babies contain a soft spot at the junction of the coronal and sagittal sutures called the *fontanelle*. Once this gap closes, the junction is called **bregma**, from the Greek word meaning "front of head." We can find bregma on a rat's skull, too, and it serves as a convenient reference point. If the animal's skull is oriented as shown in the illustration, a particular region of the brain is found in a fairly constant position relative to bregma.

A **stereotaxic atlas** contains photographs or drawings that correspond to frontal sections taken at various distances rostral and caudal to bregma. For example, the page shown in Figure 5.4 is a drawing of a slice of the brain that contains a brain structure (shown in red) that we are interested in. If we wanted to place the tip of a wire in this structure (the

FIGURE 5.3

Rat Brain and Skull. The figure shows the relation of the skull sutures to a rat's brain, and the location of a target for an electrode placement. *Top*: Dorsal view. *Bottom*: Midsagittal view.

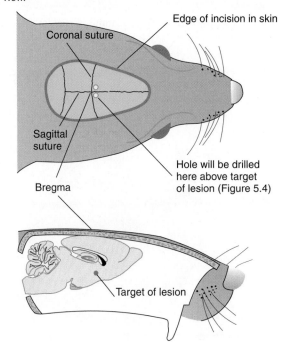

FIGURE 5.4

Stereotaxic Atlas.   This sample page from a stereotaxic atlas shows a drawing of a frontal section through the rat brain. The target (the fornix) is indicated in red. Labels have been removed for the sake of clarity.

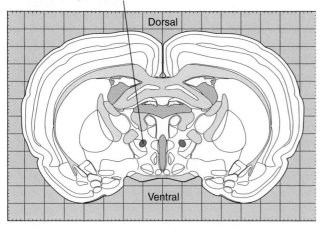

Adapted from Swanson, L. W. *Brain Maps: Structure of the Rat Brain.* New York: Elsevier, 1992.

> **stereotaxic apparatus** A device that permits a surgeon to position an electrode or cannula into a specific part of the brain.

FIGURE 5.5

Stereotaxic Apparatus.   This apparatus is used for performing brain surgery on rats.

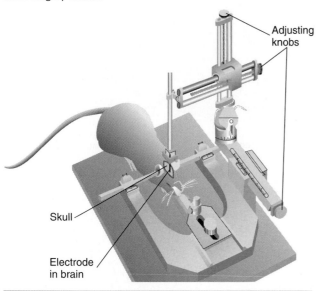

fornix), we would have to drill a hole through the skull immediately above it. (See *Figure 5.4.*) Each page of the stereotaxic atlas is labeled according to the distance of the section anterior or posterior to bregma. The grid on each page indicates distances of brain structures ventral to the top of the skull and lateral to the midline. To place the tip of a wire in the fornix, we would drill a hole above the target and then lower the electrode through the hole until the tip was at the correct depth, relative to the skull height at bregma. (Compare *Figures 5.3* and *5.4.*) Thus, by finding a neural structure (which we cannot see in our animal) on one of the pages of a stereotaxic atlas, we can determine the structure's location relative to bregma (which we can see). Note that because of variations in different strains and ages of animals, the atlas gives only an approximate location. We always have to try out a new set of coordinates, slice and stain the animal's brain, see the actual location of the lesion, correct the numbers, and try again. (Slicing and staining of brains are described later.)

The Stereotaxic Apparatus

A **stereotaxic apparatus** operates on simple principles. The device includes a head holder, which maintains the animal's skull in the proper orientation, a holder for the electrode, and a calibrated mechanism that moves the electrode holder in measured distances along the three axes: anterior–posterior, dorsal–ventral, and lateral–medial. Figure 5.5 illustrates a stereotaxic apparatus designed for small animals; various head holders can be used to outfit this device for such diverse species as rats, mice, hamsters, pigeons, and turtles. (See *Figure 5.5.*)

Once we obtain the coordinates from a stereotaxic atlas, we anesthetize the animal, place it in the apparatus, and cut the scalp open. We locate bregma, dial in the appropriate numbers on the stereotaxic apparatus, drill a hole through the skull, and lower the device into the brain by the correct amount. Now the tip of the cannula or electrode is where we want it to be, and we are ready to produce the lesion.

Of course, stereotaxic surgery may be used for purposes other than lesion production. Wires placed in the brain may be used to stimulate neurons as well as destroy them, and drugs can be injected that stimulate neurons or block specific receptors. We can attach cannulas or wires permanently by following a procedure that will be described later in this chapter. In all cases, once surgery is complete, the wound is sewn together, and the animal is taken out of the stereotaxic apparatus and allowed to recover from the anesthetic.

Stereotaxic apparatuses are also made for humans, by the way. Sometimes a neurosurgeon produces subcortical lesions—for example, to reduce the symptoms of Parkinson's disease. Usually, the surgeon uses multiple landmarks and verifies the location of the wire (or other device) inserted into the brain by taking brain scans or recording the activity of the neurons in that region before producing a brain lesion. (See *Figure 5.6.*)

Histological Methods

After producing a brain lesion and observing its effects on an animal's behavior, we must slice and stain the brain so that we can observe it under a microscope and see the location of the lesion. Brain lesions often miss the mark, so we have to verify the precise location of the brain damage after testing the animal behaviorally. To do so, we must fix, slice, stain, and examine the brain. Together, these procedures are referred to as *histological methods*. (The prefix *histo-* refers to body tissue.)

Fixation and Sectioning

If we hope to study the tissue in the form it had at the time of the organism's death, we must destroy the autolytic enzymes (*autolytic* means "self-dissolving"), which will otherwise turn the tissue into mush. The tissue must also be preserved to prevent its decomposition by bacteria or molds. To achieve both of these objectives, we place the neural tissue in a **fixative**. The most commonly used fixative is **formalin**, an aqueous solution of formaldehyde, a gas. Formalin halts autolysis, hardens the very soft and fragile brain, and kills any microorganisms that might destroy it.

Once the brain has been fixed, we must slice it into thin sections and stain various cellular structures to see anatomical details. Slicing is done with a **microtome** (literally, "that which slices small"). (See *Figure 5.7*.) Slices prepared for examination under a light microscope are typically 10 to 80 μm in thickness; those prepared for the electron microscope are generally cut at less than 1 μm. (A μm, or *micrometer*, is one-millionth of a meter, or one-thousandth of a millimeter.) For some reason, slices of brain tissue are usually referred to as *sections*.

After the tissue is cut, we attach the slices to glass microscope slides. We can then stain the tissue by putting the entire slide into various chemical solutions. Finally, we cover the stained sections with a small amount of a transparent liquid known as a *mounting medium* and place a very thin glass coverslip over the sections. The mounting medium keeps the coverslip in position. *MyPsychKit 5.1, Histological Methods* , shows these procedures.

Staining

If you looked at an unstained section of brain tissue under a microscope, you would be able to see the outlines of some large cellular masses and the more prominent fiber bundles. However, no fine details would be revealed. For this reason the study of microscopic neuroanatomy requires special histological stains. Researchers have developed many different stains to identify specific substances within and outside of cells. For verifying the location of a brain lesion, we will use one of the simplest: a cell-body stain.

In the late nineteenth century, Franz Nissl, a German neurologist, discovered that a dye known as methylene blue would stain the cell bodies of brain tissue. The material that takes up the dye, known as the *Nissl substance*, consists of RNA, DNA, and associated proteins located in the nucleus and scattered, in the form of granules, in the cytoplasm. Many dyes besides methylene blue can be used to stain cell bodies found in slices of the brain, but the most frequently used is cresyl violet. Incidentally, the dyes were not developed specifically for histological purposes but were originally formulated for use in dyeing cloth.

FIGURE 5.6

Stereotaxic Surgery on a Human Patient

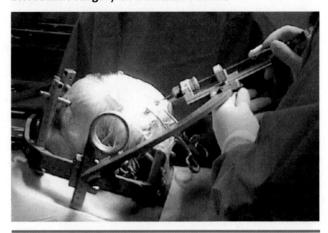

Photograph courtesy of John W. Snell, University of Virginia Health System.

fixative A chemical such as formalin; used to prepare and preserve body tissue.

formalin (*for ma lin*) The aqueous solution of formaldehyde gas; the most commonly used tissue fixative.

microtome (*my krow tome*) An instrument that produces very thin slices of body tissues.

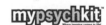

Animation 5.1
Histological Methods

FIGURE 5.7

A Microtome

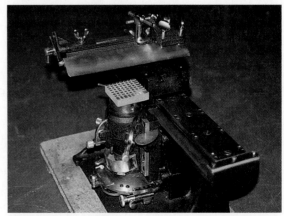

FIGURE 5.8

Cell-Body Stain. The photomicrograph shows a frontal section through a cat brain, stained with cresyl violet, a cell-body stain. The arrowheads point to *nuclei*, or groups of cell bodies.

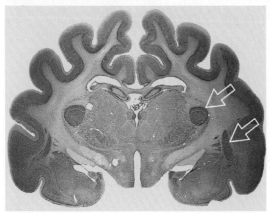

Histological material courtesy of Mary Carlson.

scanning electron microscope A microscope that provides three-dimensional information about the shape of the surface of a small object.

FIGURE 5.9

Electron Photomicrograph. The electron photomicrograph shows a section through an axodendritic synapse. Two synaptic regions are pointed out by arrows, and a circle indicates a region of pinocytosis in an adjacent terminal button, presumably representing recycling of vesicular membrane. T = terminal button; f = microfilaments; M = mitochondrion.

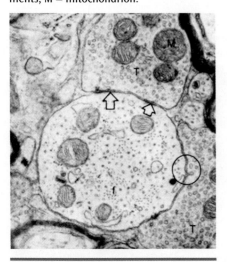

From Rockel, A. J., and Jones, E. G. *Journal of Comparative Neurology*, 1973, *147*, 61–92. Reprinted with permission.

The discovery of cell-body stains made it possible to identify nuclear masses in the brain. Figure 5.8 shows a frontal section of a cat brain stained with cresyl violet. Note that you can observe fiber bundles by their lighter appearance; they do not take up the stain. (See *Figure 5.8.*) The stain is not selective for *neural* cell bodies; all cells are stained, neurons and glia alike. It is up to the investigator to determine which is which—by size, shape, and location.

Electron Microscopy

The light microscope is limited in its ability to resolve extremely small details. Because of the nature of light itself, magnification of more than approximately 1500 times does not add any detail. To see such small anatomical structures as synaptic vesicles and details of cell organelles, investigators must use an electron microscope. A beam of electrons is passed through the tissue to be examined. A shadow of the tissue is then cast onto a sheet of photographic film, which is exposed by the electrons. Electron photomicrographs produced in this way can provide information about structural details on the order of a few tens of nanometers. (See *Figure 5.9.*)

A **scanning electron microscope** provides less magnification than a standard transmission electron microscope, which transmits the electron beam through the tissue. However, it shows objects in three dimensions. The microscope scans the tissue with a moving beam of electrons. The information received from the reflection of the beam is used to produce a remarkably detailed three-dimensional view. The scanning electron micrograph of a cut section of a nerve that you saw in Chapter 2 illustrates the detail that can be revealed by this method. (Refer to *Figure 2.3.*)

Tracing Neural Connections

Let's suppose that we were interested in discovering the neural mechanisms responsible for reproductive behavior. To start out, we wanted to study the physiology of sexual behavior of female rats. On the basis of some hints we received by reading reports of experiments by other researchers published in scientific journals, we performed stereotaxic surgery on two groups of female rats. We made a lesion in the ventromedial nucleus of the hypothalamus (VMH) of the rats in the experimental group and performed sham surgery on the rats in the control group. After a few days' recovery we placed each animal with a male rat. We found that the females in the control group responded positively to the males' attention; they engaged in courting behavior followed by copulation. However, the females with the VMH lesions rejected the males' attention and refused to copulate with them. We confirmed with histology that the VMH was indeed destroyed in the brains of the experimental animals. (One experimental rat did copulate, but we discovered later that the lesion had missed the VMH in that animal, so we discarded the data from that subject.)

The results of our experiment indicate that neurons in the VMH appear to play a role in functions required for copulatory behavior in females. (By the way, it turns out that these lesions do not affect copulatory behavior in males.) So where do we go from here? What is the next step? In fact, there are many questions that we could pursue. One question concerns the system of brain structures that participate in female copulatory behavior. Certainly, the VMH does not stand alone; it receives inputs from other structures and sends outputs to still others. Copulation requires the integration of visual, tactile, and olfactory information and the organization of patterns of movements in response to those of the partner. In addition, the entire network must be activated by the appropriate sex hormones. What is the precise role of the VMH in this complicated system?

Before we can hope to answer this question, we must know more about the connections of the VMH with the rest of the brain. What structures send their axons to the VMH, and to what structures does the VMH, in turn, send its axons? Once we know what the connections are, we can investigate the role of these structures and the nature of their interactions. (See *Figure 5.10.*)

How do we investigate the connections of the VMH? The question cannot be answered by means of histological procedures that stain all neurons, such as cell-body stains. If we look closely at a brain that has been prepared by these means, we see only a tangled mass of neurons, but in recent years researchers have developed very precise methods that make specific neurons stand out from all of the others.

Tracing Efferent Axons

Because neurons in the VMH are not directly connected to muscles, they cannot affect behavior directly. Neurons in the VMH must send axons to parts of the brain that contain neurons that are responsible for muscular movements. The pathway is probably not direct; more likely, neurons in the VMH affect neurons in other structures, which influence those in yet other structures until, eventually, the appropriate motor neurons are stimulated. To discover this system, we want to be able to identify the paths followed by axons leaving the VMH. In other words, we want to trace the *efferent axons* of this structure.

We will use an **anterograde labeling method** to trace these axons. (*Anterograde* means "moving forward.") Anterograde labeling methods employ chemicals that are taken up by dendrites or cell bodies and are then transported through the axons toward the terminal buttons.

Over the years, neuroscientists have developed several different methods for tracing the pathways followed by efferent axons. For example, to discover the destination of the efferent axons of neurons located within the VMH, we inject a minute quantity of **PHA-L** (a protein found in kidney beans) into that nucleus. (We would use a stereotaxic apparatus to do so, of course.) The molecules of PHA-L are taken up by dendrites and are transported through the soma to the axon, where they travel by means of fast axoplasmic transport to the terminal buttons. Within a few days the cells are filled in their entirety with molecules of PHA-L: dendrites, soma, axons and all their branches, and terminal buttons. Then we kill the animal, slice the brain, and mount the sections on microscope slides. A special *immunocytochemical* method is used to make the molecules of PHA-L visible, and the slides are examined under a microscope. (See *Figure 5.11.*)

Immunocytochemical methods take advantage of the immune reaction. The body's immune system has the ability to produce antibodies in response to antigens. *Antigens* are proteins (or peptides), such as those found on the surface of bacteria or viruses. *Antibodies*, which are also proteins, are produced by white blood cells to destroy invading microorganisms. Antibodies either are secreted by white blood cells or are located on their surface, in the way neurotransmitter receptors are located on the surface of neurons. When the antigens that are present on the surface of an invading microorganism come into contact with the antibodies that recognize them, the antibodies trigger an attack on the invader by the white blood cells.

Molecular biologists have developed methods for producing antibodies to any peptide or protein. The antibody molecules are attached to various types of dye molecules. Some of these dyes react with other chemicals and stain the tissue a brown color. Others are fluorescent; they glow when they are exposed to light of a

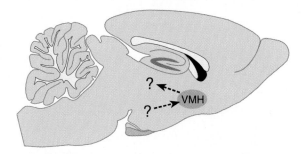

FIGURE 5.10

Tracing Neural Connections.   Once we know that a particular brain region is involved in a particular function, we may ask what structures provide inputs to the region and what structures receive outputs from it.

anterograde labeling method (*ann ter oh grade*) A histological method that labels the axons and terminal buttons of neurons whose cell bodies are located in a particular region.

PHA-L Phaseolus vulgaris leukoagglutinin; a protein derived from kidney beans and used as an anterograde tracer; taken up by dendrites and cell bodies and carried to the ends of the axons.

immunocytochemical method A histological method that uses radioactive antibodies or antibodies bound with a dye molecule to indicate the presence of particular proteins or peptides.

FIGURE 5.11

Tracing Efferent Axons.   The diagram illustrates the use of PHA-L to trace efferent axons.

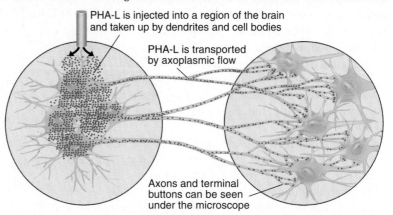

PHA-L is injected into a region of the brain and taken up by dendrites and cell bodies

PHA-L is transported by axoplasmic flow

Axons and terminal buttons can be seen under the microscope

particular wavelength. To determine where the peptide or protein (the antigen) is located in the brain, the investigator places fresh slices of brain tissue in a solution that contains the antibody/dye molecules. The antibodies attach themselves to their antigen. When the investigator examines the slices with a microscope (under light of a particular wavelength in the case of fluorescent dyes), he or she can see which parts of the brain—even which individual neurons—contain the antigen.

Figure 5.12 shows how PHA-L can be used to identify the efferents of a particular region of the brain. Molecules of this chemical were injected into the VMH. Two days later, after the PHA-L had been taken up by the neurons in this region and transported to the ends of their axons, the animal was killed. Slices of the brain were treated with an antibody to PHA-L, attached to a dye that stains the tissue a reddish brown color. Figure 5.12 shows a photomicrograph of the periaqueductal gray matter (PAG). As you can see, this region contains some labeled axons and terminal buttons (gold color), which proves that some of the efferent axons of the VMH terminate in the PAG. (See *Figure 5.12*.)

To continue our study of the role of the VMH in female sexual behavior, we would find the structures that receive information from neurons in the VMH (such as the PAG) and see what happens when each of them is destroyed. Let's suppose that damage to some of these structures also impairs female sexual behavior. We will inject these structures with PHA-L and see where *their* axons go. Eventually, we will discover the relevant pathways from the VMH to the motor neurons whose activity is necessary for copulatory behavior. (In fact, researchers have done so, and some of their results are presented in Chapter 9.)

retrograde labeling method   A histological method that labels cell bodies that give rise to the terminal buttons that form synapses with cells in a particular region.

fluorogold (*flew roh gold*)   A dye that serves as a retrograde label; taken up by terminal buttons and carried back to the cell bodies.

FIGURE 5.12

Anterograde Labeling.   PHA-L was injected into the ventromedial nucleus of the hypothalamus (VMH), where it was taken up by dendrites and carried through the cells' axons to their terminal buttons. Labeled axons and terminal buttons are seen in the periaqueductal gray matter (PAG).

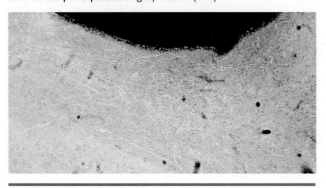

Courtesy of Kirsten Nielsen Ricciardi and Jeffrey Blaustein, University of Massachusetts.

Tracing Afferent Axons

Tracing efferent axons from the VMH will tell us only part of the story about the neural circuitry involved in female sexual behavior: the part between the VMH and the motor neurons. What about the circuits *before* the VMH? Is the VMH somehow involved in the analysis of sensory information (such as the sight, odor, or touch of the male)? Or perhaps the activating effect of a female's sex hormones on her behavior act through the VMH or through neurons whose axons form synapses there. To discover the parts of the brain that are involved in the "upstream" components of the neural circuitry, we need to find the inputs of the VMH—its afferent connections. To do so, we will employ a **retrograde labeling method**.

Retrograde means "moving backward." Retrograde labeling methods employ chemicals that are taken up by terminal buttons and carried back through the axons toward the cell bodies. The method for identifying the afferent inputs to a particular region of the brain is similar to the method used for identifying its efferents. First, we inject a small quantity of a chemical called **fluorogold** into the VMH. The chemical is taken up by terminal buttons and is transported back by means of retrograde axoplasmic transport to the cell bodies. A few days later we kill the animal, slice its brain, and examine the tissue under light of the appropriate wavelength. The molecules of fluorogold fluoresce under this light. We discover that the medial amygdala is one of the regions that provides input to the VMH. (See *Figure 5.13*.)

The anterograde and retrograde labeling methods that I have described identify a single link in a chain of neurons—neurons whose axons enter or leave a particular brain region. **Transneuronal tracing methods** identify a series of neurons that form serial synaptic connections with each other. The most effective transneuronal tracing method uses various strains of weakened rabies viruses or herpes viruses. The virus is injected directly into a brain region, is taken up by neurons there, and infects them. The virus spreads throughout the infected neurons and is eventually released, passing on the infection to other neurons that form synaptic connections with them. Depending on the type and strain of the virus, the infection is preferentially transmitted in an anterograde or a retrograde direction. After the animal is killed and the brain is sliced, immunocytochemical methods are used to localize a protein produced by the virus.

Together, anterograde and retrograde labeling methods— including transneuronal methods—enable us to discover circuits of interconnected neurons. Thus, these methods help to provide us with a "wiring diagram" of the brain. (See *Figure 5.14*.) Armed with other research methods (including some to be described later in this chapter), we can try to discover the functions of each component of this circuit.

Studying the Structure of the Living Human Brain

There are many good reasons to investigate the functions of brains of animals other than humans. For one thing, we can compare the results of studies made with different species in order to make some inferences about the evolution of various neural systems. Even if our primary interest is in the functions of the human brain, we certainly cannot ask people to submit to brain surgery for the purposes of research. But diseases and accidents do occasionally damage the human brain, and if we know where the damage occurs, we can study the people's behavior and try to make the same sorts of inferences we make with deliberately produced brain lesions in laboratory animals. The problem is, where is the lesion?

In past years a researcher might study the behavior of a person with brain damage and never find out exactly where the lesion was located. The only way to be sure was to obtain the

FIGURE 5.13

Retrograde Tracing.   Fluorogold was injected in the VMH, where it was taken up by terminal buttons and transported back through the axons to their cell bodies. The photograph shows these cell bodies, located in the medial amygdala.

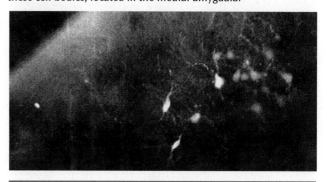

Courtesy of Yvon Delville, University of Massachusetts Medical School.

transneuronal tracing method A tracing method that identifies a series of neurons that form serial synaptic connections with each other, either in an anterograde or retrograde direction; involves infection of specific neurons with weakened forms of rabies or herpes viruses.

FIGURE 5.14

Results of Tracing Methods.   One of the inputs to the VMH and one of the outputs are revealed by anterograde and retrograde labeling methods.

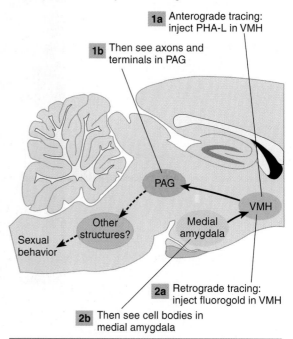

1a Anterograde tracing: inject PHA-L in VMH

1b Then see axons and terminals in PAG

PAG

Other structures?

Sexual behavior

Medial amygdala

VMH

2a Retrograde tracing: inject fluorogold in VMH

2b Then see cell bodies in medial amygdala

FIGURE 5.15

Computerized Tomography (CT) Scanner

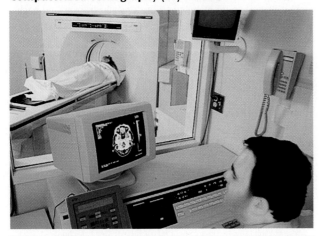

computerized tomography (CT) The use of a device that employs a computer to analyze data obtained by a scanning beam of X-rays to produce a two-dimensional picture of a "slice" through the body.

patient's brain when he or she died and examine slices of it under a microscope, but it was often impossible to do so. Sometimes the patient outlived the researcher. Sometimes the patient moved out of town. Sometimes (often, perhaps) the family refused permission for an autopsy. Because of these practical problems, study of the behavioral effects of damage to specific parts of the human brain made rather slow progress.

Recent advances in X-ray techniques and computers have led to the development of several methods for studying the anatomy of the living brain. These advances permit researchers to study the location and extent of brain damage while the patient is still living. The first method that was developed is called **computerized tomography (CT)** (from the Greek for *tomos*, "cut," and *graphein*, "to write"). This procedure, usually referred to as a *CT scan*, works as follows: The patient's head is placed in a large doughnut-shaped ring. The ring contains an X-ray tube and, directly opposite it (on the other side of the patient's head), an X-ray detector. The X-ray beam passes through the patient's head, and the detector measures the amount of radioactivity that gets through it. The beam scans the head from all angles, and a computer translates the numbers it receives from the detector into pictures of the skull and its contents. (See *Figure 5.15*.)

Figure 5.16 shows a series of these CT scans taken through the head of a patient who sustained a stroke. The stroke damaged a part of the brain involved in bodily awareness and perception of space. The patient lost her awareness of the left side of

FIGURE 5.16

CT Scans of a Lesion. The patient had a lesion in the right occipital-parietal area (scan 5). The lesion appears white because it was accompanied by bleeding; blood absorbs more radiation than does the surrounding brain tissue. Rostral is up, caudal is down; left and right are reversed. Scan 1 shows a section through the eyes and the base of the brain.

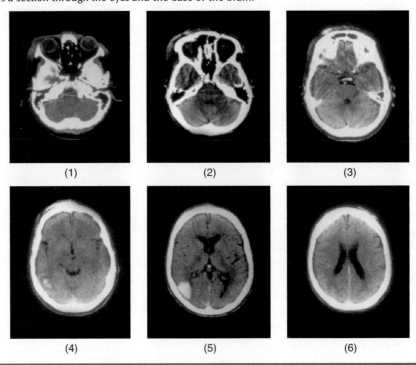

(1) (2) (3)

(4) (5) (6)

Courtesy of J. McA. Jones, Good Samaritan Hospital, Portland, Oregon.

her body and of items located on her left. You can see the damage as a white spot in the lower left corner of scan 5. (See *Figure 5.16.*)

An even more detailed, high-resolution picture of what is inside a person's head is provided by a process called **magnetic resonance imaging (MRI)**. The MRI scanner resembles a CT scanner, but it does not use X-rays. Instead, it passes an extremely strong magnetic field through the patient's head. When a person's body is placed in a strong magnetic field, the nuclei of some atoms in molecules in the body spin with a particular orientation. If a radio frequency wave is then passed through the body, these nuclei emit radio waves of their own. Different molecules emit energy at different frequencies. The MRI scanner is tuned to detect the radiation from hydrogen atoms. Because these atoms are present in different concentrations in different tissues, the scanner can use the information to prepare pictures of slices of the brain. Unlike CT scans, which are generally limited to the horizontal plane, MRI scans can be taken in the sagittal or frontal planes as well. (See *Figure 5.17.*)

As you can see in Figure 5.17, MRI scans distinguish between regions of gray matter and white matter, so major fiber bundles (such as the corpus callosum) can be seen. However, small fiber bundles are not visible on these scans. A special modification of the MRI scanner permits the visualization of even small bundles of fibers and the tracing of fiber tracts. Above absolute zero, all molecules move in random directions because of thermal agitation: the higher the temperature, the faster the random movement. **Diffusion tensor imaging (DTI)** takes advantage of the fact that the movement of water molecules in bundles of white matter will not be random, but will tend to be in a direction parallel to the axons that make up the bundles. The MRI scanner uses information about the movement of the water molecules to determine the location and orientation of bundles of axons in white matter. Figure 5.18 shows a sagittal view of some of the axons that project from the thalamus to the cerebral cortex in the human brain, as revealed by diffusion-tensor imaging. The computer adds colors to distinguish different bundles of axons. (See *Figure 5.18.*)

magnetic resonance imaging (MRI) A technique whereby the interior of the body can be accurately imaged; involves the interaction between radio waves and a strong magnetic field.

diffusion tensor imaging (DTI) An imaging method that uses a modified MRI scanner to reveal bundles of myelinated axons in the living human brain.

FIGURE 5.17

Magnetic Resonance Imaging (MRI).   This figure shows a midsagittal MRI scan of a human brain.

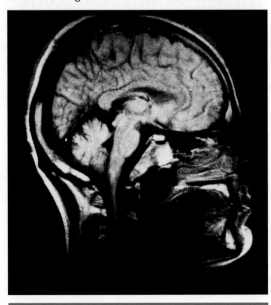

Photo courtesy of Philips Medical Systems.

FIGURE 5.18

Diffusion Tensor Imaging (DTI).   In this sagittal view, some of the axons that project from the thalamus to the cerebral cortex in the human brain are revealed by diffusion tensor imaging.

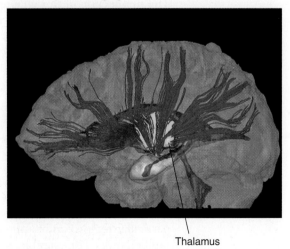

Thalamus

From Wakana, S., Jian, H., Nagae-Poetscher, L. M., van Zijl, P. C. M., and Mori, S. *Radiology*, 2004, *230*, 77–87. Reprinted with permission.

InterimSummary

Experimental Ablation

The goal of research in behavioral neuroscience is to understand the brain functions required for the performance of a particular behavior and then to learn the location of the neural circuits that perform these functions. The lesion method is the oldest one employed in such research, and it remains one of the most useful. A subcortical lesion is made under the guidance of a stereotaxic apparatus. The coordinates are obtained from a stereotaxic atlas, and the tip of an electrode or cannula is placed at the target. A lesion is made by passing radio frequency current through the electrode or infusing an excitatory amino acid through the cannula, producing an excitotoxic lesion. The advantage of excitotoxic lesions is that they destroy only neural cell bodies; axons passing through the region are not damaged.

The location of a lesion must be determined after observation of the animal's behavior. The animal is killed by humane means, and the brain is removed and placed in a fixative such as formalin. A microtome is used to slice the brain, which is usually frozen to make it hard enough to cut into thin sections. These sections are mounted on glass slides, stained with a cell-body stain, and examined under a microscope.

Light microscopes enable us to see cells and their larger organelles, but an electron microscope is needed to see small details, such as individual mitochondria and synaptic vesicles. Scanning electron microscopes provide a three-dimensional view of tissue, but at a lower magnification than transmission electron microscopes.

The next step in a research program often requires the investigator to discover the afferent and efferent connections of the region of interest with the rest of the brain. Efferent connections (those that carry information from the region in question to other parts of the brain) are revealed with anterograde tracing methods, such as the one that uses PHA-L. Afferent connections (those that bring information to the region in question from other parts of the brain) are revealed with retrograde tracing methods, such as the one that uses fluorogold. Chains of neurons that form synaptic connections are revealed by anterograde or retrograde transneuronal tracing methods, which utilized weakened forms of rabies and herpes viruses.

Although brain lesions are not deliberately made in the human brain for the purposes of research, diseases and accidents can cause brain damage, and if we know where the damage is located, we can study people's behavior and make inferences about the location of the neural circuits that perform relevant functions. If the patient dies and the brain is available for examination, ordinary histological methods can be used. Otherwise, the living brain can be examined with CT scanners and MRI scanners. Diffusion tensor imaging (DTI) uses a modified MRI scanner to visualize bundles of myelinated axons in the living human brain.

Table 5.1 summarizes the research methods presented in this section.

Recording and Stimulating Neural Activity

The first section of this chapter dealt with the anatomy of the brain and the effects of damage to particular regions. This section considers a different approach: studying the brain by recording or stimulating the activity of particular regions. Brain functions involve activity of circuits of neurons; thus, different perceptions and behavioral responses involve different patterns of activity in the brain. Researchers have devised methods to record these patterns of activity or to artificially produce them.

Recording Neural Activity

Axons produce action potentials, and terminal buttons elicit postsynaptic potentials in the membrane of the cells with which they form synapses. These electrical events can be recorded (as we saw in Chapter 2), and changes in the electrical activity of a particular region can be used to determine whether that region plays a role in various behaviors. For example, recordings can be made during stimulus presentations, decision making, or motor activities.

TABLE 5.1   Research Methods: Part I

Goal of Method	Method	Remarks
Destroy or inactivate specific brain region	Radio frequency lesion	Destroys all brain tissue near tip of electrode
	Excitotoxic lesion; uses excitatory amino acid such as kainic acid	Destroys only cell bodies near tip of cannula; spares axons passing through region
	Infusion of local anesthetic or muscimol (drug that stimulates GABA receptors)	Temporarily inactivates specific brain region; animal can serve as its own control
Place electrode or cannula in specific region within brain	Stereotaxic surgery	Consult stereotaxic atlas for coordinates
Find location of lesion	Fix brain; slice brain; stain sections	
Identify axons leaving a particular region and the terminal buttons of these axons	Anterograde tracing method, such as PHA-L	
Identify location of neurons whose axons terminate in a particular region	Retrograde tracing method, such as fluorogold	
Identify chain of neurons that are interconnected synaptically	Transneuronal tracing method; uses pseudorabies virus	Can be used for both anterograde and retrograde tracing
Find location of lesion in living human brain	Computerized tomography (CT scanner)	Slows "slice" of brain; uses X-rays
	Magnetic resonance imaging (MRI scanner)	Shows "slice" of brain; better detail than CT scan; uses a magnetic field and radio waves

Recordings can be made *chronically*, over an extended period of time after the animal recovers from surgery, or *acutely*, for a relatively short period of time during which the animal is kept anesthetized. Acute recordings, made while the animal is anesthetized, are usually restricted to studies of sensory pathways. Acute recordings seldom involve behavioral observations, since the behavioral capacity of an anesthetized animal is limited, to say the least.

If we want to record the activity of a particular region of the brain of an animal that is awake and free to move about, we would implant the electrodes by means of stereotaxic surgery. We would attach the electrodes to miniaturized electrical sockets and bond the sockets to the animal's skull, using plastics that were originally developed for the dental profession. Then, after recovery from surgery, the animal can be "plugged in" to the recording system. Laboratory animals pay no heed to the electrical sockets on their skulls and behave quite normally. (See *Figure 5.19.*)

FIGURE 5.19

Recording from a Rat's Brain.   This schematic shows a permanently attached set of electrodes, with a connecting socket cemented to the skull.

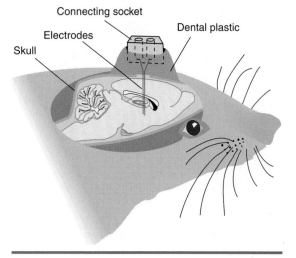

Recordings with Microelectrodes

Drugs that affect serotonergic and noradrenergic neurons also affect REM sleep. Suppose that, knowing this fact, we wondered whether the activity of serotonergic and noradrenergic neurons would vary during different stages of sleep. To find out, we would record the activity of these neurons with microelectrodes. **Microelectrodes** have a very fine tip, small enough to record the electrical activity of individual neurons. This technique is usually called **single-unit recording** (a unit refers to an individual neuron).

Because we want to record the activity of single neurons over a long period of time in unanesthetized animals, we want more durable electrodes. We can purchase arrays of very fine wires, gathered together in a bundle. The wires are insulated so that only their tips are bare.

Researchers often attach rather complex devices to the animals' skulls when they implant microelectrodes. These devices include screw mechanisms that permit the experimenter to move the electrode—or array of electrodes—deeper into the brain so that they can record from several different parts of the brain during the course of their observations.

The electrical signals detected by microelectrodes are quite small and must be amplified. Amplifiers used for this purpose work just like the amplifiers in a stereo system, converting the weak signals recorded at the brain into stronger ones. These signals can be displayed on an oscilloscope and stored in the memory of a computer for analysis at a later time.

What about the results of our recordings from serotonergic and noradrenergic neurons? As you will learn in Chapter 8, if we record the activity of these neurons during various stages of sleep, we will find that their firing rates fall almost to zero during REM sleep. This observation suggests that these neurons have an *inhibitory* effect on REM sleep. That is, REM sleep cannot occur until these neurons stop firing.

Recordings with Macroelectrodes

Sometimes, we want to record the activity of a region of the brain as a whole, not the activity of individual neurons located there. To do this, we would use macroelectrodes. **Macroelectrodes** do not detect the activity of individual neurons; rather, the records that are obtained with these devices represent the postsynaptic potentials of many thousands—or millions—of cells in the area of the electrode. These electrodes can consist of unsharpened wires inserted into the brain, screws attached to the skull, or even metal disks attached to the human scalp with a special paste that conducts electricity. Recordings taken from the scalp, especially, represent the activity of an enormous number of neurons, whose electrical signals pass through the meninges, skull, and scalp before reaching the electrodes.

Occasionally, neurosurgeons implant macroelectrodes directly into the human brain. The reason for doing so is to detect the source of abnormal electrical activity that is giving rise to frequent seizures. Once the source has been determined, the surgeon can open the skull and remove the source of the seizures—usually scar tissue caused by brain damage that occurred earlier in life. Usually, the electrical activity of a human brain is recorded through electrodes attached to the scalp and displayed on a *polygraph*.

A polygraph contains a mechanism that moves a very long strip of paper past a series of pens. These pens are essentially the pointers of large voltmeters, moving up and down in response to the electrical signal sent to them by the biologi-

microelectrode A very fine electrode, generally used to record activity of individual neurons.

single-unit recording Recording of the electrical activity of a single neuron.

macroelectrode An electrode used to record the electrical activity of large numbers of neurons in a particular region of the brain; much larger than a microelectrode.

electroencephalogram (EEG) An electrical brain potential recorded by placing electrodes on the scalp.

magnetoencephalography A procedure that detects groups of synchronously activated neurons by means of the magnetic field induced by their electrical activity; uses an array of superconducting quantum interference devices (SQUIDs).

cal amplifiers. Figure 5.20 illustrates a record of electrical activity recorded from macroelectrodes attached to various locations on a person's scalp. (See *Figure 5.20.*) Such records are called **electroencephalograms (EEGs)**, or "writings of electricity from the head." They can be used to diagnose epilepsy or study the stages of sleep and wakefulness, which are associated with characteristic patterns of electrical activity.

Another use of the EEG is to monitor the condition of the brain during surgical procedures that could potentially damage it, such as the one we encountered in the prologue to this chapter. The use of EEG monitoring during blood-vessel surgery is described in the epilogue to this chapter.

Magnetoencephalography

As you undoubtedly know, when electrical current flows through a conductor, it induces a magnetic field. This means that as action potentials pass down axons or as postsynaptic potentials pass down dendrites or sweep across the somatic membrane of a neuron, magnetic fields are also produced. These fields are exceedingly small, but engineers have developed superconducting detectors (called superconducting quantum interference devices, or SQUIDS) that can detect magnetic fields that are approximately one-billionth of the size of the earth's magnetic field. **Magnetoencephalography (MEG)** is performed with *neuromagnetometers*, devices that contain an array of several SQUIDs, oriented so that a computer can examine their output and calculate the source of particular signals in the brain. The neuromagnetometer shown in Figure 5.21 contains 275 SQUIDs. These devices can be used clinically; for example, to find the sources of seizures so that they can be removed surgically. They can also be used in experiments to measure regional brain activity that accompanies the perception of various stimuli or the performance of various behaviors or cognitive tasks. (See *Figure 5.21.*)

Recording the Brain's Metabolic and Synaptic Activity

Electrical signals are not the only signs of neural activity. If the neural activity of a particular region of the brain increases, the metabolic rate of this region increases, too, largely as a result of increased operation of transporters in the membrane of the cells. This increased metabolic rate can be measured. The experimenter injects radioactive **2-deoxyglucose (2-DG)** into the animal's bloodstream. Because this chemical resembles glucose (the principal food for the brain), it is taken into cells. Thus, the most active cells, which use glucose at the highest rate, will take up the highest concentrations of radioactive 2-DG—but unlike normal glucose, 2-DG cannot be metabolized, so it stays in the cell. The experimenter then kills the animal, removes the brain, slices it, and prepares it for *autoradiography.*

Autoradiography can be translated roughly as "writing with one's own radiation." Sections of the brain are mounted on microscope slides. The slides are then taken into a darkroom, where they are coated with a

---

FIGURE 5.20

A Record from a Polygraph

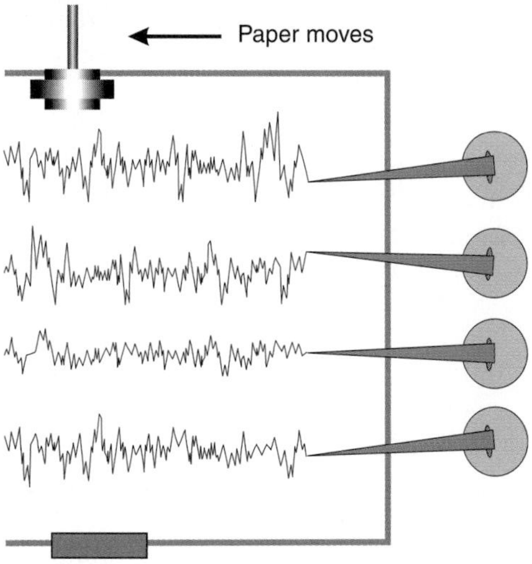

← Paper moves

2-deoxyglucose (2-DG) (*dee ox ee gloo kohss*) A sugar that enters cells along with glucose but is not metabolized.

autoradiography A procedure that locates radioactive substances in a slice of tissue; the radiation exposes a photographic emulsion or a piece of film that covers the tissue.

FIGURE 5.21

Magnetoencephalography. The neuromagnetometer is shown on the monitor to the left. The regions of increased electrical activity are shown on the monitor to the right, superimposed on an image of the brain derived from an MRI scan.

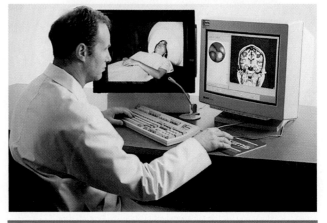

Courtesy of CTF Systems Inc.

photographic emulsion (the substance found on photographic film). Several weeks later, the slides, with their coatings of emulsion, are developed, just like photographic film. The molecules of radioactive 2-DG show themselves as spots of silver grains in the developed emulsion because the radioactivity exposes the emulsion, just as X-rays or light will do.

The most active regions of the brain contain the most radioactivity, showing this radioactivity in the form of dark spots in the developed emulsion. Figure 5.22 shows an autoradiograph of a slice of a rat brain; the dark spots at the bottom (indicated by the arrow) are nuclei of the hypothalamus with an especially high metabolic rate. Chapter 8 describes these nuclei and their function. (See *Figure 5.22*.) *MyPsychKit 5.2, Autoradiography*, shows this procedure.

Another method of identifying active regions of the brain capitalizes on the fact that when neurons are activated (for example, by the terminal buttons that form synapses with them), particular genes in the nucleus called *immediate early genes* are turned on and particular proteins are produced. These proteins then bind with the chromosomes in the nucleus. The presence of these proteins indicates that the neuron has just been activated.

One of the nuclear proteins produced during neural activation is called **Fos**. You will remember that earlier in this chapter we began an imaginary research project on the neural circuitry involved in the sexual behavior of female rats. Suppose we want to use the Fos method in this project to see what neurons are activated during a female rat's sexual activity. We place female rats with males and permit the animals to copulate. Then we remove the rats' brains, slice them, and follow a procedure that stains Fos protein. Figure 5.23 shows the results: Neurons in the medial amygdala of a female rat that has just mated show the presence of dark spots, indicating the presence of Fos protein. Thus, these neurons appear to be activated by copulatory activity—perhaps by the physical stimulation of the genitals that occurs then. As you will recall, when we injected a retrograde tracer (fluorogold) into the VMH, we found that this region receives input from the medial amygdala. (See *Figure 5.23*.)

Animation 5.2
Autoradiography

Fos (*fahs*) A protein produced in the nucleus of a neuron in response to synaptic stimulation.

FIGURE 5.22

2-DG Autoradiography.   This 2-DG autoradiogram of a rat brain (frontal section, dorsal is at top) shows especially high regions of activity in the pair of nuclei in the hypothalamus, at the base of the brain.

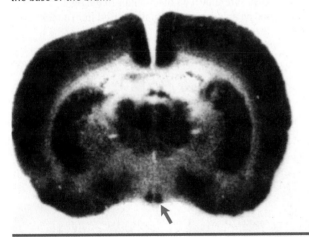

From Schwartz, W. J., and Gainer, H. *Science*, 1977, *197*, 1089–1091. Copyright © American Association for the Advancement of Sciences. Reprinted with permission.

FIGURE 5.23

Localization of Fos Protein.   The photomicrograph shows a frontal section of the brain of a female rat, taken through the medial amygdala. The dark spots indicate the presence of Fos protein, localized by means of immunocytochemistry. The synthesis of Fos protein was stimulated by permitting the animal to engage in copulatory behavior.

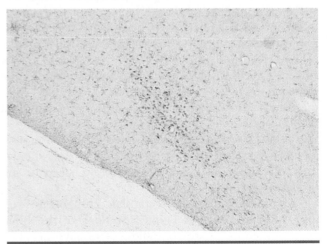

Courtesy of Marc Tetel, Wellesley College.

The metabolic activity of specific brain regions can be measured in human brains, too, by means of **functional imaging**—a computerized method of detecting metabolic or chemical changes within the brain. The first functional imaging method to be developed was **positron emission tomography (PET)**. First, the patient receives an injection of radioactive 2-DG. (Eventually, the chemical is broken down and leaves the cells. The dose given to humans is harmless.) The person's head is placed in a machine similar to a CT scanner. When the radioactive molecules of 2-DG decay, they emit subatomic particles called positrons, which are detected by the scanner. The computer determines which regions of the brain have taken up the radioactive substance, and it produces a picture of a slice of the brain, showing the activity level of various regions in that slice. (See *Figure 5.24*.)

One of the disadvantages of PET scanners is their operating cost. For reasons of safety the radioactive chemicals that are administered have very short half-lives; that is, they decay and lose their radioactivity very quickly. For example, the half-life of radioactive 2-DG is 110 minutes; the half-life of radioactive water (also used for PET scans) is only 2 minutes. Because these chemicals decay so quickly, they must be produced on site, in an atomic particle accelerator called a *cyclotron*. Therefore, to the cost of the PET scanner must be added the cost of the cyclotron and the salaries of the personnel who operate it.

The functional brain imaging method with the best spatial and temporal resolution is known as **functional MRI (fMRI)**. Engineers have devised modifications to existing MRI scanners and their software that permit the devices to acquire images that indicate regional metabolism. Brain activity is measured indirectly, by detecting levels of oxygen in the brain's blood vessels. Increased activity of a brain region stimulates blood flow to that region, which increases the local blood oxygen level. The formal name of this type of imaging is *BOLD*: blood oxygen level-dependent signal. Functional MRI scans have a higher resolution than PET scans, and they can be acquired much faster. Thus, they reveal more detailed information about the activity of particular brain regions. You will read about many functional imaging studies that employ fMRI scans in subsequent chapters of this book. (See *Figure 5.25*.)

Stimulating Neural Activity

So far, this section has been concerned with research methods that measure the activity of specific regions of the brain, but sometimes we may want to artificially change the activity of these regions to see what effects these changes have on the animal's behavior. For example, female rats will copulate with males only if certain female sex hormones are present. If we remove the rats' ovaries, the loss of these hormones will abolish their sexual behavior. We found in our earlier studies that VMH lesions disrupt this behavior. Perhaps if we *activate* the VMH, we will make up for the lack of female sex hormones and the rats will copulate again.

Electrical and Chemical Stimulation

How do we activate neurons? We can do so by electrical or chemical stimulation. Electrical stimulation simply

functional imaging A computerized method of detecting metabolic or chemical changes in particular regions of the brain.

positron emission tomography (PET) A functional imaging method that reveals the localization of a radioactive tracer in a living brain.

functional MRI (fMRI) A functional imaging method; a modification of the MRI procedure that permits the measurement of regional metabolism in the brain.

FIGURE 5.24

PET Scans.   In the top row of these human brain scans are three horizontal scans from a person at rest. The bottom row shows three scans from the same person while he was clenching and unclenching his right fist. The scans show increased uptake of radioactive 2-deoxyglucose in regions of the brain that are devoted to the control of movement, which indicates increased metabolic rate in these areas. Different computer-generated colors indicate different rates of uptake of 2-DG, as shown in the scale at the bottom.

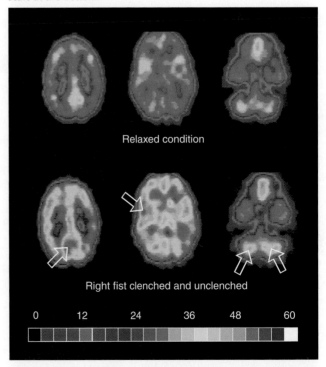

Courtesy of the Brookhaven National Laboratory and the State University of New York, Stony Brook.

FIGURE 5.25

Functional MRI Scans.   These scans of human brains show localized average increases in neural activity of males (left) and females (right) while they were judging whether pairs of written words rhymed.

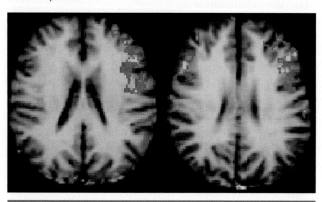

Reprinted by permission from Macmillan Publishers Ltd: *Nature*, Shaywitz, B. A., et al., Sex differences in the functional organization of the brain for language, *373*, 607–609, copyright 1995.

mypsychkit

Animation 5.3
Cannula Implantation

involves passing an electrical current through a wire inserted into the brain, as you saw in Figure 5.19. Chemical stimulation is usually accomplished by injecting a small amount of an excitatory amino acid, such as kainic acid or glutamic acid, into the brain. As you learned in Chapter 4, the principal excitatory neurotransmitter in the brain is glutamic acid (glutamate), and both of these chemicals stimulate glutamate receptors, thus activating the neurons on which these receptors are located.

Injections of chemicals into the brain can be done through an apparatus that is permanently attached to the skull so that the animal's behavior can be observed several times. We place a metal cannula (a guide cannula) in an animal's brain and cement its top to the skull. At a later date we place a smaller cannula of measured length inside the guide cannula and then inject a chemical into the brain. Because the animal is free to move about, we can observe the effects of the injection on its behavior. (See *Figure 5.26.*) *MyPsychKit 5.3, Cannula Implantation*, shows this surgical procedure.

The principal disadvantage of chemical stimulation is that it is slightly more complicated than electrical stimulation; chemical stimulation requires cannulas, tubes, special pumps or syringes, and sterile solutions of excitatory amino acids. However, it has a distinct advantage over electrical stimulation: It activates cell bodies but not axons. Because only cell bodies (and their dendrites, of course) contain glutamate receptors, we can be assured that an injection of an excitatory amino acid into a particular region of the brain excites the cells there, but not the axons of other neurons that happen to pass through the region. Thus, the effects of chemical stimulation are more localized than the effects of electrical stimulation.

FIGURE 5.26

Intracranial Cannula.   A guide cannula is permanently attached to the skull (a), and at a later time a thinner cannula can be inserted through the guide cannula into the brain (b). Chemicals can be infused into the brain through this device.

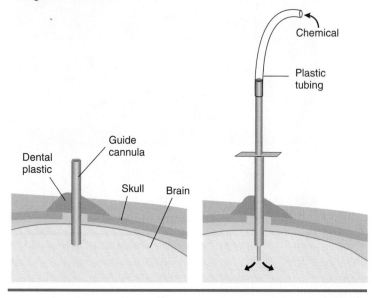

FIGURE 5.27

Transcranial Magnetic Stimulation (TMS).   Pulses of electricity through the coil produce a magnetic field that stimulates a region of the cerebral cortex under the crossing point in the middle of the figure 8.

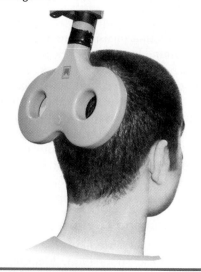

Photograph courtesy the Kastner Lab, Princeton University, Princeton, New Jersey.

You might have noticed that I just said that kainic acid, which I described earlier as a neurotoxin, can be used to stimulate neurons. These two uses are not really contradictory. Kainic acid produces excitotoxic lesions by stimulating neurons to death. Whereas large doses of a concentrated solution kill neurons, small doses of a dilute solution simply stimulate them.

What about the results of our imaginary experiment? In fact (as we shall see in Chapter 9), VMH stimulation *does* substitute for female sex hormones. Perhaps, then, the female sex hormones exert their effects in this nucleus. We will see how to test this hypothesis later in this chapter.

Transcranial Magnetic Stimulation

As we saw earlier in this chapter, neural activity induces magnetic fields that can be detected by means of magnetoencephalography. Similarly, magnetic fields can be used to stimulate neurons by inducing electrical currents in brain tissue. **Transcranial magnetic stimulation (TMS)** uses a coil of wires, usually arranged in the shape of the numeral 8, to stimulate neurons in the human cerebral cortex. The stimulating coil is placed on top of the skull so that the crossing point in the middle of the 8 is located immediately above the region to be stimulated. Pulses of electricity send magnetic fields that activate neurons in the cortex. Figure 5.27 shows an electromagnetic coil used in transcranial magnetic stimulation and its placement on a person's head. (See *Figure 5.27*.)

The effects of TMS are very similar to those of direct stimulation of the exposed brain. For example, as we shall see in Chapter 6, stimulation of a particular region of the visual association cortex will disrupt a person's ability to detect movements in visual stimuli. In addition, as we will see in Chapter 15, TMS has been used to treat the symptoms of mental disorders such as depression.

transcranial magnetic stimulation (TMS) Stimulation of the cerebral cortex by means of magnetic fields produced by passing pulses of electricity through a coil of wire placed next to the skull; interferes with the functions of the brain region that is stimulated.

Interim Summary

Recording and Stimulating Neural Activity

When circuits of neurons participate in their normal functions, their electrical activity and metabolic activity increase. Thus, by observing these processes as an animal perceives various stimuli or engages in various behaviors, we can make some inferences about the functions performed by various regions of the brain. Microelectrodes can be used to record the electrical activity of individual neurons. Chronic recordings require that the electrode be attached to an electrical socket, which is fastened to the skull with a plastic adhesive. Macroelectrodes record the activity of large groups of neurons. In rare cases macroelectrodes are placed in the depths of the human brain, but most often they are placed on the scalp and their activity is recorded on a polygraph or computer. Such records can be used in the diagnosis of epilepsy or the study of sleep.

Metabolic activity can be measured by giving an animal an injection of radioactive 2-DG, which accumulates in metabolically active neurons. The presence of the radioactivity is revealed through autoradiography: Slices of the brain are placed on microscope slides, covered with a photographic emulsion, left to sit a while, and then are developed like photographic negatives. When neurons are stimulated, they synthesize the nuclear protein Fos. The presence of Fos, revealed by a special staining method, provides another way to discover active regions of the brain. The metabolic activity of various regions of the living human brain can be revealed by the 2-DG method, but a PET scanner is used to detect the active regions. Other noninvasive methods of measuring regional brain activity are provided by functional MRI, which detects localized changes in oxygen levels, and magnetoencephalography (MEG), which detects magnetic fields produced by electrical activity of neurons.

Researchers can stimulate various regions of the brain by implanting a macroelectrode and applying mild electrical stimulation. Alternatively, they can implant a guide cannula in the brain; after the animal has recovered from the surgery, they insert a smaller cannula and inject a weak solution of an excitatory amino acid into the brain. The advantage of this procedure is that only neurons whose cell bodies are located nearby will be stimulated; axons passing through the region will not be affected. Transcranial magnetic stimulation induces electrical activity in the human cerebral cortex, which temporarily disrupts the functioning of neural circuits located there.

Table 5.2 summarizes the research methods presented in this section.

TABLE 5.2   Research Methods: Part II

Goal of Method	Method	Remarks
Record electrical activity of single neurons	Glass or metal microelectrodes	Metal microelectrodes can be implanted permanently to record neural activity as animal moves
Record electrical activity of regions of brain	Metal macroelectrodes	In humans, usually attached to the scalp with a special paste
Record magnetic fields induced by neural activity	Magnetoencephalography; uses a neuromagnetometer, which contains an array of SQUIDs	Can determine the location of a group of neurons firing synchronously
Record metabolic activity of regions of brain	2-DG autoradiography	Measures local glucose utilization
	Measurement of Fos protein	Identifies neurons that have recently been stimulated
	2-DG PET scan	Measures regional metabolic activity of human brain
	Functional magnetic resonance imaging (fMRI) scan	Measures regional metabolic activity of human brain; better spatial and temporal resolution than PET scan
Stimulate neural activity	Electrical stimulation	Stimulates neurons near the tip of the electrode and axons passing through region
	Chemical stimulation with excitatory amino acid	Stimulates only neurons near the tip of the cannula, not axons passing through region
	Transcranial magnetic stimulation	Stimulates neurons in the human cerebral cortex with an electromagnet placed on the head

Neurochemical Methods

Sometimes we are interested not in the general metabolic activity of particular regions of the brain, but in the location of neurons that possess particular types of receptors or produce particular types of neurotransmitters or neuromodulators. We might also want to measure the amount of these chemicals secreted by neurons in particular brain regions during particular circumstances.

Finding Neurons that Produce Particular Neurochemicals

Suppose we learn that a particular drug affects behavior. How would we go about discovering the neural circuits that are responsible for the drug's effects? To answer this question, let's take a specific example. Physicians discovered several years ago that farm workers who had been exposed to certain types of insecticides (the organophosphates) had particularly intense and bizarre dreams and even reported having hallucinations while awake. A plausible explanation for these symptoms is that the drug stimulates the neural circuits responsible for REM sleep—the phase of sleep during which dreaming occurs. (After all, dreams are hallucinations that we have while sleeping.)

The first question to ask relates to how the organophosphate insecticides work. Pharmacologists have the answer: These drugs are acetylcholinesterase inhibitors. As you learned in Chapter 4, acetylcholinesterase inhibitors are potent acetylcholine agonists. By inhibiting AChE, the drugs prevent the rapid destruction of ACh after it is released by terminal buttons and thus prolong the postsynaptic potentials at acetylcholinergic synapses.

Now that we understand the action of the insecticides, we know that these drugs act at acetylcholinergic synapses. What neurochemical methods should we use to discover the sites of action of the drugs in the brain? There are three possibilities: We could look for neurons that contain acetylcholine, we could look for the enzyme acetylcholinesterase (which must be present in the postsynaptic membranes of cells that receive synaptic input from acetylcholinergic neurons), or we could look for acetylcholine receptors. Let's see how these three methods work.

First, let's consider methods by which we can localize particular neurochemicals, such as neurotransmitters and neuromodulators. (In our case we are interested in acetylcholine.) There are two basic ways of localizing neurochemicals in the brain: localizing the chemicals themselves or the enzymes that produce them.

Peptides (or proteins) can be localized directly by means of immunocytochemical methods, which were described in the first section of this chapter. Slices of brain tissue are exposed to an antibody for the peptide, linked to a dye (usually, a fluorescent dye). The slices are then examined under a microscope using light of a particular wavelength. For example, Figure 5.28 shows the location of axons in the forebrain that contain vasopressin, a peptide neurotransmitter. Two sets of axons are shown. One set, which forms a cluster around the third ventricle at the base of the brain, shows up as a rusty color. The other set, scattered through the lateral septum, looks like strands of gold fibers. (As you can see, a properly stained brain section can be beautiful. See *Figure 5.28.*)

But we are interested in acetylcholine, which is not a peptide. Therefore, we cannot use immunocytochemical methods to find this neurotransmitter. However, we can use these methods to localize the enzyme that produces it. The synthesis of acetylcholine is made possible by the enzyme choline acetyltransferase (ChAT). Thus, neurons that contain this enzyme almost certainly secrete ACh. Figure 5.29 shows acetylcholinergic neurons in the pons that have been identified by means of immunocytochemistry; the brain tissue was exposed to an antibody to ChAT attached to a fluorescent dye. In fact, research using many of the methods described in this chapter indicate that these neurons play a role in controlling REM sleep. (See *Figure 5.29.*)

Localizing Particular Receptors

As we saw in Chapter 4, neurotransmitters, neuromodulators, and hormones convey their messages to their target cells by binding with receptors located on or in these cells. The location of these receptors can be determined by two different procedures.

The first procedure uses autoradiography. We expose slices of brain tissue to a solution containing a radioactive ligand for a particular receptor. Next, we rinse the slices so that the only radioactivity remaining in them is that of the molecules of the ligand bound to their receptors. Finally, we use autoradiographic methods to localize the radioactive ligand—and thus the receptors. Figure 5.30 shows an example of the results of this procedure. We see an autoradiogram of a slice of a rat's brain that was soaked in a solution that contained radioactive morphine, which bound with the brain's opiate receptors. (See *Figure 5.30.*)

FIGURE 5.28

Localization of a Peptide.   The peptide is revealed by means of immunocytochemistry. The photomicrograph shows a portion of a frontal section through the rat forebrain. The gold- and rust-colored fibers are axons and terminal buttons that contain vasopressin, a peptide neurotransmitter.

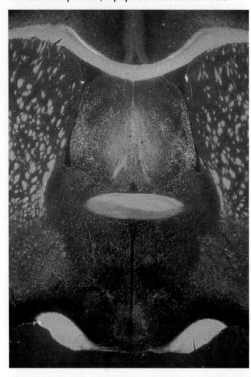

Courtesy of Geert DeVries, University of Massachusetts.

FIGURE 5.29

Localization of an Enzyme.   An enzyme responsible for the synthesis of a neurotransmitter is revealed by immunocytochemistry. The photomicrograph shows a section through the pons. The orange neurons contain choline acetyltransferase, which implies that they produce (and thus secrete) acetylcholine.

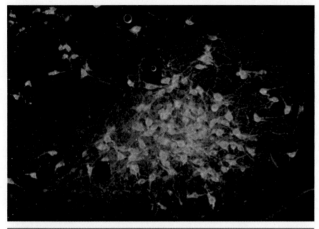

Courtesy of David A. Morilak and Roland Ciaranello, Nancy Pritzker Laboratory of Developmental and Molecular Neurobiology, Department of Psychiatry and Behavioral Sciences, Stanford University School of Medicine.

FIGURE 5.30

Autoradiogram.   This autoradiogram of a rat brain (horizontal section, rostral is at top); was incubated in a solution containing radioactive morphine, a ligand for opiate receptors. The receptors are indicated by white areas.

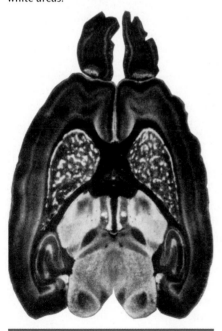

From Herkenham, M. A., and Pert, C. B. *Journal of Neuroscience*, 1982, *2*, 1129–1149. Reprinted with permission.

The second procedure uses immunocytochemistry. Receptors are proteins; therefore, we can produce antibodies against them. We expose slices of brain tissue to the appropriate antibody (labeled with a fluorescent dye) and look at the slices with a microscope under light of a particular wavelength.

Let's apply the method for localizing receptors to the first line of investigation we considered in this chapter: the role of the ventromedial hypothalamus (VMH) in the sexual behavior of female rats. As we saw, lesions of the VMH abolish this behavior. We also saw that the behavior does not occur if the rat's ovaries are removed but that it can be activated by stimulation of the VMH with electricity or an excitatory amino acid. These results suggest that the sex hormones produced by the ovaries act on neurons in the VMH.

This hypothesis suggests two experiments. First, we could use the procedure shown in Figure 5.26 to place a small amount of the appropriate sex hormone directly into the VMH of female rats whose ovaries we had previously removed. As we shall see in Chapter 9, this procedure works; the hormone *does* reactivate the animals' sexual behavior. The second experiment would use autoradiography to look for the receptors for the sex hormone. We would expose slices of rat brain to the radioactive hormone, rinse them, and perform autoradiography. If we did so, we would indeed find radioactivity in the VMH. (And if we compared slices from the brains of female and male rats, we would find evidence of more hormone receptors in the females' brains.) We could also use immunocytochemistry to localize the hormone receptors, and we would obtain the same results.

Measuring Chemicals Secreted in the Brain

The previous two subsections described methods that permit researchers to identify the location of chemicals within cells or in cell membranes, but sometimes we might want to measure the concentration of particular chemicals secreted in particular regions of the brain. For example, we know that cocaine—a particularly addictive drug—blocks the reuptake of dopamine, which suggests that the extracellular concentration of dopamine increases in some parts of the brain when a person takes cocaine. To measure the amount of dopamine in particular regions of an animal's brain, we would use a procedure called **microdialysis**.

Dialysis is a process in which substances are separated by means of an artificial membrane that is permeable to some molecules but not others. A microdialysis probe consists of a small metal tube that introduces a solution into a section of dialysis tubing—a piece of artificial membrane shaped in the form of a cylinder, sealed at the bottom. Another small metal tube leads the solution away after it has circulated through the pouch. A drawing of such a probe is shown in *Figure 5.31*.

We use stereotaxic surgery to place a microdialysis probe in a rat's brain so that the tip of the probe is located in the region we are interested in. We pump a small amount of a solution similar to extracellular fluid through one of the small metal tubes into the dialysis tubing. The fluid circulates through the dialysis tubing and passes through the second metal tube, from which it is taken for analysis. As the fluid passes through the dialysis tubing, it collects molecules from the extracellular fluid of the brain, which are pushed across the membrane by the force of diffusion.

We analyze the contents of the fluid that has passed through the dialysis tubing by an extremely sensitive analytical method. This method is so sensitive that it can detect neurotransmitters (and their breakdown products) that have been released by the terminal buttons and have escaped from the synaptic cleft into the rest of the extracellular fluid. We find that the amount of dopamine present in the extracellular fluid of the nucleus accumbens, located in the basal forebrain, *does* increase when we give a rat an injection of cocaine. In fact, we find that the amount of dopamine in this region increases when we administer any addictive drug, such as heroin, nicotine, or alcohol. We even see an increased dopamine secretion when the animal participates in a pleasurable activity such as eating when hungry, drinking when thirsty, or engaging in sexual activity. Such observations support the conclusion that the release of dopamine in the nucleus accumbens plays a role in reinforcement.

In a few special cases (for example, in monitoring brain chemicals of people with intracranial hemorrhages or head trauma), the microdialysis procedure has been applied to study of the human brain, but ethical reasons prevent us from doing so for research purposes. Fortunately, there is a noninvasive way to measure neurochemicals in the human brain. Although PET scanners are expensive machines, they are also versatile. They can be used to localize *any* radioactive substance that emits positrons.

As we saw in the prologue to Chapter 4, several years ago, several people injected themselves with an illicit drug that was contaminated with a chemical that destroyed their dopaminergic neurons. As a result they suffered from severe parkinsonism. Recently, neurosurgeons used stereotaxic procedures to transplant fetal dopaminergic neurons into the basal ganglia of some of these patients. **Figure 5.32**

microdialysis A procedure for analyzing chemicals present in the interstitial fluid through a small piece of tubing made of a semipermeable membrane that is implanted in the brain.

FIGURE 5.31

Microdialysis.   A dilute salt solution is slowly infused into the microdialysis tube, where it picks up molecules that diffuse in from the extracellular fluid. The contents of the fluid are then analyzed.

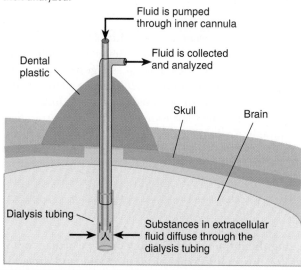

Adapted from Hernandez, L., Stanley, B. G., and Hoebel, B. G. *Life Sciences*, 1986, *39*, 2629–2637.

FIGURE 5.32

PET Scans of a Patient with Parkinsonian Symptoms.
The scans show uptake of radioactive L-DOPA in the basal ganglia of a patient with parkinsonian symptoms, which were induced by a toxic chemical, who later received a transplant of fetal dopaminergic neurons. (a) Preoperative scan. (b) Scan taken 13 months postoperatively. The increased uptake of L-DOPA indicates that the fetal transplant was secreting dopamine.

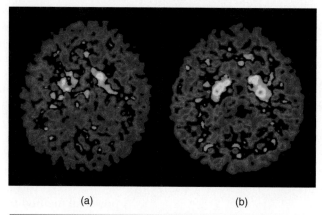

(a)   (b)

Adapted from Widner, H., Tetrud, J., Rehncrona, S., Snow, B., Brundin, P., Gustavii, B., Björklund, A., Lindvall, O., and Langston, J. W. *New England Journal of Medicine*, 1992, *327*, 1556–1563. Scans reprinted with permission.

shows PET scans of the brain of one of them. The patient was given an injection of radioactive L-DOPA 1 hour before each scan was made. As you learned in Chapter 4, L-DOPA is taken up by the terminals of dopaminergic neurons, where it is converted to dopamine; thus, the radioactivity shown in the scans indicates the presence of dopamine-secreting terminals in the basal ganglia. The scans show the amount of radioactivity before (part a) and after (part b) the patient received the transplant, which greatly diminished his symptoms. (See *Figure 5.32*.)

I wish I could say that the fetal transplantation procedure has cured people stricken with Parkinson's disease and those whose brains were damaged with the contaminated drug. Unfortunately, as we will see in Chapter 14, the therapeutic effects of the transplant are often temporary, and with time, serious side effects often emerge.

InterimSummary

Neurochemical Methods

Neurochemical methods can be used to determine the location of an enormous variety of substances in the brain. They can identify neurons that secrete a particular neurotransmitter or neuromodulator and those that possess receptors that respond to the presence of these substances. Peptides and proteins can be directly localized, through immunocytochemical methods; the tissue is exposed to an antibody that is linked to a molecule that fluoresces under light of a particular wavelength. Other substances can be detected by immunocytochemical localization of an enzyme that is required for their synthesis.

Receptors for neurochemicals can be localized by two means. The first method uses autoradiography to reveal the distribution of a radioactive ligand to which the tissue has been exposed. The second method uses immunocytochemistry to detect the presence of the receptors themselves, which are proteins.

The secretions of neurotransmitters and neuromodulators can be measured by implanting the tip of a microdialysis probe in a particular region of the brain. A PET scanner can be used to perform similar observations of the human brain. People are given an injection of a radioactive tracer such as a drug that binds with a particular receptor or a chemical that is incorporated into a particular neurotransmitter, and a PET scanner reveals the location of the tracer in the brain.

Table 5.3 summarizes the research methods presented in this section.

Genetic Methods

All behavior is determined by interactions between an individual's brain and his or her environment. Many behavioral characteristics—such as talents, personality variables, and mental disorders—seem to run in families. This fact suggests that genetic factors may play a role in the development of physiological differences that are ultimately responsible for these characteristics. In some cases the genetic link is very clear: A defective gene interferes with brain development, and a neurological abnormality causes behavioral deficits. In other cases the links between heredity and behavior are much more subtle, and special genetic methods must be used to reveal them.

Twin Studies

A powerful method for estimating the influence of heredity on a particular trait is to compare the *concordance rate* for this trait in pairs of monozygotic and dizygotic twins. Monozygotic twins (identical twins) have identical genotypes—that is, their chromosomes, and the genes they contain, are identical. In contrast, the genetic

TABLE 5.3   Research Methods: Part III

Goal of Method	Method	Remarks
Measure neurotransmitters and neuromodulators released by neurons	Microdialysis	A wide variety of substances can be analyzed
Measure neurochemicals in the living human brain	PET scan	Can localize any radioactive substance taken up in the human brain
Identify neurons producing a particular neurotransmitter or neuromodulator	Immunocytochemical localization of peptide or protein	Requires a specific antibody
	Immunocytochemical localization of enzyme responsible for synthesis of substance	Useful if substance is not a peptide or protein
Identify neurons that contain a particular type of receptor	Autoradiographic localization of radioactive ligand	
	Immunocytochemical localization of receptor	Requires a specific antibody
Genetic methods	Twin studies	Comparison of concordance rates of monozygotic and dizygotic twins estimates heritability of trait
	Adoption studies	Similarity of offspring and adoptive and biological parents estimates heritability of trait
	Targeted mutations	Inactivation, insertion, or increased expression of a gene
	Antisense oligonucleotides	Bind with messenger RNA; prevent synthesis of protein

similarity between dizygotic twins (fraternal twins) is, on the average, 50 percent. Investigators study records to identify pairs of twins in which at least one member has the trait; for example, a diagnosis of a particular mental disorder. If both twins have been diagnosed with this disorder, they are said to be *concordant.* If only one has received this diagnosis, the twins are said to be *discordant.* Thus, if a disorder has a genetic basis, the percentage of monozygotic twins who are concordant for the diagnosis will be higher than the percentage of dizygotic twins. For example, as we will see in Chapter 15, the concordance rate for schizophrenia in twins is at least four times higher for monozygotic twins than for dizygotic twins, a finding that provides strong evidence that schizophrenia is a heritable trait. Twin studies have found that many individual characteristics, including personality traits, prevalence of obesity, incidence of alcoholism, and a wide variety of mental disorders, are influenced by genetic factors.

Adoption Studies

Another method for estimating the heritability of a particular behavioral trait is to compare people who were adopted early in life with their biological and adoptive

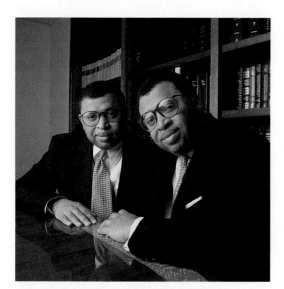

Twin studies provide a powerful method for estimating the relative roles of heredity and environment in the development of particular behavioral traits.

parents. All behavioral traits are affected to some degree by hereditary factors, environmental factors, and an interaction between hereditary and environmental factors. Environmental factors are both social and biological in nature. For example, the mother's health, nutrition, and drug-taking behavior during pregnancy are prenatal environmental factors, and the child's diet, medical care, and social environment (both inside and outside the home) are postnatal environmental factors. If a child is adopted soon after birth, the genetic factors will be associated with the biological parents, the prenatal environmental factors will be associated with the biological mother, and most of the postnatal environmental factors will be associated with the adoptive parents.

Adoption studies require that the investigator know the identity of the parents of the people being studied and be able to measure the behavioral trait in the biological and adoptive parents. If the people being studied strongly resemble their biological parents, we conclude that the trait is probably influenced by genetic factors. To be certain, we will have to rule out possible differences in the prenatal environment of the adopted children. If, instead, the people resemble their adoptive parents, we conclude that the trait is influenced by environmental factors. (It would take further study to determine just what these environmental factors might be.) Of course, it is possible that both hereditary and environmental factors play a role, in which case the people being studied will resemble both their biological and adoptive parents.

Targeted Mutations

A recently developed method has put a powerful tool in the hands of neuroscientists. **Targeted mutations** are mutated genes produced in the laboratory and inserted into the chromosomes of mice. These mutated genes (also called knockout genes) are defective: They fail to produce a functional protein. In many cases the target of the mutation is an enzyme that controls a particular chemical reaction. For example, we will see in Chapter 12 that lack of a particular enzyme interferes with learning. This result suggests that the enzyme is partly responsible for changes in the structure of synapses required for learning to occur. In other cases the target of the mutation is a protein that itself serves useful functions in the cell. For example, we will see in Chapter 16 that a particular type of cannabinoid receptor is involved in the reinforcing and analgesic effects of opiates. Researchers can even produce *conditional knockouts* that cause the animal's genes to stop expressing a particular gene when the animal is given a particular drug. This permits the targeted gene to express itself normally during the animal's development and then be knocked out at a later time.

Investigators can also use methods of genetic engineering to insert genes into the DNA of mice. These genes can cause increased production of proteins normally found in the host species, or they can produce entirely new proteins.

Antisense Oligonucleotides

Another genetic method involves the production of molecules that block the production of proteins encoded by particular genes by injecting **antisense oligonucleotides**. The most common type of antisense oligonucleotide are modified strands of RNA or DNA that will bind with specific molecules of messenger RNA and prevent them from producing their protein. Once the molecules of mRNA are trapped this way, they are destroyed by enzymes present in the cell. The term *antisense* refers to the fact that the synthetic oligonucleotides contain a sequence of bases complementary to those contained by a particular gene or molecule of mRNA.

targeted mutation A mutated gene (also called a "knockout gene") produced in the laboratory and inserted into the chromosomes of mice; fails to produce a functional protein.

antisense oligonucleotide (*oh li go new klee oh tide*) A modified strand of RNA or DNA that binds with a specific molecule of messenger RNA and prevents it from producing its particular protein.

InterimSummary

Genetic Methods

Because genes direct an organism's development, genetic methods are very useful in studies of the physiology of behavior. Twin studies compare the concordance rates of monozygotic (identical) and dizygotic (fraternal) twins for a particular trait. A higher concordance rate for monozygotic twins provides evidence that the trait is influenced by heredity. Adoption studies compare people who were adopted during infancy with their biological and adoptive parents. If the people resemble their biological parents, evidence is seen for genetic factors. If the people resemble their adoptive parents, evidence is seen for a role of factors in the family environment.

Targeted mutations permit neuroscientists to study the effects of a lack of a particular protein—for example, an enzyme, structural protein, or receptor—on an animal's physiological and behavioral characteristics. Genes that cause the production of foreign proteins or increase production of native proteins can be inserted into the genome of strains of animals. Antisense oligonucleotides can be used to block the production of particular proteins.

Thought Questions

1. You have probably read news reports about studies of the genetics of human behavioral traits or seen them on television. What does it really mean when a laboratory reports the discovery of, say, a "gene for shyness"?

2. Most rats do not appear to like the taste of alcohol, but researchers have bred some rats that will drink alcohol in large quantities. Can you think of ways to use these animals to investigate the possible role of genetic factors in alcoholism in humans?

EPILOGUE   Watch the Brain Waves

What went wrong? Why did Mrs. H.'s "successful" surgery cause a neurological problem? And can anything be done for her?

First, let's consider the cause of the problem. As you will recall, an artificial heart circulated Mrs. H.'s blood while the surgeon was removing two of her coronary arteries and replacing them with veins taken from her leg. The output of the machine is adjustable; that is, the person operating it can control the patient's blood pressure. The surgeon tries to keep the blood pressure just high enough to sustain the patient but not so high as to interfere with the delicate surgery on the coronary arteries. Unfortunately, Mrs. H.'s coronary arteries were not the only blood vessels to be partially blocked; the arteries in her brain, too, contained atherosclerotic plaque. When the machine took over the circulation of her blood, some parts of her brain received an inadequate blood flow, and the cells in these regions were damaged.

If Mrs. H.'s blood pressure had been maintained at a slightly higher level during the surgery, her brain damage might have been prevented. For most patients, the blood pressure would have been sufficient, but in her case it was not. Mrs. H.'s brain damage is irreversible. But are there steps that can be taken to prevent others from sharing her fate?

The answer is yes. The solution is to use a method described in this chapter: electroencephalography. What we need is a warning system to indicate that the brain is not receiving a sufficient blood flow so that the surgeon can adjust the machine and increase the patient's blood pressure. That warning can be provided by an EEG. For many years, clinical electroencephalographers (specialists who perform EEGs to diagnose neurological disorders) have known that diffuse, widespread brain damage caused by various poisons, anoxia, or extremely low levels of blood glucose produces slowing of the regular rhythmic pattern of the EEG. Fortunately, this pattern begins right away, as soon as the damage commences. Thus, if EEG leads are attached to a patient undergoing cardiac surgery, an electroencephalographer can watch the record coming off the polygraph and warn the surgeon if the record shows slowing. If it does, the patient's blood flow can be increased until the EEG reverts to normal, and brain damage can be averted.

Mrs. H. was operated on over 20 years ago, at a time when only a few cardiac surgeons had their patient's brain waves monitored. Today, the practice is common, and it is used during other surgical procedures that may reduce blood flow to the brain. For example, when the carotid arteries (the vessels that provide most of the brain's blood supply) become obstructed by atherosclerotic plaque, a surgeon can cut open the arteries and remove the plaque. During this procedure, called *carotid endarterectomy*, clamps must be placed on the carotid artery, completely stopping the blood flow. Some patients can tolerate the temporary clamping of one carotid artery without damage; others cannot. If the EEG record shows no slowing while the artery is clamped, the surgeon can proceed. If it does, the surgeon must place the ends of a plastic tube into the artery above and below the clamped region to maintain a constant blood flow. This procedure introduces a certain amount of additional risk to the patient, so most surgeons would prefer to do it only if necessary. The EEG provides the essential information.

Key Concepts

EXPERIMENTAL ABLATION

1. Neuroscientists produce brain lesions to try to infer the functions of the damaged region from changes in the animal's behavior.
2. Brain lesions may be produced in the depths of the brain by passing electrical current through an electrode placed there or by infusing an excitatory amino acid; the latter method kills cells but spares axons that pass through the region.
3. The behavior of animals with brain lesions must be compared with that of a control group consisting of animals with sham lesions.
4. A stereotaxic apparatus is used to place electrodes or cannulas in particular locations in the brain. The coordinates are obtained from a stereotaxic atlas.
5. The location of a lesion is verified by means of histological methods, which include fixation, slicing, staining, and examination of the tissue under a microscope.
6. Special histological methods have been devised to trace the afferent and efferent connections of a particular brain region.
7. The structure of the living human brain can be revealed through CT scans or MRI scans.

RECORDING AND STIMULATING NEURAL ACTIVITY

8. The electrical activity of single neurons can be recorded with microelectrodes, and that of entire regions of the brain can be recorded with macroelectrodes. EEGs are recorded on polygraphs and recorded from macroelectrodes pasted on a person's scalp.
9. Metabolic activity of particular parts of animals' brains can be assessed by means of 2-DG autoradiography or by measurement of the production of Fos protein. The metabolic activity of specific regions of the human brain can be revealed through PET scans or functional MRI scans.
10. Neurons can be stimulated electrically, through electrodes, or chemically, by infusing dilute solutions of excitatory amino acids through cannulas.

NEUROCHEMICAL METHODS

11. Immunocytochemical methods can be used to localize peptides in the brain or localize the enzymes that produce substances other than peptides.
12. Receptors can be localized by exposing the brain tissue to radioactive ligands and assessing the results with autoradiography or immunocytochemistry.
13. Microdialysis permits a researcher to measure the secretion of particular chemicals in specific regions of the brain. PET scans can be used to reveal the location of particular chemicals in the human brain.

GENETIC METHODS

14. Twin studies and adoption studies enable investigators to estimate the role of hereditary factors in a particular physiological characteristic or behavior.
15. Targeted mutations are artificially produced mutations that interfere with the action of one or more genes, which enables investigators to study the effects of the lack of a particular gene product.
16. Genes that cause the production of foreign proteins or increase production of native proteins can be inserted into the genome of strains of animals, and antisense oligonucleotides can be used to block the production of particular proteins

Suggested Readings

STEREOTAXIC ATLASES

Paxinos, G., and Watson, C. *The Rat Brain in Stereotaxic Coordinates*, 4th ed. San Diego, CA: Academic Press, 1998.

Slotnick, B. M., and Leonard, C. M. *A Stereotaxic Atlas of the Albino Mouse Forebrain*. Rockville, MD: Public Health Service, 1975. (U.S. Government Printing Office Stock Number 017-024-00491-0.)

Snider, R. S., and Niemer, W. T. *A Stereotaxic Atlas of the Cat Brain*. Chicago: University of Chicago Press, 1961.

Swanson, L. W. *Brain Maps: Structure of the Rat Brain*. Amsterdam: Elsevier, 1992.

HISTOLOGICAL METHODS

Heimer, L., and Záborsky, L. *Neuroanatomical Tract-Tracing Methods 2: Recent Progress*. New York: Plenum Press, 1989.

BRAIN IMAGING

Raichle, M. E. A brief history of human brain mapping. *Trends in Neuroscience*, 2008, *32*, 118–126.

Additional Resources

Visit www.mypsychkit.com for additional review and practice of the material covered in this chapter. Within MyPsychKit, you can take practice tests and receive a customized study plan to help you review. Dozens of animations, tutorials, and Web links are also available. You can even review using the interactive electronic version of this textbook. You will need to register for MyPsychKit. See www.mypsychkit.com for complete details.

chapter 6 : Vision

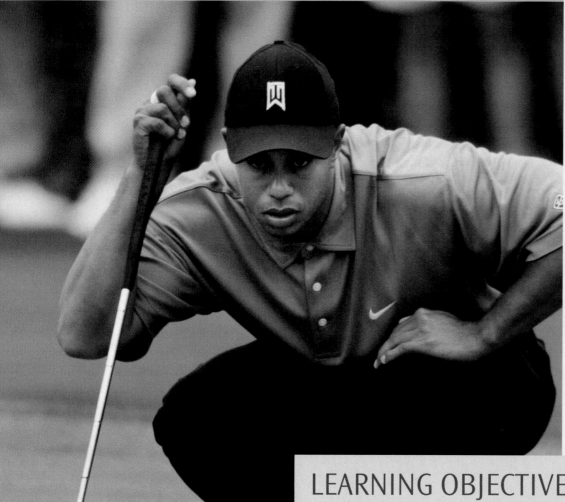

LEARNING OBJECTIVES

1. Describe the characteristics of light and color, outline the anatomy of the eye and its connections with the brain, and describe the process of transduction of visual information.

2. Describe the coding of visual information by photoreceptors and ganglion cells in the retina.

3. Describe the striate cortex and discuss how its neurons respond to orientation, movement, spatial frequency, retinal disparity, and color.

4. Describe the anatomy of the visual association cortex and discuss the location and functions of the two streams of visual analysis that take place there.

5. Discuss the perception of color and the analysis of form by neurons in the ventral stream.

6. Describe the role of the visual association cortex in the perception of objects, faces, body parts, and places.

7. Describe the role of the visual association cortex in the perception of movement.

8. Describe the role of the visual association cortex in the perception of spatial location.

:PROLOGUE Seeing Without Perceiving

Dr. L., a young neuropsychologist, was presenting the case of Mrs. R. to a group of medical students doing a rotation in the neurology department at the medical center. The chief of the department had shown them Mrs. R.'s MRI scans, and now Dr. L was addressing the students. He told them that Mrs. R.'s stroke had not impaired her ability to talk or to move about, but it had affected her vision.

A nurse ushered Mrs. R. into the room and helped her find a seat at the end of the table.

"How are you, Mrs. R.?" asked Dr. L.

"I'm fine. I've been home for a month now, and I can do just about everything that I did before I had my stroke."

"Good. How is your vision?"

"Well, I'm afraid that's still a problem."

"What seems to give you the most trouble?"

"I just don't seem to be able to recognize things. When I'm working in my kitchen, I know what everything is as long as no one moves anything. A few times my husband tried to help me by putting things away, and I couldn't see them any more." She laughed. "Well, I could see them, but I just couldn't say what they were."

Dr. L. took some objects out of a paper bag and placed them on the table in front of her.

"Can you tell me what these are?" he asked. "No," he said, "please don't touch them."

Mrs. R. stared intently at the objects. "No, I can't rightly say what they are."

Dr. L. pointed to one of them, a wristwatch. "Tell me what you see here," he said.

Mrs. R. looked thoughtful, turning her head one way and then the other. "Well, I see something round, and it has two things attached to it, one on the top and one on the bottom." She continued to stare at it. "There are some things inside the circle, I think, but I can't make out what they are."

"Pick it up."

She did so, made a wry face, and said, "Oh. It's a wristwatch." At Dr. L.'s request, she picked up the rest of the objects, one by one, and identified each of them correctly.

"Do you have trouble recognizing people, too?" asked Dr. L.

"Oh, yes!" she sighed. "While I was still in the hospital, my husband and my son both came in to see me, and I couldn't tell who was who until my husband said something—then I could tell which direction his voice was coming from. Now I've trained myself to recognize my husband. I can usually see his glasses and his bald head, but I have to work at it. And I've been fooled a few times." She laughed. "One of our neighbors is bald and wears glasses, too, and one day when he and his wife were visiting us, I thought he was my husband, so I called him 'honey.' It was a little embarrassing at first, but everyone understood."

"What does a face look like to you?" asked Dr. L.

"Well, I know that it's a face, because I can usually see the eyes, and it's on top of a body. I can see a body pretty well, by how it moves." She paused a moment. "Oh, yes, I forgot, sometimes I can recognize a person by how he moves. You know, you can often recognize friends by the way they walk, even when they're far away. I can still do that. That's funny, isn't it? I can't see people's faces very well, but I can recognize the way they walk."

Dr. L. made some movements with his hands. "Can you tell what I'm pretending to do?" he asked.

"Yes, you're mixing something—like some cake batter."

He mimed the gestures of turning a key, writing, and dealing out playing cards, and Mrs. R. recognized them without any difficulty.

"Do you have any trouble reading?" he asked.

"Well, a little, but I don't do too badly."

Dr. L. handed her a magazine, and she began to read the article aloud—somewhat hesitantly but accurately. "Why is it," she asked, "that I can see the *words* all right but have so much trouble with *things* and with people's faces?"

A s we saw in Chapter 3, the brain performs two major functions: It controls the movements of the muscles, producing useful behaviors, and it regulates the body's internal environment. To perform both these tasks, the brain must be informed about what is happening both in the external environment and within the body. Such information is received by the sensory systems. This chapter and the next are devoted to a discussion of the ways in which sensory organs detect changes in the environment and the ways in which the brain interprets neural signals from these organs.

We receive information about the environment from **sensory receptors**—specialized neurons that detect a variety of physical events. (Do not confuse *sensory receptors* with receptors for neurotransmitters, neuromodulators, and hormones. Sensory receptors are specialized neurons, and the other types of receptors are specialized proteins that bind with certain molecules.) Stimuli impinge on the receptors and alter their membrane potentials. This process is known as

sensory receptor A specialized neuron that detects a particular category of physical events.

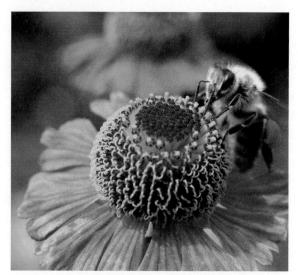

Some insects, such as this honeybee, can detect wavelengths of electromagnetic radiation that are invisible to people.

sensory transduction because sensory events are *transduced* ("transferred") into changes in the cells' membrane potential. These electrical changes are called **receptor potentials**. These potentials affect the release of neurotransmitters and hence modify the pattern of firing in neurons with which sensory receptors form synapses. Ultimately, the information reaches the brain.

This chapter considers vision, the sensory modality that receives the most attention from psychologists, anatomists, and physiologists. One reason for this attention derives from the fascinating complexity of the sensory organs of vision and the relatively large proportion of the brain that is devoted to the analysis of visual information. Approximately 20 percent of the cerebral cortex plays a direct role in the analysis of visual information (Wandell, Dumoulin, and Brewer, 2007). Another reason, I am sure, is that vision is so important to us as individuals. A natural fascination with such a rich source of information about the world leads to curiosity about how this sensory modality works. Chapter 7 deals with the other sensory modalities: audition, the vestibular senses, the somatosenses, gustation, and olfaction.

The Stimulus

As we all know, our eyes detect the presence of light. For humans, light is a narrow band of the spectrum of electromagnetic radiation. Electromagnetic radiation with a wavelength of between 380 and 760 nm (a nanometer, nm, is one-billionth of a meter) is visible to us. (See *Figure 6.1*.) Other animals can detect different ranges of electromagnetic radiation. For example, honeybees can detect differences in ultraviolet radiation reflected by flowers that appear white to us. The range of wavelengths we call *light* is not qualitatively different from the rest of the electromagnetic spectrum; it is simply the part of the continuum that we humans can see.

The perceived color of light is determined by three dimensions: *hue, saturation,* and *brightness*. Light travels at a constant speed of approximately 300,000 kilometers (186,000 miles) per second. Thus, if the frequency of oscillation of the wave varies, the distance between the peaks of the waves will vary similarly, but in inverse fashion. Slower oscillations lead to longer wavelengths, and faster ones lead to shorter wavelengths. Wavelength determines the first of the three perceptual dimensions of

sensory transduction The process by which sensory stimuli are transduced into slow, graded receptor potentials.

receptor potential A slow, graded electrical potential produced by a receptor cell in response to a physical stimulus.

FIGURE 6.1

The Electromagnetic Spectrum

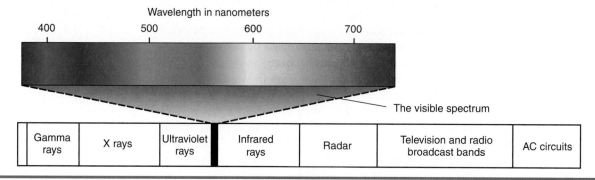

light: **hue**. The visible spectrum displays the range of hues that our eyes can detect.

Light can also vary in intensity, which corresponds to the second perceptual dimension of light: **brightness**. The third dimension, **saturation**, refers to the relative purity of the light that is being perceived. If all the radiation is of one wavelength, the perceived color is pure, or fully saturated. Conversely, if the radiation contains all wavelengths, it produces no sensation of hue—it appears white. Colors with intermediate amounts of saturation consist of different mixtures of wavelengths. Figure 6.2 shows some color samples, all with the same hue but with different levels of brightness and saturation. (See *Figure 6.2*.)

Anatomy of the Visual System

For an individual to see, an image must be focused on the retina, the inner lining of the eye. This image causes changes in the electrical activity of millions of neurons in the retina, which results in messages being sent through the optic nerves to the rest of the brain. (I said "the rest" because the retina is actually part of the brain; it and the optic nerve are in the central—not peripheral—nervous system.) This section describes the anatomy of the eyes, the photoreceptors in the retina that detect the presence of light, and the connections between the retina and the brain.

The Eyes

The eyes are suspended in the *orbits*, bony pockets in the front of the skull. They are held in place and moved by six extraocular muscles attached to the tough, white outer coat of the eye called the *sclera*. Normally, we cannot look behind our eyeballs and see these muscles, because their attachments to the eyes are hidden by the *conjunctiva*. These mucous membranes line the eyelid and fold back to attach to the eye (thus preventing a contact lens that has slipped off the cornea from "falling behind the eye"). Figure 6.3 illustrates the anatomy of the eye. (See *Figure 6.3*.)

When you scan the scene in front of you, your gaze does not roam slowly and steadily across its features. Instead, your eyes make jerky **saccadic movements**—you shift your gaze abruptly from one point to another. (*Saccade* comes from the French word for "jerk.") When you read a line in this book, your eyes stop several times, moving very quickly between each stop. You cannot consciously control the speed of movement between stops; during each *saccade* the eyes move as fast as they can. Only by performing a **pursuit movement**—say, by looking at your finger while you move it around—can you make your eyes move more slowly.

The white outer layer of most of the eye, the sclera, is opaque and does not permit entry of light. However, the cornea, the outer layer at the front of the eye, is transparent and admits light. The amount of light that enters is regulated by the size of the pupil, which is an opening in the iris, the pigmented ring of muscles situated behind the

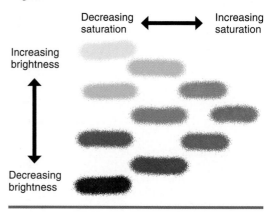

Saturation and Brightness. This figure shows examples of colors with the same dominant wavelength (hue) but different levels of saturations or brightness.

Decreasing saturation ⟷ Increasing saturation

Increasing brightness

Decreasing brightness

hue One of the perceptual dimensions of color; the dominant wavelength.

brightness One of the perceptual dimensions of color; intensity.

saturation One of the perceptual dimensions of color; purity.

saccadic movement (*suh **kad** ik*) The rapid, jerky movement of the eyes used in scanning a visual scene.

pursuit movement The movement that the eyes make to maintain an image of a moving object on the fovea.

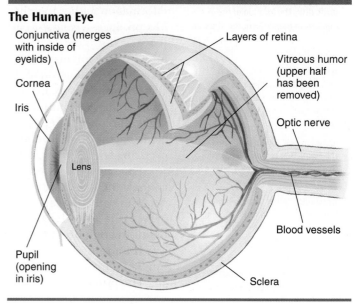

The Human Eye

Conjunctiva (merges with inside of eyelids)

Cornea

Iris

Lens

Pupil (opening in iris)

Layers of retina

Vitreous humor (upper half has been removed)

Optic nerve

Blood vessels

Sclera

TABLE 6.1   Locations and Response Characteristics of Photoreceptors

Cones	Rods
Most prevalent in the central retina; found in the fovea	Most prevalent in the peripheral retina; not found in the fovea
Sensitive to moderate-to-high levels of light	Sensitive to low levels of light
Provide information about hue	Provide only monochromatic information
Provide excellent acuity	Provide poor acuity

accommodation Changes in the thickness of the lens of the eye, accomplished by the ciliary muscles, that focus images of near or distant objects on the retina.

retina The neural tissue and photo-receptive cells located on the inner surface of the posterior portion of the eye.

rod One of the receptor cells of the retina; sensitive to light of low intensity.

cone One of the receptor cells of the retina; maximally sensitive to one of three different wavelengths of light and hence encodes color vision.

photoreceptor One of the receptor cells of the retina; transduces photic energy into electrical potentials.

fovea (*foe vee a*) The region of the retina that mediates the most acute vision of birds and higher mammals. Color-sensitive cones constitute the only type of photoreceptor found in the fovea.

optic disk The location of the exit point from the retina of the fibers of the ganglion cells that form the optic nerve; responsible for the blind spot.

bipolar cell A bipolar neuron located in the middle layer of the retina, conveying information from the photoreceptors to the ganglion cells.

ganglion cell A neuron located in the retina that receives visual information from bipolar cells; its axons give rise to the optic nerve.

horizontal cell A neuron in the retina that interconnects adjacent photoreceptors and the outer processes of the bipolar cells.

amacrine cell (*amm a krin*) A neuron in the retina that interconnects adjacent ganglion cells and the inner processes of the bipolar cells.

cornea. The lens, situated immediately behind the iris, consists of a series of transparent, onion-like layers. Its shape can be altered by contraction of the *ciliary muscles*, a set of muscle fibers attached to the outer edge of the lens. These changes in shape permit the eye to focus images of near or distant objects on the retina—a process called **accommodation**.

After passing through the lens, light traverses the main part of the eye, which is filled with *vitreous humor* ("glassy liquid"), a clear, gelatinous substance. Light then falls on the **retina**, the interior lining of the back of the eye. In the retina are located the receptor cells, the **rods** and **cones** (named for their shapes), collectively known as **photoreceptors**.

The human retina contains approximately 120 million rods and 6 million cones. Although they are greatly outnumbered by rods, cones provide us with most of the information about our environment. In particular, they are responsible for our daytime vision. They provide us with information about small features in the environment and thus are the source of vision of the highest sharpness, or *acuity* (from *acus*, "needle"). The **fovea**, or central region of the retina, which mediates our most acute vision, contains only cones. Cones are also responsible for color vision—our ability to discriminate light of different wavelengths. Although rods do not detect different colors and provide vision of poor acuity, they are more sensitive to light. In a very dimly lighted environment, we use our rod vision; therefore, in dim light we are color-blind and lack foveal vision. (See *Table 6.1*.)

Another feature of the retina is the **optic disk**, where the axons conveying visual information gather together and leave the eye through the optic nerve. The optic disk produces a *blind spot* because no receptors are located there. We do not normally perceive our blind spots, but their presence can be demonstrated. If you have not found yours, you may want to try the exercise described in *Figure 6.4*.

Close examination of the retina shows that it consists of several layers of neuron cell bodies, their axons and dendrites, and the photoreceptors. Figure 6.5 illustrates a cross section through the primate retina, which is divided into three main layers: the photoreceptive layer, the bipolar cell layer, and the ganglion cell layer. Note that the photoreceptors are at the *back* of the retina; light must pass through the overlying layers (which are transparent, of course) to get to them. (See *Figure 6.5*.)

The photoreceptors form synapses with **bipolar cells**, neurons whose two arms connect the shallowest and deepest layers of the retina. In turn, these neurons form synapses with the **ganglion cells**, neurons whose axons travel through the optic nerves (the second cranial nerves) and carry visual information into the rest of the brain. In addition, the retina contains **horizontal cells** and **amacrine cells**, both of which transmit information in a direction parallel to the surface of the retina and thus combine messages from adjacent photoreceptors. (See *Figure 6.5*.)

The primate retina contains approximately fifty-five different types of neurons: one type of rod, three types of cones, two types of horizontal cells, ten types of bipo-

FIGURE 6.4

A Test for the Blind Spot.   With your left eye closed, look at the plus sign with your right eye and move the page nearer to and farther from you. When the page is about 20 cm (8 in) from your face, the green circle disappears because its image falls on the blind spot of your right eye.

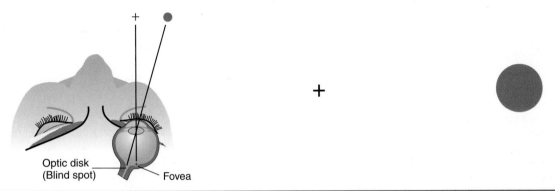

Optic disk
(Blind spot)   Fovea

lar cells, twenty-four to twenty-nine types of amacrine cells, and ten to fifteen types of ganglion cells (Masland, 2001).

Photoreceptors

Rods and cones consist of an outer segment connected by a cilium to an inner segment, which contains the nucleus. (See *Figure 6.5*.) The outer segment contains several hundred **lamellae**, or thin plates of membrane. (*Lamella* is the diminutive form of *lamina*, "thin layer.")

Let's consider the nature of transduction of visual information. The first step in the chain of events that leads to visual perception involves a special chemical called a photopigment. **Photopigments** are special molecules embedded in the membrane of the lamellae; a single human rod contains approximately ten million of them. The molecules consist of two parts: an **opsin** (a protein) and **retinal** (a lipid). There

FIGURE 6.5

Details of Retinal Circuitry

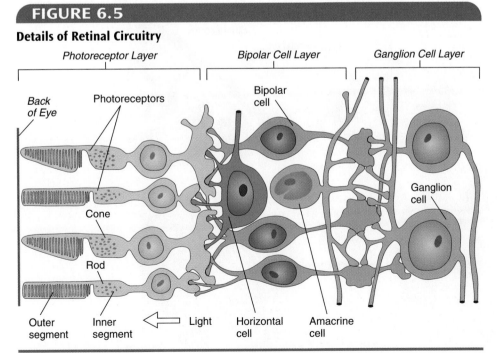

Photoreceptor Layer   *Bipolar Cell Layer*   *Ganglion Cell Layer*

Back of Eye   Photoreceptors

Bipolar cell

Ganglion cell

Cone

Rod

Outer segment   Inner segment   ⇦ Light   Horizontal cell   Amacrine cell

Adapted from Dowling, J. E., and Boycott, B. B. *Proceedings of the Royal Society of London, B*, 1966, *166*, 80–111.

lamella A layer of membrane containing photopigments; found in rods and cones of the retina.

photopigment A protein dye bonded to retinal, a substance derived from vitamin A; responsible for transduction of visual information.

opsin (***opp*** *sin*) A class of protein that, together with retinal, constitutes the photopigments.

retinal (***rett*** *i nahl*) A chemical synthesized from vitamin A; joins with an opsin to form a photopigment.

rhodopsin (*roh dopp sin*) A particular opsin found in rods.

dorsal lateral geniculate nucleus (LGN) A group of cell bodies within the lateral geniculate body of the thalamus; receives inputs from the retina and projects to the primary visual cortex.

magnocellular layer One of the inner two layers of neurons in the dorsal lateral geniculate nucleus; transmits information necessary for the perception of form, movement, depth, and small differences in brightness to the primary visual cortex.

parvocellular layer One of the four outer layers of neurons in the dorsal lateral geniculate nucleus; transmits information necessary for perception of color and fine details to the primary visual cortex.

koniocellular sublayer (*koh nee oh sell yew lur*) One of the sublayers of neurons in the dorsal lateral geniculate nucleus found ventral to each of the magnocellular and parvocellular layers; transmits information from short-wavelength ("blue") cones to the primary visual cortex.

are several forms of opsin; for example, the photopigment of human rods, **rhodopsin**, consists of *rod opsin* plus retinal. (*Rhod-* refers to the Greek *rhodon*, "rose," not to *rod*. Before it is bleached by the action of light, rhodopsin has a pinkish hue.) Retinal is synthesized from vitamin A, which explains why carrots, which are rich in this vitamin, are said to be good for your eyesight.

When a molecule of rhodopsin is exposed to light, it breaks into its two constituents: rod opsin and retinal. When that happens, the opsin changes from its rosy color to a pale yellow; hence, we say that the light *bleaches* the photopigment. The splitting of the photopigment produces the receptor potential: a change in the membrane potential of the photoreceptor. The receptor potential affects the release of neurotransmitter by the photoreceptor, which alters the firing rate of the bipolar cells with which the photoreceptors communicates. This information is passed on to the ganglion cells. (See *Figure 6.5*.)

Connections Between Eye and Brain

The axons of the retinal ganglion cells bring information to the rest of the brain. They ascend through the optic nerves and reach the **dorsal lateral geniculate nucleus (LGN)** of the thalamus. This nucleus receives its name from its resemblance to a bent knee (*genu* is Latin for "knee"). It contains six layers of neurons, each of which receives input from only one eye. The neurons in the two inner layers contain cell bodies that are larger than those in the outer four layers. For this reason, the inner two layers are called the **magnocellular layers**, and the outer four layers are called the **parvocellular layers** (*parvo-* refers to the small size of the cells). A third set of neurons in the **koniocellular sublayers** are found ventral to each of the magnocellular and par-

---

FIGURE 6.6

Lateral Geniculate Nucleus (LGN).   The photomicrograph shows a section through the lateral geniculate nucleus and striate cortex of a rhesus monkey (cresyl violet stain). Layers 1, 4, and 6 of the lateral geniculate nucleus receive input from the contralateral eye, and layers 2, 3, and 5 receive input from the ipsilateral eye. Layers 1 and 2 are the magnocellular layers; layers 3–6 are the parvocellular layers. The koniocellular sublayers are found ventral to each of the parvocellular and magnocellular layers. The receptive fields of all six principal layers are in almost perfect registration; cells located along the line of the unlabeled arrow have receptive fields centered on the same point. The ends of the striate cortex are shown by arrows.

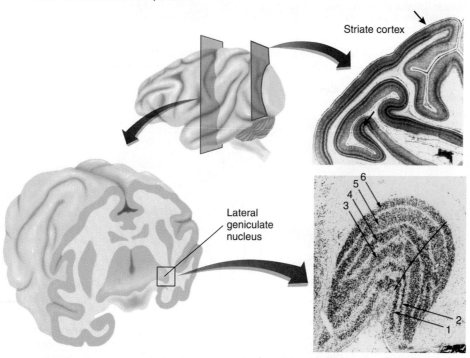

Photomicrograph from Hubel, D. H., Wiesel, T. N., and Le Vay, S. *Philosophical Transactions of the Royal Society of London, B*, 1977, *278*, 131–163.

vocellular layers. (*Konis* is the Greek word for "dust." we will see later, these three sets of layers belong to different systems, which are responsible for the analysis of different types of visual information. They receive input from different types of retinal ganglion cells. (See *Figure 6.6*.)

The neurons in the dorsal lateral geniculate nucleus send their axons through a pathway known as the *optic radiations* to the primary visual cortex—the region surrounding the **calcarine fissure** (*calcarine* means "spur shaped"), a horizontal fissure located in the medial and posterior occipital lobe. The primary visual cortex is often called the **striate cortex** because it contains a dark-staining layer (*striation*) of cells. (See *Figure 6.6*.)

Figure 6.7 shows a diagrammatical view of a horizontal section of the human brain. The optic nerves join together at the base of the brain to form the X-shaped **optic chiasm** (*khiasma* means "cross"). There, axons from ganglion cells serving the inner halves of the retina (the nasal sides) cross through the chiasm and ascend to the dorsal lateral geniculate nucleus of the opposite side of the brain. The axons from the outer halves of the retina (the temporal sides) remain on the same side of the brain. (See *Figure 6.7*.) The lens inverts the image of the world projected on the retina (and similarly reverses left and right). Therefore, because the axons from the nasal halves of the retinas cross to the other side of the brain, each hemisphere receives information from the contralateral half (opposite side) of the visual scene. That is, if a person looks straight ahead, the right hemisphere receives information from the left half of the visual field, and the left hemisphere receives information from the right. It is *not* correct to say that each hemisphere receives visual information solely from the contralateral eye. (See *Figure 6.7*.)

Besides the primary retino-geniculo-cortical pathway, several other pathways are taken by fibers from the retina. For example, one pathway to the hypothalamus synchronizes an animal's activity cycles to the 24-hour rhythms of day and night. (We will study this system in Chapter 8.) Other pathways, especially those that travel to the optic tectum and other midbrain nuclei, coordinate eye movements, control the muscles of the iris (and thus the size of the pupil) and the ciliary muscles (which control the lens), and help to direct our attention to sudden movements that occur in the periphery of our visual field.

FIGURE 6.7

The Primary Visual Pathway

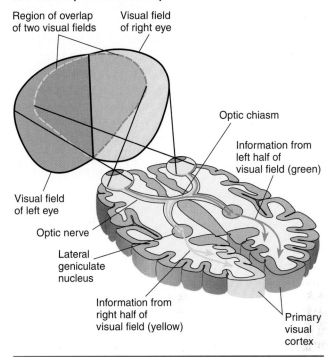

Region of overlap of two visual fields

Visual field of right eye

Optic chiasm

Information from left half of visual field (green)

Visual field of left eye

Optic nerve

Lateral geniculate nucleus

Information from right half of visual field (yellow)

Primary visual cortex

---

calcarine fissure (*kal ka rine*) A horizontal fissure on the inner surface of the posterior cerebral cortex; the location of the primary visual cortex.

striate cortex (*stry ate*) The primary visual cortex.

optic chiasm A cross-shaped connection between the optic nerves, located below the base of the brain, just anterior to the pituitary gland.

InterimSummary

The Stimulus and Anatomy of the Visual System

Light consists of electromagnetic radiation, similar to radio waves but of a different frequency and wavelength. Color can vary in three perceptual dimensions: hue, brightness, and saturation, which correspond to the physical dimensions of wavelength, intensity, and purity.

The photoreceptors in the retina—the rods and the cones—detect light. Muscles move the eyes so that images of particular parts of the environment fall on the retina. Accommodation is accomplished by the ciliary muscles, which change the shape of the lens.

Photoreceptors communicate with bipolar cells, which communicate with ganglion cells whose axons send visual information to the rest of the brain. In addition, horizontal cells and amacrine cells combine messages from adjacent photoreceptors.

When light strikes a molecule of photopigment in a photoreceptor, the retinal molecule detaches from the opsin molecule, a process known as bleaching. This event causes a receptor potential, which changes the rate of firing of the ganglion cell, signaling the detection of light.

Visual information from the retina reaches the striate cortex surrounding the calcarine fissure after being relayed through the magnocellular, parvocellular, and koniocellular layers of the LGN. Several other regions of the brain, including the hypothalamus and the tectum, also receive visual information. These regions help to regulate activity during the day–night cycle, coordinate eye and head movements, regulate the size of the pupils, and control attention to visual stimuli.

Thought Question

People who try to see faint, distant lights at night are often advised to look just to the side of the location where they expect to see the lights. Can you explain the reason for this advice?

Coding of Visual Information in the Retina

This section describes the way in which cells of the retina encode information they receive from the photoreceptors.

Coding of Light and Dark

One of the methods for studying the physiology of the visual system is the use of microelectrodes to record the electrical activity of single neurons. As we saw in the previous section, some ganglion cells become excited when light falls on the photoreceptors that communicate with them. The **receptive field** of a neuron in the visual system is the part of the visual field that an individual neuron "sees"; that is, the place in which a visual stimulus must be located to produce a response in that neuron. Obviously, the location of the receptive field of a particular neuron depends on the location of the photoreceptors that provide it with visual information. If a neuron receives information from photoreceptors located in the fovea, its receptive field will be at the fixation point—the point at which the eye is looking. If the neuron receives information from photoreceptors located in the periphery of the retina, its receptive field will be located off to one side.

At the periphery of the retina many individual receptors converge on a single ganglion cell, bringing information from a relatively large area of the retina—and hence a relatively large area of the visual field. However, the fovea contains approximately equal numbers of ganglion cells and cones. These receptor-to-axon relationships explain the fact that our foveal (central) vision is very acute but our peripheral vision is much less precise. (See *Figure 6.8.*)

Kuffler (1952, 1953), recording from ganglion cells in the retina of the cat, discovered that their receptive field consists of a roughly circular center, surrounded by a ring. Stimulation of the center or surrounding fields had contrary effects: ON cells were excited by light falling in the central field (*center*) and were inhibited by light falling in the surrounding field (*surround*), whereas OFF cells responded in the opposite manner. ON/OFF ganglion cells were briefly excited when light was turned on or off. In primates these ON/OFF cells project to the superior colliculus, which is primarily involved in visual

receptive field That portion of the visual field in which the presentation of visual stimuli will produce an alteration in the firing rate of a particular neuron.

FIGURE 6.8

Central Versus Peripheral Acuity. Ganglion cells in the fovea receive input from a smaller number of photoreceptors than in the periphery and hence provide more acute visual information.

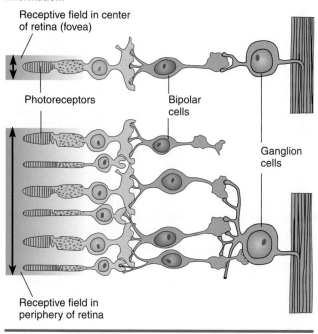

Receptive field in center of retina (fovea)

Photoreceptors

Bipolar cells

Ganglion cells

Receptive field in periphery of retina

FIGURE 6.9

ON and OFF Ganglion Cells. This figure shows responses of ON and OFF ganglion cells to stimuli presented in the center or the surround of the receptive field.

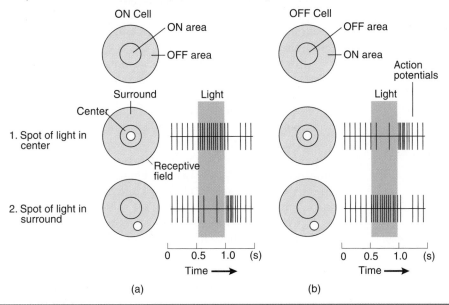

Adapted from Kuffler, S. W. *Cold Spring Harbor Symposium for Quantitative Biology*, 1952, *17*, 281–292.

reflexes (Schiller and Malpeli, 1977), which suggests that they do not play a direct role in form perception. (See *Figure 6.9*.)

Coding of Color

So far, we have been examining the monochromatic properties of ganglion cells—that is, their responses to light and dark. But, of course, objects in our environment selectively absorb some wavelengths of light and reflect others, which, to our eyes, gives them different colors. The retinas of humans, apes, Old World monkeys, and one species of New World monkey contain three different types of cones, which provides them (and us) with the most elaborate form of color vision (Jacobs, 1996; Hunt et al., 1998). Although monochromatic (black-and-white) vision is perfectly adequate for most purposes, color vision gave our primate ancestors the ability to distinguish ripe fruit from unripe fruit and made it more difficult for other animals to hide themselves by means of camouflage (Mollon, 1989). In fact, the photopigments of primates with three types of cones seem well suited for distinguishing red and yellow fruits against a background of green foliage (Regan et al., 2001).

Photoreceptors: Trichromatic Coding

Various theories of color vision have been proposed for many years—long before it was possible to disprove or validate them by physiological means. In 1802 Thomas Young, a British physicist and

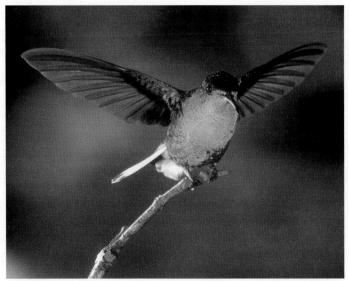

Birds have full, three-cone color vision; thus, this green breast can be perceived by rival males of this hummingbird.

FIGURE 6.10

Absorbance of Light by Rods and Cones.   The graph shows the relative absorbance of light of various wavelengths by rods and the three types of cones in the human retina.

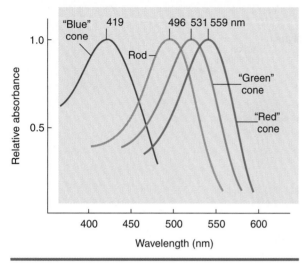

physician, proposed that the eye detected different colors because it contained three types of receptors, each sensitive to a single hue. His theory was referred to as the *trichromatic (three-color) theory*. It was suggested by the fact that for a human observer any color can be reproduced by mixing various quantities of three colors judiciously selected from different points along the spectrum.

I must emphasize that *color mixing* is different from *pigment mixing*. If we combine yellow and blue pigments (as when we mix paints), the resulting mixture is green. Color mixing refers to the addition of two or more light sources. However, if we shine a beam of red light and a beam of bluish green light together on a white screen, we will see yellow light. When white light appears on a color television screen or computer monitor, it actually consists of a blend of tiny red, blue, and green pixels. If you look closely at one of these screens with a strong magnifying glass, you will see these colored pixels.

Physiological investigations of retinal photoreceptors in higher primates have found that Young was right: Three different types of photoreceptors (three different types of cones) are responsible for color vision. Investigators have studied the absorption characteristics of individual photoreceptors, determining the amount of light of different wavelengths that is absorbed by the photopigments. These characteristics are controlled by the particular opsin a photoreceptor contains; different opsins absorb particular wavelengths more readily. The peak sensitivities of the three types of cones are approximately 420 nm (blue-violet), 530 nm (green), and 560 nm (yellow-green). The peak sensitivity of the short-wavelength cone is actually 440 nm in the intact eye because the lens absorbs some short-wavelength light. For convenience the short-, medium-, and long-wavelength cones are traditionally called "blue," "green," and "red" cones, respectively. The relative number of "red" and "green" cones varies considerably from person to person. Amazingly, even large differences in the relative numbers of these cones has no measurable effect on a person's color vision. The retina contains a much smaller number of "blue" cones—approximately 8 percent of the total. (See ***Figure 6.10.***)

Genetic defects in color vision appear to result from anomalies in one or more of the three types of cones (Boynton, 1979; Wissinger and Sharpe, 1998; Nathans, 1999). The first two kinds of defective color vision described here involve genes on the X chromosome; thus, because males have only one X chromosome, they are much more likely to have this disorder. (Females are likely to have a normal gene on one of their X chromosomes, which compensates for the defective one.) People with **protanopia** ("first-color defect") confuse red and green. They see the world in shades of yellow and blue; both red and green look yellowish to them. Their visual acuity is normal, which suggests that their retinas do not lack "red" or "green" cones. This fact, and their sensitivity to lights of different wavelengths, suggests that their "red" cones are filled with "green" cone opsin. People with **deuteranopia** ("second-color defect") also confuse red and green and also have normal visual acuity. Their "green" cones appear to be filled with "red" cone opsin.

Tritanopia ("third-color defect") is rare, affecting fewer than 1 in 10,000 people. This disorder involves a faulty gene that is not located on an X chromosome; thus, it is equally prevalent in males and females. People with tritanopia have difficulty with hues of short wavelengths and see the world in greens and reds. To them a clear blue sky is a bright green, and yellow looks pink. Their retinas lack "blue" cones. Because the retina contains so few of these cones, their absence does not noticeably affect visual acuity.

protanopia (*pro tan **owe** pee a*) An inherited form of defective color vision in which red and green hues are confused; "red" cones are filled with "green" cone opsin.

deuteranopia (*dew ter an **owe** pee a*) An inherited form of defective color vision in which red and green hues are confused; "green" cones are filled with "red" cone opsin.

tritanopia (*try tan **owe** pee a*) An inherited form of defective color vision in which hues with short wavelengths are confused; "blue" cones are either lacking or faulty.

Retinal Ganglion Cells: Opponent-Process Coding

At the level of the retinal ganglion cell, the three-color code gets translated into an opponent-color system. Daw (1968) and Gouras (1968) found that these neurons respond specifically to pairs of primary colors: red versus green and yellow versus blue. Thus, the retina contains two kinds of color-sensitive ganglion cells: *red-green* cells and *yellow-blue* cells. Some color-sensitive ganglion cells respond in a center-surround fashion. For example, a cell might be excited by red and inhibited by green in the center of their receptive fields while showing the opposite response in the surrounding ring. (See *Figure 6.11.*) Other ganglion cells that receive input from cones do not respond differentially to different wavelengths but simply encode relative brightness in the center and surround. These cells serve as "black-and-white detectors."

The response characteristics of retinal ganglion cells to light of different wavelengths are obviously determined by the particular circuits that connect the three types of cones with the two types of ganglion cells. These circuits involve different types of bipolar cells, amacrine cells, and horizontal cells. For example, a red-green ganglion cell is excited by activation of "red" cones and inhibited by activation of "green" cones.

The opponent-color system employed by the ganglion cells explains why we cannot perceive a reddish green or a bluish yellow: An axon that signals red or green (or yellow or blue) can either increase or decrease its rate of firing; it cannot do both at the same time. A reddish green would have to be signaled by a ganglion cell firing slowly and rapidly at the same time, which is obviously impossible. *MyPsychKit 6.1, Complementary Colors*, demonstrates an interesting phenomenon that emerges from opponent-process coding.

FIGURE 6.11

Receptive Fields of Color-Sensitive Ganglion Cells. When a portion of the receptive field is illuminated with the color shown, the cell's rate of firing increases. When a portion is illuminated with the complementary color, the cell's rate of firing decreases.

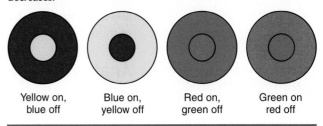

Yellow on, blue off   Blue on, yellow off   Red on, green off   Green on red off

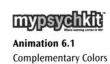

Animation 6.1
Complementary Colors

Interim Summary

Coding of Visual Information in the Retina

Recordings of the electrical activity of single neurons in the retina indicate that each ganglion cell receives information from photoreceptors—just one in the fovea and many more in the periphery. The receptive field of most retinal ganglion cells consists of two concentric circles; the cells become excited when light falls in one region and become inhibited when it falls in the other. ON cells are excited by light in the center, and OFF cells are excited by light in the surround.

Color vision occurs as a result of information provided by three types of cones, each of which is sensitive to light of a certain wavelength: long, medium, or short. The absorption characteristics of the cones are determined by the particular opsin that their photopigment contains. Most forms of defective color vision appear to be caused by alterations in cone opsins. The "red" cones of people with protanopia are filled with "green" cone opsin, and the "green" cones of people with deuteranopia are filled with "red" cone opsin. The retinas of people with tritanopia appear to lack "blue" cones.

Most color-sensitive ganglion cells respond in an opposing center-surround fashion to the pairs of primary colors: red and green, and blue and yellow. The responses of these neurons are determined by the retinal circuitry connecting them with the photoreceptors.

Thought Questions

Why is color vision useful? Birds, some fish, and some primates have full, three-cone color vision. Considering our own species, what other benefits (besides the ability to recognize ripe fruit, mentioned in the previous section) might come from the evolution of color vision?

simple cell An orientation-sensitive neuron in the striate cortex whose receptive field is organized in an opponent fashion.

complex cell A neuron in the visual cortex that responds to the presence of a line segment with a particular orientation located within its receptive field, especially when the line moves perpendicularly to its orientation.

hypercomplex cell A neuron in the visual cortex that responds to the presence of a line segment with a particular orientation that ends at a particular point within the cell's receptive field.

sine-wave grating A series of straight parallel bands varying continuously in brightness according to a sine-wave function, along a line perpendicular to their lengths.

spatial frequency The relative width of the bands in a sine-wave grating, measured in cycles per degree of visual angle.

Analysis of Visual Information: Role of the Striate Cortex

The retinal ganglion cells encode information about the relative amounts of light falling on the center and surround regions of their receptive field and, in many cases, about the wavelength of that light. The striate cortex performs additional processing of this information, which it then transmits to the visual association cortex.

Anatomy of the Striate Cortex

The striate cortex consists of six principal layers (and several sublayers), arranged in bands parallel to the surface. These layers contain the nuclei of cell bodies and dendritic trees that show up as bands of light or dark in sections of tissue that have been dyed with a cell-body stain. (See *Figure 6.12*.)

If we consider the striate cortex of one hemisphere as a whole—if we imagine that we remove it and spread it out on a flat surface—we find that it contains a map of the contralateral half of the visual field. (Remember that each side of the brain sees the opposite side of the visual field.) The map is distorted; approximately 25 percent of the striate cortex is devoted to the analysis of information from the fovea, which represents a small part of the visual field. (The area of the visual field seen by the fovea is approximately the size of a large grape held at arm's length.)

The pioneering studies of David Hubel and Torsten Wiesel at Harvard University during the 1960s began a revolution in the study of the physiology of visual perception (see Hubel and Wiesel, 1977, 1979). Hubel and Wiesel discovered that neurons in the visual cortex did not simply respond to spots of light; they selectively responded to specific *features* of the visual world. That is, the neural circuitry within the visual cortex combines information from several sources (for example, from axons carrying information received from several different ganglion cells) in such a way as to detect features that are larger than the receptive field of a single ganglion cell or a single cell in the LGN. The following subsections describe the visual characteristics that researchers have studied so far: orientation and movement, spatial frequency, retinal disparity, and color.

Orientation and Movement

Most neurons in the striate cortex are sensitive to *orientation*. That is, if a line or an edge (the border of a light and a dark region) is positioned in the cell's receptive field and rotated around its center, the cell will respond best when the line is in a particular position—a particular orientation. Some neurons respond best to a vertical line, some to a horizontal line, and some to a line oriented somewhere in between. Figure 6.13 shows the responses of a neuron in the striate cortex when lines were presented at various orientations. As you can see, this neuron responded best when a vertical line was presented in its receptive field. (See *Figure 6.13*.)

Some orientation-sensitive neurons have receptive fields organized in an opponent fashion. Hubel and Wiesel referred to them as **simple cells**. For example, a line of a particular orientation (say, a dark 45° line against a white background) might excite a cell if placed

---

FIGURE 6.12

The Six Layers of the Striate Cortex. This photomicrograph of a small section of the striate cortex shows the six principal layers. The letter W refers to the white matter that underlies the visual cortex; beneath the white matter is layer VI of the striate cortex on the opposite side of the gyrus.

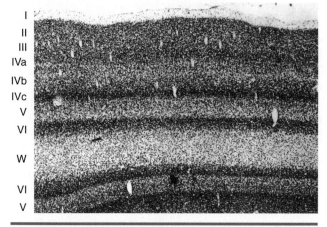

I
II
III
IVa
IVb
IVc
V
VI
W
VI
V

From Hubel, D. H., and Wiesel, T. N. *Proceedings of the Royal Society of London, B*, 1977, *198*, 1–59. Reprinted with permission.

in the center of the receptive field but inhibit it if moved away from the center. (See *Figure 6.14a*.) Another type of neuron, which the researchers referred to as a **complex cell**, also responded best to a line of a particular orientation but did not show an inhibitory surround; that is, it continued to respond while the line was moved within the receptive field. In fact, many complex cells increased their rate of firing when the line was moved perpendicular to its angle of orientation—often only in one direction. Thus, these neurons also served as movement detectors. In addition, complex cells responded equally well to white lines against black backgrounds and black lines against white backgrounds. (See *Figure 6.14b*.) Finally, **hypercomplex cells** responded to lines of a particular orientation but had an inhibitory region at the end (or ends) of the lines, which meant that the cells detected the location of *ends* of lines of a particular orientation. (See *Figure 6.14c*.)

Spatial Frequency

Although the early studies by Hubel and Wiesel suggested that neurons in the primary visual cortex detected lines and edges, subsequent research found that they actually responded best to sine-wave gratings (De Valois, Albrecht, and Thorell, 1978). Figure 6.15 compares a sine-wave grating with a more familiar square-wave grating. A square-wave grating consists of a simple set of rectangular bars that vary in brightness; the brightness along the length of a line perpendicular to them would vary in a stepwise (square-wave) fashion. (See *Figure 6.15a*.) A **sine-wave grating** looks like a series of fuzzy, unfocused parallel bars. Along any line perpendicular to the long axis of the grating, the brightness varies according to a sine-wave function. (See *Figure 6.15b*.)

A sine-wave grating is designated by its spatial frequency. We are accustomed to the expression of frequencies (for example, of sound waves or radio waves) in terms of time or distance (such as cycles per second or wavelength in cycles per meter). However, because the image of a stimulus on the retina varies in size according to how close it is to the eye, the visual angle is generally used instead of the physical distance between adjacent cycles. Thus, the **spatial frequency** of a sine-wave grating is its variation in brightness measured in cycles per degree of visual angle. (See *Figure 6.16*.)

Most neurons in the striate cortex respond best when a sine-wave grating of a particular spatial frequency is placed in the appropriate part of the visual field. But what is the point of having neural circuits that analyze spatial frequency? A complete answer requires some rather complicated mathematics, so I will give a simplified one here. (If you are interested, you can consult a classic book by De Valois and De Valois, 1988.) Consider the types of information provided by high and low spatial frequencies. Small objects, details within a large object, and large objects with sharp edges provide a signal rich in high frequencies, whereas large areas of light and dark are represented by low frequencies. An image that is deficient in

FIGURE 6.13

Orientation Sensitivity. An orientation-sensitive neuron in the striate cortex will become active only when a line of a particular orientation appears within its receptive field. For example, the neuron depicted in this figure responds best to a bar that is vertically oriented.

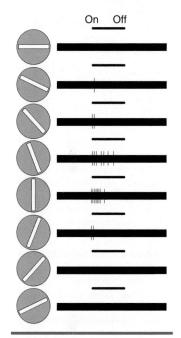

From Hubel, D. H., and Wiesel, T. N. *Journal of Physiology* (London), 1959, *148*, 574–591. Reprinted with permission by Blackwell Science Ltd.

FIGURE 6.14

Types of Orientation-Sensitive Neurons. The figure illustrates the response characteristics of three types of orientation-sensitive neurons in the primary visual cortex: (a) simple cell, (b) complex cell, and (c) hypercomplex cell.

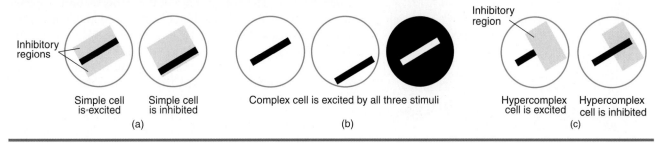

FIGURE 6.15

Parallel Gratings.   Two kinds of gratings are compared in this figure: (a) square-wave grating and (b) sine-wave grating.

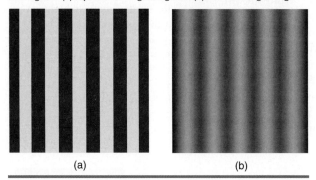

(a)   (b)

high-frequency information looks fuzzy and out of focus, like the image seen by a nearsighted person who is not wearing corrective lenses. This image still provides much information about forms and objects in the environment; thus, the most important visual information is that contained in *low spatial frequencies*. When low-frequency information is removed, the shapes of images are very difficult to perceive. (As we will see, the evolutionarily older magnocellular system provides low-frequency information.)

Retinal Disparity

We perceive depth by many means, most of which involve cues that can be detected monocularly, by one eye alone. For example, perspective, relative retinal size, loss of detail through the effects of atmospheric haze, and relative apparent movement of retinal images as we move our heads all contribute to depth perception and do not require binocular vision. However, binocular vision provides a vivid perception of depth through the process of stereoscopic vision, or *stereopsis*. If you have used a stereoscope (such as a View-Master) or have seen a 3-D movie, you know what I mean. Stereopsis is particularly important in the visual guidance of fine movements of the hands and fingers, such as we use when we thread a needle.

Most neurons in the striate cortex are *binocular*—that is, they respond to visual stimulation of either eye. Many of these binocular cells, especially those found in a layer that receives information from the magnocellular system, have response patterns that appear to contribute to the perception of depth (Poggio and Poggio, 1984). In most cases the cells respond most vigorously when each eye sees a stimulus in a slightly *different* location. That is, the neurons respond to **retinal disparity**, a stimulus that produces images on slightly different parts of the retina of each eye. This is exactly the information that is needed for stereopsis; each eye sees a three-dimensional scene slightly differently, and the presence of retinal disparity indicates differences in the distance of objects from the observer.

retinal disparity The fact that points on objects located at different distances from the observer will fall on slightly different locations on the two retinas; provides the basis for stereopsis.

cytochrome oxidase (CO) blob The central region of a module of the primary visual cortex, revealed by a stain for cytochrome oxidase; contains wavelength-sensitive neurons; part of the parvocellular system.

Color

In the striate cortex, information from color-sensitive ganglion cells is transmitted, through the parvocellular and koniocellular layers of the LGN, to special cells grouped together in **cytochrome oxidase (CO) blobs**. CO blobs were discovered by Wong-Riley (1978), who found that a stain for cytochrome oxidase, an enzyme that is present in mitochondria, showed a patchy distribution. (The presence of high levels of cytochrome oxidase in a cell indicates that the cell normally has a high rate of metabolism.) Subsequent research with the stain (Horton and Hubel, 1980; Humphrey and Hendrickson, 1980) revealed the presence of a polka-dot pattern of dark columns extending through layers 2 and 3 and (more faintly) layers 5 and 6. The columns are oval in cross section, approximately 150×200 μm in diameter, and spaced at 0.5-mm intervals (Fitzpatrick, Itoh, and Diamond, 1983; Livingstone and Hubel, 1987).

Figure 6.17 shows a photomicrograph of a slice through the striate cortex (also called V1 because it is the first area of visual cortex) and an adjacent area of visual association cortex (area V2) of a macaque monkey. The visual cortex has been flattened out and stained for the mitochondrial enzyme. You can clearly see the CO blobs within the striate cortex. The

FIGURE 6.16

Visual Angle and Spatial Frequency.   Angles are drawn between the sine waves, with the apex at the viewer's eye. This figure shows that the *visual angle* between adjacent sine waves is smaller when the waves are closer together.

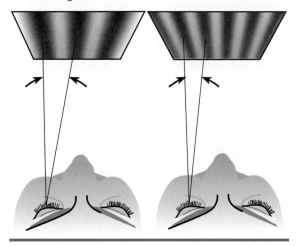

distribution of CO-rich neurons in area V2 consists of three kinds of stripes: *thick stripes, thin stripes,* and *pale stripes.* The thick and thin stripes stain heavily for cytochrome oxidase; the pale stripes do not. (See *Figure 6.17.*)

Until recently, researchers believed that the parvocellular system transmitted all information pertaining to color to the striate cortex. However, we now know that the parvocellular system receives information only from "red" and "green" cones; additional information from "blue" cones is transmitted through the koniocellular system (Hendry and Yoshioka, 1994; Chatterjee and Callaway, 2003).

To summarize, neurons in the striate cortex respond to several different features of a visual stimulus, including orientation, movement, spatial frequency, retinal disparity, and color. Now let us turn our attention to the way in which this information is organized within the striate cortex.

Modular Organization of the Striate Cortex

Most investigators believe that the brain is organized in modules, which probably range in size from a hundred thousand to a few million neurons. Each module receives information from other modules, performs some calculations, and then passes the results to other modules. In recent years investigators have been learning the characteristics of the modules that are found in the visual cortex.

The striate cortex is divided into approximately 2500 modules, each approximately 0.5 × 0.7 mm and containing approximately 150,000 neurons. The neurons in each module are devoted to the analysis of various features contained in one very small portion of the visual field. Collectively, these modules receive information from the entire visual field, the individual modules serving like the tiles in a mosaic mural.

The modules actually consist of two segments, each surrounding a CO blob. Neurons located within the blobs have a special function: Most of them are sensitive to color, and all of them are sensitive to low spatial frequencies but relatively insensitive to other visual features. Outside the CO blob, neurons show sensitivity to orientation, movement, spatial frequency, and binocular disparity, but most do not respond to color (Livingstone and Hubel, 1984; Born and Tootell, 1991; Edwards, Purpura, and Kaplan, 1995). Each half of the module receives input from only one eye, but the circuitry within the module combines the information from both eyes, which means that most of the neurons are binocular. If we insert a microelectrode straight down into an interblob region of the striate cortex (that is, in a location in a module outside one of the CO blobs), we will find that all of the orientation-sensitive cells will respond to lines of the same orientation. (See *Figure 6.18.*)

FIGURE 6.17

Blobs and Stripes in the Visual Cortex. A photomicrograph (actually, a montage of several different tissue sections) shows a slice through the primary visual cortex (area V1) and a region of visual association cortex (V2) of a macaque monkey, stained for cytochrome oxidase. Area V1 shows spots ("blobs"), and area V2 shows three types of stripes: thick, thin (both dark), and pale.

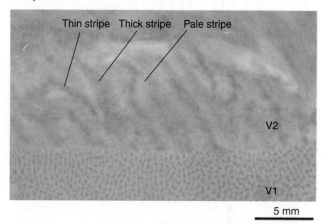

From Sincich, L. C., and Horton, J. C. *Annual Review of Neuroscience,* 2005, *28,* 303–326. By Annual Reviews at www.annualreviews.org.

FIGURE 6.18

One Module of the Primary Visual Cortex

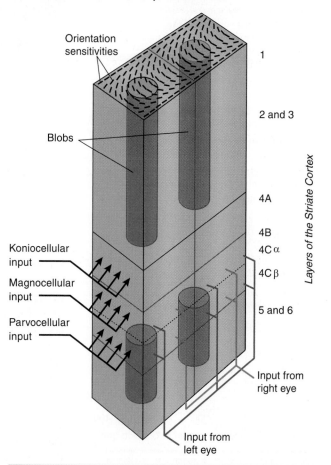

How does spatial frequency fit into this organization? Edwards, Purpura, and Kaplan (1995) found that neurons within the CO blobs responded to low spatial frequencies but were sensitive to small differences in brightness. Outside the blobs, sensitivity to spatial frequency varied with the distance from the center of the nearest blob. Higher frequencies were associated with greater distances. (See *Figure 6.19*.)

InterimSummary

Analysis of Visual Information: Role of the Striate Cortex

The striate cortex (area V1) consists of six layers and several sublayers. Visual information is received from the magnocellular, parvocellular, and koniocellular layers of the LGN. Information from V1 is sent to area V2, the first region of the visual association cortex. The magnocellular system is phylogenetically older, color-blind, and sensitive to movement, depth, and small differences in brightness. The parvocellular and koniocellular systems evolved more recently. The parvocellular system receives information from "red" and "green" cones and is able to discriminate finer details. The koniocellular system provides additional information about color, received from "blue" cones.

The striate cortex is organized into modules, each surrounding a pair of CO blobs, which are revealed by a stain for cytochrome oxidase, an enzyme found in mitochondria. Each half of a module receives information from one eye, but because information is shared, most of the neurons respond to information from both eyes. The neurons in the CO blobs are sensitive to color and to low-frequency sine-wave gratings, whereas those between the blobs are sensitive to sine-wave gratings of higher spatial frequencies, orientation, retinal disparity, and movement.

Thought Question

Look at the scene in front of you and try to imagine how its features are encoded by neurons in your striate cortex. Try to picture how the objects you see can be specified by an analysis of orientation, spatial frequency, and color.

extrastriate cortex A region of the visual association cortex; receives fibers from the striate cortex and from the superior colliculi and projects to the inferior temporal cortex.

FIGURE 6.19

Organization of Responses to Spatial Frequency.   Optimal spatial frequency of neurons in the striate cortex is shown here as a function of the distance of the neuron from the center of the nearest cytochrome oxidase blob.

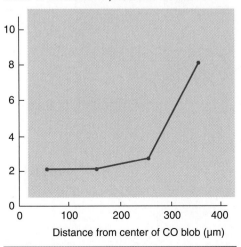

Adapted from Edwards, D. P., Purpura, K. P., and Kaplan, E. *Vision Research*, 1995, *35*, 1501–1523.

Analysis of Visual Information: Role of the Visual Association Cortex

Although the striate cortex is necessary for visual perception, perception of objects and of the totality of the visual scene does not take place there. Each module of the striate cortex sees only what is happening in one tiny part of the visual field. Thus, for us to perceive objects and entire visual scenes, the information from these individual modules must be combined. That combination takes place in the visual association cortex.

Two Streams of Visual Analysis

Visual information received from the striate cortex is analyzed in the visual association cortex. Neurons in the striate cortex send axons to the **extrastriate cortex**, the region of the visual association cortex that surrounds the striate cortex (Zeki and Shipp, 1988). The primate extrastriate cortex consists of several regions, each of which contains one or more independent maps of the visual field. Each region is specialized, containing neurons that respond to a particular feature of visual information, such as orientation, movement, spatial frequency, retinal disparity, or color. So far, investigators have identified over two dozen distinct regions and subregions of the visual cortex of the rhesus monkey. These regions are arranged hierarchically, beginning with the striate cortex (Grill-Spector and Malach, 2004; Wandell, Dumoulin, and Brewer, 2007). Most of the information passes up the hierarchy; each region receives information from regions located beneath it in the hierarchy (closer to the striate cortex), analyzes the information, and passes the results on to "higher" regions for further analysis.

The results of a functional-imaging study by Murray, Boyaci, and Kersten (2006) demonstrate a phenomenon that owes its existence to information that follows pathways that travel up the hierarchy, from regions of the visual association cortex back to the striate cortex. First, try the following demonstration. Stare at an object (for example, an illuminated light bulb) that has enough contrast with the background to produce an afterimage. Then look at a nearby surface, such as the back of your hand. Before the afterimage fades away, look at a more distant surface, such as the far wall of the room (assuming you are inside). You will see that the afterimage looks much larger when it is seen against a distant background. The investigators presented subjects with stimuli like those shown in Figure 6.20: spheres positioned against a background in locations that made them look closer to or farther from the observer. Although the spheres were actually the same size, their location on the background made the one that was apparently farther away look larger than the other one. (See *Figure 6.20.*)

Murray and his colleagues used functional imaging to record activation of the striate cortex while the subjects looked at the spheres. They found that looking at the sphere that appeared to be larger activated a larger area of the striate cortex. We know that perception of apparent distance in a background like that shown in Figure 6.20 cannot take place in the striate cortex, but requires neural circuitry found in the visual association cortex. This fact means that computations made in higher levels of the visual system can act back on the striate cortex and modify the activity taking place there.

Figure 6.21 shows the location of the striate cortex and several regions in the extrastriate cortex of the human brain. The views of a brain in Figures 6.21(a) and 6.21(b) are nearly normal in appearance. Figures 6.21(c) and 6.21(d) show "inflated" cortical surfaces, enabling us to see regions that are normally hidden in the depths of sulci and fissures. The hidden regions are shown in dark gray, while regions that are normally visible (the surfaces of gyri) are shown in light gray. Figure 6.21(e) shows an unrolling of the cortical surface caudal to the dotted red line and green lines in Figure 6.21(c) and 6.21(d). (See *Figure 6.21.*)

As we saw in the previous subsection, most of the outputs of the striate cortex (area V1) are sent to area V2, a region of the extrastriate cortex just adjacent to V1.

FIGURE 6.20

Effect of Perceived Distance on Perceived Size.   The ball that appears to be farther away looks larger than the closer one, even though the images they cast on the retina are exactly the same size.

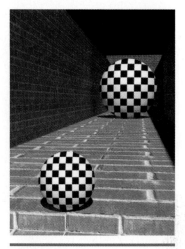

Courtesy of Scott Murray.

FIGURE 6.21

The Striate Cortex and Regions of the Extrastriate Cortex.   These views of a human brain show (a) a nearly normal lateral view, (b) a nearly normal midsagittal view, (c) an "inflated" lateral view, (d) an "inflated" midsagittal view, and (e) an unrolling of the cortical surface caudal to the dotted red line and green lines shown in (c) and (d).

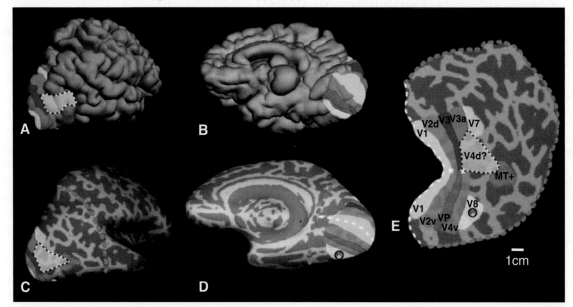

From Tootell, B. H., and Hadjikhani, N. *Cerebral Cortex*, 2001, *11*, 298–311. Reprinted with permission.

FIGURE 6.22

The Human Visual System. The figure shows the human visual system from the eye to the two streams of the visual association cortex.

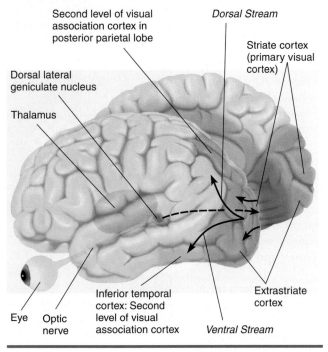

Second level of visual association cortex in posterior parietal lobe

Dorsal lateral geniculate nucleus

Thalamus

Dorsal Stream

Striate cortex (primary visual cortex)

Eye Optic nerve

Inferior temporal cortex: Second level of visual association cortex

Ventral Stream

Extrastriate cortex

At this point, the visual association cortex divides into two pathways. On the basis of their own research and a review of the literature, Ungerleider and Mishkin (1982) concluded that the visual association cortex contains two streams of analysis: the **dorsal stream** and the **ventral stream**. One stream continues forward toward a series of regions that constitute the ventral stream, terminating in the inferior temporal cortex. The other stream ascends into regions of the dorsal stream, terminating in the posterior parietal cortex. Some axons conveying information received from the magnocellular system bypass area V2: They project from area V1 directly to a region of the extrastriate cortex devoted to the analysis of movement. The ventral stream recognizes *what* an object is and what color it has, and the dorsal stream recognizes *where* the object is located and, if it is moving, its speed and direction of movement. (See *Figure 6.22*.)

As we saw, the parvocellular, koniocellular, and magnocellular systems provide different kinds of information. The magnocellular system is found in all mammals, whereas the parvocellular and koniocellular systems are found only in some species of primates. Only the cells in the parvocellular and koniocellular system analyze information concerning color. Cells in the parvocellular system also show high spatial resolution and low temporal resolution; that is, they are able to detect very fine details, but their response is slow and prolonged. The koniocellular system receives information only from "blue" cones and does not provide information about fine details. Neurons in the magnocellular system are color-blind and are not able to detect fine details, but can detect smaller contrasts between light and dark. They are also especially sensitive to movement. (See *Table 6.2*.) The dorsal stream receives mostly magnocellular input, but the ventral stream receives approximately equal input from the magnocellular and parvocellular/koniocellular systems.

Perception of Color

As we saw earlier, neurons within the CO blobs in the striate cortex respond to colors. Like the ganglion cells in the retina (and the parvocellular and koniocellular neurons in the LGN), these neurons respond in opponent fashion. This information is analyzed by the regions of the visual association cortex that constitute the ventral stream.

Studies with Laboratory Animals

Zeki (1980) found that neurons in a region of the extrastriate cortex called *V4* respond to a variety of wavelengths, not just those that correspond to red, green, yellow, and blue. This region appears to perform an important role in perception of color. The appearance of the colors of objects remains much the same whether we observe them under artificial light, under an overcast sky, or at noon on a cloudless day. This phenomenon is known as **color constancy**. Our visual system does not simply respond according to the wavelength of the light reflected by objects in each part of the visual field; instead, it compensates for the source of the light by comparing the color composition of each point in the visual field with the average color of the entire scene. If the scene contains a particularly high level of long-wavelength

dorsal stream A system of interconnected regions of visual cortex involved in the perception of spatial location, beginning with the striate cortex and ending with the posterior parietal cortex.

ventral stream A system of interconnected regions of visual cortex involved in the perception of form, beginning with the striate cortex and ending with the inferior temporal cortex.

color constancy The relatively constant appearance of the colors of objects viewed under varying lighting conditions.

cerebral achromatopsia (*ay krohm a top see a*) Inability to discriminate among different hues; caused by damage to area V8 of the visual association cortex.

TABLE 6.2   Properties of the Magnocellular, Parvocellular, and Koniocellular Divisions of the Visual System

Property	Magnocellular Division	Parvocellular Division	Koniocellular Division
Color	No	Yes (from "red" and "green" cones)	Yes (from "blue" cones)
Sensitivity to contrast	High	Low	Low
Spatial resolution (ability to detect fine details)	Low	High	low
Temporal resolution	Fast (transient response)	Slow (sustained response)	Slow (sustained response)

light (as it would if an object were illuminated by the light of a setting sun), then some long-wavelength light is "subtracted out" of the perception of each point in the scene. This compensation helps us to see what is actually out there. Electrical recording of the activity of neurons in area V4 of the monkey extrastriate cortex indicates that this region appears to contain the neural circuits that carry out this analysis (Schein and Desimone, 1990). Walsh et al. (1993) confirmed this prediction; damage to area V4 does disrupt color constancy, but not the ability to discriminate between different colors. *MyPsychKit 6.2, Color Constancy*, illustrates the effects of the color of overall illumination on color perception.

A study by Conway, Moeller, and Tsao (2007) performed a detailed analysis of the responsiveness of neurons in a large region of the visual association cortex in monkeys, including area V4. Using fMRI, the investigators identified color "hot-spots"—small scattered regions that were strongly activated by changes in the color of visual stimuli. Next, they used microelectrodes to record the response characteristics of neurons inside and outside these spots, which they called *globs*. (I'm sure the similarity between the terms "blobs" and "globs" was intentional.) They found that glob neurons were indeed responsive to colors and had only weak sensitivity to shapes. In contrast, interglob neurons (those located outside globs) did not respond to colors, but were strongly selective to shape. The fact that color-sensitive globs are spread across a wide area of visual association cortex probably explains the fact that only rather large brain lesions cause severe disruptions in perception of color.

Studies with Humans

Lesions of a region of the human visual association cortex can cause loss of color vision without disrupting visual acuity. The patients describe their vision as resembling a black-and-white film. In addition, they cannot even imagine colors or remember the colors of objects they saw before their brain damage occurred (Damasio et al., 1980; Heywood and Kentridge, 2003). The condition is known as **cerebral achromatopsia** ("vision without color"). If the brain damage is unilateral, people will lose color vision in only half of the visual field.

A functional MRI study by Hadjikhani et al. (1998) found a color-sensitive region in the inferior temporal cortex, which they called area V8. An analysis of ninety-two cases of cerebral achromatopsia by Bouvier and Engel (2006) confirmed that damage to this region (which is adjacent to and partly overlaps the *fusiform face area*, discussed later in this chapter) disrupts color vision. (See *Figure 6.23*.)

An interesting functional imaging study by Zeki and Marini (1998) found that although multicolored stimuli activated areas V1, V2, and V4, the color-sensitive region in the inferior temporal cortex that we now call area V8 was activated only when the subjects saw color photographs of real objects. In fact, photographs that showed objects in unnatural colors did *not* activate area V8. (See *Figure 6.23*.) These

mypsychkit

Animation 6.2
Color Constancy

FIGURE 6.23

Natural and Unnatural Colors.   Neurons in color-sensitive area V8 responded to photographs of objects in their natural colors (a) but not to those of objects in unnatural colors (b).

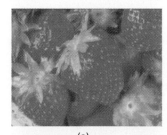

(a)

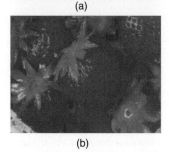

(b)

From Zeki, S., and Marini, L. *Brain*, 1998, *121*, 1669–1685.

results suggest that area V8 is involved not only with color perception, but also with the memories of colors of particular objects.

Our ability to perceive different colors helps us to perceive different objects in our environment. Thus, for us to perceive and understand what is in front of us, information about color must be combined with other forms of information. Some people with brain damage lose the ability to perceive shapes but can still perceive colors. For example, Zeki et al. (1999) described a patient who could identify colors but was otherwise blind. Patient P. B. had received an electrical shock that caused both cardiac and respiratory arrest. He was revived, but the period of anoxia caused extensive damage to his extrastriate cortex. As a result, he lost all form perception. However, even though he could not recognize objects presented on a video monitor, he could still identify their colors.

Perception of Form

The analysis of visual information that leads to the perception of form begins with neurons in the striate cortex that are sensitive to orientation and spatial frequency. These neurons send information to area V2 that is then relayed to the subregions of the visual association cortex that constitute the ventral stream.

Studies with Laboratory Animals

In primates the recognition of visual patterns and identification of particular objects take place in the inferior temporal cortex, located on the ventral part of the temporal lobe. This region of the visual association cortex is located at the end of the ventral stream. It is here that analyses of form and color are put together and perceptions of three-dimensional objects and backgrounds are achieved. Damage to this region causes severe deficits in visual discrimination (Mishkin, 1966; Gross, 1973; Dean, 1976).

In general, neurons in the inferior temporal cortex respond best to specific three-dimensional objects (or photographs of them). They respond poorly to simple stimuli such as spots, lines, or sine-wave gratings. Most of them continue to respond even when complex stimuli are moved to different locations, are changed in size, are placed against a different background, or are partially occluded by other objects (Rolls and Baylis, 1986; Kovács, Vogels, and Orban, 1995). Thus, they appear to participate in the recognition of objects rather than the analysis of specific features. The fact that neurons in the primate inferior temporal cortex respond to very specific complex shapes indicates that the development of the circuits responsible for detecting them must involve learning. The role of the inferior temporal cortex in visual learning is discussed in greater detail in Chapter 12.

Studies with Humans

Study of people who have sustained brain damage to the visual association cortex has told us much about the organization of the human visual system. In recent years, our knowledge has been greatly expanded by functional imaging studies.

Visual Agnosia   Damage to the human visual association cortex can cause a category of deficits known as **visual agnosia**. *Agnosia* ("failure to know") refers to an inability to perceive or identify a stimulus by means of a particular sensory modality, even though its details can be detected by means of that modality and the person retains relatively normal intellectual capacity.

Mrs. R., whose case was described in the opening of this chapter, had visual agnosia caused by damage to the ventral stream of her visual association cortex. As we saw, she could not identify common objects by sight, even though she had relatively normal visual acuity. However, she could still read—even small print, which indicates that reading involves different brain regions than object perception does.

visual agnosia (*ag no* zha) Deficits in visual form perception in the absence of blindness; caused by brain damage.

(Chapter 13 discusses research that has identified brain regions involved in visual recognition of letters and words.) When she was permitted to hold an object that she could not recognize visually, she could immediately recognize it by touch and say what it was, which proved that she had not lost her memory for the object or simply forgotten how to say its name.

Analysis of Specific Categories of Visual Stimuli   Visual agnosia is caused by damage to those parts of the visual association cortex that contribute to the ventral stream. In fact, damage to specific regions of the ventral stream can impair the ability to recognize specific categories of visual stimuli. Of course, even if specific regions of the visual association cortex are involved in analyzing specific categories of stimuli, the boundaries of brain lesions will seldom coincide the boundaries of brain regions with particular functions.

With the advent of functional imaging, investigators have studied the responses of the normal human brain and have discovered several regions of the ventral stream that are activated by the sight of particular categories of visual stimuli. For example, functional imaging studies have identified regions of the inferior temporal and lateral occipital cortex that are specifically activated by categories such as animals, tools, cars, flowers, letters and letter strings, faces, bodies, and scenes. (See Tootell, Tsao, and Vanduffel, 2003, and Grill-Spector and Malach, 2004 for a review.) However, not all of these findings have been replicated, and, of course, people can learn to recognize shapes that do not fall into these categories. A relatively large region of the ventral stream of the visual association cortex, the **lateral occipital complex (LOC)**, appears to respond to a wide variety of objects and shapes.

A common symptom of visual agnosia is **prosopagnosia**, the inability to recognize particular faces (*prosopon* is Greek for "face"). That is, patients with this disorder can recognize that they are looking at a face, but they cannot say whose face it is—even if it belongs to a relative or close friend. They see eyes, ears, a nose, a mouth, but they cannot recognize the particular configuration of these features that identifies an individual face. They still remember who these people are and will usually recognize them when they hear their voice. As one patient said, "I have trouble recognizing people from just faces alone. I look at their hair color, listen to their voices. . . . I use clothing, voice, and hair. I try to associate something with a person one way or another . . . what they wear, how their hair is worn" (Buxbaum, Glosser, and Coslett, 1999, p. 43).

Studies with brain-damaged people and functional imaging studies suggest that these special face-recognizing circuits are found in the **fusiform face area (FFA)**, located in the fusiform gyrus on the base of the temporal lobe. For example, Grill-Spector, Knouf, and Kanwisher (2004) obtained fMRI scans of the brains of people who looked at pictures of faces and several other categories of objects. Figure 6.24 shows the results, projected on an "inflated" ventral view of the cerebral cortex. The black outlines show the regions of the fusiform cortex that were activated by viewing faces, drawn on all images of the brain for comparison with the activation produced by other categories of objects. As you can see, images of faces activated the regions indicated by these outlines better than other categories of visual stimuli. (See ***Figure 6.24***.)

Most cases of prosopagnosia occur as a result of damage to the brain of a person who previously had no difficulty recognizing faces. In contrast, *developmental prosopagnosia* (also known as *congenital prosopagnosia*) refers to difficulty recognizing faces that becomes apparent as children develop. A diffusion tensor imaging (DTI) study by Thomas et al. (2009) found that the fiber bundles that transmit visual information to the FFA were smaller in people with developmental prosopagnosia. As Figure 6.25 shows, the right inferior longitudinal fasciculus (ILF) of people with developmental prosopagnosia contained fewer axons than those of people with normal ability to recognize faces. (The ILF connects the FFA with regions of the ventral stream in the temporal cortex.) In fact, Thomas et al. found that the number of

lateral occipital complex (LOC) A region of the extrastriate cortex, involved in perception of objects other than people's bodies and faces.

prosopagnosia (*prah soh pag **no** zha*) Failure to recognize particular people by the sight of their faces.

fusiform face area (FFA) A region of the visual association cortex located in the inferior temporal; involved in perception of faces.

FIGURE 6.24

Responses to Categories of Visual Stimuli.   These functional MRI scans are of people looking at six categories of visual stimuli. Neural activity is shown on "inflated" ventral views of the cerebral cortex. The fusiform face area is shown as a black outline, derived from the responses to faces shown in the upper left scan.

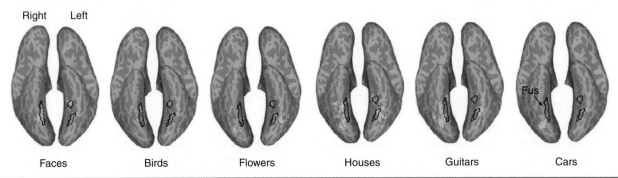

Reprinted by permission from Macmillan Publishers Ltd: *Nature Neuroscience*, Grill-Spector, K., Knouf, N., and Knawisher, N. The fusiform face perception, not generic within-category identification, *7*, 555–561, copyright 2004.

FIGURE 6.25

Perception of Faces and Bodies.   The fusiform face area (FFA) and the extrastriate body area (EBA) were activated by images of faces, headless bodies, body parts, and assorted objects.

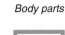

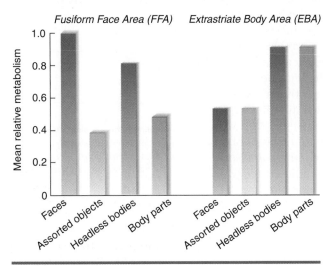

Adapted from Schwarzlose, R. F., Baker, C. I., and Kanwisher, N. *Journal of Neuroscience*, 2005, *23*, 11055–11059.

axons in the ILF was correlated with this ability. In support this finding, Yamasaki et al. (2004) reported a case of prosopagnosia in a patient with multiple sclerosis that was caused by damage to the ILF.

Another interesting region of the ventral stream is the **extrastriate body area (EBA)**, which is just posterior to the FFA and partly overlaps it. Downing et al. (2006) found that this region was specifically activated by photographs, silhouettes, or stick drawings of human bodies or body parts and not by control stimuli such as photographs or drawings of tools, scrambled silhouettes, or scrambled stick drawings of human bodies. Figure 6.25 shows the magnitude of the fMRI response in the nonoverlapping regions of the FFA and EBA to several categories of stimuli (Schwarzlose, Baker, and Kanwisher, 2005). As you can see, the FFA responded to faces more than any of the other categories, and the EBA showed the greatest response to headless bodies and body parts. (See *Figure 6.25*.)

Urgesi, Berlucchi, and Aglioti (2004) used transcranial magnetic stimulation to temporarily disrupt the normal neural activity of the EBA. (As we saw in Chapter 5, the TMS procedure applies a strong localized magnetic field to the brain by passing an electrical current through a coil of wire placed on the scalp.) The investigators found that the disruption temporarily impaired people's ability to recognize photographs of body parts, but not parts of faces or motorcycles.

As we will see in Chapter 12, the hippocampus and nearby regions of the medial temporal cortex are involved in spatial perception and memory. Several studies have identified a **parahippocampal place area (PPA)**, located in a region of limbic cortex bordering the ventromedial temporal lobe, that is activated by the sight of scenes and backgrounds. For example, Steeves et al. (2004) studied Patient D. F., a 47-year-old woman who had sustained brain damage caused by accidental carbon monoxide poisoning 14 years earlier. Bilateral damage to her lateral occipital cortex (an important part of the ventral stream) caused a profound visual agnosia for objects. However, she was able to recognize both natural and human-made scenes (beaches, forests, deserts, cities, markets, and rooms). Functional imaging showed activation of her intact PPA. These results suggest that scene recognition does not depend on recognition of particular objects found within the scene, because D. F. was incapable of recognizing these objects.

By the way, there are three basic ways that we can recognize individual faces: differences in features (for example, the size and shape of the eyes, nose, and mouth), differences in contour (the all-over shape of the face), and differences in configuration of features (for example, the spacing of the eyes, nose, and mouth). Figure 6.26 illustrates these differences in a series of composite faces (Le Grand et al., 2003). You can see that the face on the left is the same in each of the rows. The faces in the top row contain different features: eyes and mouths from photos of different people. (The noses are all the same.) The faces in the middle row are all of the same person, but the contours of the faces have different shapes. The faces in the bottom row contain different configurations of features from one individual. In these faces, the spacing between the eyes and between the eyes and the mouth has been altered. Differences in configuration are the most difficult to detect. (See *Figure 6.26*.)

As we will see in Chapter 16, people with autistic disorder fail to develop normal social relations with other people. Indeed, in severe cases they give no signs that they recognize that other people exist. Grelotti, Gauthier, and Schultz (2002) found that people with autistic disorder showed a deficit in the ability to recognize faces and that looking at faces failed to activate the fusiform gyrus. The authors speculated that the lack of interest in other people, caused by the brain abnormalities responsible for autism, resulted in a lack of motivation that normally promotes the acquisition of expertise in recognizing faces as a child grows up. Chapter 16 discusses autistic disorder in greater detail.

Perception of Movement

We need to know not only what things are, but also where they are and if they are moving, where they are going. Without the ability to perceive the direction and velocity of movement of objects, we would have no way to predict where they will be. We would be unable to catch them (or avoid letting them catch us). This section examines the perception of movement; the final section examines the perception of location.

Studies with Laboratory Animals

One of the regions of the extrastriate cortex—area V5, also known as area MT, for *medial temporal*—contains neurons that respond to movement. Damage to this region severely disrupts a monkey's ability to perceive moving stimuli (Siegel and Andersen, 1986). Area V5 receives input directly from the striate cortex and from several regions of the extrastriate cortex. It also receives input from the superior colliculus, which is involved in visual reflexes, including reflexive control of eye movements.

A region adjacent to area V5 (sometimes called V5a but more often referred to as MST, for *medial superior temporal*) receives information about movement from V5 and performs a further analysis. MST neurons respond to complex patterns of movement, including radial, circular, and spiral motion (see Vaina, 1998, for a

FIGURE 6.26

Composite Faces.   The faces in the top row contain different features: eyes and mouths from photos of different people. The middle row of faces are all of the same person, but the contours of the faces have different shapes. The faces in the bottom row contain different configurations of features from one individual: The spacing between the eyes and between the eyes and the mouth have been altered.

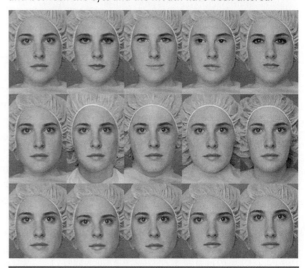

Reprinted by permission from Macmillan Publishers Ltd: *Nature Neuroscience*, Le Grand, R., Mondloch, C. J., Maurer, D., and Brent, H. P., Expert face processing requires visual input to the right hemisphere during infancy, 6, 1108–1112, copyright 2003.

extrastriate body area (EBA) A region of the visual association cortex located in the lateral occipitotemporal cortex; involved in perception of the human body and body parts other than faces.

parahippocampal place area (PPA) A region of the medial temporal cortex; involved in perception of particular places ("scenes").

FIGURE 6.27

Location of Visual Area V5. The location of visual area V5 (also called MT/MST or MT+) in the human brain was identified by a stain that showed the presence of a dense projection of thick, heavily myelinated axons. LOS = lateral occipital sulcus, IOS = inferior occipital sulcus.

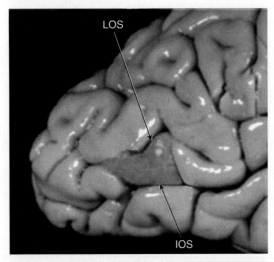

From Annese, J., Gazzaniga, M. S., and Toga, A. W., Localization of the Human Cortical Visual Area MT Based on Computer Aided Histological Analysis, *Cerebral Cortex*, 2005, *15*, 7, 1044–1053, by permission of Oxford University Press.

review). One important function of this region—in particular, the dorsolateral MST, or MSTd—appears to be analysis of **optic flow**. As we move around in our environment or as objects in our environment move in relation to us, the sizes, shapes, and locations of environmental features on our retinas change. Imagine the image seen by a video camera as you walk along a street, pointing the lens of the camera straight in front of you. Suppose your path will pass just to the right of a mailbox. The image of the mailbox will slowly get larger. Finally, as you pass it, it will veer to the left and disappear. Points on the sidewalk will move downward, and branches of trees that you pass under will move upward. Analysis of the relative movement of the visual elements of your environment—the optic flow—will tell you where you are heading, how fast you are approaching different items in front of you, and whether you will pass to the left or right (or under or over) these items. The point toward which we are moving does not move, but all other points in the visual scene move away from it. Therefore, this point is called the *center of expansion*. If we keep moving in the same direction, we will eventually bump into an object that lies at the center of expansion. We can also use optic flow to determine whether an object approaching us will hit us or pass us by. Britten and van Wezel (1998) found that electrical stimulation of MSTd disrupted monkeys' ability to perceive the apparent direction in which they were heading; thus, these neurons do indeed seem to play an essential role in heading estimation derived from optic flow.

Studies with Humans

Perception of Motion Functional imaging studies suggest that a motion-sensitive area (usually called MT/MST) is found within the inferior temporal sulcus of the human brain (Dukelow et al., 2001). However, a more recent study suggests that this region is located in the lateral occipital cortex, between the lateral and inferior occipital sulci (Annese, Gazzaniga, and Toga, 2005). Annese and his colleagues examined sections of the brains of deceased subjects that had been stained for the presence of myelin. Area V5 receives a dense projection of thick, heavily myelinated axons, and the location of this region was revealed by the myelin stain. (See *Figure 6.27*.)

Bilateral damage to the human brain that includes the motion-sensitive area produces an inability to perceive movement—**akinetopsia**. For example, Zihl et al. (1991) reported the case of a woman with bilateral lesions that damaged area MT/MST.

optic flow The complex motion of points in the visual field caused by relative movement between the observer and environment; provides information about the relative distance of objects from the observer and of the relative direction of movement.

akinetopsia Inability to perceive movement, caused by damage to area V5 (also called MST) of the visual association cortex.

Patient L. M. had an almost total loss of movement perception. She was unable to cross a street without traffic lights, because she could not judge the speed at which cars were moving. Although she could perceive movements, she found moving objects very unpleasant to look at. For example, while talking with another person, she avoided looking at the person's mouth because she found its movements very disturbing. When the investigators asked her to try to detect movements of a visual target in the laboratory, she said, "First the target is completely at rest. Then it suddenly jumps upwards and downwards" (Zihl et al., 1991, p. 2244). She was able to see that the target was constantly changing its position, but she was unaware of any sensation of movement.

Walsh and Devlin (1998) used transcranial magnetic stimulation (TMS) to temporarily inactivate area MT/MST in normal human subjects. The investigators found that during the stimulation, people were unable to detect which of several objects displayed on a computer screen was moving. When the current was off, the subjects had no trouble detecting the motion. The current had no effect on the subjects' ability to recognize stimuli with different shapes. (*MyPsychKit 6.3, Motion Aftereffects*, illustrates an interesting movement-related phenomenon.)

Optic Flow   As we saw in the previous subsection, neurons in area MSTd of the monkey brain respond to optic flow, an important source of information about the direction in which the animal is heading. A functional imaging study by Peuskens et al. (2001) found that the corresponding area in the human brain became active when people judged their heading while viewing a display showing optic flow. Vaina and her colleagues (Jornales et al., 1997; Vaina, 1998) found that people with damage to this region were able to perceive motion but could not perceive heading from optic flow.

Form from Motion   Perception of movement can even help us to perceive three-dimensional forms—a phenomenon known as *form from motion.* Johansson (1973) demonstrated just how much information we can derive from movement. He dressed actors in black and attached small lights to several points on their bodies, such as their wrists, elbows, shoulders, hips, knees, and feet. He made movies of the actors in a darkened room while they were performing various behaviors, such as walking, running, jumping, limping, doing push-ups, and dancing with a partner who was also equipped with lights. Even though observers who watched the films could see only a pattern of moving lights against a dark background, they could readily perceive the pattern as belonging to a moving human and could identify the behavior the actor was performing. Subsequent studies (Kozlowski and Cutting, 1977; Barclay, Cutting, and Kozlowski, 1978) showed that people could even tell, with reasonable accuracy, the sex of the actor wearing the lights. The cues appeared to be supplied by the relative amounts of movement of the shoulders and hips as the person walked.

A functional imaging study by Grossman et al. (2000) found that when people viewed a video that showed form from motion, a small region on the ventral bank of the posterior end of the superior temporal sulcus became active. More activity was seen in the right hemisphere, whether the images were presented to the left or right visual field. Grossman and Blake (2001) found that this region became active even when people *imagined* that they were watching points of light representing form from motion. (See *MyPsychKit 6.4, Form from Motion.*)

Perception of form from motion might not seem like a phenomenon that has any importance outside the laboratory. However, this phenomenon does occur under natural circumstances, and it appears to involve brain mechanisms different from those involved in normal object perception. For example, as we saw in the prologue to this chapter, people with visual agnosia can often still perceive *actions* (such as someone pretending to stir something in a bowl or deal out some playing cards) even though they cannot recognize objects by sight. They may be able to recognize friends by the way they walk, even though they cannot recognize their faces. As we saw earlier in this chapter, neurons in the extrastriate body area (EBA) are activated by the sight of human body parts. A functional imaging study by Pelphrey et al. (2005) observed activation of a brain region just anterior to the EBA when subjects viewed people's hand, eye, and mouth movements.

Lê et al. (2002) reported the case of patient S. B., a 30-year-old man whose ventral stream was damaged extensively bilaterally by encephalitis when he was 3 years old. As a result, he was unable to recognize objects, faces, textures, or colors. However, he could perceive movement and could even catch a ball that was thrown to him. Furthermore, he could recognize other people's arm and hand movements that mimed common activities such as cutting something with a knife or brushing one's teeth, and he could recognize people he knew by their gait.

mypsychkit
Animation 6.3
Motion Aftereffects

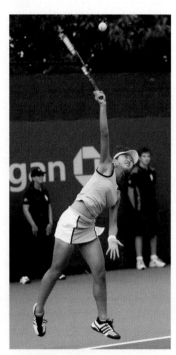

Tracking moving objects by the visual system is an important role in many skill activities.

mypsychkit
Animation 6.4
Form from Motion

FIGURE 6.28

The Posterior Parietal Cortex. An "inflated" dorsal view of the left hemisphere of a human brain shows the anatomy of the posterior parietal cortex.

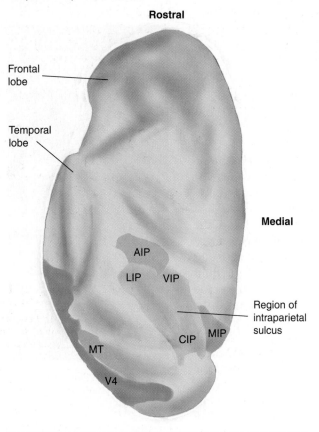

Rostral

Frontal lobe

Temporal lobe

Medial

AIP

LIP   VIP

Region of intraparietal sulcus

MT   CIP   MIP

V4

Adapted from Astafiev, S. V., Shulman, G. L., Stanley, C. M., Snyder, A. Z., Van Essen, D. C., and Corbetta, M. *Journal of Neuroscience*, 2003, *23*, 4689–4699.

intraparietal sulcus (IPS) The end of the dorsal stream of the visual association cortex; involved in perception of location, visual attention, and control of eye and hand movements.

Perception of Spatial Location

The parietal lobe is involved in spatial and somatosensory perception, and it receives visual, auditory, somatosensory, and vestibular information to perform these tasks. Damage to the parietal lobes disrupts performance on a variety of tasks that require perceiving and remembering the locations of objects and controlling movements of the eyes and the limbs. The dorsal stream of the visual association cortex terminates in the posterior parietal cortex.

The anatomy of the posterior parietal cortex is shown in Figure 6.28. We see an "inflated" dorsal view of the left hemisphere of a human brain. Five regions within the **intraparietal sulcus (IPS)** are of particular interest: AIP, LIP, VIP, CIP, and MIP (anterior, lateral, ventral, caudal, and medial IPS) are indicated. (See *Figure 6.28.*)

Single-unit studies with monkeys and functional imaging studies with humans indicate that neurons in the IPS are involved in visual attention and control of saccadic eye movements (LIP and VIP), visual control of reaching and pointing (VIP and MIP), visual control of grasping and manipulating hand movements (AIP), and perception of depth from stereopsis (CIP) (Snyder, Batista, and Andersen, 2000; Culham and Kanwisher, 2001; Astafiev et al., 2003; Tsao et al., 2003; Frey et al., 2005).

Goodale and his colleagues (Goodale and Milner, 1992; Goodale et al., 1994; Goodale and Westwood, 2004) suggested that the primary function of the dorsal stream of the visual cortex is to guide actions rather than simply to perceive spatial locations. As Ungerleider and Mishkin (1982) originally put it, the ventral and dorsal streams tell us "what" and "where." Goodale and his colleagues suggested that the better terms are "what" and "*how*." They cited the case of a woman with bilateral lesions of the posterior parietal cortex who had no difficulty recognizing line drawings (that is, her ventral stream was intact) but who had trouble picking up objects (Jakobson et al., 1991). The patient could easily perceive the difference in size of wooden blocks that were set out before her, but she failed to adjust the distance between her thumb and forefinger to the size of the block she was about to pick up. In contrast, a patient with profound visual agnosia caused by damage to the ventral stream could not distinguish between wooden blocks of different sizes but *could* adjust the distance between her thumb and forefinger when she picked them up. She made this adjustment by means of vision, before she actually touched them (Milner et al., 1991; Goodale et al., 1994). A functional imaging study of this patient (James et al., 2003) showed normal activity in the dorsal stream while she was picking up objects—especially in the anterior intraparietal sulcus (AIP), which is involved in manipulating and grasping.

The suggestion by Goodale and his colleagues seems a reasonable one. Certainly, the dorsal stream is involved in perception of the location of object's space—but then, if its primary role is to direct movements, it *must* be involved in location of these objects, or else how could it direct movements toward them? In addition, it must contain information about the size and shape of objects, or else how could it control the distance between thumb and forefinger?

A fascinating (and delightful) study with young children demonstrates the importance of communication between the dorsal and ventral streams of the visual system (DeLoache, Uttal, and Rosengren, 2004). The experimenters let children play with large toys: an indoor slide that they could climb and slide down, a chair that they could sit on, and a toy car that they could enter. After the children played in and on the large toys, the children were brought out of the room, the large toys were replaced with identical miniature versions, and the children were then brought back into the room. When the children played with the miniature toys, they acted as if they were the large versions: They tried to climb onto the slide, climb into the car, and sit on the chair. *MyPsychKit 6.5, Dissociation of Perception and Action* shows a video of a 2-year-old child trying to climb into the toy car. He says "In!" several times, and calls for his mother, apparently asking her to help him. The authors suggest that this behavior reflects incomplete maturation of connections between the dorsal and ventral streams. The ventral stream recognizes the identity of the objects and the dorsal stream recognizes their size, but the information is not adequately shared between these two systems.

The importance of the visual system is shown by the fact that approximately 25 percent of our cerebral cortex is devoted to this sense modality and by the many discoveries being made by the laboratories that are busy discovering interesting things about vision. *Figure 6.29* shows the location of the regions that make up the ventral stream and some of the dorsal stream. (The rest of the dorsal stream lies in the intraparietal sulcus, which is illustrated in Figure 6.29.) *Table 6.3* lists these regions and summarizes their major functions.

FIGURE 6.29

Components of the Ventral and Dorsal Streams of the Visual Cortex.   The figure shows some major components of the ventral stream and some of the dorsal stream of the visual cortex. The view is similar to that seen in Figure 6.21(e).

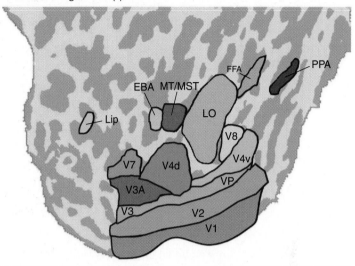

Adapted from Tootell, R. B. H., Tsao, D., and Vanduffel, W. *Journal of Neuroscience*, 2003, *23*, 3981–3989.

mypsychkit

Animation 6.5
Dissociation of Perception and Action

InterimSummary

Analysis of Visual Information: Role of the Visual Association Cortex

The visual cortex consists of the striate cortex and two streams of visual association cortex. The ventral stream, which ends with the inferior temporal cortex, is involved with perception of objects. The dorsal stream, which ends with the posterior parietal cortex, is involved with perception of movement, location, visual attention, and control of eye and hand movements. There are at least two dozen different subregions of the visual cortex, arranged in a hierarchical fashion. Each region analyzes a particular characteristic of visual information and passes the results of this analysis to other regions in the hierarchy. Damage to area V4 abolishes color constancy (accurate perception of color under different lighting conditions), and damage to area V8 causes cerebral achromatopsia, a loss of color vision but not of form perception.

Functional imaging studies indicate that specific regions of the cortex are involved in perception of form, movement, and color, and these studies are enabling us to discover the correspondences between the anatomy of the human visual system and that of labora-

tory animals. Studies of humans who have sustained damage to the ventral stream of visual association cortex sustain a perceptual impairment known as visual agnosia.

Prosopagnosia—failure to recognize faces—is caused by damage to the fusiform face area, a region on the medial surface of the extrastriate cortex on the base of the brain. The fusiform face region fails to develop in people with autism, presumably because of insufficient motivation to become expert in recognizing other people's faces. Other specialized regions of the visual association cortex are involved in the recognition of body parts and environmental scenes.

Damage to area V5 (also called area MT/MST) disrupts an animal's ability to perceive movement, and damage to the posterior parietal cortex disrupts perception of the spatial location of objects. Damage to the human visual association cortex corresponding to area V5 disrupts perception of movement, producing a disorder known as akinetopsia. In addition, transcranial magnetic stimulation of V5 causes a temporary disruption of perception of motion,

TABLE 6.3   Regions of the Human Visual Cortex and Their Functions

Region of Human Visual Cortex	Name of Region (If Different)	Function
V1	Striate cortex	Small modules that analyze orientation, movement, spatial frequency, retinal disparity, and color
V2		Further analysis of information from V1
Ventral Stream		
V3 and VP		Further analysis of information from V2
V3A		Processing of visual information across entire visual field of contralateral eye
V4d/V4v	V4 dorsal/ventral	Analysis of form
		Processing of color constancy
		V4v = upper visual field, V4d = lower visual field
V8	Lateral occipital complex	Color perception
LOC	Fusiform face area	Object recognition
FFA		Face recognition, object recognition by experts ("flexible fusiform area")
	Parahippocampal place area	
PPA	Extrastriate body area	Recognition of particular places and scenes
EBA		Perception of body parts other than face
Dorsal Stream		
V7		Visual attention
		Control of eye movements
V5 (also called MT/MST or MT+)	Medial temporal/medial superior temporal (named for locations in monkey brain)	Perception of motion
		Perception of biological motion and optic flow in specific subregions
LIP	Lateral intraparietal area	Visual attention
		Control of saccadic eye movements
VIP	Ventral intraparietal area	Control of visual attention to particular locations
		Control of eye movements
		Visual control of pointing
AIP	Anterior intraparietal area	Visual control of hand movements: grasping, manipulation
MIP	Middle intraparietal area	Visual control of reaching
	Parietal reach region (monkeys)	
CIP	Caudal intraparietal area	Perception of depth from stereopsis
	Caudal parietal disparity region	

and functional imaging studies show that perception of moving stimuli activate this region. In both monkeys and humans, area MSTd, a region of extrastriate cortex adjacent to area V5, appears to be specialized for perceiving optic flow, one of the cues we use to perceive the direction in which we are heading. The ability to perceive form from motion—recognition of complex movements of people indicated by lights attached to parts of their body—is probably related to the ability to recognize people by the way they walk. This ability apparently depends on a region of cerebral cortex on the ventral bank of the posterior end of the superior temporal sulcus.

Most of the visual association cortex at the end of the dorsal stream is located in the intraparietal sulcus: LIP and VIP are involved in visual attention and control of saccadic eye movements,

VIP and MIP are involved in visual control of reaching and pointing, AIP is involved in visual control of grasping and manipulating, and CIP is involved in perception of depth from stereopsis.

Goodale and his colleagues suggest that the primary function of the dorsal stream of the visual association cortex is better characterized as "how" rather than "what"; the role of the posterior parietal cortex in control of reaching, grasping, and manipulation requires visually derived information of movement, depth, and location.

Thought Question

Some psychologists are interested in "top-down" processes in visual perception—that is, the effects of context on perceiving ambiguous stimuli. For example, if you are in a dimly lighted kitchen and see a shape that could be either a loaf of bread or a country mailbox, you will be more likely to perceive the object as a loaf of bread. Where in the brain might contextual information affect perception?

⋮ EPILOGUE   Case Studies

The discussion of Mrs. R. in the prologue raises an issue about research that I would like to address: the issue of making generalizations from the study of an individual patient. Some researchers have argued that because no two people are alike, we cannot make generalizations from a single individual such as Mrs. R. They say that valid inferences can be made only from studies that involve *groups* of people, so that individual differences can be accounted for statistically. Is this criticism valid?

The careful, detailed investigation of the abilities and disabilities of a single person is called a *case study*. In my opinion, case studies of people with brain damage can provide very useful information. In the first place, even if we were not able to make firm conclusions from the study of one person, a careful analysis of the pattern of deficits shown by an individual patient might give us some useful ideas for further research, and sources of good ideas for research should not be neglected. However, under some circumstances we *can* draw conclusions from a single case.

Before describing what kinds of inferences we can and cannot make from case studies, let me review what we hope to accomplish by studying the behavior of people with brain damage. The brain seems to be organized in modules. A given module receives information from other modules, performs some kinds of analysis, and sends the results on to other modules with which it communicates. In some cases, the wiring of the module may change. That is, synaptic connections may be modified so that in the future the module will respond differently to its inputs. (As you will see in Chapter 12, the ability of modules to modify their synaptic connections serves as the basis for the ability to learn and remember.)

If we want to understand how the brain works, we have to know what the individual modules do. A particular module is not *responsible* for a behavior; instead, it performs one of the many functions that are necessary for a set of behaviors. For example, as I sit here typing this epilogue, I am using modules that perform functions related to posture and balance, to the control of eye movements, to memories related to the topic I am writing about, to memories of English words and their spellings, to control of finger movements . . . well, you get the idea. We would rarely try to analyze such a complex task as sitting and writing an epilogue, but we might try to analyze how we spell a familiar English word. Possibly, we use modules that perform functions normally related to hearing: We use these modules to "hear" the word in our head and then use other modules to convert the sounds into the appropriate patterns of letters. Alternatively, we may picture the word we want to spell, which would use modules that perform functions related to vision. I do not want to go into the details of spelling and writing here (they will be covered in Chapter 13), but I do want you to see why it is important to try to understand the functions performed by groups of modules located in particular parts of the brain. In practice, this means studying and analyzing the pattern of deficits shown by people with brain damage.

What kinds of conclusions can we make by studying a single individual? We *cannot* conclude that because two behaviors are impaired, the deficit is caused by damage to a set of common modules needed for both behaviors. Instead, it could be that behavior X is impaired by damage to module A and behavior Y is impaired by damage to module B and it just happens that modules A and B were both damaged by the brain lesion. However, we *can* conclude that if a brain lesion causes a loss of behavior X but not of behavior Y, then the functions performed by the damaged modules are not required to perform behavior Y. The study of a single patient permits us to make this conclusion.

You can see that although case studies do not permit us to make sweeping conclusions, under the right circumstances we can properly draw firm if modest conclusions that help us to understand the organization of the brain and suggest hypotheses to test with further research.

Key Concepts

THE STIMULUS

1. Light, a form of electromagnetic radiation, can vary in wavelength, intensity, and purity; it can thus give rise to differences in perceptions of hue, brightness, and saturation.

ANATOMY OF THE VISUAL SYSTEM

2. The eyes are complex sensory organs that focus an image of the environment on the retina. The retina consists of three layers: the photoreceptor layer (rods and cones), the bipolar cell layer, and the ganglion cell layer.

3. Information from the eye is sent to the parvocellular, koniocellular, and magnocellular layers of the dorsal lateral geniculate nucleus and then to the primary visual cortex (striate cortex).

CODING OF VISUAL INFORMATION IN THE RETINA

4. When light strikes a molecule of photopigment in a photoreceptor, the molecule splits and initiates a receptor potential.

5. Ganglion cells of the retina respond in an opposing center/surround fashion.

6. Colors are detected by three types of cones, and the code is changed into an opponent-process system by the time it reaches the retinal ganglion cells.

ANALYSIS OF VISUAL INFORMATION: ROLE OF THE STRIATE CORTEX

7. Neurons in the striate cortex are organized in modules, each containing two blobs. Neurons within the blobs respond to color; those outside the blobs respond to orientation, movement, spatial frequency, and retinal disparity.

8. Visual information is processed by two parallel systems: the magnocellular system and the parvocellular/koniocellular system.

ANALYSIS OF VISUAL INFORMATION: ROLE OF THE VISUAL ASSOCIATION CORTEX

9. Specific regions of the extrastriate cortex receive information about specific features of the visual scene from the striate cortex, analyze it, and send their information on to higher levels of visual association cortex.

10. The association cortex of the inferior temporal lobe (ventral stream) recognizes the shape of objects, whereas the parietal cortex (dorsal stream) recognizes their location.

11. Damage to the visual association cortex can disrupt visual perception. The fusiform gyrus on the base of the occipital lobe is involved in perception of faces. An adjacent region is involved in perception of bodies and body parts, and the parahippocampal gyrus contains a region involved in perception of environmental scenes. A region located in the extrastriate cortex (V8) is involved in color vision.

12. The region corresponding to area V5 is involved in perception of movement, and a nearby region (MSTd) is involved in perception of optic flow. Five regions within the intraparietal sulcus are involved in visual attention; control of eye movements; visual control of reaching, pointing, grasping, and manipulating; and perception of depth from stereopsis.

Suggested Readings

Gregory, R. L. *Eye and Brain: The Psychology of Seeing,* 5th ed. Princeton, NJ: Princeton University Press, 1997.

Grill-Spector, K., and Malach, R. The human visual cortex. *Annual Review of Neuroscience,* 2002, *27,* 649–677.

Jacobs, G. H., and Nathans, J. The evolution of primate color vision. *Scientific American,* 2009, *300,* 56–63.

Oyster, C. W. *The Human Eye: Structure and Function.* Sunderland, MA: Sinauer Associates, 1999.

Purves, D., and Lotto, R. B. *Why We See What We Do: An Empirical Theory of Vision.* Sunderland, MA: Sinauer Associates, 2002.

Rodieck, R. W. *The First Steps in Seeing.* Sunderland, MA: Sinauer Associates, 1998.

Solomon, S. G., and Lennie, P. The machinery of colour vision. *Nature Reviews: Neuroscience,* 2007, *8,* 276–286.

Wandell, B. A. *Foundations of Vision: Behavior, Neuroscience, and Computation.* Sunderland, MA: Sinauer Associates, 1995.

Additional Resources

Visit www.mypsychkit.com for additional review and practice of the material covered in this chapter. Within MyPsychKit, you can take practice tests and receive a customized study plan to help you review. Dozens of animations, tutorials, and Web links are also available. You can even review using the interactive electronic version of this textbook. You will need to register for MyPsychKit. See www.mypsychkit.com for complete details.

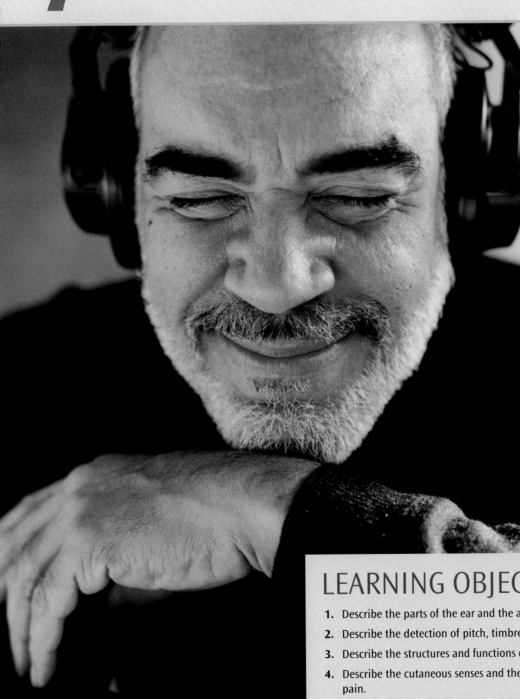

chapter 7

- Audition, the Body
- Senses, and the
- Chemical Senses

LEARNING OBJECTIVES

1. Describe the parts of the ear and the auditory pathway.

2. Describe the detection of pitch, timbre, and the location of the source of a sound.

3. Describe the structures and functions of the vestibular system.

4. Describe the cutaneous senses and their response to touch, temperature, and pain.

5. Describe the somatosensory pathways and the perception of pain.

6. Describe the five taste qualities, the anatomy of the taste buds and how they detect taste, and the gustatory pathway and neural coding of taste.

7. Describe the major structures of the olfactory system, explain how odors are detected, and describe the patterns of neural activity produced by these stimuli.

PROLOGUE   All in Her Head?

Melissa, a junior at the state university, had volunteered to be a subject in an experiment at the dental school. She had been told that she might feel a little pain but that everything was under medical supervision and no harm would come to her. She didn't particularly like the idea of pain, but she would be well paid, and she saw in the experience an opportunity to live up to her own self-image as being as brave as anyone.

She entered the reception room, where she signed consent forms saying that she agreed to participate in the experiment and knew that a physician would be giving her a drug and that her reaction to pain would be measured. The experimenter greeted her, led her to a room, and asked her to be seated in a dental chair. He inserted a needle attached to a plastic tube into a vein in her right arm so that he could inject drugs.

"First," he said, "we want to find out how sensitive you are to pain." He showed her a device that looked something like an electric toothbrush with a metal probe on the end. "This device will stimulate nerves in the pulp of your tooth. Do you have some fillings?" She nodded. "Have you ever bitten on some aluminum foil?" She winced and nodded again. "Good, then you will know what to expect." He adjusted a dial on the stimulator, touched the tip of it to a tooth, and pressed the button. No response. He turned the dial and stimulated the tooth again. Still no response. He turned the dial again, and this time, the stimulation made her gasp and wince. He recorded the voltage setting in his notebook.

"Okay, now we know how sensitive this tooth is to pain. Now I'm going to give you a drug we are testing. It should decrease the pain quite a bit." He injected the drug and after a short while said, "Let's try the tooth again." The drug apparently worked; he had to increase the voltage considerably before she felt any pain.

"Now," he said, "I want to give you some more of the drug to see if we can make you feel even less pain." He gave another injection and, after a little wait, tested her again. But the drug had not further decreased her pain sensitivity; instead, it had

increased it; she was now as sensitive as she had been before the first injection.

After the experiment was over, the experimenter walked with Melissa into a lounge. "I want to tell you about the experiment you were in, but I'd like to ask you not to talk about it with other people who might also serve as subjects." She nodded her head in agreement.

"Actually, you did not receive a painkiller. The first injection was pure salt water."

"It was? But I thought it made me less sensitive to pain."

"It did. When an innocuous substance such as an injection of salt water or a sugar pill has an effect like that, we call it a placebo effect."

"You mean that it was all in my mind? That I only *thought* that the shock hurt less?"

"No. Well, that is, it was necessary for you to think that you had received a painkiller. But the effect was a physiological one. We know that, because the second injection contained a drug that counteracts the effects of opiates."

"Opiates? You mean like morphine or heroin?"

"Yes." He saw her start to protest, shook his head, and said, "No, I'm sure you don't take drugs. But your brain makes them. For reasons we still do not understand, your believing that you had received a painkiller caused some cells in your brain to release a chemical that acts the way opiates do. The chemical acts on other neurons in your brain and decreases your sensitivity to pain. When I gave you the second injection—the drug that counteracts opiates—your sensitivity to pain came back."

"But then, did my mind or my brain make the placebo effect happen?"

"Well, think about it. Your mind and your brain are not really separate. Experiences can change the way your brain functions, and these changes can alter your experiences. Mind and brain have to be studied together, not separately."

One chapter was devoted to vision, but the rest of the sensory modalities must share a chapter. This unequal allocation of space reflects the relative importance of vision to our species and the relative amount of research that has been devoted to it. This chapter is divided into five major sections, which discuss audition, the vestibular system, the somatosenses, gustation, and olfaction.

Audition

For most people audition is the second most important sense. The value of verbal communication makes it even more important than vision in some respects; for example, a blind person can join others in conversation more easily than a deaf person can. (Of course, deaf people can use sign language to converse with others.) Acoustic stimuli also provide information about things that are hidden from view, and our ears work just as well in the dark. This section describes the nature of the stimulus, the sensory receptors, the brain mechanisms devoted to audition, and some of the details of the physiology of auditory perception.

The Stimulus

We hear sounds, which are produced by objects that vibrate and set molecules of air into motion. When an object vibrates, its movements cause molecules of air surrounding it alternately to condense and rarefy (pull apart), producing waves that travel away from the object at approximately 700 miles per hour. If the vibration ranges between approximately 30 and 20,000 times per second, these waves will stimulate receptor cells in our ears and will be perceived as sounds. (See **Figure 7.1.**)

In Chapter 6 we saw that light has three perceptual dimensions—hue, brightness, and saturation—that correspond to three physical dimensions. Similarly, sounds vary in their pitch, loudness, and timbre. The perceived **pitch** of an auditory stimulus is determined by the frequency of vibration, which is measured in **hertz (Hz)**, or cycles per second. (The term honors Heinrich Hertz, a nineteenth-century German physicist.) **Loudness** is a function of intensity—the degree to which the condensations and rarefactions of air differ from each other. More vigorous vibrations of an object produce more intense sound waves and hence louder ones. **Timbre** provides information about the nature of the particular sound—for example, the sound of an oboe or a train whistle. Most natural acoustic stimuli are complex, consisting of several different frequencies of vibration. The particular mixture determines the sound's timbre. (See **Figure 7.2.**)

Anatomy of the Ear

Figure 7.3 shows a section through the ear and auditory canal and illustrates the apparatus of the middle and inner ear. (See **Figure 7.3.**) Sound is funneled via the *pinna* (external ear) through the ear canal to the **tympanic membrane** (eardrum), which vibrates with the sound.

The *middle ear* consists of a hollow region behind the tympanic membrane, approximately 2 ml in volume. It contains the bones of the middle ear, called the **ossicles**, which are set into vibration by the tympanic membrane. The **malleus** (hammer) connects with the tympanic membrane and transmits vibrations via the **incus** (anvil) and **stapes** (stirrup) to the **cochlea**, the structure that contains the receptors. The baseplate of the stapes presses against the membrane behind the **oval window**, the opening in the bony process surrounding the cochlea. (See **Figure 7.3.**)

pitch A perceptual dimension of sound; corresponds to the fundamental frequency.

hertz (Hz) Cycles per second.

loudness A perceptual dimension of sound; corresponds to intensity.

timbre (*tim* ber or *tamm* ber) A perceptual dimension of sound; corresponds to complexity.

tympanic membrane The eardrum.

ossicle (*ahss i kul*) One of the three bones of the middle ear.

malleus The "hammer"; the first of the three ossicles.

incus The "anvil"; the second of the three ossicles.

stapes (*stay* peez) The "stirrup"; the last of the three ossicles.

cochlea (*cock lee uh*) The snail-shaped structure of the inner ear that contains the auditory transducing mechanisms.

oval window An opening in the bone surrounding the cochlea that reveals a membrane, against which the baseplate of the stapes presses, transmitting sound vibrations into the fluid within the cochlea.

FIGURE 7.1

Sound Waves. Changes in air pressure from sound waves move the eardrum in and out. Air molecules are closer together in regions of higher pressure and farther apart in regions of lower pressure.

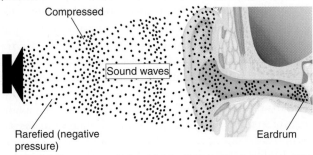

Compressed

Sound waves

Rarefied (negative pressure)

Eardrum

FIGURE 7.2

Physical and Perceptual Dimensions of Sound Waves

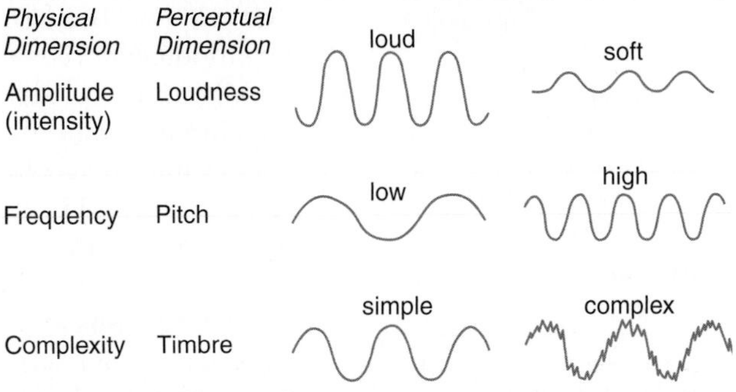

Physical Dimension	Perceptual Dimension		
Amplitude (intensity)	Loudness	loud	soft
Frequency	Pitch	low	high
Complexity	Timbre	simple	complex

FIGURE 7.3

The Auditory Apparatus

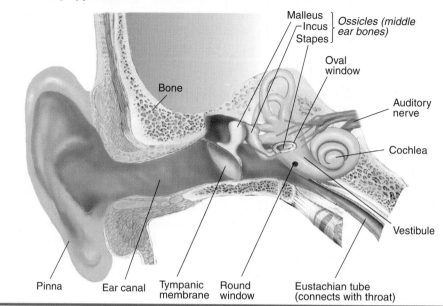

The cochlea is part of the *inner ear*. It is filled with fluid; therefore, sounds transmitted through the air must be transferred into a liquid medium. This process normally is very inefficient—99.9 percent of the energy of airborne sound would be reflected away if the air impinged directly against the oval window of the cochlea. The chain of ossicles serves as an extremely efficient means of energy transmission. The bones provide a mechanical advantage, with the baseplate of the stapes making smaller but more forceful excursions against the oval window than the tympanic membrane makes against the malleus.

The name *cochlea* comes from the Greek word *kokhlos*, or "land snail." It is indeed snail-shaped, consisting of two and three-quarters turns of a gradually tapering cylinder, 35 mm (1.37 in.) long. The cochlea is divided longitudinally into three sections, the *scala vestibuli* ("vestibular stairway"), the *scala media* ("middle stairway"), and the *scala tympani* ("tympanic stairway"), as shown in *Figure 7.4*. The receptive organ, known as the **organ of Corti**, consists of the *basilar membrane*, the *hair cells*, and the *tectorial membrane*. The auditory receptor cells are called **hair cells**, and they are anchored, via rodlike **Deiters's cells**, to the **basilar membrane**. The cilia of the hair cells pass through the *reticular membrane*, and the ends of some of them attach to the fairly rigid **tectorial membrane**, which projects overhead like a shelf. (See *Figure 7.4*.) Sound waves cause the basilar membrane to move relative to the tectorial membrane, which bends the cilia of the hair cells. This bending produces receptor potentials.

Figure 7.5 shows this process in a cochlea that has been partially straightened. If the cochlea were a closed system, no vibration would be transmitted through the oval window, because liquids are essentially incompressible. However, there is a membrane-covered opening, the **round window**, that allows the fluid inside the cochlea to move back and forth. The baseplate of the stapes vibrates against the membrane behind the oval window and introduces sound waves of high or low frequency into the cochlea. The vibrations cause part of the basilar membrane to flex back and forth. Pressure changes in the fluid underneath the basilar membrane are transmitted to the membrane of the round window, which moves in and out in a manner opposite to the movements of the oval window. That is, when the baseplate of the stapes pushes in, the membrane behind the round window bulges out. As we will see in a later subsection, different frequencies of sound vibrations cause different portions of the basilar membrane to flex. (See *Figure 7.5*.)

organ of Corti The sensory organ on the basilar membrane that contains the auditory hair cells.

hair cell The receptive cell of the auditory apparatus.

Deiters's cell (*dye terz*) A supporting cell found in the organ of Corti; sustains the auditory hair cells.

basilar membrane (*bazz i ler*) A membrane in the cochlea of the inner ear; contains the organ of Corti.

tectorial membrane (*tek torr ee ul*) A membrane located above the basilar membrane; serves as a shelf against which the cilia of the auditory hair cells move.

round window An opening in the bone surrounding the cochlea of the inner ear that permits vibrations to be transmitted, via the oval window, into the fluid in the cochlea.

FIGURE 7.4

The Cochlea.   A cross section through the cochlea, shows the organ of Corti.

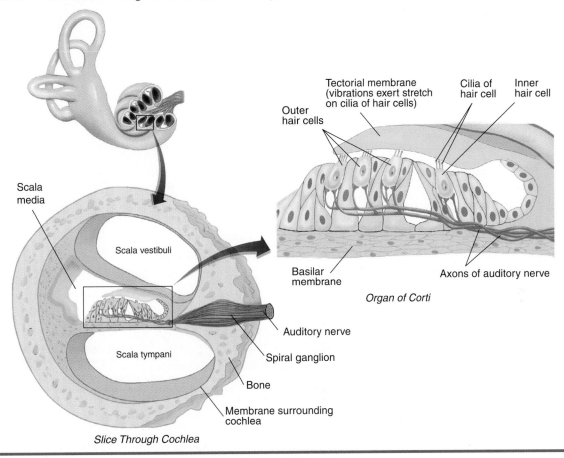

Scala media

Scala vestibuli

Scala tympani

Auditory nerve

Spiral ganglion

Bone

Membrane surrounding cochlea

Slice Through Cochlea

Tectorial membrane (vibrations exert stretch on cilia of hair cells)

Outer hair cells

Cilia of hair cell

Inner hair cell

Basilar membrane

Axons of auditory nerve

Organ of Corti

Some people suffer from a middle ear disease that causes the bone to grow over the round window. Because their basilar membrane cannot easily flex back and forth, these people have a severe hearing loss. However, their hearing can be restored by a surgical procedure called *fenestration* ("window making"), in which a tiny hole is drilled in the bone where the round window should be.

Auditory Hair Cells and the Transduction of Auditory Information

Two types of auditory receptors, *inner* and *outer* auditory hair cells, are located on the basilar membrane. Hair cells contain **cilia** ("eyelashes"), fine hairlike appendages, arranged in rows according to height. The human cochlea contains approximately 3500 inner hair cells and 12,000 outer hair cells. The hair cells form synapses with dendrites of bipolar neurons whose axons bring auditory information to the brain. (Refer to *Figure 7.4*.)

Sound waves cause both the basilar membrane and the tectorial membrane to flex up and down. These movements bend the cilia of the hair cells in one direction or the other. The tips of the cilia of outer hair cells are attached directly to the tectorial membrane. The cilia of the inner hair cells do not touch the overlying tectorial membrane, but the relative movement of the two membranes causes the fluid within the cochlea to flow past them, making them bend back and forth too.

Cilia contain a core of actin filaments surrounded by myosin filaments, and these proteins make the cilia stiff and rigid (Flock, 1977). Adjacent cilia are linked to each other by elastic filaments known as **tip links**. Each tip link is attached to the

cilium (plural: cilia) A hairlike appendage of a cell involved in movement or in transducing sensory information; found on the receptors in the auditory and vestibular system.

tip link An elastic filament that attaches the tip of one cilium to the side of the adjacent cilium.

FIGURE 7.5

Responses to Sound Waves.   When the stapes pushes against the membrane behind the oval window, the membrane behind the round window bulges outward. Different high-frequency and medium-frequency sound vibrations cause flexing of different portions of the basilar membrane. In contrast, low-frequency sound vibrations cause the tip of the basilar membrane to flex in synchrony with the vibrations.

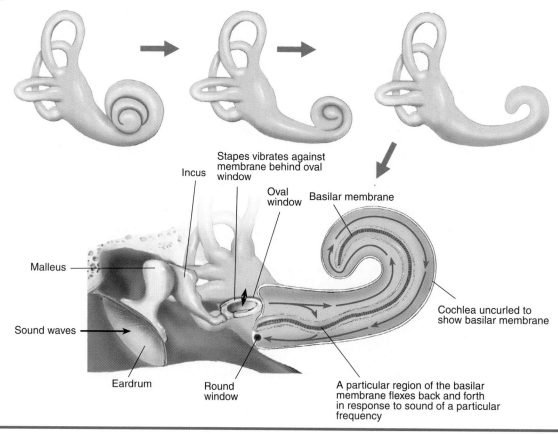

end of one cilium and to the side of an adjacent cilium. The points of attachment, known as **insertional plaques**, look dark under an electron microscope. As we will see, receptor potentials are triggered at the insertional plaques. (See *Figure 7.6*.)

Normally, tip links are slightly stretched, which means that they are under a small amount of tension. Thus, movement of the bundle of cilia in the direction of the tallest of them further stretches these linking fibers, whereas movement in the opposite direction relaxes them. Each insertional plaque contains a single ion channel, which opens and closes according to the amount of stretch exerted by the tip links. Thus, bending of the bundle of cilia produces receptor potentials (Pickles and Corey, 1992; Hudspeth and Gillespie, 1994; Gillespie, 1995; Jaramillo, 1995). Corey et al. (2004) identified the ion channels as TRPA1, a member of the *transient receptor potential cation channel*, subfamily A, type 1. (I mention the TRP family of receptors because, as we shall see later in this chapter, this family includes receptors involved in perception of touch, temperature, and taste.)

The Auditory Pathway

Connections with the Cochlear Nerve

The organ of Corti sends auditory information to the brain by means of the **cochlear nerve**, a branch of the auditory nerve (eighth cranial nerve). Approximately 95 percent of these axons receive information from the inner hair cells. These axons are thick and myelinated. Even though the outer hair cells are much

insertional plaque The point of attachment of a tip link to a cilium.

cochlear nerve The branch of the auditory nerve that transmits auditory information from the cochlea to the brain.

more numerous, they send information through only 5 percent of the sensory axons in the cochlear nerve, and these axons are thin and unmyelinated. These facts suggest that inner hair cells are of primary importance in the transmission of auditory information to the central nervous system.

Physiological and behavioral studies confirm this suggestion: The inner hair cells are necessary for normal hearing. In fact, Deol and Gluecksohn-Waelsch (1979) found that a mutant strain of mice whose cochleas contain *only* outer hair cells apparently cannot hear at all. Subsequent research indicates that the outer hair cells are *effector* cells, involved in altering the mechanical characteristics of the basilar membrane and thus influencing the effects of sound vibrations on the inner hair cells. I will discuss the role of outer hair cells in the section on place coding of pitch.

The Central Auditory System

The anatomy of the subcortical components of the auditory system is more complicated than that of the visual system. Rather than giving a detailed verbal description of the pathways, I will refer you to *Figure 7.7*. Note that axons enter the **cochlear nucleus** of the medulla and synapse there. Most of the neurons in the cochlear nucleus send axons to the **superior olivary complex**, also located in the medulla. Axons of neurons in these nuclei pass through a large fiber bundle called the **lateral lemniscus** to the inferior colliculus, located in the dorsal midbrain. Neurons there send their axons to the medial geniculate nucleus of the thalamus, which sends its axons to the auditory cortex of the temporal lobe. As you can see, there are many synapses along the way that complicate the story. Each hemisphere receives information from both ears but primarily from the contralateral one. Auditory information is relayed to the cerebellum and reticular formation as well.

If we unrolled the basilar membrane into a flat strip and followed afferent axons serving successive points along its length, we would reach successive points in the nuclei of the auditory system and ultimately successive points along the surface of the primary auditory cortex. The *basal* end of the basilar membrane (the end toward the oval window) is represented most medially in the auditory cortex, and the *apical* end is represented most laterally there. Because, as we will see, different parts of the basilar membrane respond best to different frequencies of sound, this relationship between cortex and basilar membrane is referred to as **tonotopic representation** (*tonos* means "tone," and *topos* means "place").

Neurons in the primary auditory cortex send axons to the auditory association cortex. In Chapter 3 we saw that most of the primary auditory cortex lies hidden on the inside of the lateral fissure and that the auditory association cortex lies on the superior part of the temporal lobe. Like the visual cortex, the auditory cortex is arranged in two streams, dorsal and ventral. The dorsal stream, which terminates in the posterior parietal cortex, is involved with sound localization; the ventral stream, which terminates in the parabelt region of the anterior temporal lobe, is involved with analysis of complex sounds (Rauschecker and Tian, 2000). Research on the functions of these streams is described later.

Perception of Pitch

As we have seen, the perceptual dimension of pitch corresponds to the physical dimension of frequency. The cochlea detects frequency by two means: moderate to

FIGURE 7.6

Transduction Apparatus in Hair Cells. These electron micrographs are of the transduction apparatus in hair cells: (a) a longitudinal section through three adjacent cilia. Tip links, elastic filaments attached to insertional plaques, link adjacent cilia. (b) A cross section through several cilia, showing an insertional plaque.

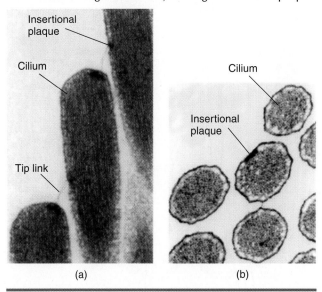

(a) (b)

From Hudspeth, A. J., and Gillespie, P. G. *Neuron*, 1994, *12*, 1–9.

cochlear nucleus One of a group of nuclei in the medulla that receive auditory information from the cochlea.

superior olivary complex A group of nuclei in the medulla; involved with auditory functions, including localization of the source of sounds.

lateral lemniscus A band of fibers running rostrally through the medulla and pons; carries fibers of the auditory system.

tonotopic representation (*tonn oh top ik*) A topographically organized mapping of different frequencies of sound that are represented in a particular region of the brain.

FIGURE 7.7

Pathways of the Auditory System. The major pathways are indicated by heavy arrows.

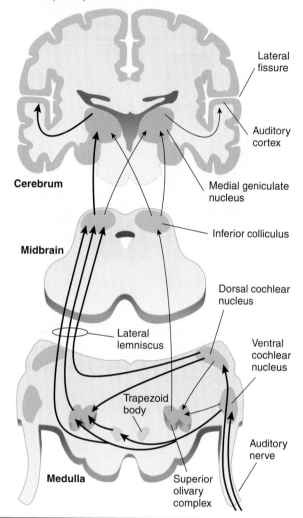

Lateral fissure

Auditory cortex

Medial geniculate nucleus

Inferior colliculus

Dorsal cochlear nucleus

Ventral cochlear nucleus

Lateral lemniscus

Cerebrum

Midbrain

Trapezoid body

Auditory nerve

Medulla

Superior olivary complex

place code The system by which information about different frequencies is coded by different locations on the basilar membrane.

cochlear implant An electronic device surgically implanted in the inner ear that can enable a deaf person to hear.

high frequencies by place coding and low frequencies by rate coding. These two types of coding are described next.

Place Coding

Because of the mechanical construction of the cochlea and basilar membrane, acoustic stimuli of different frequencies cause different parts of the basilar membrane to flex back and forth. Figure 7.8 illustrates the amount of deformation along the length of the basilar membrane produced by stimulation with tones of various frequencies. Note that higher frequencies produce more displacement at the basal end of the membrane (the end closest to the stapes). (See *Figure 7.8.*)

These results suggest that at least some frequencies of sound waves are detected by means of a **place code**. In this context a code represents a means by which neurons can represent information. Thus, if neurons at one end of the basilar membrane are excited by higher frequencies and those at the other end are excited by lower frequencies, we can say that the frequency of the sound is *coded* by the particular neurons that are active. In turn, the firing of particular axons in the cochlear nerve tells the brain about the presence of particular frequencies of sound.

Good evidence for place coding of pitch in humans comes from the effectiveness of cochlear implants. **Cochlear implants** are devices that are used to restore hearing in people with deafness caused by damage to the hair cells. The external part of a cochlear implant consists of a microphone and a miniaturized electronic signal processor. The internal part contains a very thin, flexible array of electrodes, which the surgeon carefully inserts into the cochlea in such a way that it follows the snail-like curl and ends up resting along the entire length of the basilar membrane. Each electrode in the array stimulates a different part of the basilar membrane. Information from the signal processor is passed to the electrodes by means of flat coils of wire, implanted under the skin. (See *Figure 7.9.*)

The primary purpose of a cochlear implant is to restore a person's ability to understand speech. Because most of the important acoustical information in speech is contained in frequencies that are too high to be accurately represented by a rate code, the multichannel electrode was developed in an attempt to duplicate the place coding of pitch on the basilar membrane (Copeland and Pillsbury, 2004). When different regions of the basilar membrane are stimulated, the person perceives sounds with different pitches. The signal processor in the external device analyzes the sounds detected by the microphone and sends separate signals to the appropriate portions of the basilar membrane. This device can work well; most people with cochlear implants can understand speech well enough to use a telephone (Shannon, 2007).

As mentioned earlier, the brain receives auditory information solely from the axons of inner hair cells. What role, then, do outer hair cells play? These cells contain contractile proteins, just as muscle fibers do. When they are exposed to an electrical current, outer hair cells contract by up to 10 percent of their length (Brownell et al., 1985; Zenner, Zimmermann, and Schmitt, 1985).

FIGURE 7.8

Anatomical Coding of Pitch. Stimuli of different frequencies maximally deform different regions of the basilar membrane.

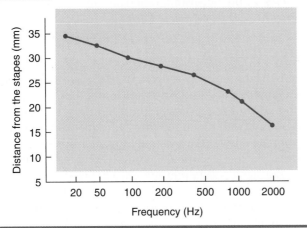

From von Békésy, G. *Journal of the Acoustical Society of America*, 1949, *21*, 233–245.

FIGURE 7.9

A Child with a Cochlear Implant. The microphone and processor are worn over the ear and the headpiece contains a coil that transmits signals to the implant.

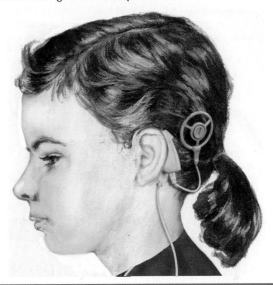

When the basilar membrane vibrates, movement of the cilia of the outer hair cells opens and closes ion channels, causing changes in the membrane potential. These changes cause movements of the contractile proteins, thus lengthening and shortening the cells. These changes in length amplify the vibrations of the basilar membrane. As a consequence, the signal that is received by inner hair cells is enhanced, which greatly increases the sensitivity of the inner ear to sound waves.

Figure 7.10 illustrates the importance of outer hair cells to the sensitivity and frequency selectivity of inner hair cells (Fettiplace and Hackney, 2006). The three V-shaped *tuning curves* indicate the sensitivity of individual inner hair cells, as shown by the response of individual afferent auditory nerve axons to pure tones. The low points of the three solid curves indicate that the hair cells will respond to a faint sound only if it is of a specific frequency—for these cells, either 0.5 kHz (red curve), 2.0 kHz (green curve), or 8.0 kHz (blue curve). If the sound is louder, the cells will respond to frequencies above and below their preferred frequencies. The dotted line indicates the response of the "blue" neuron after the outer hair cells have been destroyed. As you can see, this cell loses both sensitivity and selectivity: It will respond only to loud sounds, but to a wide range of frequencies. (See *Figure 7.10*.)

Rate Coding

We have seen that the frequency of a sound can be detected by place coding. However, the lowest frequencies do not appear to be accounted for in this manner. Kiang (1965) was unable to find any cells that responded best to frequencies of less than 200 Hz. How, then, can animals distinguish low frequencies? It appears that lower frequencies are detected by neurons that fire in synchrony to the movements of the apical end of the basilar membrane. Thus, lower frequencies are detected by means of **rate coding**.

The most convincing evidence of rate coding of pitch also comes from studies of people with cochlear implants. Pijl and Schwarz (1995a, 1995b) found that stimulation of a single electrode with pulses of electricity produced sensations of pitch that were proportional to the frequency of the stimulation. In fact, the subjects could even recognize familiar tunes produced by modulating the pulse frequency.

rate coding The system by which information about different frequencies is coded by the rate of firing of neurons in the auditory system.

FIGURE 7.10

Tuning Curves.   The figure shows the responses of single axons in the cochlear nerve that receive information from inner hair cells on different locations of the basilar membrane. The cells are more frequency selective at lower sound intensities. The dotted line shows the loss of sensitivity and selectivity of the high-frequency neuron after destruction of the outer hair cells.

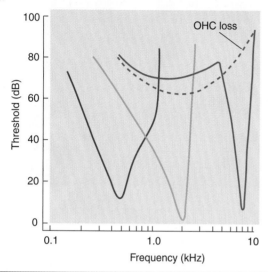

Adapted from Fettiplace, R., and Hackney, C. M. *Nature Reviews: Neuroscience,* 2006, *7*, 19–29.

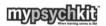

Animation 7.1
Perception of Pitch

fundamental frequency The lowest, and usually most intense, frequency of a complex sound; most often perceived as the sound's basic pitch.

overtone The frequency of complex tones that occurs at multiples of the fundamental frequency.

(The subjects had become deaf later in life, after they had already learned to recognize the tunes.) As we would expect, the subjects' perceptions were best when the tip of the basilar membrane was stimulated, and only low frequencies could be distinguished by this method. (See *MyPsychKit 7.1, Perception of Pitch.*)

Perception of Timbre

Although laboratory investigations of the auditory system often employ pure sine waves as stimuli, these waves are seldom encountered outside the laboratory. Instead, we hear sounds with a rich mixture of frequencies—sounds of complex timbre. For example, consider the sound of a clarinet playing a particular note. If we hear it, we can easily say that it is a clarinet and not a flute or a violin. The reason we can do so is that these three instruments produce sounds of different timbre, which our auditory system can distinguish.

Figure 7.11 shows the waveform from a clarinet playing a steady note (*top*). The shape of the waveform repeats itself regularly at the **fundamental frequency**, which corresponds to the perceived pitch of the note. A Fourier analysis of the waveform shows that it actually consists of a series of sine waves that includes the fundamental frequency and many **overtones**, multiples of the fundamental frequency. Different instruments produce overtones with different intensities. (See *Figure 7.11.*) Electronic synthesizers simulate the sounds of real instruments by producing a series of overtones of the proper intensities, mixing them, and passing them through a loudspeaker.

When the basilar membrane is stimulated by the sound of a clarinet, different portions respond to each of the overtones. This response produces a unique anatomically coded pattern of activity in the cochlear nerve, which is subsequently identified by circuits in the auditory association cortex.

Actually, the recognition of complex sounds is not quite that simple. Figure 7.11 shows the analysis of a *sustained* sound of a clarinet, but most sounds (including those produced by a clarinet) are dynamic; that is, their beginning, middle, and end are different from each other. The beginning of a note played on a clarinet (the *attack*) contains frequencies that appear and disappear in a few milliseconds. At the end of the note (the *decay*), some harmonics disappear before others. If we are to recognize different sounds, the auditory cortex must analyze a complex sequence of multiple frequencies that appear, change in amplitude, and disappear. When you consider the fact that we can listen to an orchestra and identify several instruments that are playing simultaneously, you can appreciate the complexity of the analysis performed by the auditory system. We will revisit this process later in this chapter.

Perception of Spatial Location

So far, I have discussed coding of pitch and timbre only (the last of which is actually a complex frequency analysis). The auditory system also responds to other qualities of acoustic stimuli. For example, our ears are very good at determining whether the source of a sound is to the right or left of us. Two separate physiological mechanisms detect the location of sound sources: We use phase differences for low frequencies (less than approximately 3000 Hz) and intensity differences for high frequencies. In addition, we use another mechanism—analysis of timbre—to determine the height of the source of a sound and whether it is in front of us or behind us.

If we are blindfolded, we can still determine with rather good accuracy the location of a stimulus that emits a click. We do so because neurons respond selectively to different *arrival times* of the sound waves at the left and right ears. If the source of the click is to the right or left of the midline, the sound pressure wave will reach one ear sooner and initiate action potentials there first. Only if the stimulus is straight ahead will the ears be stimulated simultaneously. Neurons in the superior olivary complex of the medulla detect differences in arrival times of sound waves produced by clicks.

Of course, we can hear continuous sounds as well as clicks, and we can also perceive the location of their source. We detect the source of continuous low-pitched sounds by means of phase differences. **Phase differences** refer to the simultaneous arrival, at each ear, of different portions (phases) of the oscillating sound wave. For example, if we assume that sound travels at 700 miles per hour through the air, adjacent cycles of a 1000-Hz tone are 12.3 inches apart. Thus, if the source of the sound is located to one side of the head, one eardrum is pulled out while the other is pushed in. The movement of the eardrums will reverse, or be 180° *out of phase*. If the source were located directly in front of the head, the movements would be perfectly in phase (0° out of phase). (See *Figure 7.12*.) Because some auditory neurons respond only when the eardrums (and thus the bending of the basilar membrane) are at least somewhat out of phase, neurons in the superior olivary complex in the brain are able to use the information they provide to detect the source of a continuous sound. (See *MyPsychKit 7.2, Sound Localization*.)

The auditory system cannot readily detect binaural phase differences of high-frequency stimuli; the differences in phases of such rapid sine waves are simply too short to be measured by the neurons. However, high-frequency stimuli that occur to the right or left of the midline stimulate the ears unequally. The head absorbs high frequencies, producing a "sonic shadow," so the ear closest to the source of the sound receives the most intense stimulation. Some neurons in the superior olivary complex respond differentially to binaural stimuli of different intensity in each ear, which means that they provide information that can be used to detect the source of tones of high frequency.

How can we determine the elevation of the source of a sound and perceive whether it is in front of us or behind us? One answer is that we can turn and tilt our heads, thus transforming the discrimination into a left–right decision. However, we have another means by which we can determine elevation and distinguish front from back: analysis of timbre. If you look at someone's external ear (pinna), you will see that it contains several folds and ridges. Most of the sound waves that we hear bounce off the folds and ridges of the pinna before they enter the ear canal. Depending on the angle at which the sound waves strike these folds and ridges, different frequencies will be enhanced or attenuated. In other words, the pattern of reflections will change with the location of the source of the sound, which will alter

FIGURE 7.11

Sound Wave from a Clarinet. The figure shows the shape of a sound wave from a clarinet (*top*) and the individual frequencies into which it can be analyzed.

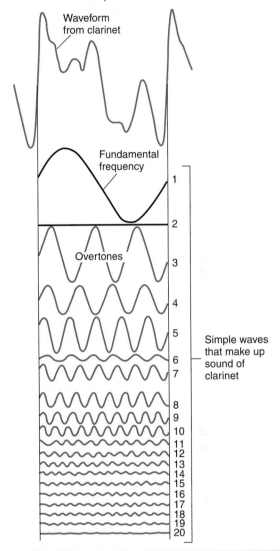

Reprinted from *Stereo Review*, copyright © 1977 by Diamandis Communications Inc.

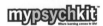

Animation 7.2
Sound Localization

phase difference The difference in arrival times of sound waves at each of the eardrums.

FIGURE 7.12

Sound Localization.   This method localizes the source of low-frequency and medium-frequency sounds through phase differences. (a) Source of a 1000-Hz tone to the right. The pressure waves on each eardrum are out of phase; one eardrum is pushed in while the other is pushed out. (b) Source of a sound directly in front. The vibrations of the eardrums are synchronized (in phase).

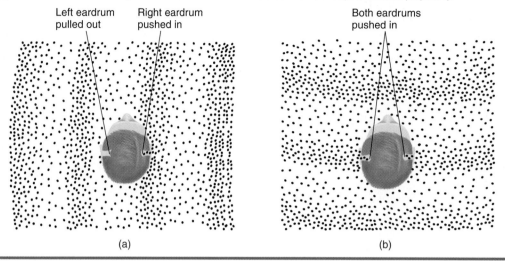

(a)   (b)

the timbre of the sound that is perceived. Because people's ears differ in shape, each individual must learn to recognize the subtle changes in the timbre of sounds that originate in locations in front of the head, behind it, above it, or below it. The neural circuits that accomplish this task are not genetically programmed—they must be acquired as a result of experience.

Figure 7.13 shows the effects of elevation on the intensity of sounds of various frequencies received at an ear (Oertel and Young, 2004). The experimenters placed a small microphone in a cat's ear and recorded the sound produced by an auditory stimulus presented at various elevations relative to the cat's head. They used a computer to plot the ear's *transfer functions*—a graph that compares the intensity of various frequencies of sound received by the ear to the intensity of these frequencies received by a microphone in open air. What is important in Figure 7.13 is not the shape of the transfer functions, but the fact that these functions varied with the elevation of the source of the sound. The transfer function for a sound directly in front of the cat (0° of elevation) is shown in green. This curve is shown at the 60°, 30°, and −30° positions as well, so that they can be compared with the curves obtained with the sound source at these locations, too (red, orange, and blue, respectively). That sounds complicated, I know, but if you look at the figure, you will clearly see that the timbre of sounds that reaches the cat's ear changed along with elevation of the source of the sound. (See *Figure 7.13*.)

Perception of Complex Sounds

Hearing has three primary functions: to detect sounds, to determine the location of their sources, and to recognize the identity of these sources—and thus their meaning and relevance to us (Heffner and Heffner, 1990; Yost, 1991). Let us consider the third function: recognizing the identity of a sound source. Unless you are in a completely silent location, pay attention to what you can hear. Right now, I am sitting in an office and can hear the sound of a fan in a computer, the tapping of the keys as I write this, the footsteps of someone passing outside the door, and the voices of some people talking in the hallway. How can I recognize these sources? The axons in my cochlear nerve contain a constantly changing pattern of activity corresponding to the constantly changing mixtures of frequencies that strike my eardrums. Somehow, the auditory system of my brain recognizes particular patterns that belong to particular sources, and I perceive each of them as an independent entity.

Perception of Environmental Sounds and Their Location

The task of the auditory system in identifying sound sources, then, is one of *pattern recognition*. The auditory system must recognize that particular patterns of constantly changing activity belong to different sound sources. Few patterns are simple mixtures of fixed frequencies. Consider the complexity of sounds that occur in the environment: cars honking, birds chirping, people coughing, doors slamming, and so on. (See *MyPsychKit 7.3, Perception of Environmental Sounds.*) (I will discuss speech recognition—an even more complicated task—in Chapter 13.)

As mentioned earlier in this chapter, the auditory cortex, like the visual cortex, is organized into two streams: a dorsal stream, involved in perception of location, and a ventral stream, involved in perception of particular complex sounds. A review of thirty-eight functional imaging studies with human subjects (Arnott et al., 2004) reported a consistent result: perception of the identity of sounds activated the ventral stream of the auditory cortex and perception of the location of sounds activated the dorsal stream. An fMRI study by Alain, He, and Grady (2008) supports this conclusion. The investigators presented people with sounds of animals, humans, and musical instruments (for example, the bark of a dog, a cough, and the sound of a flute) in one of three locations: 90° to the left, straight ahead, or 90° to the right. On some blocks of trials the subjects were asked to press a button when they heard two sounds of any kind from the same location. On other blocks of trials they were asked to indicate when they heard the same kind of sound twice in a row, regardless of its location. As Figure 7.14 shows, judgments of location (blue) activated dorsal regions ("where"), and judgments of the nature of a sound (orange) activated ventral regions ("what"). (See *Figure 7.14.*)

FIGURE 7.13

Changes in Timbre of Sounds with Changes in Elevation.
The graphs are transfer functions, which compare the intensity of various frequencies of sound received by the ear to the intensity of these frequencies received by a microphone in open air. For ease of comparison, the 0° transfer function (green) is superimposed on the transfer functions obtained at 60° (red), 30° (orange), and −30° (blue). The differences in the transfer functions at various elevations provide cues that aid in perception of the location of a sound source.

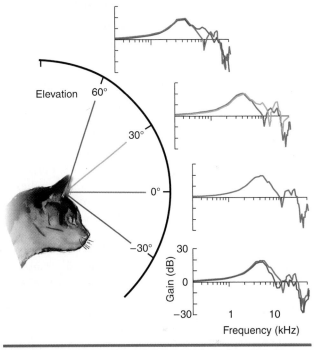

Adapted from Oertel, D., and Young, E. D. *Trends in Neuroscience*, 2004, *27*, 104–110.

Animation 7.3
Perception of Environmental Sounds

Patient I. R., a right-handed woman in her early forties, sustained bilateral damage during surgical treatment of an abnormal blood vessel in her brain. Ten years after her surgery, Peretz and her colleagues studied the effects of her brain damage on her musical ability (Peretz, Gagnon, and Bouchard, 1998). Although Patient I. R. had normal hearing, could understand speech and converse normally, and could recognize environmental sounds, she showed a nearly complete **amusia**—loss of the ability to perceive or produce melodic or rhythmic aspects of music. She had been raised in a musical environment: Both her grandmother and brother were professional musicians. After her surgery, she lost the ability to recognize melodies that she had been familiar with previously, including simple pieces such as "Happy Birthday." She was no longer able to sing.

Remarkably, despite her inability to recognize melodic and rhythmic aspects of music, she insisted that she still enjoyed listening to music. Peretz and her colleagues discovered that I. R. was still able to recognize emotional aspects of music. Although she could not recognize pieces that the experimenters played for her, she recognized whether the music sounded happy or sad. She could also recognize happiness, sadness, fear, anger, surprise, and disgust in a person's tone of voice. Her

amusia (*a mew* zia) Loss or impairment of musical abilities, produced by hereditary factors or brain damage.

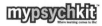

Animation 7.4
Emotion and Dissonance in Music

ability to recognize emotion in music contrasts with her inability to recognize dissonance in music—a quality that normal listeners find intensely unpleasant. Peretz and her colleagues (2001) discovered that I. R. was totally insensitive to changes in music that irritate normal listeners. Even 4-month-old babies prefer consonant music to dissonant music, which shows that recognition of dissonance develops very early in life (Zentner and Kagan, 1998). You can listen to music that varies in emotional content (happy, sad, peaceful, and scary) and dissonance in *MyPsychKit 7.4, Emotion and Dissonance in Music.* I find it fascinating that I. R. could not distinguish between the dissonant and consonant versions but could still identify happy and sad music.

Perception of Music

Perception of music is a special form of auditory perception. Music consists of sounds of various pitches and timbres played in a particular sequence with an underlying rhythm. Particular combinations of musical notes played simultaneously are perceived as consonant or dissonant, pleasant or unpleasant. The intervals between notes of musical scales follow specific rules, which may vary in the music of different cultures. In Western music, melodies played using notes that follow one set of rules (the major mode) usually sound happy, while those played following another set of rules (the minor mode) generally sound sad. In addition, a melody is recognized by the relative intervals between its notes, not by their absolute value. A melody is perceived as unchanging even when it is played in different keys; that is, when the pitches of all the notes are raised or lowered without changing the relative intervals between them. Thus, musical perception requires recognition of sequences of notes, their adherence to rules that govern permissible pitches, harmonic combinations of notes, and rhythmical structure. Because the duration of musical pieces is several seconds to many minutes, musical perception involves a substantial memory capacity. Thus, the neural mechanisms required for musical perception must obviously be complex.

Different regions of the brain are involved in different aspects of musical perception (Peretz and Zatorre, 2005). For example, the inferior frontal cortex appears to be involved in recognition of harmony, the right auditory cortex appears to be involved in perception of the underlying beat in music, and the left auditory cortex appears to be involved in perception of rhythmic patterns that are superimposed on the rhythmic beat. (Think of a drummer indicating the regular, underlying beat by operating the foot pedal of the bass drum and superimposing a more complex pattern of beats on smaller drums with the drumsticks.) In addition, the cerebellum and basal ganglia are involved in timing of musical rhythms, as they are in the timing of movements.

Everyone learns a language, but only some people become musicians. Musical training obviously makes changes in the brain—changes in motor systems involved in singing or playing an instrument, and changes in the auditory system involved in recognizing subtle complexities of harmony, rhythm, and other characteristics of musical structure. Here, I will consider aspects of musical expertise related to audition. Some of the effects of musical training can be seen in changes in the structure or activity of portions of the auditory system of the brain. For example, a study by Schneider et al. (2002) found that the volume of the primary auditory cortex of musicians was 130 percent larger than that of nonmusicians, and the neural response in this area to musical tones was 102 percent greater in musicians. Moreover, both of these measures were positively related to a person's musical aptitude.

FIGURE 7.14

"Where" Versus "What." This figure shows regional brain activity in response to judgments of category (blue) and location (red) of sounds. IFG = inferior frontal gyrus, IPL = inferior parietal lobule, MFG = middle frontal gyrus, SFG = superior frontal gyrus, SPL = superior parietal lobule.

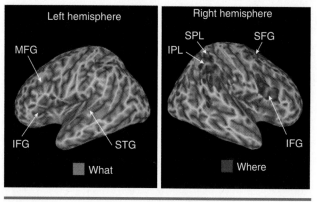

From Alain, C., He, Y., and Grady, C. *Journal of Cognitive Neuroscience*, 2008, *20*, 285–295. Reprinted with permission.

InterimSummary

Audition

The receptive organ for audition is the organ of Corti, located on the basilar membrane. When sound strikes the tympanic membrane, it sets the ossicles into motion, and the baseplate of the stapes pushes against the membrane behind the oval window. Pressure changes thus applied to the fluid within the cochlea cause a portion of the basilar membrane to flex, causing the basilar membrane to move laterally with respect to the tectorial membrane that overhangs it. This movement pulls directly on the cilia of the outer hair cells and changes their membrane potential. This change causes contractions or relaxations of contractile proteins within the cell, which amplify movements of the basilar membrane and sharpen their focus. These events cause movements in the fluid within the cochlea, which, in turn, causes the cilia of the inner hair cells to wave back and forth. These mechanical forces open cation channels in the tips of the hair cells and thus produce receptor potentials.

The inner hair cells send auditory information to the brain via the cochlear branch of the eighth cranial nerve. The central auditory system involves several brain stem nuclei, including the cochlear nuclei, superior olivary complex, and inferior colliculi. The medial geniculate nucleus relays auditory information to the primary auditory cortex on the medial surface of the temporal lobe. The primary auditory cortex is surrounded by the auditory association cortex. As we saw in Chapter 6, the visual association cortex is divided into two streams, one analyzing color and form, and the other analyzing location and movement. Similarly, the auditory association cortex is organized into streams that analyze the nature of sounds and the location of their sources.

Pitch is encoded by two means. High-frequency sounds cause the base of the basilar membrane (near the oval window) to flex; low-frequency sounds cause the apex (opposite end) to flex. Because high and low frequencies thus stimulate different groups of auditory hair cells, frequency is encoded anatomically. The lowest frequencies cause the apex of the basilar membrane to flex back and forth in time with the acoustic vibrations. The outer hair cells act as motive elements rather than as sensory transducers, contracting in response to activity of the efferent axons and modifying the mechanical properties of the basilar membrane.

The auditory system is analytical in its operation. That is, it can discriminate between sounds with different timbres by detecting the individual overtones that constitute the sounds and producing unique patterns of neural firing in the auditory system.

Left–right localization is performed by analyzing binaural differences in arrival time, in phase relations, and in intensity. The left/right location of the sources of brief sounds (such as clicks) and sounds of frequencies below approximately 3000 Hz is detected by neurons in the superior olivary complex, which respond most vigorously when one ear receives the click first or when the phase of a sine wave received by one ear leads that received by the other. The left/right location of the sources of high-frequency sounds is detected by another group of neurons in the superior olivary complex, which respond most vigorously when one organ of Corti is stimulated more intensely than the other. Localization of the elevation of the sources of sounds can be accomplished by turning the head or by perception of subtle differences in the timbre of sounds coming from different directions. The folds and ridges in the external ear (pinna) reflect different frequencies into the ear canal, changing the timbre of the sound according to the location of its source.

To recognize the source of sounds, the auditory system must recognize the constantly changing patterns of activity received from the axons in the cochlear nerve. Like the visual cortex, the auditory cortex is organized into two streams. The ventral stream is involved in the analysis of the sound, and the dorsal stream is involved in perception of its location. Recognition of complex environmental sounds activates a region of the left posterior middle temporal gyrus.

Perception of music requires recognition of sequences of notes, their adherence to rules governing permissible pitches, harmonic combinations of notes, and rhythmical structure. Perception of pitch activates regions of the superior temporal gyrus rostral and lateral to the primary auditory cortex. Other regions of the brain—especially in the right hemisphere—are involved in perception of the underlying beat of music and the specific rhythmic patterns of a particular piece. Musical training appears to increase the size and responsiveness of the primary auditory cortex. A case study indicates that recognition of emotion in music involves some brain mechanisms independent of those that recognize dissonance.

Thought Question

A naturalist once noted that when a male bird stakes out his territory, he sings with a very sharp, staccato song that says, in effect, "Here I am, and stay away!" In contrast, if a predator appears in the vicinity, many birds will emit alarm calls that consist of steady whistles that start and end slowly. Knowing what you do about the two means of localizing sounds, why do these two types of calls have different characteristics?

Vestibular System

The vestibular system has two components: the vestibular sacs and the semicircular canals. They represent the second and third components of the *labyrinths* of the inner ear. (We just studied the first component, the cochlea.) The **vestibular sacs**

vestibular sac One of a set of two receptor organs in each inner ear that detects changes in the tilt of the head.

respond to the force of gravity and inform the brain about the head's orientation. The **semicircular canals** respond to angular acceleration—changes in the rotation of the head—but not to steady rotation. They also respond (but rather weakly) to changes in position or to linear acceleration.

The functions of the vestibular system include balance, maintenance of the head in an upright position, and adjustment of eye movement to compensate for head movements. Vestibular stimulation does not produce any readily definable sensation; certain low-frequency stimulation of the vestibular sacs can produce nausea, and stimulation of the semicircular canals can produce dizziness and rhythmic eye movements (*nystagmus*). However, we are not directly aware of the information received from these organs. This section describes the vestibular system: the vestibular apparatus, the receptor cells, and the vestibular pathway in the brain.

Anatomy of the Vestibular Apparatus

Figure 7.15 shows the labyrinths of the inner ear, which include the cochlea, the semicircular canals, and the two vestibular sacs: the **utricle** ("little pouch") and the **saccule** ("little sack"). (See *Figure 7.15*.) The semicircular canals approximate the

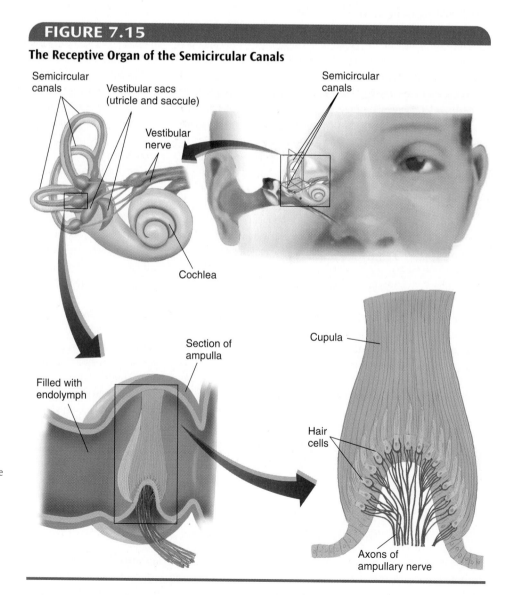

FIGURE 7.15

The Receptive Organ of the Semicircular Canals

Semicircular canals

Vestibular sacs (utricle and saccule)

Vestibular nerve

Semicircular canals

Cochlea

Section of ampulla

Filled with endolymph

Cupula

Hair cells

Axons of ampullary nerve

semicircular canal One of the three ringlike structures of the vestibular apparatus that detect changes in head rotation.

utricle (*you* trih kul) One of the vestibular sacs.

saccule (*sak* yule) One of the vestibular sacs.

FIGURE 7.16

The Receptive Tissue of The Vestibular Sacs: The Utricle and the Saccule

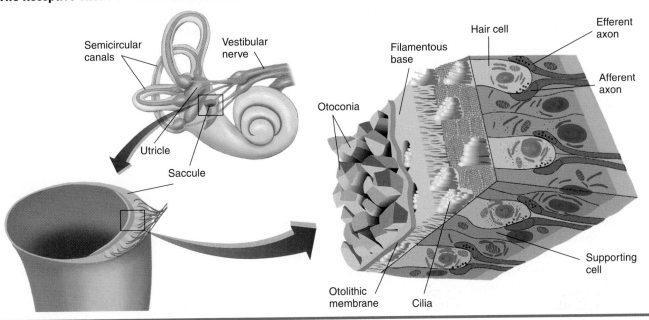

three major planes of the head: sagittal, transverse, and horizontal. Receptors in each canal respond maximally to sudden turning movements of the head in one particular plane. The semicircular canal consists of a membranous canal floating within a bony one; the membranous canal contains a fluid called *endolymph*. An enlargement called the **ampulla** contains the organ in which the sensory receptors reside. The sensory receptors are hair cells similar to those found in the cochlea. Their cilia are embedded in a gelatinous mass called the **cupula**, which blocks part of the ampulla. Rotation of the head causes the fluid in the semicircular canals to rotate in the opposite direction which pushes against the cupula, triggering receptor potentials in the hair cells located there. (See *Figure 7.15*.)

The vestibular sacs (the utricle and saccule) work very differently. These organs are roughly circular, and each contains a patch of receptive tissue. The receptive tissue is located on the "floor" of the utricle and on the "wall" of the saccule when the head is in an upright position. The receptive tissue, like that of the semicircular canals and cochlea, contains hair cells. The cilia of these receptors are embedded in an overlying gelatinous mass, which contains something rather unusual: *otoconia*, which are small crystals of calcium carbonate. (See *Figure 7.16*.) The weight of the crystals causes the gelatinous mass to shift in position as the orientation of the head changes. Thus, movement produces a shearing force on the cilia of the receptive hair cells.

The Vestibular Pathway

The vestibular and cochlear nerves constitute the two branches of the eighth cranial nerve (auditory nerve). The bipolar cell bodies that give rise to the afferent axons of the vestibular nerve (a branch of the eighth cranial nerve) are located in the **vestibular ganglion**, which appears as a nodule on the vestibular nerve.

Most of the axons of the vestibular nerve synapse within the vestibular nuclei in the medulla, but some axons travel directly to the cerebellum. Neurons of the vestibular nuclei send their axons to the cerebellum, spinal cord, medulla, and pons. There also appear to be vestibular projections to the temporal cortex, but the precise pathways have not been determined. Most investigators believe that the cortical

ampulla (*am **pull** uh*) An enlargement in a semicircular canal; contains the cupula and the crista.

cupula (*kew pew luh*) A gelatinous mass found in the ampulla of the semicircular canals; moves in response to the flow of the fluid in the canals.

vestibular ganglion A nodule on the vestibular nerve that contains the cell bodies of the bipolar neurons that convey vestibular information to the brain.

projections are responsible for feelings of dizziness; the activity of projections to the lower brain stem can produce the nausea and vomiting that accompany motion sickness. Projections to brain stem nuclei controlling neck muscles are clearly involved in maintaining an upright position of the head and in producing eye movements to compensate for sudden head movements. Without this compensatory mechanism, our vision of the world would become a blur whenever we walked or ran.

InterimSummary

Vestibular System

The semicircular canals are filled with fluid. When the head begins rotating or comes to rest after rotation, inertia causes the fluid to push the cupula to one side or the other. This movement exerts a shearing force on the cupula, the organ containing the vestibular hair cells. The vestibular sacs contain a patch of receptive tissue that contains hair cells whose cilia are embedded in a gelatinous mass. The weight of the otoconia in the gelatinous mass shifts when the head tilts, causing a shearing force on some of the cilia of the hair cells.

Each hair cell contains one long cilium and several shorter ones. These cells form synapses with dendrites of bipolar neurons whose axons travel through the vestibular nerve. The receptors also receive efferent terminal buttons from neurons located in the cerebellum and medulla, but the function of these connections is not known. Vestibular information is received by the vestibular nuclei in the medulla, which relay it on to the cerebellum, spinal cord, medulla, pons, and temporal cortex. These pathways are responsible for control of posture, head movements, and eye movements and the puzzling phenomenon of motion sickness.

Thought Questions

Why can slow, repetitive vestibular stimulation cause nausea and vomiting? Obviously, there are connections between the vestibular system and the area postrema, which (as you learned in Chapter 2) controls vomiting. Can you think of any useful functions that might be served by these connections?

Somatosenses

The somatosenses provide information about what is happening on the surface of our body and inside it. The **cutaneous senses** (skin senses) include several submodalities commonly referred to as *touch*. **Proprioception** and **kinesthesia** provide information about body position and movement. The **organic senses** arise from receptors in and around the internal organs. Because the cutaneous senses are the most studied of the somatosenses, both perceptually and physiologically, I will devote most of my discussion to them.

The Stimuli

The cutaneous senses respond to several different types of stimuli: pressure, vibration, heating, cooling, and events that cause tissue damage (and hence pain). Feelings of pressure are caused by mechanical deformation of the skin. Vibration is produced in the laboratory or clinic by tuning forks or mechanical devices, but it more commonly occurs when we move our fingers across a rough surface. Thus, we use vibration sensitivity to judge an object's roughness. Obviously, sensations of warmth and coolness are produced by objects that change skin temperature from normal. Sensations of pain can be caused by many different types of stimuli, but it appears that most cause at least some tissue damage.

Kinesthesia is provided by stretch receptors in skeletal muscles that report changes in muscle length to the central nervous system and by stretch receptors in tendons that measure the force being exerted by the muscles. Receptors within joints between adjacent bones respond to the magnitude and direction of limb

cutaneous sense (*kew tane ee us*) One of the somatosenses; includes sensitivity to stimuli that involve the skin.

proprioception Perception of the body's position and posture.

kinesthesia Perception of the body's own movements.

organic sense A sense modality that arises from receptors located within the inner organs of the body.

glabrous skin (*glab russ*) Skin that does not contain hair; found on the palms and the soles of the feet.

Ruffini corpuscle A vibration-sensitive organ located in hairy skin.

movement. Muscle length detectors, located within the muscles, do not give rise to conscious sensations; their information is used to help control movement.

Anatomy of the Skin and Its Receptive Organs

The skin is a complex and vital organ of the body—one that we tend to take for granted. We cannot survive without it; extensive skin burns are fatal. Our cells, which must be bathed by a warm fluid, are protected from the hostile environment by the skin's outer layers. The skin participates in thermoregulation by producing sweat, thus cooling the body, or by restricting its circulation of blood, thus conserving heat. Its appearance varies widely across the body, from mucous membrane to hairy skin to the smooth, hairless skin of the palms and the soles of the feet.

Skin consists of subcutaneous tissue, dermis, and epidermis and contains various receptors scattered throughout these layers. Figure 7.17 shows cross sections through hairy and **glabrous skin** (hairless skin, found on our fingertips and palms and on the bottoms of our toes and feet). Hairy skin contains unencapsulated (free) nerve endings; **Ruffini corpuscles**, which respond to indentation of the skin; and **Pacinian corpuscles**, which respond to rapid vibrations. Pacinian corpuscles are the largest sensory end organs in the body. Their size, approximately 0.5×1.0 mm, makes them visible to the naked eye. They consist of up to seventy onion-like layers wrapped around the dendrite of a single myelinated axon. Free nerve endings, which detect painful stimuli and changes in temperature, are found just below the surface of the skin. Other free nerve endings are found in a basketwork around the base of hair follicles and around the emergence of hair shafts from the skin. These fibers detect movement of hairs. (See *Figure 7.17.*)

Glabrous skin contains a more complex mixture of free nerve endings and axons that terminate within specialized end organs (Iggo and Andres, 1982). The increased complexity reflects the fact that we use the palms of our hands and the inside surfaces of our fingers to explore the environment actively: We use them to hold and touch objects. In contrast, the rest of our body most often contacts the environment passively; that is, other things come into contact with it.

Glabrous skin, like hairy skin, contains free nerve endings, Ruffini corpuscles, and Pacinian corpuscles. (Pacinian corpuscles are also found in the joints and in various internal organs.) Glabrous skin also contains **Meissner's corpuscles**, which are found in *papillae* ("nipples"), small elevations of the dermis that project up into the epidermis. These end organs are innervated by between two and six axons. They respond to low-frequency vibration or to brief taps on the skin. **Merkel's disks**, which respond to indentation of the skin, are found at the base of the epidermis, in the same general locations as Meissner's corpuscles, adjacent to sweat ducts. (See *Figure 7.17.*)

Perception of Cutaneous Stimulation

The three most important qualities of cutaneous stimulation are touch, temperature, and pain. These qualities are described in the sections that follow.

Touch

Sensitivity to pressure and vibration is caused by movement of the skin, which moves the dendrites of mechanoreceptors. Most investigators believe that the

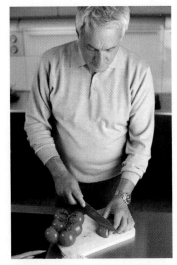

After wearing a wristwatch for several minutes, a person wearing a watch can no longer feel it unless it moves on the wrist.

Pacinian corpuscle (*pa chin ee un*) A specialized, encapsulated somatosensory nerve ending that detects mechanical stimuli, especially vibrations.

Meissner's corpuscle The touch-sensitive end organs located in the papillae, small elevations of the dermis that project up into the epidermis.

Merkel's disk The touch-sensitive end organs found at the base of the epidermis, adjacent to sweat ducts.

FIGURE 7.17

Cutaneous Receptors

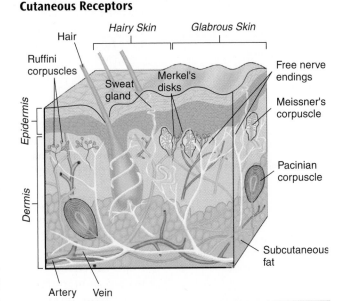

encapsulated nerve endings serve only to modify the physical stimulus transduced by the dendrites that reside within them. But what is the mechanism of transduction? How does movement of the dendrites of mechanoreceptors produce changes in membrane potentials? It appears that the movement causes ion channels to open, and the flow of ions into or out of the dendrite causes a change in the membrane potential.

Most information about tactile sensation is precisely localized; that is, we can perceive the location on our skin where we are being touched. In the past, neuroscientists believed that in humans this information was transmitted to the central nervous system only by fast-conducting myelinated axons. However, a study by Olausson et al. (2002) discovered a new category of tactile sensation that is transmitted by small-diameter unmyelinated axons.

At age 31, patient G. L., a 54-year-old woman, "suffered a permanent and specific loss of large myelinated afferents after episodes of acute polyradiculitis and polyneuropathy that affected her whole body below the nose. A sural nerve biopsy indicated a complete loss of large-diameter myelinated fibers. . . . Before the present study, she denied having any touch sensibility below the nose, and she lost the ability to perceive tickle when she became ill. She states that her perceptions of temperature, pain and itch are intact" (Olausson et al., 2002, pp. 902–903).

G. L. could indeed detect the stimuli that are normally attributed to small-diameter unmyelinated axons—temperature, pain, and itch—but she could not detect vibratory or normal tactile stimuli. But when the hairy skin on her forearm or the back of her hand was stroked with a soft brush, she reported a faint, pleasant sensation. However, she could not determine the direction of the stroking or its precise location. Functional MRI (fMRI) analysis showed that this stimulation activated the insular cortex, a region that is known to be associated with emotional responses. The somatosensory cortex was not activated. When regions of hairy skin of control subjects were stimulated this way, fMRI showed activation of the primary and secondary somatosensory cortex as well as the insular cortex because the stimulation activated both large and small axons. The glabrous skin on the palm of the hand is served only by large-diameter, myelinated axons. When this region was stroked with a brush, G. L. reported no sensation at all, presumably because of the absence of these axons.

The investigators concluded that besides conveying information about noxious and thermal stimuli, small-diameter unmyelinated axons constitute a "system for limbic touch that may underlie emotional, hormonal and affiliative responses to caresslike, skin-to-skin contact between individuals" (Olausson et al., 2002, p. 900).

Studies of people who make especially precise use of their fingertips show changes in the regions of somatosensory cortex that receive information from this part of the body. For example, violinists must make very precise movements of the four fingers of their left hand, which are used to play notes by pressing the strings against the fingerboard. Tactile and proprioceptive feedback are very important in accurately moving and positioning these fingers so that sounds of the proper pitch are produced. In contrast, placement of the thumb, which slides along the bottom of the neck of the violin, is less critical. In a study of violin players, Elbert et al. (1995) found that the portions of their right somatosensory cortex that receive information from the four fingers of their left hand were enlarged relative to the corresponding parts of the left somatosensory cortex. The amount of somatosensory cortex that receives information from the thumb was not enlarged.

Temperature

There are two categories of thermal receptors: those that respond to warmth and those that respond to coolness. Cold sensors in the skin are located just beneath the epidermis, and warmth sensors are located more deeply in the skin. Information from cold sensors is conveyed to the CNS by thinly myelinated Aδ fibers, and information from warmth sensors is conveyed by unmyelinated C fibers. We can detect thermal stimuli over a very wide range of temperatures, from less than 8°C (noxious cold) to over 52°C. (noxious heat). Investigators have long believed that no single receptor could detect such a range of temperatures, and recent research indicates that this belief was correct. At present, we know of six mammalian thermoreceptors—all members of the TRP family (Bandell, Macpherson, and Patapoutian, 2007; Romanovsky, 2007). (See *Figure 7.18* and *Table 7.1*.)

Some of the thermal receptors respond to particular chemicals as well as to changes in temperature. For example, the *M* in TRPM8 stands for menthol, a compound found in the leaves of many members of the mint family. As you undoubtedly know, peppermint tastes cool in the mouth, and menthol is added to some cigarettes to make the smoke feel cooler (and perhaps to try to delude smokers into thinking that the smoke is less harsh and damaging to the lungs). Menthol provides a cooling sensation because it binds with and stimulates the TRPM8 receptor and produces neural activity that the brain interprets as coolness. As we will see in the next subsection, chemicals can produce the sensation of heat also.

Pain

Pain reception, like thermoreception, is accomplished by the networks of free nerve endings in the skin. There appears to be at least three types of pain receptors (usually referred to as *nociceptors,* or "detectors of noxious stimuli"). High-threshold mechanoreceptors are free nerve endings that respond to intense pressure, which might be caused by something striking, stretching, or pinching the skin. A second type of free nerve ending appears to respond to extremes of heat, to acids, and to the presence of *capsaicin,* the active ingredient in chile peppers. (Note that we say that chile peppers make food taste "hot.") This type of fiber contains TRPV1 receptors (Kress and Zeilhofer, 1999). The *V* stands for *vanilloid*—a group of chemicals of which capsaicin is a member. Caterina et al. (2000) found that mice with a knockout of the gene for the TRPV1 receptor showed less sensitivity to painful high-temperature stimuli and would drink water to which capsaicin had been added. The mice responded normally to noxious mechanical stimuli. Presumably, the TRPV1 receptor is responsible for pain produced by burning of the skin. It also appears to play a role in regulation of body temperature. In addition, Ghilardi et al. (2005) found that a drug that blocks TRPV1 receptors reduced pain in patients with bone cancer, which is apparently caused by the production of acid by the tumors.

Another type of nociceptive fiber contains TRPA1 receptors which, as we saw earlier in this chapter, are found in the cilia of auditory and vestibular hair cells. These

FIGURE 7.18

Activity of TRP Channels.   The activity of cold-activated (blue) and heat-activated (orange) temperature-sensitive TRP channels are shown as a function of temperature.

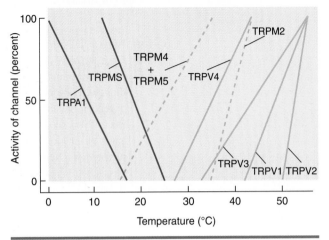

Adapted from Romanovsky, A. A. *American Journal of Physiology,* 2007, *292,* R37–R46.

TABLE 7.1   Categories of Mammalian Thermal Receptors

Name of Receptor	Type of Stimulus	Temperature Range
TRPV2	noxious heat	above 52°C
TRPV1	heat	above 43°C
TRPV3	warmth	above 31°C
TRPV4	warmth	above 25°C
TRPM8	coolness	below 28°C
TRPA1	cold (also found in cilia of auditory and vestibular hair cells)	below 18°C

receptors are sensitive to pungent irritants found in mustard oil, wintergreen oil, horseradish, and garlic, and to a variety of environmental irritants, including those found in vehicle exhaust and tear gas (Bautista et al., 2006; Nilius et al., 2007). The primary function of this receptor appears to provide information about the presence of chemicals that produce inflammation.

Pain can be extremely unpleasant, but it provides useful information that can help us avoid injury. Cox et al. (2006) studied three families from northern Pakistan whose members included several people with a complete absence of pain and discovered the location of the gene responsible for this disorder. The gene, an autosomal recessive allele located on chromosome 2, encodes for a voltage-dependent sodium channel, $Na_x1.7$. The case that brought the families to their attention was a 10-year-old boy who performed a "street theater" during which he would thrust knives through his arms and walk on burning coals without feeling any pain. He died just before his fourteenth birthday after jumping off of the roof of a house. All six of the affected people in the three families had injuries to their lips or tongues caused by self-inflicted bites. They all suffered from bruises and cuts, and many sustained bone fractures that they did not notice until the injuries impaired their mobility. Despite their total lack of pain from any type of noxious stimulus, they had normal sensations of touch, warmth, coolness, proprioception, tickle, and pressure.

The Somatosensory Pathways

Somatosensory axons from the skin, muscles, or internal organs enter the central nervous system via spinal nerves. Those located in the face and head primarily enter through the trigeminal nerve (fifth cranial nerve). The cell bodies of the unipolar neurons are located in the dorsal root ganglia and cranial nerve ganglia. Axons that convey precisely localized information, such as fine touch, ascend through the *dorsal columns* in the white matter of the spinal cord to nuclei in the lower medulla. From there axons cross the brain and ascend through the *medial lemniscus* to the *ventral posterior nuclei of the thalamus*, the relay nuclei for somatosensation. Axons from the thalamus project to the primary somatosensory cortex, which in turn sends axons to the secondary somatosensory cortex. In contrast, axons that convey poorly localized information, such as pain or temperature, form synapses with other neurons as soon as they enter the spinal cord. The axons of these neurons cross to the other side of the spinal cord and ascend through the *spinothalamic tract* to the ventral posterior nuclei of the thalamus. (See *Figure 7.19.*)

As we saw in Chapter 6, damage to the visual association cortex can cause visual agnosia, and as we saw earlier in this chapter, damage to the auditory association cortex can cause auditory agnosia. You will not be surprised to learn that damage to the somatosensory association cortex can cause tactile agnosia. Reed, Caselli, and Farah (1996) described patient E. C., a woman with left parietal lobe damage who was unable to recognize common objects by touch. For example, the patient identified a pine cone as a brush, a ribbon as a rubber band, and a snail shell as a bottle cap. The deficit was not due to a simple loss of tactile sensitivity; the patient was still sensitive to light touch and to warm and cold objects, and she could easily discriminate objects by their size, weight, and roughness.

Recognition of objects by touch requires cooperation between the somatosensory and motor systems. When we attempt to identify objects by touch alone, we explore them with moving fingers. Valenza et al. (2001) reported the case of a patient with brain damage to the right hemisphere that produced a disorder they called tactile apraxia. (Apraxia refers to a difficulty in carrying out purposeful movements in the absence of paralysis or muscular weakness.) When the experimenters gave the patient objects to identify by touch with her left hand, the patient explored it with her fingers in a disorganized fashion. (Exploration and identification using her right hand were normal.) If the experimenters guided the patient's fingers and explored the object the way people normally do, she was able to recognize the object's shape. Thus, her deficit was caused by a movement disorder and not by damage to brain mechanisms involved in tactile perception.

Perception of Pain

Pain is a curious phenomenon. It is more than a mere sensation; it can be defined only by some sort of withdrawal reaction or, in humans, by verbal report. Pain can be modified by opiates, by hypnosis, by the administration of pharmacologically inert sugar pills, by emotions, and even by other forms of stimulation, such as acupuncture. Recent research efforts have made remarkable progress in discovering the physiological bases of these phenomena.

Pain appears to have three different perceptual and behavioral effects (Price, 2000). First is the sensory component—the pure perception of the intensity of a painful stimulus. The second component is the immediate emotional consequences of pain—the unpleasantness or degree to which the individual is bothered by the painful stimulus. The third component is the long-term emotional implications of chronic pain—the threat that such pain represents to one's future comfort and well-being.

These three components of pain appear to involve different brain mechanisms. The purely sensory component of pain is mediated by a pathway from the spinal cord to the ventral posterolateral thalamus to the primary and secondary somatosensory cortex. The immediate emotional component of pain appears to be mediated by pathways that reach the anterior cingulate cortex (ACC) and insular cortex. The long-term emotional component appears to be mediated by pathways that reach the prefrontal cortex. (See *Figure 7.20*.)

Rainville et al. (1997) produced pain sensations in human subjects by having them put their arms in ice water. Under one condition the researchers used hypnosis to diminish the unpleasantness of the pain. The hypnosis worked; the subjects said that the pain was less unpleasant, even though it was still as intense. Meanwhile, the investigators used a PET scanner to measure regional activation of the brain. They found that the painful stimulus increased the activity of both the primary somatosensory cortex and the ACC. When the subjects were hypnotized and found the pain less unpleasant, the activity of the ACC decreased—but the activity of the primary somatosensory cortex remained high. Presumably, the primary somatosensory cortex is involved in the perception of pain, and the ACC is involved in its immediate emotional effects—its unpleasantness. (See *Figure 7.21*.)

Several functional imaging studies have shown that under certain conditions, stimuli associated with pain can activate the ACC even when no actual painful stimulus is applied. In a test of romantically involved couples, Singer et al. (2004) found that when women received a painful electrical shock to the back of their hand, their ACC, anterior insular cortex, thalamus, and somatosensory cortex became active. When they saw their partners receive a painful shock but did not receive one themselves, the same regions (except for the somatosensory cortex) became active. Thus, the emotional component of pain—in this case, a vicarious experience of pain, provoked by empathy with the feelings of someone a person loved—caused responses in the brain similar to the ones caused by actual pain. Just as we saw in the study by

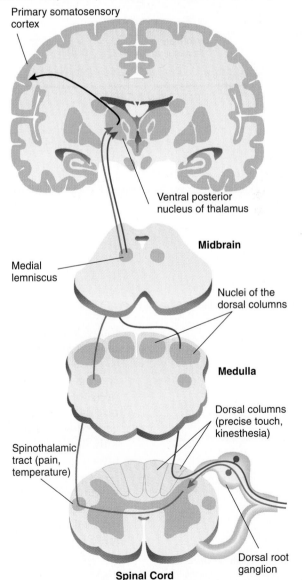

FIGURE 7.19

The Somatosensory Pathways. The figure shows the somatosensory pathways from the spinal cord to the somatosensory cortex. Note that precisely localized information (such as fine touch) and imprecisely localized information (such as pain and temperature) are transmitted by different pathways.

FIGURE 7.20

The Three Components of Pain.   A simplified, schematic diagram shows the brain mechanisms involved in the three components of pain: the sensory component, the immediate emotional component, and the long-term emotional component.

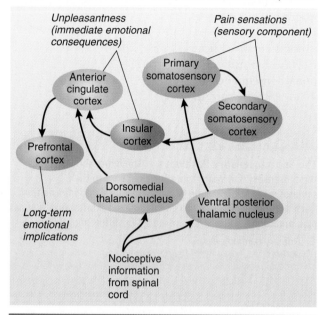

Adapted from Price, D. B. *Science*, 2000, *288*, 1769–1772.

FIGURE 7.21

Sensory and Emotional Components of Pain.   The PET scans show regions of the brain that respond to sensory and emotional components of pain. *Top*: Dorsal views of the brain. Activation of the primary somatosensory cortex (circled in red) by a painful stimulus was not affected by a hypnotically suggested reduction in unpleasantness of a painful stimulus, indicating that this region responded to the sensory component of pain. *Bottom*: Midsagittal views of the brain. The anterior cingulate cortex (circled in red) showed much less activation when the unpleasantness of the painful stimulus was reduced by hypnotic suggestion.

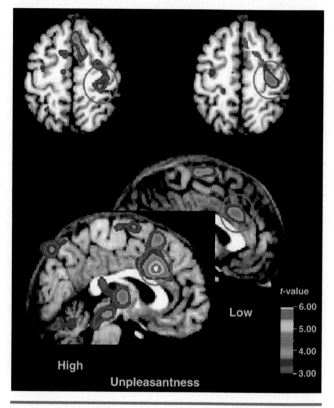

From Rainville, P., Duncan, G. H., Price, D. D., Carrier, Benoit, and Bushnell, M. C. *Science*, 1997, *277*, 968–971. Copyright © 1997. Reprinted with permission from AAAS.

Rainville et al. (1997), the somatosensory cortex is activated only by an actual noxious stimulus.

The third component of pain—the emotional consequences of chronic pain—appears to involve the prefrontal cortex. As we will see in Chapter 10, damage to the prefrontal cortex impairs people's ability to make plans for the future and to recognize the personal significance of situations in which they are involved. Along with the general lack of insight, people with prefrontal damage tend not to be concerned with the implications of chronic conditions—including chronic pain—for their future.

A particularly interesting form of pain sensation occurs after a limb has been amputated. After the limb is gone, up to 70 percent of amputees report that they feel as though the missing limb still existed and that it often hurts. This phenomenon is referred to as the **phantom limb** (Melzak, 1992). People with feelings of phantom limbs report that the limb feels very real, and they often say that if they try to reach out with it, it feels as though it were responding. Sometimes, they perceive it as sticking out, and they may feel compelled to avoid knocking it against the side of a doorframe or sleeping in a position that would make it come between them and the

phantom limb Sensations that appear to originate in a limb that has been amputated.

mattress. People have reported all sorts of sensations in phantom limbs, including pain, pressure, warmth, cold, wetness, itching, sweatiness, and prickliness.

Interim Summary

Somatosenses

Cutaneous sensory information is provided by specialized receptors in the skin. Pacinian corpuscles provide information about vibration. Ruffini corpuscles, similar to Pacinian corpuscles but considerably smaller, respond to indentation of the skin. Meissner's corpuscles, found in papillae and innervated by several axons, respond to low-frequency vibration or to brief taps on the skin. Merkel's disks, also found in papillae, consist of single, flattened dendritic endings next to specialized epithelial cells. These receptors respond to pressure. Painful stimuli and changes in temperature are detected by free nerve endings.

When the dendrites of mechanoreceptors bend, ion channels open, producing a receptor potential. A member of the transient receptor potential (TRP) family of receptors, TRPC1, controls the ion channel. Although most tactile information is transmitted to the CNS via fast-conducting myelinated axons, gentle stroking produces a pleasant sensation mediated by small, unmyelinated axons. This information is received by the insular cortex, a region associated with emotional responses.

Transduction of different ranges of temperatures is accomplished by six members of the TRP (transient receptor potential) family of receptors. One of the coolness receptors, TRPM8, also responds to menthol, and is involved in responsiveness to environmental cold. There are at least three different types of pain receptors: high-threshold mechanoreceptors; fibers with capsaicin receptors (TRPV1 receptors), which detect extremes of heat, acids, and the presence of capsaicin; and fibers with TRPA1 receptors, which are sensitive to chemical irritants and inflammation.

Precise, well-localized somatosensory information is conveyed by a pathway through the dorsal columns and their nuclei and the medial lemniscus, connecting the dorsal column nuclei with the ventral posterior nuclei of the thalamus. Information about pain and temperature ascends the spinal cord through the spinothalamic system. Damage to the somatosensory association cortex can disrupt the ability to recognize common objects by touch—a condition known as tactile agnosia. Tactile apraxia is a movement disorder that impairs the ability to explore objects with the finger.

Pain perception is not a simple function of stimulation of pain receptors; it is a complex phenomenon with sensory and emotional components that can be modified by experience and the immediate environment. The sensory component is mediated by the primary and secondary somatosensory cortex, the immediate emotional component appears to be mediated by the anterior cingulate cortex and the insular cortex, and the long-term emotional component appears to be mediated by the prefrontal cortex. The phantom limb phenomenon, which often accompanies limb amputation, is characterized by a variety of sensory events, including pain.

Thought Questions

Our fingertips and our lips are the most sensitive parts of our bodies; relatively large amounts of the primary somatosensory cortex are devoted to analyzing information from these parts of the body. It is easy to understand why our fingertips are so sensitive: We use them to explore object by touch. But why are our lips so sensitive? Does it have something to do with eating?

Gustation

The stimuli that we have encountered so far produce receptor potentials by imparting physical energy: thermal, photic (involving light), or kinetic. However, the stimuli received by the last two senses to be studied—gustation and olfaction—interact with their receptors chemically. This section discusses the first of them: gustation.

The Stimuli

Gustation is clearly related to eating; this sense modality helps us to determine the nature of things we put in our mouths. For a substance to be tasted, molecules of it must dissolve in the saliva and stimulate the taste receptors on the tongue. Tastes of different substances vary, but much less than we generally realize. There are only five qualities of taste: *bitterness, sourness, sweetness, saltiness,* and *umami.* You are familiar with the first four qualities, and I will explain the fifth one later. Flavor, as opposed to taste, is a composite of olfaction and gustation. Much of the flavor of food

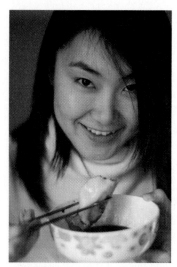

In the past, researchers believed that humans possessed four kinds of taste receptors that are sensitive to sweetness, sourness, bitterness, and saltiness. Now we know that the umami receptor, discovered by Japanese neuroscientists, can detect the savory taste of glutamate, which accounts for the flavor-enhancing effect of MSG.

depends on its odor; *anosmic* people (who lack the sense of smell) or people whose nostrils are stopped up have difficulty distinguishing between different foods by taste alone.

Most vertebrates possess gustatory systems that respond to all five taste qualities. (An exception is the cat family; lions, tigers, leopards, and house cats do not detect sweetness—but then, none of the food they normally eat is sweet.) Clearly, sweetness receptors are food detectors. Most sweet-tasting foods, such as fruits and some vegetables, are safe to eat (Ramirez, 1990). Saltiness receptors detect the presence of sodium chloride. In some environments inadequate amounts of this mineral are obtained from the usual source of food, so sodium chloride detectors help the animal to detect its presence. Injuries that cause bleeding deplete an organism of its supply of sodium rapidly, so the ability to find it quickly can be critical. Researchers now recognize the existence of a fifth taste quality: *umami*. **Umami**, a Japanese word that means "good taste," refers to the taste of monosodium glutamate (MSG), a substance that is often used as a flavor enhancer in Asian cuisine (Kurihara, 1987; Scott and Plata-Salaman, 1991). The umami receptor detects the presence of glutamate, an amino acid found in proteins. Presumably, the umami receptor provides the ability to taste proteins, an important nutrient.

Most species of animals will readily ingest substances that taste sweet or somewhat salty. Similarly, they are attracted to foods that are rich in amino acids, which explains the use of MSG as a flavor enhancer. However, they will tend to avoid substances that taste sour or bitter. Because of bacterial activity, many foods become acidic when they spoil. In addition, most unripe fruits are acidic. Acidity tastes sour and causes an avoidance reaction. (Of course, we have learned to make highly preferred mixtures of sweet and sour, such as lemonade.) Bitterness is almost universally avoided and cannot easily be improved by adding some sweetness. Many plants produce poisonous alkaloids, which protect them from being eaten by animals. Alkaloids taste bitter; thus, the bitterness receptor undoubtedly serves to warn animals away from these chemicals.

Anatomy of the Taste Buds and Gustatory Cells

The tongue, palate, pharynx, and larynx contain approximately 10,000 taste buds. Most of these receptive organs are arranged around *papillae*, small protuberances of the tongue. Taste buds consist of groups of twenty to fifty receptor cells, specialized neurons arranged somewhat like the segments of an orange. Cilia are located at the end of each cell and project through the opening of the taste bud (the pore) into the saliva that coats the tongue. Tight junctions between adjacent taste cells prevent substances in the saliva from diffusing freely into the taste bud itself. Figure 7.22 shows the appearance of a papilla; a cross section through the trench that surrounds it contains a taste bud. (See *Figure 7.22*.)

Taste receptor cells form synapses with dendrites of bipolar neurons whose axons convey gustatory information to the brain through the seventh, ninth, and tenth cranial nerves. The receptor cells have a life span of only 10 days. They quickly wear out, being directly exposed to a rather hostile environment. As they degenerate, they are replaced by newly developed cells; the dendrite of the bipolar neuron is passed on to the new cell (Beidler, 1970).

Perception of Gustatory Information

Transduction of taste is similar to the chemical transmission that takes place at synapses: The tasted molecule binds with the receptor and produces changes in membrane permeability that cause receptor potentials. Different substances bind with different types of receptors, producing different taste sensations. In this section I will describe what we know about the nature of the molecules with particular tastes and the receptors that detect their presence.

umami (*oo mah mee*) The taste sensation produced by glutamate; identify the presence of amino acids in foods.

To taste salty, a substance must ionize. Although the best stimulus for saltiness receptors is sodium chloride (NaCl), a variety of salts containing metallic cations (such as Na^+, K^+, and Li^+) with a small anion (such as Cl^-, Br^-, SO_4^{2-}, or NO_3^-) taste salty. The receptor for saltiness seems to be a simple sodium channel. When present in the saliva, sodium enters the taste cell and depolarizes it, triggering action potentials that cause the cell to release neurotransmitter (Avenet and Lindemann, 1989; Kinnamon and Cummings, 1992).

Sourness receptors respond to the hydrogen ions present in acidic solutions. However, because the sourness of a particular acid is not simply a function of the concentration of hydrogen ions, the anions must have an effect as well. Bitter and sweet substances are difficult to characterize. The typical stimulus for bitterness is a plant alkaloid such as quinine; for sweetness it is a sugar such as glucose or fructose. The fact that some molecules elicit both sensations suggested to early researchers that bitterness and sweetness receptors may be similar. For example, the Seville orange rind contains a glycoside (complex sugar) that tastes extremely bitter; the addition of a hydrogen ion to the molecule makes it taste intensely sweet (Horowitz and Gentili, 1974). Some amino acids taste sweet. Indeed, the commercial sweetener aspartame consists of just two amino acids: aspartate and phenylalanine.

Two different receptors are responsible for detection of sweet tastes. Bitterness is detected by members of a family of about thirty different receptors (Matsunami, Montmayeur, and Buck, 2000; Scott, 2004). The existence of so many different bitterness receptors suggests that although different bitter compounds share a common taste quality, they are detected by different means. As we saw, many compounds found in nature that taste bitter to us are poisonous. Rather than entrusting detection of these compounds to a single receptor, the process of evolution has given us the ability to detect a wide variety of compounds with different molecular shapes.

We saw earlier that cats are insensitive to sweet tastes. Li et al. (2005) discovered the reason for the absence of sweet sensitivity: The DNA of members of the cat family (the investigators tested domestic cats, tigers, and cheetahs) lacks functional genes that produce a class of proteins that form an essential part of sweet receptors. The investigators concluded that this mutation was probably an important event in the evolution of cats' carnivorous behavior.

For many years, researchers have known that many species of animals (including our own) show a distinct preference for high-fat foods. Because there is not a distinct taste that is associated with the presence of fat, most investigators concluded that we detected fat by its odor and texture ("mouth feel"). However, Fukuwatari et al. (2003) found that rats whose olfactory sense was destroyed continued to show a preference for a liquid diet containing a long-chain fatty acid, one of the breakdown products of fat. Laugerette et al. (2005) reported that a fatty acid transporter found in the papillae of the tongue appears to serve as a fatty-acid detector. The investigators found that in contrast to normal mice, mice with a knockout of the gene for this transporter showed no preference for fatty acids. When fats reach the tongue, some of these molecules are broken down by an enzyme called *lingual lipase*, which is found in the vicinity of taste buds. The activity of lingual lipase ensures that fatty acid detectors are stimulated when food containing fat enters the mouth.

The Gustatory Pathway

Gustatory information is transmitted through cranial nerves 7, 9, and 10. The first relay station for taste is the **nucleus of the solitary tract**, located in the medulla. In primates the taste-sensitive neurons of this nucleus send their axons to the ventral

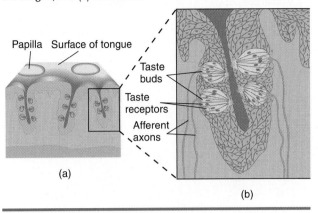

FIGURE 7.22

The Tongue.   The figure shows (a) papillae on the surface of the tongue, and (b) taste buds.

Papilla   Surface of tongue

Taste buds
Taste receptors
Afferent axons

(a)

(b)

nucleus of the solitary tract A nucleus of the medulla that receives information from visceral organs and from the gustatory system.

FIGURE 7.23

Neural Pathways of the Gustatory System

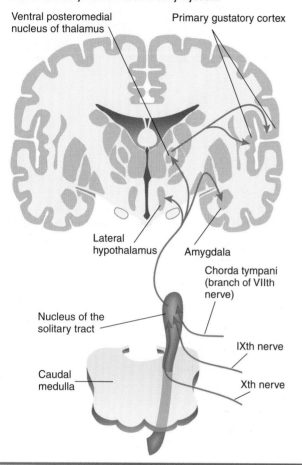

FIGURE 7.24

Activation in the Primary Gustatory Cortex. Functional MRI images of six subjects show that the responsive regions varied between subjects but were stable for each subject.

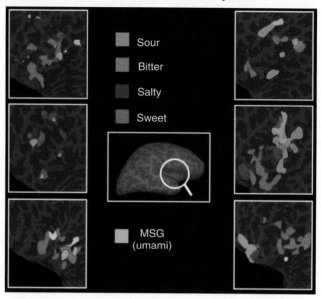

Reprinted from *NeuroScience, 127*, Schoenfeld, M. A., Neuer, G., Tempelmann, C., Schussler, K., Noesselt, T., Hopf, J.-M., and Heinze, H.-J., Functional Magnetic Resonance Tomography Correlates of Taste Perception in the Human Primary Taste Cortex, 347–353, Copyright 2004, with permission from Elsevier.

posteromedial thalamic nucleus, a nucleus that also receives somatosensory information received from the trigeminal nerve (Beckstead, Morse, and Norgren, 1980). Thalamic taste-sensitive neurons send their axons to the primary gustatory cortex, which is located in the base of the frontal cortex and in the insular cortex (Pritchard et al., 1986). Neurons in this region project to the secondary gustatory cortex, located in the caudolateral orbitofrontal cortex (Rolls, Yaxley, and Sienkiewicz, 1990). Unlike most other sense modalities, taste is ipsilaterally represented in the brain; that is, the right side of the tongue projects to the right side of the brain, and the left projects to the left. (See *Figure 7.23*.)

In a functional imaging study, Schoenfeld et al. (2004) had people sip water that was flavored with sweet, sour, bitter, and umami tastes. The investigators found that tasting each flavor activated different regions in the primary gustatory area of the insular cortex. Although the locations of the taste-responsive regions differed from subject to subject, the same pattern was seen when a subject was tested on different occasions. Thus, the representation of tastes in the gustatory cortex is idiosyncratic but stable. (See *Figure 7.24*.)

Gustatory information also reaches the amygdala and the hypothalamus and adjacent basal forebrain (Nauta, 1964; Russchen, Amaral, and Price, 1986). Many investigators believe that the hypothalamic pathway plays a role in mediating the reinforcing effects of sweet, umami, and slightly salty tastes. In fact, some neurons in the hypothalamus respond to sweet stimuli only when the animal is hungry (Rolls et al., 1986).

Olfaction

Olfaction, the second chemical sense, helps us to identify food and avoid food that has spoiled and is unfit to eat. It helps the members of many species to track prey or

InterimSummary

Gustation

Taste receptors detect only five sensory qualities: bitterness, sourness, sweetness, saltiness, and umami (umaminess?). Bitter foods often contain plant alkaloids, many of which are poisonous. Sour foods have usually undergone bacterial fermentation, which can produce toxins. On the other hand, sweet foods (such as fruits) are usually nutritious and safe to eat, and salty foods contain an essential cation: sodium. The fact that people in affluent cultures today tend to ingest excessive amounts of sweet and salty foods suggests that these taste qualities are naturally reinforcing. Umami, the taste of glutamate, identifies proteins.

Saltiness receptors appear to be simple sodium channels. Sourness receptors appear to detect the presence of hydrogen ions, but various anions also affect these receptors. The umami receptor detects the presence of glutamate. Two receptors are responsible for detection of sweet tastes, and thirty receptors detect bitterness.

Gustatory information is transmitted from the tongue through cranial nerves 7, 9, and 10 to the nucleus of the solitary tract (located in the medulla) and is relayed by the ventral posteromedial thalamus to the primary gustatory cortex in the basal frontal and insular areas. Different tastes activate different regions of the primary gustatory cortex. The caudolateral orbitofrontal cortex contains the secondary gustatory cortex. Gustatory information is also sent to the amygdala, hypothalamus, and basal forebrain.

Thought Questions

Bees and birds can taste sweet substances, but cats cannot. Obviously, the ability to taste particular substances is related to the range of foods a species eats. If, through the process of evolution, a species develops a greater range of foods, what do you think comes first: the food or the receptor? Would a species start eating something with a new taste (say, something sweet) and later develop the appropriate taste receptors, or would the taste receptors evolve first and then lead the animal to a new taste?

---

detect predators and to identify friends, foes, and receptive mates. For humans, olfaction is the most enigmatic of all sensory modalities. Odors have a peculiar ability to evoke memories, often vague ones that seem to have occurred in the distant past—a phenomenon that Marcel Proust vividly described in his book *Remembrance of Things Past*. Although people can discriminate among many thousands of different odors, we lack a good vocabulary to describe them. It is relatively easy to describe sights we have seen or sounds we have heard, but the description of an odor is difficult. At best, we can say that it smells like something else. Thus, the olfactory system appears to be specialized for *identifying things*, not for analyzing particular qualities.

For years I have told my students that one reason for the difference in sensitivity between our olfactory system and those of other mammals is that other mammals put their noses where odors are the strongest—just above the ground. For example, a dog following an odor trail sniffs along the ground, where the odors of a passing animal may have clung. Even a bloodhound's nose would not be very useful if it were located 5 or 6 feet above the ground, as ours is. I was gratified to learn that a scientific study established the fact that when people sniff the ground like dogs do, their olfactory system works much better. Porter et al. (2007) prepared a scent trail—a string moistened with essential oil of chocolate and laid down in a grassy field. The subjects were blindfolded and wore earmuffs, kneepads, and gloves, which prevented them from using anything other than their noses to follow the scent trail. They did quite well, and they adopted the same zigzag strategy used by dogs. (See *Figure 7.25*.) As the authors wrote, these findings ". . . suggest that the poor reputation of human olfaction may reflect, in part, behavioral demands rather than ultimate abilities" (Porter et al., 2006, p. 27).

FIGURE 7.25

Scent-Tracking Behavior. The path followed by a dog and a human during scent tracking is shown in red.

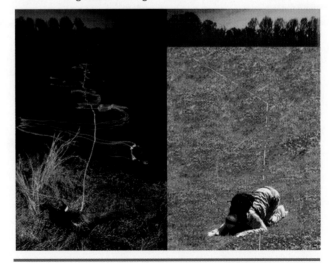

From (*left*) Louie Psihoyos/Science Faction; (*right*) Reprinted by permission from Macmillan Publishers Ltd: *Nature Neuroscience,* Porter, J., Craven, B., Khan, R. M., Chang, S.-J., Kang, I., Judkewitz, B., Volpe, J., Settles, G., and Sobel, N., Mechanisms of scent-tracking in humans, *10,* 27–29, copyright 2007.

The Stimulus

The stimulus for odor (known formally as *odorants*) consists of volatile substances that have a molecular weight in the range of approximately 15 to 300. Almost all odorous compounds are lipid soluble and of organic origin. However, many substances that meet these criteria have no odor at all, so we still have much to learn about the nature of odorants.

Anatomy of the Olfactory Apparatus

Our six million olfactory receptor cells reside within two patches of mucous membrane (the **olfactory epithelium**), each having an area of about 1 square inch. The olfactory epithelium is located at the top of the nasal cavity, as shown in *Figure 7.26*. Less than 10 percent of the air that enters the nostrils reaches the olfactory epithelium; a sniff is needed to sweep air upward into the nasal cavity so that it reaches the olfactory receptors.

The inset in Figure 7.26 illustrates a group of olfactory receptor cells, along with their supporting cells. (See *inset, Figure 7.26*.) Olfactory receptor cells are bipolar neurons whose cell bodies lie within the olfactory mucosa that lines the *cribriform plate*, a bone at the base of the rostral part of the brain. There is a constant production of new olfactory receptor cells, but their life is considerably longer than those of gustatory receptor cells. Supporting cells contain enzymes that destroy odorant

olfactory epithelium The epithelial tissue of the nasal sinus that covers the cribriform plate; contains the cilia of the olfactory receptors.

FIGURE 7.26

The Olfactory System

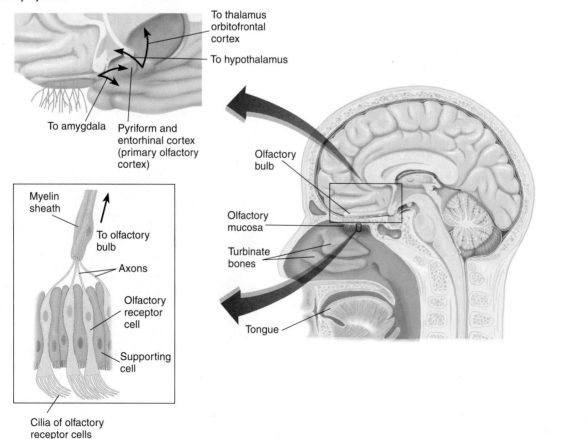

To thalamus orbitofrontal cortex

To hypothalamus

To amygdala

Pyriform and entorhinal cortex (primary olfactory cortex)

Olfactory bulb

Olfactory mucosa

Turbinate bones

Tongue

Myelin sheath

To olfactory bulb

Axons

Olfactory receptor cell

Supporting cell

Cilia of olfactory receptor cells

molecules and thus help to prevent them from damaging the olfactory receptor cells.

Olfactory receptor cells send a process toward the surface of the mucosa, which divides into ten to twenty cilia that penetrate the layer of mucus. Odorous molecules must dissolve in the mucus and stimulate receptor molecules on the olfactory cilia. Approximately thirty-five bundles of axons, ensheathed by glial cells, enter the skull through small holes in the cribriform ("perforated") plate. The olfactory mucosa also contains free nerve endings of trigeminal nerve axons; these nerve endings presumably mediate sensations of pain that can be produced by sniffing some irritating chemicals, such as ammonia.

The **olfactory bulbs** lie at the base of the brain on the ends of the stalk-like olfactory tracts. Each olfactory receptor cell sends a single axon into an olfactory bulb, where it forms synapses with dendrites of **mitral cells** (named for their resemblance to a bishop's miter, a form of ceremonial headgear). These synapses take place in the complex axonal and dendritic arborizations called **olfactory glomeruli** (from *glomus*, "ball"). There are approximately 10,000 glomeruli, each of which receives input from a bundle of approximately 2000 axons. The axons of the mitral cells travel to the rest of the brain through the olfactory tracts. Some of these axons terminate in other regions of the ipsilateral forebrain; others cross the brain and terminate in the contralateral olfactory bulb.

Olfactory tract axons project directly to the amygdala and to two regions of the limbic cortex: the piriform cortex and the entorhinal cortex. (See *Figure 7.26*.) The amygdala sends olfactory information to the hypothalamus, the entorhinal cortex sends it to the hippocampus, and the piriform cortex sends it to the hypothalamus and to the orbitofrontal cortex, via the dorsomedial nucleus of the thalamus (Buck, 1996; Shipley and Ennis, 1996). As you may recall, the orbitofrontal cortex also receives gustatory information; thus, it may be involved in the combining of taste and olfaction into flavor. The hypothalamus also receives a considerable amount of olfactory information, which is probably important for the acceptance or rejection of food and for the olfactory control of reproductive processes seen in many species of mammals.

Most mammals have another organ that responds to chemicals in the environment: the *vomeronasal organ*. Because it plays an important role in animals' responses to pheromones, chemicals produced by other animals that affect reproductive physiology and behavior, its structure and function are described in Chapter 9.

Transduction of Olfactory Information

For many years researchers have recognized that olfactory cilia contain receptors that are stimulated by molecules of odorants, but the nature of the receptors was unknown. Buck and Axel (1991), using molecular genetics techniques, discovered a family of genes that code for a family of olfactory receptor proteins (and in 2004 won a Nobel Prize for doing so). So far, olfactory receptor genes have been isolated in more than twelve species of vertebrates, including mammals, birds, and amphibians (Mombaerts, 1999). Humans have 339 different olfactory receptor genes, and mice have 913 (Malnic, Godfrey, and Buck, 2004; Godfrey, Malnic, and Buck, 2004). Molecules of odorant bind with olfactory receptors, and the G proteins coupled to these receptors open sodium channels and produce depolarizing receptor potentials.

Perception of Specific Odors

Recognition of specific odors has been an enigma for many years. Humans can recognize up to ten thousand different odorants, and other animals can probably recognize even more of them (Shepherd, 1994). Even with 339 different olfactory

olfactory bulb The protrusion at the end of the olfactory tract; receives input from the olfactory receptors.

mitral cell A neuron located in the olfactory bulb that receives information from olfactory receptors; axons of mitral cells bring information to the rest of the brain.

olfactory glomerulus (*glow mare you luss*) A bundle of dendrites of mitral cells and the associated terminal buttons of the axons of olfactory receptors.

receptors, many odors remain unaccounted for—and every year, chemists synthesize new chemicals, many with odors unlike those that anyone has previously detected. How can we use a relatively small number of receptors to detect so many different odorants?

Before I answer this question, we should look more closely at the relation between receptors, olfactory neurons, and the glomeruli to which the axons of these neurons project. First, the cilia of each olfactory neuron contain only one type of receptor (Nef et al., 1992; Vassar, Ngai, and Axel, 1993). As we saw, each glomerulus receives information from many individual olfactory receptor cells. Ressler, Sullivan, and Buck (1994) discovered that although a given glomerulus receives information from many olfactory receptor cells, each of these cells contains the same type of receptor molecule. Thus, there are as many types of glomeruli as there are types of receptor molecules. Furthermore, the location of particular types of glomeruli (defined by the type of receptor that sends information to them) appears to be the same in each of the olfactory bulbs in a given animal and may even be the same from one animal to another. (See *Figure 7.27*.)

Now let's get back to the question I just posed: How can we use a relatively small number of receptors to detect so many different odorants? The answer is that a particular odorant binds to more than one receptor. Thus, because a given glomerulus receives information from only one type of receptor, different odorants produce different *patterns* of activity in different glomeruli. Recognizing a particular odor, then, is a matter of recognizing a particular pattern of activity in the glomeruli. The task of chemical recognition is transformed into a task of spatial recognition.

Figure 7.28 illustrates this process (Malnic et al., 1999). The left side of the figure shows the shapes of eight hypothetical odorants. The right side shows four hypothetical odorant receptor molecules. If a portion of the odorant molecule fits the binding site of the receptor molecule, it will activate it and stimulate the olfactory neuron.

FIGURE 7.27

Connections of Olfactory Receptor Cells with Glomeruli.   Each glomerulus receives information from only one type of receptor cell. Olfactory receptor cells of different colors contain different types of receptor molecules.

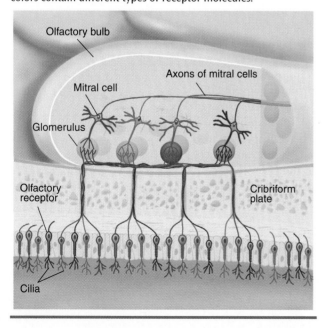

FIGURE 7.28

Coding of Olfactory Information.   A hypothetical explanation of coding of olfactory information shows that different odorant molecules attach to different combinations of receptor molecules. (Activated receptor molecules are shown in blue.) Unique patterns of activation represent particular odorants.

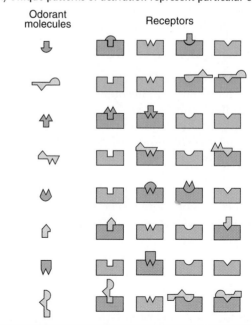

Adapted from Malnic, B., Hirono, J, Sato, T., and Buck, L. B. *Cell*, 1999, *96*, 713–723.

As you can see, each odorant molecule fits the binding site of at least one of the receptors and in most cases fits more than one of them. Notice also that the *pattern* of receptors activated by each of the eight odorants is different, which means that if we know which pattern of receptors is activated, we know which odorant is present. Of course, even though a particular odorant might bind with several different types of receptor molecules, it might not bind equally well with each of them. For example, it might bind very well with one receptor molecule, moderately well with another, weakly with another, and so on. (See *Figure 7.28*.) As we just saw, the spatial pattern of "olfacto-topic" information is maintained in the olfactory cortex. Presumably, the brain recognizes particular odors by recognizing different patterns of activation there.

Although we can often identify individual components of mixtures of odors, some odors have the ability to mask others. (The existence of the deodorant and air-freshener industries depends on this fact.) Cooks in various cultures have long known that as long as it is not too strong, the unpleasant, rancid off-flavor of spoiled food can be masked by the spices fennel and clove. Takahashi, Nagayama, and Mori (2004) mapped the regions of the olfactory bulb that responded to bad odorants (alkyl-amines and aliphatic aldehydes) and to the odors of fennel and clove. They found that responses to the bad odors was suppressed by the presence of the spice odors, indicating that the masking took place in the olfactory bulbs. Presumably, the glomeruli that responded to the spice odors inhibited those that responded to the rancid ones.

InterimSummary

Olfaction

The olfactory receptors consist of bipolar neurons located in the olfactory epithelium that lines the roof of the nasal sinuses, on the bone that underlies the frontal lobes. The receptors send processes toward the surface of the mucosa, which divide into cilia. The membranes of these cilia contain receptors that detect aromatic molecules dissolved in the air that sweeps past the olfactory mucosa. The axons of the olfactory receptors pass through the perforations of the cribriform plate into the olfactory bulbs, where they form synapses in the glomeruli with the dendrites of the mitral cells. These neurons send axons through the olfactory tracts to the brain, principally to the amygdala, the piriform cortex, and the entorhinal cortex. The hippocampus, hypothalamus, and orbitofrontal cortex receive olfactory information indirectly.

Aromatic molecules produce membrane potentials by interacting with a newly discovered family of receptor molecules, which in humans contains 339 members. Each glomerulus receives information from only one type of olfactory receptor, and "olfactotopic" coding is maintained all the way to the olfactory cortex. This means that the task of detecting different odors is a spatial one; the brain recognizes odors by means of the patterns of activity created in the olfactory cortex.

Thought Questions

As mentioned in the preceding section, odors have a peculiar ability to evoke memories, a phenomenon that Marcel Proust vividly described in his book *Remembrance of Things Past*. Have you ever encountered an odor that you knew was somehow familiar, but you couldn't say exactly why? Can you think of any explanations? Might this phenomenon have something to do with the fact that the sense of olfaction developed very early in our evolutionary history?

⋮ EPILOGUE Natural Analgesia

The brain contains neural circuitry through which certain types of stimuli can produce analgesia, primarily through the release of the endogenous opiates. What functions does this system perform? Most researchers believe that it prevents pain from disrupting behavior in situations in which pain is unavoidable and in which the damaging effect of the painful stimuli are less important than the goals of the behavior. For example, males fighting for access to females during mating season will fail to pass on their genes if pain elicits withdrawal responses that interfere with fighting. Indeed, these conditions (fighting or mating) *do* diminish pain.

Komisaruk and Larsson (1971) found that genital stimulation produced analgesia. They gently probed the cervix of female rats with a glass rod and found that the procedure diminished the animals' sensitivity to pain. It also increased the activity of neurons in the periaqueductal gray matter and decreased the pain response in the thalamus (Komisaruk and Steinman, 1987). The phenomenon also occurs in humans; Whipple and Komisaruk (1988) found that self-administered vaginal stimulation reduces women's sensitivity to painful stimuli but not to neutral tactile stimuli. Presumably, copulation also triggers analgesic mechanisms. The adaptive significance of this phenomenon is clear: Painful stimuli that are encountered during the course of copulation are less likely to cause the behavior to be interrupted; thus, the chances of pregnancy are increased. (As you will recall, passing on one's genes is the ultimate criterion of the adaptive significance of a trait.)

Pain can also be reduced, at least in some people, by administering a pharmacologically inert placebo. When some people take a medication that they believe will reduce pain, it triggers the release of endogenous opioids and actually does reduce pain sensations. This effect is eliminated if the people are given an injection of naloxone, a drug that blocks opiate receptors (Benedetti, Arduino, and Amanzio, 1999). Thus, for some people a placebo is not pharmacologically inert—it has a physiological effect. The experimenter in the chapter prologue used this drug when he blocked the analgesic effect of Melissa's own endogenous opiates. The placebo effect may be mediated through connections of the frontal cortex with the periaqueductal gray matter—a region of the midbrain that modulates the transmission of pain information to the brain.

A functional-imaging study by Zubieta et al. (2005) found that placebo-induced analgesia did indeed cause the release of endogenous opiates. They used a PET scanner to detect the presence of μ-opioid neurotransmission in the brains of people who responded to the effects of a placebo. As Figure 7.29 shows, several regions of the brain, including the anterior cingulate cortex and insular cortex, showed evidence of increased endogenous opioid activity. (See *Figure 7.29*.)

The endogenous opiates were first discovered by scientists who were investigating the perception of pain; thus, many of the studies using these peptides have examined their role in mechanisms of analgesia. However, their role in other functions may be even more important. As you will see in subsequent chapters, the endogenous opiates may even be involved in learning, especially in mechanisms of reinforcement. This connection should not come as a surprise; as you know, many people have found injections of opiates such as morphine or heroin to be extremely pleasurable.

FIGURE 7.29

Effects of a Placebo on μ-Opioid Neurotransmission.
The figure shows scans of people who responded to a placebo with the release of endogenous opioids and analgesia. ACC = anterior cingulate cortex, DLPFC = dorsolateral prefrontal cortex, NAC = nucleus accumbens.

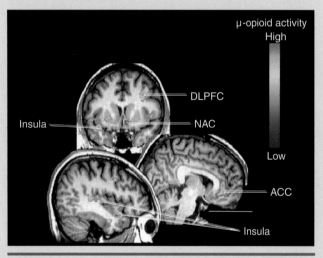

From Zubieta, J.-K., Bueller, J. A., Jackson, L. R., Scott, D. J., et al. *Journal of Neuroscience*, 2005, *25*, 7754–7762. Reprinted with permission.

Key Concepts

AUDITION

1. The bones of the middle ear transmit sound vibrations from the eardrum to the cochlea, which contains the auditory receptors the hair cells.
2. The hair cells send information through the eighth cranial nerve to nuclei in the brain stem; it is then relayed to the medial geniculate nucleus and finally to the primary auditory cortex.
3. The ear is analytical; it detects individual frequencies by means of place coding and rate coding.

Left–right localization is also accomplished by two means: arrival time (phase differences) and binaural differences in intensity.

VESTIBULAR SYSTEM

4. The vestibular system helps us to maintain our balance and makes compensatory eye movements to help us maintain fixation when our head moves. The semicircular canals detect head rotations and the vestibular sacs detect changes in the tilt of the head.

SOMATOSENSES

5. Cutaneous receptors in the skin provide information about touch, pressure, vibration, changes in temperature, and stimuli that cause tissue damage.

6. Pain perception helps to protect us from harmful stimuli. The sensory component of pain involves the thalamus and the somatosensory cortex, the immediate emotional component of pain involves the anterior cingulate cortex and insular cortex, and the long-term emotional component involves the prefrontal cortex.

GUSTATION

7. Taste receptors on the tongue respond to bitterness, sourness, sweetness, saltiness, and umami (the taste of glutamate, used to identify proteins). Together with olfactory information, gustation provides us with information about complex flavors.

OLFACTION

8. The olfactory system detects the presence of aromatic molecules. A family of several hundred different receptors is involved in olfactory discrimination. Patterns of activation of these receptors lead to perception of different odorants.

Suggested Readings

AUDITION

Copeland, B. J., and Pillsbury, H. C. Cochlear implantation for the treatment of deafness. *Annual Review of Medicine*, 2004, *55*, 157–167.

Ehret, G., and Romand, R. *The Central Auditory System.* New York: Oxford University Press, 1997.

Fettiplace, R., and Hackney, C. M. The sensory and motor roles of auditory hair cells. *Nature Reviews: Neuroscience*, 2006, *7*, 19–29.

Peretz, I., and Zatorre, R. J. Brain organization for music processing. *Annual Review of Psychology*, 2005, *56*, 89–114.

Stewart, L., von Kriegstein, K., Warren, J. D., and Griffiths, T. D. Music and the brain: Disorders of musical listening. *Brain*, 2006, *129*, 2533–2553.

Yost, W. A. *Fundamentals of Hearing: An Introduction*, 4th ed. San Diego: Academic Press, 2000.

Zatorre, R. J., Chen, J. L., and Penhune, V. B. When the brain plays music: Auditory–motor interactions in music perception and production. *Nature Reviews: Neuroscience*, 2007, *8*, 547–558.

VESTIBULAR SYSTEM

Cohen, B., Tomko, D. L., and Guedry, F. E. *Sensing and Controlling Motion: Vestibular and Sensorimotor Function.* New York: New York Academy of Sciences, 1992.

SOMATOSENSES

Benedetti, F., Mayberg, H. S., Wager, T. D., Stohler, C. S., and Zubieta, J.-K. Neurobiological mechanisms of the placebo effect. *Journal of Neuroscience*, 2005, *25*, 10390–10402.

Dhaka, A., Viswanath, V., and Patapoutian, A. TRP ion channels and temperature sensation. *Annual Review of Neuroscience*, 2006, *29*, 135–161.

García-Añoveros, J., and Corey, D. P. The molecules of mechanosensation. *Annual Review of Neuroscience*, 1997, *20*, 567–594.

Ikoma, A., Steinhoff, M., Ständer, S., Yosipovitch, G., and Schmelz, M. The neurobiology of itch. *Nature Reviews: Neuroscience*, 2006, *7*, 535–547.

Kruger, L. *Pain and Touch: Handbook of Perception and Cognition*, 2nd ed. San Diego: Academic Press, 1996.

Melzak, R. Phantom limbs. *Scientific American*, 1992, *266(4)*, 120–126.

OLFACTION AND GUSTATION

Lledo, P.-M., Gheusi, G., and Vincert, J.-D. Information processing in the mammalian olfactory system. *Physiological Reviews*, 2005, *85*, 281–317.

Simon, S. A., de Araujo, I. E., Gutierrez, R., and Nicolelis, M. A. L. The neural mechanisms of gustation: A distributed processing code. *Nature Reviews: Neuroscience*, 2006, *7*, 890–901.

Wilson, R. L., and Mainen, Z. F. Early events in olfactory processing. *Annual Review of Neuroscience*, 2006, *29*, 163–201.

Additional Resources

Visit www.mypsychkit.com for additional review and practice of the material covered in this chapter. Within MyPsychKit, you can take practice tests and receive a customized study plan to help you review. Dozens of animations, tutorials, and Web links are also available. You can even review using the interactive electronic version of this textbook. You will need to register for MyPsychKit. See www.mypsychkit.com for complete details.

chapter 8 : Sleep and Biological Rhythms

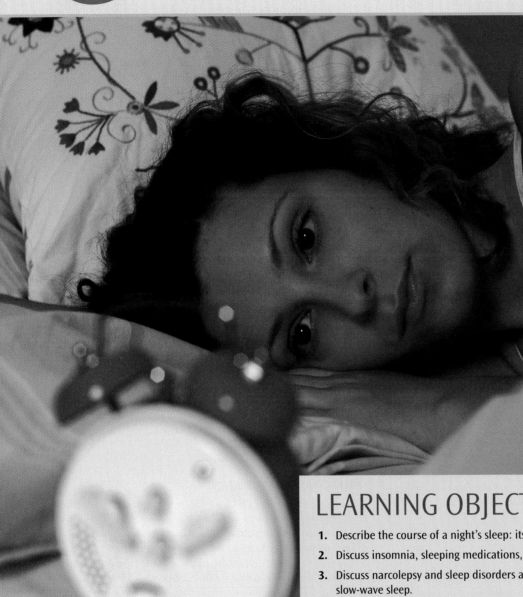

LEARNING OBJECTIVES

1. Describe the course of a night's sleep: its stages and their characteristics.

2. Discuss insomnia, sleeping medications, and sleep apnea.

3. Discuss narcolepsy and sleep disorders associated with REM sleep and slow-wave sleep.

4. Review the hypothesis that sleep serves as a period of restoration by discussing the effects of sleep deprivation, exercise, and mental activity.

5. Discuss research on the effects of REM sleep and slow-wave sleep on learning.

6. Evaluate evidence that the onset and amount of sleep is chemically controlled, and describe the neural control of arousal.

7. Discuss the neural control of slow-wave sleep, including the sleep/waking flip-flop and the role of orexinergic neurons.

8. Discuss the neural control of REM sleep, including the REM sleep flip-flop.

9. Describe circadian rhythms and discuss research on the neural and physiological bases of these rhythms.

PROLOGUE   Waking Nightmares

Lately, Michael felt almost afraid of going to bed because of the unpleasant experiences he had been having. His dreams seemed to have become more intense in a rather disturbing way. Several times in the past few months, he felt as if he were paralyzed as he lay in bed, waiting for sleep to come. It was a strange feeling. Was he *really* paralyzed, or was he just not trying hard enough to move? He always fell asleep before he was able to decide. A couple of times he woke up just before it was time for his alarm to go off and felt unable to move. Then the alarm would ring, and he would quickly shut it off. That meant that he really wasn't paralyzed, didn't it? Was he going crazy?

Last night brought the worst experience of all. As he was falling asleep, he felt again as if he were paralyzed. Then he saw his old roommate enter his bedroom. But that wasn't possible! Since the time he graduated from college, he had lived alone, and he always locked the door. He tried to say something, but he could not. His roommate was holding a hammer. He walked up to his bed, stood over Michael, and suddenly raised the hammer, as if to smash in his forehead. When he awoke in the morning, he shuddered with the remembrance. It had seemed so real! It must have been a dream, but he didn't think he was asleep. He was in bed. Can a person really dream that he is lying in bed, not yet asleep?

That day at the office, he had trouble concentrating on his work. He forced himself to review his notes, because he had to present the details of the new project to the board of directors. This was his big chance; if the project were accepted, he would certainly be chosen to lead it, and that would mean a promotion and a substantial raise. Naturally, with so much at stake, he felt

nervous when he entered the boardroom. His boss introduced Michael and asked him to begin. Michael glanced at his notes and opened his mouth to talk. Suddenly, he felt his knees buckle. All his strength seemed to slip away. He fell heavily to the floor. He could hear people running over and asking what had happened. He couldn't move anything except his eyes. His boss got down on his knees, looked into Michael's face, and asked, "Michael, are you all right?" Michael looked at his boss and tried to answer, but he couldn't say a thing. A few seconds later, he felt his strength coming back. He opened his mouth and said, "I'm okay." He struggled to his knees and then sat in a chair, feeling weak and frightened.

"You undoubtedly have a condition known as narcolepsy," said the doctor whom Michael visited. "It's a problem that concerns the way your brain controls sleep. I'll have you spend a night in the sleep clinic and get some recordings done to confirm my diagnosis, but I'm sure that I'll be proved correct. You told me that lately you've been taking short naps during the day. What were these naps like? Were you suddenly struck by an urge to sleep?" Michael nodded. "I just had to put my head on the desk, even though I was afraid that my boss might see me. But I don't think I slept more than 5 minutes or so." "Did you still feel sleepy when you woke?" "No," he replied, "I felt fine again." The doctor nodded. "All the symptoms you have reported—the sleep attacks, the paralysis you experienced before sleeping and after waking up, the spell you had today—they all fit together. Fortunately, we can usually control narcolepsy with medication. In fact, we have a new one that does an excellent job. I'm sure we'll have you back to normal, and there is no reason why you can't continue with your job. If you'd like, I can talk with your boss and reassure him, too."

Why do we sleep? Why do we spend at least one-third of our lives doing something that provides most of us with only a few fleeting memories? I will attempt to answer this question in several ways. In the first two parts of this chapter I will describe what is known about the phenomenon of sleep and its disorders, including insomnia, narcolepsy, sleepwalking, and other sleep-related disorders. In the third part I will discuss research on the functions performed by sleep. In the fourth part I will describe the search for the chemicals and the neural circuits that control sleep and wakefulness. In the final part of the chapter I will discuss the brain's biological clock—the mechanism that controls daily rhythms of sleep and wakefulness.

A Physiological and Behavioral Description of Sleep

Sleep is a behavior. That statement might seem peculiar, because we usually think of behaviors as activities that involve movements, such as walking or talking. Except for

FIGURE 8.1

A Subject Prepared for a Night's Sleep in a Sleep Laboratory

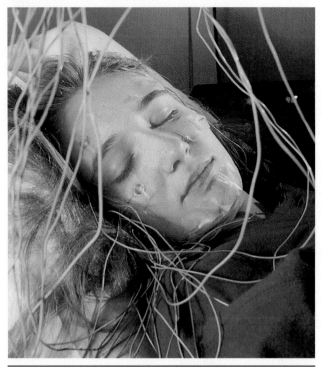

Philippe Platilly/Science Photo Library/Photo Researchers Inc.

electromyogram (EMG) (*my oh gram*) An electrical potential recorded from an electrode placed on or in a muscle.

electro-oculogram (EOG) (*ah kew loh gram*) An electrical potential from the eyes, recorded by means of electrodes placed on the skin around them; detects eye movements.

alpha activity Smooth electrical activity of 8–12 Hz recorded from the brain; generally associated with a state of relaxation.

beta activity Irregular electrical activity of 13–30 Hz recorded from the brain; generally associated with a state of arousal.

theta activity EEG activity of 3.5–7.5 Hz that occurs intermittently during early stages of slow-wave sleep and REM sleep.

the rapid eye movements that accompany a particular stage, sleep is not distinguished by movement. What characterizes sleep is that the insistent urge of sleepiness forces us to seek out a quiet, warm, comfortable place, lie down, and remain there for several hours. Because we remember very little about what happens while we sleep, we tend to think of sleep more as a state of consciousness than as a behavior. The change in consciousness is undeniable, but it should not prevent us from noticing the behavioral changes.

The best research on human sleep is conducted in a sleep laboratory. A sleep laboratory, usually located at a university or medical center, consists of one or several small bedrooms adjacent to an observation room, where the experimenter spends the night (trying to stay awake). The experimenter prepares the sleeper for electrophysiological measurements by attaching electrodes to the scalp to monitor the electroencephalogram (EEG) and to the chin to monitor muscle activity, recorded as the **electromyogram (EMG)**. Electrodes attached around the eyes monitor eye movements, recorded as the **electro-oculogram (EOG)**. In addition, other electrodes and transducing devices can be used to monitor autonomic measures such as heart rate, respiration, and changes in the ability of the skin to conduct electricity. (See *Figure 8.1*.)

During wakefulness the EEG of a normal person shows two basic patterns of activity: *alpha activity* and *beta activity*. **Alpha activity** consists of regular, medium-frequency waves of 8–12 Hz. The brain produces this activity when a person is resting quietly, not particularly aroused or excited and not engaged in strenuous mental activity (such as problem solving). Although alpha waves sometimes occur when a person's eyes are open, they are much more prevalent when the eyes are closed. The other type of waking EEG pattern, **beta activity**, consists of irregular, mostly low-amplitude waves of 13–30 Hz. Beta activity shows *desynchrony*; it reflects the fact that many different neural circuits in the brain are actively processing information. Desynchronized activity occurs when a person is alert and attentive to events in the environment or is thinking actively. (See *Figure 8.2*.)

Let us look at a typical night's sleep of a female college student in a sleep laboratory. (Of course, we would obtain similar results from a male, with one exception, which is noted later.) The experimenter attaches the electrodes, turns the lights off, and closes the door. Our subject becomes drowsy and soon enters stage 1 sleep, marked by the presence of some **theta activity** (3.5–7.5 Hz), which indicates that the firing of neurons in the neocortex is becoming more synchronized. This stage is actually a transition between sleep and wakefulness; if we watch our volunteer's eyelids, we will see that from time to time they slowly open and close and that her eyes roll upward and downward. (See *Figure 8.2*.) About 10 minutes later she enters stage 2 sleep. The EEG during this stage is generally irregular but contains periods of theta activity, *sleep spindles*, and *K complexes*. Sleep spindles are short bursts of waves of 12–14 Hz that occur between two and five times a minute during stages 1–4 of sleep. K complexes are sudden, sharp waveforms that, unlike sleep spindles, are usually found only during stage 2 sleep. They spontaneously occur at the rate of approximately one per minute but often can be triggered by noises—especially unexpected noises. A functional MRI study by Czisch et al. (2004) indicated that K complexes, triggered by an auditory stimulus, represent an inhibitory mechanism that presumably protects the sleeper from awakening. As we will see, K complexes appear to be the forerunner of delta waves, which appear in the deepest levels of sleep. (See *Figure 8.2*.)

The subject is sleeping soundly now; but if awakened, she might report that she has not been asleep. This phenomenon often is reported by nurses who awaken loudly snoring patients early in the night (probably to give them a sleeping pill) and find that the patients insist that they were lying there awake all the time. About 15 minutes later the subject enters stage 3 sleep, signaled by the occurrence of high-amplitude **delta activity** (slower than 3.5 Hz). (See *Figure 8.2*.) The distinction between stage 3 and stage 4 is not clear-cut; stage 3 contains 20–50 percent delta activity, and stage 4 contains more than 50 percent. Because slow-wave EEG activity predominates during sleep stages 3 and 4, they are collectively referred to as **slow-wave sleep**. (See *Figure 8.2*.)

About 90 minutes after the beginning of sleep (and about 45 minutes after the onset of stage 4 sleep), we notice an abrupt change in a number of physiological measures recorded from our subject. The EEG suddenly becomes mostly desynchronized, with a sprinkling of theta waves, very similar to the record obtained during stage 1 sleep. (See *Figure 8.2*.) We also note that her eyes are rapidly darting back and forth beneath her closed eyelids. We can see this activity in the EOG, recorded from electrodes attached to the skin around her eyes, or we can observe the eye movements directly—the cornea produces a bulge in the closed eyelids that can be seen to move about. We also see that the EMG becomes silent; there is a profound loss of muscle tone. In fact, physiological studies have shown that, aside from occasional twitching, a person actually becomes paralyzed during REM sleep. This peculiar stage of sleep is quite distinct from the quiet sleep we saw earlier. It is usually referred to as **REM sleep** (for the **r**apid **e**ye **m**ovements that characterize it).

By most criteria, stage 4 is the deepest stage of sleep; only loud noises will cause a person to awaken, and when awakened, the person acts groggy and confused. During REM sleep a person might not react to noises, but he or she is easily aroused by meaningful stimuli, such as the sound of his or her name. Also, when awakened from REM sleep, a person appears alert and attentive.

If we arouse our volunteer during REM sleep and ask her what was going on, she will almost certainly report that she had been dreaming. The dreams of REM sleep tend to be narrative in form, with a story-like progression of events. If we wake her during slow-wave sleep and ask, "Were you dreaming?" she will most likely say, "No." However, if we question her more carefully, she might report the presence of a thought, an image, or some emotion.

During the rest of the night our subject's sleep alternates between periods of REM and non-REM sleep. Each cycle is approximately 90 minutes long, containing a 20- to 30-minute bout of REM sleep. Thus, an 8-hour sleep will contain four or five periods of REM sleep. Figure 8.3 shows a graph of a typical night's sleep. The vertical axis indicates the EEG activity that is being recorded; thus REM sleep and stage 1 sleep are placed on the same line because similar patterns of EEG activity occur at these times. Note that most slow-wave sleep (stages 3 and 4) occurs during the first half of night. Subsequent bouts of non-REM sleep contain more and more stage 2 sleep, and bouts of REM sleep (indicated by the horizontal bars) become more prolonged. (See *Figure 8.3*.)

As we saw, during REM sleep we become paralyzed; most of our spinal and cranial motor neurons are strongly inhibited. (Obviously, the ones that control respiration and eye movements are spared.) At the same time the brain is very active.

FIGURE 8.2

EEG Recording of the Stages of Sleep

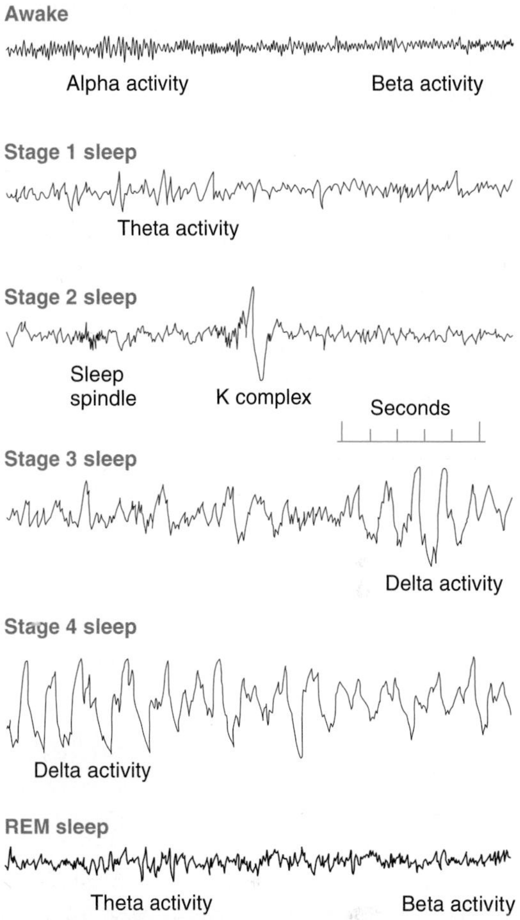

Awake

Alpha activity   Beta activity

Stage 1 sleep

Theta activity

Stage 2 sleep

Sleep spindle   K complex   Seconds

Stage 3 sleep

Delta activity

Stage 4 sleep

Delta activity

REM sleep

Theta activity   Beta activity

From Horne, J. A. *Why We Sleep: The Functions of Sleep in Humans and Other Mammals.* Oxford, England: Oxford University Press, 1988. Reprinted with permission.

delta activity Regular, synchronous electrical activity of less than 4 Hz recorded from the brain; occurs during the deepest stages of slow-wave sleep.

slow-wave sleep Non-REM sleep, characterized by synchronized EEG activity during its deeper stages.

REM sleep A period of desynchronized EEG activity during sleep, at which time dreaming, rapid eye movements, and muscular paralysis occur; also called *paradoxical sleep.*

FIGURE 8.3

Sleep Stages During a Single Night. In this typical pattern of sleep stages, the dark blue shading indicates REM sleep.

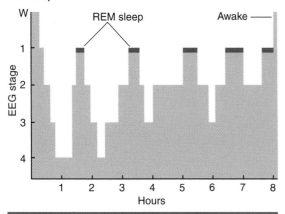

Cerebral blood flow and oxygen consumption are accelerated. In addition, during most periods of REM sleep, a male's penis will become at least partially erect, and a female's vaginal secretions will increase. However, Fisher, Gross, and Zuch (1965) found that in males, genital changes do not signify that the person is experiencing a dream with sexual content. (Of course, people can have dreams with frank sexual content. In males some dreams culminate in ejaculation—the so-called nocturnal emissions, or "wet dreams." Females, too, sometimes experience orgasm during sleep.)

The fact that penile erections occur during REM sleep, independent of sexual arousal, has been used clinically to assess the causes of impotence (Karacan, Salis, and Williams, 1978; Singer and Weiner, 1996). A subject sleeps in the laboratory with a device attached to his penis that measures its circumference. If penile enlargement occurs during REM sleep, then his failure to obtain an erection during attempts at intercourse is not caused by physiological problems such as nerve damage or a circulatory disorder. (A neurologist told me that there is a less-expensive way to gather the same data: The patient obtains a strip of postage stamps, moistens them, and applies them around his penis before going to bed. In the morning he checks to see whether the perforations are broken.)

The important differences between REM and slow-wave sleep are listed in *Table 8.1*.

TABLE 8.1 Principal Characteristics of REM and Slow-Wave Sleep	
REM Sleep	**Slow-Wave Sleep**
EEG desynchrony (rapid, irregular waves)	EEG synchrony (slow waves)
Lack of muscle tonus	Moderate muscle tonus
Rapid eye movements	Slow or absent eye movements
Penile erection or vaginal secretion	Lack of genital activity
Dreams	

InterimSummary

A Physiological and Behavioral Description of Sleep

Sleep is generally regarded as a state, but it is nevertheless a behavior. The stages of non-REM sleep, stages 1–4, are defined by EEG activity. Slow-wave sleep (stages 3 and 4) includes the two deepest stages. Alertness consists of desynchronized beta activity (13–30 Hz); relaxation and drowsiness consist of alpha activity (8–12 Hz); stage 1 sleep consists of alternating periods of alpha activity, irregular fast activity, and theta activity (3.5–7.5 Hz); the EEG of stage 2 sleep lacks alpha activity but contains sleep spindles (short periods of 12–14 Hz activity) and occasional K complexes; stage 3 sleep consists of 20–50 percent delta activity (less than 3.5 Hz); and stage 4 sleep consists of more than 50 percent delta activity. About 90 minutes after the beginning of sleep, people enter REM sleep. Cycles of REM and slow-wave sleep alternate in periods of approximately 90 minutes.

REM sleep consists of rapid eye movements, a desynchronized EEG, sensitivity to external stimulation, muscular paralysis, genital activity, and dreaming. Mental activity can accompany slow-wave sleep too, but most narrative dreams occur during REM sleep.

Thought Questions

1. Have you ever been resting quietly and suddenly heard someone tell you that you had obviously been sleeping because you were

snoring? Did you believe them, or were you certain that you were really awake? Do you think it was likely that you had actually entered stage 1 sleep?

2. What is accomplished by dreaming? Some researchers believe that the subject matter of a dream does not matter; it is the REM sleep itself that is important. Others believe that the subject matter *does* count. Some researchers believe that if we remember a dream, then the dream failed to accomplish all of

its functions; others say that remembering dreams is useful because it can give us some insights into our problems. What do you think of these controversies?

3. Some people report that they are "in control" of some of their dreams, that they feel as if they determine what comes next and are not simply swept along passively. Have you ever had this experience? Have you ever had a "lucid dream," in which you were aware of the fact that you were dreaming?

Disorders of Sleep

Because we spend about one-third of our lives sleeping, sleep disorders can have a significant impact on our quality of life. They can also affect the way we feel while we are awake.

Insomnia

Insomnia is a problem that is said to affect approximately 25 percent of the population occasionally and 9 percent regularly (Ancoli-Israel and Roth, 1999), but we need to define *insomnia* carefully. First, there is no single definition of insomnia that can apply to all people. The amount of sleep that individuals require is quite variable. A short sleeper may feel fine with 5 hours of sleep; a long sleeper may still feel unrefreshed after 10 hours of sleep. Insomnia must be defined in relation to a person's particular sleep needs.

The second consideration in defining insomnia is the unreliability of self-reports. Most patients who receive a prescription for a sleeping medication are given one on the basis of their own description of their symptoms. That is, they tell their physician that they sleep very little at night, and the drug is prescribed on the basis of this testimony. Very few patients are observed during a night's sleep in a sleep laboratory; thus, insomnia is one of the few medical problems that physicians treat without having direct clinical evidence for its existence. However, studies on the sleep of people who complain of insomnia show that most of them grossly underestimate the amount of time they actually sleep.

For many years the goal of sleeping medication was to help people fall asleep, and when drug companies evaluated potential medications, they concentrated on that property. However, if we think about the ultimate goal of sleeping medication, it is to make the person feel more refreshed the next day. If a medication puts people to sleep right away but produces a hangover of grogginess and difficulty concentrating the next day, it is worse than useless. In fact, many drugs that were traditionally used to treat insomnia had just this effect. More recently, researchers have recognized that the true evaluation of a sleeping medication must be made during wakefulness the following day, and "hangover-free" drugs are finally being developed (Hajak et al., 1995; Ramakrishnan and Scheid, 2007).

A particular form of insomnia is caused by an inability to sleep and breathe at the same time. Patients with this disorder, called **sleep apnea**, fall asleep and then cease to breathe. (Nearly all people, especially people who snore, have occasional episodes of sleep apnea, but not to the extent that it interferes with sleep.) During a period of sleep apnea the level of carbon dioxide in the blood stimulates chemoreceptors (neurons that detect the presence of certain chemicals), and the person wakes up, gasping for air. The oxygen level of the blood returns to normal, the person falls asleep, and the whole cycle begins again. Because sleep is disrupted, people with this disorder typically feel sleepy and groggy during the day. Fortunately, many cases of sleep apnea are caused by an obstruction of the airway that can be

sleep apnea (*app nee a*) Cessation of breathing while sleeping.

corrected surgically or relieved by a device that attaches to the sleeper's face and provides pressurized air that keeps the airway open (Sher, 1990; Piccirillo, Duntley, and Schotland, 2000).

Narcolepsy

Narcolepsy (*narke* means "numbness," and *lepsis* means "seizure") is a neurological disorder characterized by sleep (or some of its components) at inappropriate times. The symptoms can be described in terms of what we know about the phenomena of sleep. The primary symptom of narcolepsy is the **sleep attack**. The narcoleptic sleep attack is an overwhelming urge to sleep that can happen at any time but occurs most often under monotonous, boring conditions. Sleep (which appears to be entirely normal) generally lasts for 2–5 minutes. The person usually wakes up feeling refreshed.

Another symptom of narcolepsy—in fact, the most striking one—is **cataplexy** (from *kata*, "down," and *plexis*, "stroke"). During a cataplectic attack a person will sustain varying amounts of muscle weakness. In some cases, the person will become completely paralyzed and slump down to the floor. The person will lie there, *fully conscious*, for a few seconds to several minutes. What apparently happens is that one of the phenomena of REM sleep—muscular paralysis—occurs at an inappropriate time. As we saw, this loss of tonus is caused by massive inhibition of motor neurons in the spinal cord. When this happens during waking, the victim of a cataplectic attack loses control of his or her muscles. (As in REM sleep, the person continues to breathe and is able to control eye movements.)

Cataplexy is quite different from a narcoleptic sleep attack; cataplexy is usually precipitated by strong emotional reactions or by sudden physical effort, especially if the patient is caught unaware. Laughter, anger, or an effort to catch a suddenly thrown object can trigger a cataplectic attack. In fact, as Guilleminault, Wilson, and Dement (1974) noted, even people who do not have cataplexy sometimes lose muscle strength after a bout of intense laughter. (Perhaps that is why we say a person can become "weak from laughter.") Common situations that bring on cataplexy are attempting to discipline one's children and making love (an awkward time to become paralyzed!). Michael, the man described in the opener to this chapter, had his first cataplectic attack when he was addressing the board of directors of the company he worked for. Wise (2004) notes that patients with narcolepsy often try to avoid thoughts and situations that are likely to evoke strong emotions because they know that these emotions are likely to trigger cataplectic attacks.

REM sleep paralysis sometimes intrudes into waking at a time that does not present any physical danger—just before or just after normal sleep, when a person is already lying down. This symptom of narcolepsy is referred to as **sleep paralysis**, an inability to move just before the onset of sleep or upon waking in the morning. A person can be snapped out of sleep paralysis by being touched or by hearing someone call his or her name. Sometimes, the mental components of REM sleep intrude into sleep paralysis; that is, the person dreams while lying awake, paralyzed. These episodes, called **hypnagogic hallucinations**, are often alarming or even terrifying. (The term *hypnagogic* comes from the Greek words *hupnos*, "sleep," and *agogos*, "leading.") During a hypnagogic hallucination Michael thought that his former roommate was trying to attack him with a hammer.

Narcoleptic patients often have difficulty staying awake, and aspects of REM sleep sometimes intrude into the waking state. In addition, they often skip the slow-wave sleep that normally begins a night's sleep and go directly into REM sleep from waking. Finally, their sleep is often fragmented—disrupted by periods of wakefulness.

Fortunately, human narcolepsy is relatively rare, with an incidence of approximately one in 2000 people. This hereditary disorder appears to involve a gene found on chromosome 6, but it is strongly influenced by unknown environmental

narcolepsy (*nahr ko lep see*) A sleep disorder characterized by periods of irresistible sleep, attacks of cataplexy, sleep paralysis, and hypnagogic hallucinations.

sleep attack A symptom of narcolepsy; an irresistible urge to sleep during the day, after which the person awakens feeling refreshed.

cataplexy (*kat a plex ee*) A symptom of narcolepsy; complete paralysis that occurs during waking.

sleep paralysis A symptom of narcolepsy; paralysis occurring just before a person falls asleep.

hypnagogic hallucination (*hip na gah jik*) A symptom of narcolepsy; vivid dreams that occur just before a person falls asleep; accompanied by sleep paralysis.

FIGURE 8.4

A Dog Undergoing a Cataplectic Attack. The attack was triggered by the dog's excitement at finding some food on the floor. (a) The dog sniffs the food. (b) Muscles begin to relax. (c) The dog is temporarily paralyzed, as it would be during REM sleep.

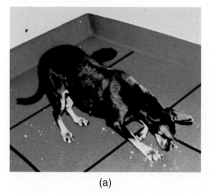
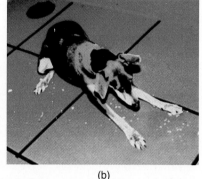
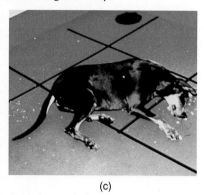

(a)   (b)   (c)

Photos courtesy of the Sleep Disorders Foundation, Stanford University.

factors (Mignot, 1998; Mahowald and Schenck, 2005; Nishino, 2007). Years ago, researchers began a program to maintain breeds of dogs that are afflicted with narcolepsy, with the hopes that discovery of the causes of canine narcolepsy would further our understanding of the causes of human narcolepsy. (See *Figure 8.4*.) Eventually, this research paid off. Lin et al. (1999) discovered that a mutation of a specific gene is responsible for canine narcolepsy. The product of this gene is a receptor for a peptide neurotransmitter called *hypocretin* by some researchers, and as *orexin* by others. The name "hypocretin" comes from the fact that the lateral *hypo*thalamus contains the cell bodies of all of the neurons that se*crete* this peptide. The name "orexin" comes from the role this peptide plays in the control of eating and metabolism, which are discussed in greater detail in Chapter 11. (*Orexis* means "appetite" in Greek.) Most researchers appear to have settled on the word **orexin**, so I will use this term also. There are two orexin receptors. Lin and his colleagues discovered that the mutation responsible for canine narcolepsy involves the orexin B receptor.

Chemelli et al. (1999) prepared a targeted mutation in mice against the orexin gene and found that the animals showed symptoms of narcolepsy. Like human patients with narcolepsy, they went directly into REM sleep from waking and showed periods of cataplexy while they were awake. (Videos of narcoleptic dogs, mice, and people are shown in *MyPsychKit 8.1, Narcolepsy*.) Gerashchenko et al. (2001, 2003) prepared a toxin that attacked only orexinergic neurons, which they then administered to rats. The destruction of the orexin system produced the symptoms of narcolepsy.

In humans, narcolepsy appears to be caused by a hereditary autoimmune disorder (Nishino et al., 2000). Most patients with narcolepsy are born with orexinergic neurons, but during adolescence the immune system attacks these neurons, and the symptoms of narcolepsy begin.

The symptoms of narcolepsy can be treated with drugs. Sleep attacks can be diminished by stimulants such a methylphenidate (Ritalin), a catecholamine agonist (Vgontzas and Kales, 1999). The REM sleep phenomena (cataplexy, sleep paralysis, and hypnagogic hallucinations) have traditionally been treated with antidepressant drugs, which facilitate both serotonergic and noradrenergic activity (Mitler, 1994; Hublin, 1996). More recently, modafinil, a stimulant drug whose precise site of action is still unknown, has been used to treat narcolepsy (Fry, 1998; Nishino, 2007). (Michael, the man discussed in the prologue, is now taking this drug.)

The connections of orexinergic neurons with other regions of the brain is discussed later in this chapter.

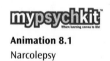

Animation 8.1
Narcolepsy

Orexin A peptide, also known as *hypocretin*, produced by neurons whose cell bodies are located in the hypothalamus; their destruction causes narcolepsy.

REM Sleep Behavior Disorder

Several years ago, Schenck et al. (1986) reported the existence of an interesting disorder: **REM sleep behavior disorder**. As you now know, REM sleep is accompanied by paralysis. Although the motor cortex and subcortical motor systems are extremely active during REM sleep (McCarley and Hobson, 1979), people are unable to move at this time.

The fact that people are paralyzed while they dream suggests the possibility that but for the paralysis, they would act out their dreams. Indeed, they would. The behavior of people who exhibit REM sleep behavior disorder corresponds with the contents of their dreams. Consider the following case:

> I was a halfback playing football, and after the quarterback received the ball from the center he lateraled it sideways to me and I'm supposed to go around the end and cut back over tackle and—this is very vivid—as I cut back over tackle there is this big 280-pound tackle waiting, so I, according to football rules, was to give him my shoulder and bounce him out of the way . . . when I came to I was standing in front of our dresser and I had [gotten up out of bed and run and] knocked lamps, mirrors and everything off the dresser, hit my head against the wall and my knee against the dresser. (Schenck et al., 1986, p. 294)

Like narcolepsy, REM sleep behavior disorder appears to be a neurodegenerative disorder with at least some genetic component (Schenck, Hurwitz, and Mahowald, 1993). It is often associated with better-known neurodegenerative disorders such as Parkinson's disease (Boeve et al., 2007). The symptoms of REM sleep behavior disorder are the opposite of those of cataplexy; that is, rather than exhibiting paralysis outside REM sleep, patients with REM sleep behavior disorder *fail* to exhibit paralysis *during* REM sleep. As you might expect, the drugs that are used to treat the symptoms of cataplexy will aggravate the symptoms of REM sleep behavior disorder (Schenck and Mahowald, 1992). REM sleep behavior disorder is usually treated by clonazepam, a benzodiazepine (Schenck, Hurwitz, and Mahowald, 1993).

Problems Associated with Slow-Wave Sleep

Some maladaptive behaviors occur during slow-wave sleep, especially during its deepest phase, stage 4. These behaviors include bedwetting (*nocturnal enuresis*), sleepwalking (*somnambulism*), and night terrors (*pavor nocturnus*). All three events occur most frequently in children. Often bedwetting can be cured by training methods, such as having a special electronic circuit ring a bell when the first few drops of urine are detected in the bed sheet (a few drops usually precede the ensuing flood). Night terrors consist of anguished screams, trembling, a rapid pulse, and usually no memory of what caused the terror. Night terrors and somnambulism usually cure themselves as the child gets older. Neither of these phenomena is related to REM sleep; a sleepwalking person is *not* acting out a dream. Especially when it occurs in adulthood, sleepwalking appears to have a genetic component (Hublin et al., 1997).

Sometimes, people can engage in complex behaviors while sleepwalking. Consider the following cases:

> One evening Ed Weber got up from a nap on the sofa, polished off a half-gallon of chocolate chip ice cream, then dozed off again. He woke up an hour later and went looking for the ice cream, summoning his wife to the kitchen and insisting, to her astonishment, that someone else must have eaten it.

REM sleep behavior disorder A neurological disorder in which the person does not become paralyzed during REM sleep and thus acts out dreams.

[T]elevision talk show host Montel Williams . . . told viewers he had removed raw foods from his refrigerator because "I wake up in the morning and there's a pack of chicken and there's a bite missing out of it. . . . I can take a whole pound of ham or bologna . . . and then wake up in the morning and not realize that I had [eaten] it and ask, 'Who ate my lunch meat?' " (Boodman, 2004, p. HE01)

Schenck et al. (1991) reported nineteen cases of people with histories of eating during the night while they were asleep, which the researchers labeled **sleep-related eating disorder**. Almost half of the patients had become overweight from night eating. Once patients realize that they are eating in their sleep, they often employ such stratagems as keeping their food under lock and key or setting alarms that will awaken them when they try to open their refrigerator.

Sleep-related eating disorder usually responds well to dopaminergic agonists, anxiolytic drugs, or antianxiety drugs. An increased incidence of nocturnal eating in family members of people with this disorder suggests that heredity may play a role (De Ocampo et al., 2002). Preliminary evidence suggests that nocturnal eating may be associated with the use of some sleeping medications used to treat insomnia (Morgenthaler and Silber, 2002; Najjar, 2007).

Interim Summary

Disorders of Sleep

Although many people believe that they have insomnia—that they do not obtain as much sleep as they would like—insomnia is not a disease. Insomnia can be caused by depression, mania, pain, illness, or even excited anticipation of a pleasurable event. Sometimes, insomnia is caused by sleep apnea, which can often be corrected surgically or treated by wearing a mask that delivers pressurized air.

Narcolepsy is characterized by four symptoms. *Sleep attacks* consist of overwhelming urges to sleep for a few minutes. *Cataplexy* is sudden paralysis, during which the person remains conscious. *Sleep paralysis* is similar to cataplexy, but it occurs just before sleep or on waking. *Hypnagogic hallucinations* are dreams that occur during periods of sleep paralysis, just before a night's sleep. Sleep attacks are treated with stimulants such as amphetamine, and the other symptoms are treated with serotonin agonists. Studies with narcoleptic dogs and humans indicate that this disorder is caused by pathologies in a system of neurons that secrete a neuropeptide known as orexin (also known as hypocretin). REM sleep behavior disorder is a neurodegenerative disease that damages brain mechanisms that produce paralysis during REM sleep. As a result, the patient acts out his or her dreams.

During slow-wave sleep, especially during stage 4, some people are afflicted by bedwetting (nocturnal enuresis), sleepwalking (somnambulism), or night terrors (pavor nocturnus). These problems are most common in children, who usually outgrow them. People with sleep-related eating disorder seek and consume food while sleepwalking.

Thought Question

Suppose you spent the night at a friend's house and, hearing a strange noise during the night, got out of bed and found your friend walking around, still asleep. How would you tell whether your friend was sleepwalking or had REM sleep behavior disorder?

Why Do We Sleep?

We all know how insistent the urge to sleep can be and how uncomfortable we feel when we have to resist it and stay awake. With the exception of the effects of severe pain and the need to breathe, sleepiness is probably the most insistent drive that we can experience. People can commit suicide by refusing to eat or drink, but even the most stoical person cannot indefinitely defy the urge to sleep. Sleep will come, sooner or later, no matter how hard a person tries to stay awake. Although the issue is not yet settled, most researchers believe that the primary function of slow–wave sleep is to permit the brain to rest. In addition, slow-wave sleep and REM sleep

sleep-related eating disorder A disorder in which the person leaves his or her bed and seeks out and eats food while sleepwalking, usually without a memory for the episode the next day.

promote different types of learning, and REM sleep appears to promote brain development.

Functions of Slow-Wave Sleep

Sleep is a universal phenomenon among vertebrates. As far as we know, all mammals and birds sleep (Durie, 1981). Reptiles also sleep, and fish and amphibians enter periods of quiescence that probably can be called sleep. However, only warm-blooded vertebrates (mammals and birds) exhibit unequivocal REM sleep, with muscular paralysis, EEG signs of desynchrony, and rapid eye movements.

Sleep appears to be essential to survival. Evidence for this assertion comes from the fact that sleep is found in some species of mammals that would seem to be better off without it. For example, some species of marine mammals have developed an extraordinary pattern of sleep: The cerebral hemispheres take turns sleeping, presumably because that strategy always permits at least one hemisphere to be alert and keep the animal from sinking and drowning. In addition, the eye contralateral to the active hemisphere remains open. Some birds (for example, mallard ducks) can also sleep with only one hemisphere, keeping the opposite eye open to watch for predators (Rattenborg, Lima, and Amlaner, 1999). The bottlenose dolphin (*Tursiops truncatus*) and the porpoise (*Phocoena phocoena*) both sleep with one hemisphere at a time (Mukhametov, 1984). Figure 8.5 shows the EEG recordings from the two hemispheres; note that slow-wave sleep occurs independently in the left and right hemispheres. (See *Figure 8.5*.)

Effects of Sleep Deprivation

When we are forced to miss a night's sleep, we become very sleepy. The fact that sleepiness is so motivating suggests that sleep is a necessity of life. If so, it should be possible to deprive people of sleep and see what functions are disrupted. We should then be able to infer the role that sleep plays. The results of sleep deprivation studies suggest that the restorative effects of sleep are more important for the brain than for the rest of the body.

Sleep deprivation studies with human subjects have provided little evidence that sleep is needed to keep the body functioning normally. Horne (1978) reviewed over fifty experiments in which people had been deprived of sleep. He reported that most of the studies found that sleep deprivation did not interfere with people's ability to perform physical exercise. In addition, the studies found no evidence of a physiological stress response to sleep deprivation. Thus, the primary role of sleep does not seem to be rest and recuperation of the body. However, people's cognitive abilities were affected; some people reported perceptual distortions or even hallucinations and had trouble concentrating on mental tasks. Perhaps sleep provides the opportunity for the brain to rest.

During slow-wave sleep, both cerebral metabolic rate and cerebral blood flow decline, falling to about 75 percent of the waking level during stage 4 sleep (Sakai et al., 1979; Buchsbaum et al., 1989; Maquet, 1995). In particular, the regions that have the highest levels of activity during waking show the highest levels of delta waves—and the lowest levels of metabolic activity—during slow-wave sleep. Thus, the presence of slow-wave activity in a particular region of the brain appears to indicate that that region is resting. As we know from behavioral observation, people are unreactive to all but intense stimuli during slow-wave sleep and, if awakened, act groggy and

FIGURE 8.5

Sleep in a Dolphin. The two hemispheres sleep independently, presumably so that the animal remains behaviorally alert.

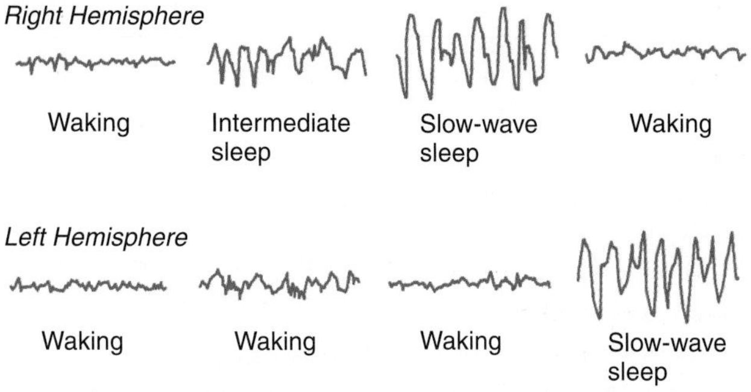

Right Hemisphere

Waking   Intermediate sleep   Slow-wave sleep   Waking

Left Hemisphere

Waking   Waking   Waking   Slow-wave sleep

Adapted from Mukhametov, L. M., in *Sleep Mechanisms*, edited by A. A. Borbély and J. L. Valatx. Munich: Springer-Verlag, 1984.

confused, as if their cerebral cortex has been shut down and has not yet resumed its functioning. In addition, several studies have shown that missing a single night's sleep impairs people's cognitive abilities; presumably, the brain needs sleep to function at peak efficiency (Harrison and Horne, 1998, 1999). These observations suggest that during slow-wave sleep the brain is indeed resting.

An inherited neurological disorder called **fatal familial insomnia** results in damage to portions of the thalamus (Sforza et al., 1995; Gallassi et al., 1996; Montagna et al., 2003). The symptoms of this disease, which is related to Creutzfeldt-Jakob disease and bovine spongiform encephalopathy ("mad cow disease"), include deficits in attention and memory, followed by a dreamlike, confused state; loss of control of the autonomic nervous system and the endocrine system; and insomnia. The first signs of sleep disturbances are reductions in sleep spindles and K complexes. As the disease progresses, slow-wave sleep completely disappears, and only brief episodes of REM sleep (without the accompanying paralysis) remain. As the name indicates, the disease is fatal. Whether the insomnia, caused by the brain damage, contributes to the other symptoms and to the patient's death is not known.

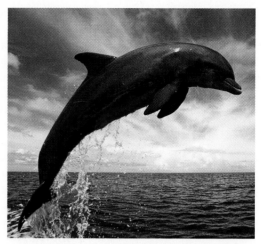

The two cerebral hemispheres of some species of porpoises take turns sleeping—although probably not when the animals are as active as the one shown here.

Schenkein and Montagna (2006a, 2006b) describe the case of a man diagnosed with a form of fatal familial insomnia that usually causes death within 12 months. Because several relatives had died of this disorder, the man knew what to expect, and he enlisted the aid of several physicians to administer drugs and treatments designed to help him sleep. For several months, the treatments did help him sleep, and the man survived about a year longer than would have been expected. Further studies will be needed to determine whether his increased survival time was a direct result of the increased sleep. In any event, his quality of life during most of the period of his illness was much improved.

Effects of Exercise on Slow-Wave Sleep

Sleep deprivation studies with humans suggest that the brain may need slow-wave sleep in order to recover from the day's activities. Another way to determine whether sleep is needed for restoration of physiological functioning is to look at the effects of daytime activity on nighttime sleep. If the function of sleep is to repair the effects on the body of physical activity during waking hours, then we should expect that sleep and exercise are related. That is, we should sleep more after a day of vigorous exercise than after a day spent quietly at an office desk.

However, the relationship between sleep and exercise is not very compelling. For example, Ryback and Lewis (1971) found no changes in slow-wave or REM sleep of healthy subjects who spent 6 weeks resting in bed. If sleep repairs wear and tear, we would expect these people to sleep less. Adey, Bors, and Porter (1968) studied the sleep of almost completely immobile quadriplegics and paraplegics and found only a small decrease in slow-wave sleep as compared with uninjured people. Thus, although sleep certainly provides the body with rest, its primary function appears to be something else.

Functions of REM Sleep

Clearly, REM sleep is a time of intense physiological activity. The eyes dart about rapidly, the heart rate shows sudden accelerations and decelerations, breathing becomes irregular, and the brain becomes more active. It would be unreasonable to expect that REM sleep has the same functions as slow-wave sleep. An early report on the effects of REM sleep deprivation (Dement, 1960) observed that as the deprivation progressed, subjects had to be awakened from REM sleep more frequently; the

fatal familial insomnia A fatal inherited disorder characterized by progressive insomnia.

"pressure" to enter REM sleep built up. Furthermore, after several days of REM sleep deprivation, subjects would show a **rebound phenomenon** when permitted to sleep normally; they spent a much greater-than-normal percentage of the recovery night in REM sleep. This rebound suggests that there is a need for a certain amount of REM sleep—that REM sleep is controlled by a regulatory mechanism. If selective deprivation causes a deficiency in REM sleep, the deficiency is made up later, when uninterrupted sleep is permitted.

Researchers have long been struck by the fact that the highest proportion of REM sleep is seen during the most active phase of brain development. Perhaps, then, REM sleep plays a role in this process (Siegel, 2005). Infant animals born with a well-developed brain spend less time in REM sleep than animals born with an immature brain. For example, guinea pigs, which are born with teeth, claws, and fur and are able to walk within an hour of birth, spend around 1 hour in REM sleep each day (Jouvet-Mounier, Astic, and Lacote, 1970). In contrast, ferrets, which are born with less-developed brains, spend around 6 hours in REM sleep each day (Jha, Coleman, and Frank, 2006). Humans, too, are born with immature brains. Studies of human fetuses and infants born prematurely indicate that REM sleep begins to appear 30 weeks after conception and peaks at around 40 weeks (Roffwarg, Muzio, and Dement, 1966; Petre-Quadens and De Lee, 1974; Inoue et al., 1986). Approximately 70 percent of a newborn infant's sleep is REM sleep. By 6 months of age this proportion has declined to approximately 30 percent. By 8 years of age it has fallen to approximately 22 percent, and by late adulthood it is less than 15 percent. Clearly, there is a relation between brain development and REM sleep.

But if the function of REM sleep is to promote brain development, why do adults have REM sleep? One possibility is that REM sleep facilitates the massive changes in the brain that occur during development but also some of the more modest changes responsible for learning that occur later in life. As we will see in the next subsection, evidence does suggest that REM sleep facilitates learning—but so does slow-wave sleep.

Sleep and Learning

Research with both humans and laboratory animals indicates that sleep does more than allow the brain to rest: It also aids in the consolidation of long-term memories (Marshall and Born, 2007). In fact, slow-wave sleep and REM sleep play different roles in memory consolidation.

As we will see in Chapter 12, there are two major categories of long-term memory: *declarative memory* (also called *explicit memory*) and *nondeclarative memory* (also called *implicit memory*). Declarative memories include those that people can talk about, such as memories of past episodes in their lives. They also include memories of the relationships between stimuli or events, such as the spatial relationships between landmarks that permit us to navigate around our environment. Nondeclarative memories include those gained through experience and practice that do not necessarily involve an attempt to "memorize" information, such as learning to drive a car, throw and catch a ball, or recognize a person's face. Research has found that slow-wave sleep and REM sleep play different roles in the consolidation of declarative and nondeclarative memories.

Before I tell you about the results of this research, let's review the consciousness of a person engaged in each of these stages of sleep. During REM sleep, people normally have a high level of consciousness. If we awaken people during REM sleep, they will be alert and clear-headed and will almost always be able to describe the details of a dream that they were having. However, if we awaken people during slow-wave sleep, they will be groggy and confused, and will usually tell us that nothing was happening. So which stages of sleep do you think aid in the consolidation of declarative and nondeclarative memories?

rebound phenomenon The increased frequency or intensity of a phenomenon after it has been temporarily suppressed; for example, the increase in REM sleep seen after a period of REM sleep deprivation.

I would have thought that REM sleep would be associated with declarative memories and slow-wave sleep with nondeclarative memories. However, just the opposite is true. Let's look at evidence from two studies that looked at the effects of a nap on memory consolidation. Mednick, Nakayama, and Stickgold (2003) had subjects learn a nondeclarative visual discrimination task at 9:00 A.M. The subjects' ability to perform the task was tested 10 hours later, at 7:00 P.M. Some, but not all, of the subjects took a 90-minute nap during the day between training and testing. The investigators recorded the EEGs of the sleeping subjects to determine which of them engaged in REM sleep and which of them did not. (Obviously, all of them engaged in slow-wave sleep, because this stage of sleep always comes first in healthy people.) The investigators found that the performance of subjects who did not take a nap was worse when they were tested at 7:00 P.M. than it had been at the end of training. The subjects who engaged only in slow-wave sleep did about the same during testing as they had done at the end of training. However, the subjects who engaged in REM sleep performed significantly better. Thus, REM sleep strongly facilitated the consolidation of a nondeclarative memory. (See *Figure 8.6*.)

In the second study, Tucker et al. (2006) trained subjects on two tasks: a declarative task (learning a list of paired words) and a nondeclarative task (learning to trace a pencil-and-paper design while looking at the paper in a mirror). Afterwards, some of subjects were permitted to take a nap lasting for about 1 hour. Their EEGs were recorded, and they were awakened before they could engage in REM sleep. The subjects' performance on the two tasks was then tested 6 hours after the original training. The investigators found that compared with subjects who stayed awake, a nap consisting of just slow-wave sleep increased the subjects' performance on the declarative task but had no effect on performance of the nondeclarative task. (See *Figure 8.7*.) So these two experiments (and many others I have not described) indicate that REM sleep facilitates consolidation of nondeclarative memories, and slow-wave sleep facilitates consolidation of declarative memories.

One last experiment on this topic: Peigneux et al. (2004) had human subjects learn their way around a computerized virtual-reality town. This task is very similar to what people do when they learn their way around a real town. They must learn the relative locations of landmarks and streets that connect them so that they can find particular locations when the experimenter "placed" them at various starting points. As we will see in Chapter 12, the hippocampus plays an essential role in learning of this kind. Peigneux and his colleagues used functional brain imaging to measure regional brain activity and found that the same regions of the hippocampus were activated during route learning and during slow-wave sleep the following night. These patterns were *not* seen during REM sleep. Thus, although people awakened during slow-wave sleep seldom report that they had been dreaming, the sleeping brain apparently rehearses information that was acquired during the previous day.

Many studies with laboratory animals have directly recorded the activity of individual neurons in the animals' brains. These studies, too, indicate that the brain

FIGURE 8.6

REM Sleep and Learning.   The graph shows the role of REM sleep in learning a nondeclarative visual discrimination task. Only after a 90-minute nap that included both slow-wave sleep and REM sleep did the subjects' performance improve.

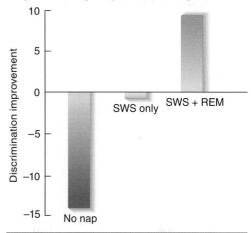

Adapted from Mednick, S., Nakayama, K., and Stickgold, R. *Nature Neuroscience*, 2003, 6, 697–698.

FIGURE 8.7

Slow-Wave Sleep and Learning.   Subjects learned a declarative learning task (list of paired words) and a nondeclarative learning task (mirror tracing). After a nap that included just slow-wave sleep, only subjects who learned the declarative learning task showed improved performance, compared with subjects who stayed awake.

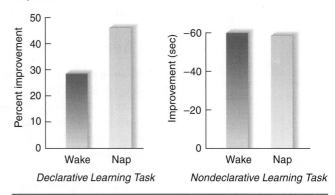

Adapted from Tucker, M. A., Hirota, Y., Wamsley, E. J., Lau, H., Chaklader, A., and Fishbein, W. *Neurobiology of Learning and Memory*, 2006, 86, 241–247.

appears to rehearse newly learned information during slow-wave sleep. Chapter 12 reviews this evidence and describes research on the relevant brain mechanisms.

InterimSummary

Why Do We Sleep?

The fact that all vertebrates sleep, including some that would seem to be better off without it, suggests that sleep performs some important functions. In humans the effects of several days of sleep deprivation include perceptual distortions and (sometimes) mild hallucinations and difficulty performing tasks that require prolonged concentration. These effects suggest that sleep deprivation impairs cerebral functioning. Deep slow-wave sleep appears to be the most important stage, and perhaps its function is to permit the brain to recuperate. Fatal familial insomnia is an inherited disease that results in degeneration of parts of the thalamus, deficits in attention and memory, a dreamlike state, loss of control of the autonomic nervous system and the endocrine system, insomnia, and death.

The primary function of sleep does not seem to be to provide an opportunity for the body to repair the wear and tear that occurs during waking hours. Changes in a person's level of exercise do not significantly alter the amount of sleep the person needs the following night. Instead, the most important function of slow-wave sleep seems to be to lower the brain's metabolism and permit the brain to rest. In support of this hypothesis, research has shown that slow-wave sleep does indeed reduce the brain's metabolic rate.

The functions of REM sleep are even less understood than those of slow-wave sleep. REM sleep may promote brain development. Both REM sleep and slow-wave sleep promote learning: REM sleep facilitates nondeclarative learning, and slow-wave sleep facilitates declarative learning.

Thought Questions

The evidence presented in this section suggests that the primary function of sleep is to permit the brain to rest—but could sleep also have some other functions? For example, could sleep serve as an adaptive response, keeping animals out of harm's way *as well as* provide some cerebral repose? Sleep researcher William Dement pointed out that one of the functions of the lungs is communication. Obviously, the *primary* function of our lungs is to provide oxygen and rid the body of carbon dioxide, and this function explains the evolution of the respiratory system, but we can also use our lungs to vibrate our vocal cords and provide sounds used to talk, so they play a role in communication, too. Other functions of our lungs are to warm our cold hands (by breathing on them), to kindle fires by blowing on hot coals, and to blow out candles. With this perspective in mind, can you think of some other useful functions of sleep?

Physiological Mechanisms of Sleep and Waking

So far, I have discussed the nature of sleep, problems associated with it, and its functions. Now it is time to examine what researchers have discovered about the physiological mechanisms that are responsible for the behavior of sleep and for its counterpart, alert wakefulness.

Chemical Control of Sleep

As we have seen, sleep is *regulated*; that is, if an organism is deprived of slow-wave sleep or REM sleep, the organism will make up at least part of the missed sleep when permitted to do so. In addition, the amount of slow-wave sleep that a person obtains during a daytime nap is deducted from the amount of slow-wave sleep he or she obtains the next night (Karacan et al., 1970). These facts suggest that some physiological mechanism monitors the amount of sleep that an organism needs—in other words, keeps track of the sleep debt we incur during hours of wakefulness.

The simplest explanation would be that the body produces a sleep-promoting substance that accumulates during wakefulness and is destroyed during sleep. The longer someone is awake, the longer he or she has to sleep to deactivate this substance. If such a substance exists, it does not appear to be found in the general circulation of the body. As we saw earlier, the cerebral hemispheres of some species of animals can sleep at different times (Mukhametov, 1984). If sleep were controlled by chemicals in the blood, the hemispheres should sleep at the same time. This observation suggests that if sleep is controlled by chemicals, these chemicals are produced within the brain and act there. In support of this suggestion, Oleksenko et al. (1992) obtained evidence that indicates that each hemisphere of the brain incurs its own sleep debt. The researchers deprived a bottlenose dolphin of sleep in only one hemisphere by waking the animal whenever that hemisphere entered a sleep state. When they allowed the animal to sleep normally, they saw a rebound of slow-wave sleep only in the deprived hemisphere.

Benington, Kodali, and Heller (1995) suggested that **adenosine**, a nucleoside neuromodulator, might play a primary role in the control of sleep, and subsequent studies have supported this suggestion. Astrocytes maintain a small stock of nutrients in the form of glycogen, an insoluble carbohydrate that is also stocked by the liver and the muscles. In times of increased brain activity, this glycogen is converted into fuel for neurons; thus, prolonged wakefulness causes a decrease in the level of glycogen in the brain (Kong et al., 2002). A fall in the level of glycogen causes an increase in the level of extracellular adenosine, which has an inhibitory effect on neural activity. This accumulation of adenosine serves as a sleep-promoting substance. During slow-wave sleep, neurons in the brain rest, and the astrocytes renew their stock of glycogen (Basheer et al., 2004; Wigren et al., 2007). If wakefulness is prolonged, even more adenosine accumulates, which inhibits neural activity and produces the cognitive and emotional effects that are seen during sleep deprivation. (As we saw in Chapter 4, caffeine blocks adenosine receptors. I don't need to tell you the effect that caffeine has on sleepiness.)

Rétey et al. (2005) found that in humans, alleles of the gene for the enzyme that destroys adenosine are associated with depth and duration of slow-wave sleep. Rétey and her colleagues found that people whose chromosomes contained at least one copy of the G/A allele, which breaks down adenosine more slowly than the more common and more effective G/G allele, engaged in a higher percentage of deep slow-wave sleep. In other words, higher levels of adenosine were associated with increased deep sleep. In addition, Halassa et al. (2009) observed a significant decrease in slow-wave sleep in mice with a targeted mutation that reduced the secretion of adenosine by astrocytes. Halassa and his colleagues also found that injection into the cerebral ventricles of a drug that blocks adenosine receptors had the same effect: reduction of slow-wave sleep. These findings support the conclusion that adenosine promotes slow-wave sleep.

The role of adenosine as a sleep-promoting factor is discussed in greater detail later in this chapter, in a section devoted to the neural control of sleep.

Neural Control of Arousal

As we have seen, sleep is not a unitary condition but consists of several different stages with very different characteristics. The waking state, too, is nonuniform; sometimes we are alert and attentive, and sometimes we fail to notice much about what is happening around us. Of course, sleepiness has an effect on wakefulness; if we are fighting to stay awake, the struggle might impair our ability to concentrate on other things. But everyday observations suggest that even when we are not sleepy, our alertness can vary. For example, when we observe something very interesting (or frightening or simply surprising), we become more alert and aware of our surroundings.

Circuits of neurons that secrete at least five different neurotransmitters play a role in some aspect of an animal's level of alertness and wakefulness—what is commonly called arousal: acetylcholine, norepinephrine, serotonin, histamine, and orexin (Wada et al., 1991; McCormick, 1992; Marrocco, Witte, and Davidson, 1994; Hungs and Mignot, 2001).

adenosine (*a den* oh *seen*) A neuromodulator that is released by neurons engaging in high levels of metabolic activity, may play a primary role in the initiation of sleep.

Acetylcholine and the Sleep–Waking Cycle.   The graphs show the release of acetylcholine from the cortex and hippocampus during the sleep–waking cycle. SWS = slow-wave sleep, QW = quiet waking, AW = active waking.

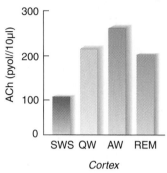

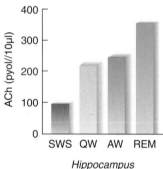

Adapted from Marrosu, F., Portas, C., Mascia, M. S., el al. *Brain Research*, 1995, *671*, 329–332.

locus coeruleus (*sa roo lee us*) A dark-colored group of noradrenergic cell bodies located in the pons near the rostral end of the floor of the fourth ventricle; involved in arousal and vigilance.

raphe nuclei (*ruh fay*) A group of nuclei located in the reticular formation of the medulla, pons, and midbrain, situated along the midline; contain serotonergic neurons.

Acetylcholine

One of the most important neurotransmitters involved in arousal—especially of the cerebral cortex—is acetylcholine. Two groups of ACh neurons, one in the dorsal pons and one located in the basal forebrain, produce activation and cortical desynchrony when they are stimulated (Jones, 1990; Steriade, 1996).

Researchers have long known that ACh agonists increase EEG signs of cortical arousal and that ACh antagonists decrease them (Vanderwolf, 1992). Marrosu et al. (1995) used microdialysis probes to measure the release of acetylcholine in the hippocampus and neocortex—two regions whose activity is closely related to an animal's alertness and behavioral arousal. They found that the levels of ACh in these regions were high during both waking and REM sleep—periods during which the EEG displayed desynchronized activity—but low during slow-wave sleep. (See **Figure 8.8.**) In addition, Rasmusson, Clow, and Szerb (1994) electrically stimulated a region of the dorsal pons and found that the stimulation activated the cerebral cortex and increased the release of acetylcholine there by 350 percent (as measured by microdialysis probes). A group of ACh neurons located in the basal forebrain forms an essential part of the pathway that is responsible for this effect. If these neurons were deactivated by infusing a local anesthetic or drugs that blocked synaptic transmission, the activating effects of the pontine stimulation were abolished.

Norepinephrine

Investigators have long known that catecholamine agonists such as amphetamine produce arousal and sleeplessness. These effects appear to be mediated primarily by the noradrenergic system of the **locus coeruleus**, located in the dorsal pons. Neurons of the locus coeruleus give rise to axons that branch widely, releasing norepinephrine (from axonal varicosities) throughout the neocortex, hippocampus, thalamus, cerebellar cortex, pons, and medulla; thus, they potentially affect widespread and important regions of the brain.

Aston-Jones and Bloom (1981) recorded from noradrenergic neurons of the locus coeruleus (LC) across the sleep–waking cycle in unrestrained rats. As Figure 8.9 shows, these neurons exhibited a close relationship to behavioral arousal. Note the decline in firing rate before and during sleep and the abrupt increase when the animal wakes. In addition, the rate of firing of neurons in the locus coeruleus falls almost to zero during REM sleep and increases dramatically when the animal wakes. (See **Figure 8.9.**) Most investigators believe that activity of noradrenergic LC neurons increases an animal's vigilance—its ability to pay attention to stimuli in the environment. In fact, a study by Aston-Jones et al. (1994) found that the moment-to-moment activity of noradrenergic LC neurons was directly related to the animals' current performance on a task that required vigilance.

Serotonin

A third neurotransmitter, serotonin (5-HT) also appears to play a role in activating behavior. Almost all of the brain's serotonergic neurons are found in the **raphe nuclei**, which are located in the medullary and pontine regions of the reticular formation. The axons of these neurons project to many parts of the brain, including the thalamus, hypothalamus, basal ganglia, hippocampus, and neocortex. Stimulation of the raphe nuclei causes locomotion and cortical arousal (as measured by the EEG), whereas PCPA, a drug that blocks the synthesis of serotonin, reduces cortical arousal (Peck and Vanderwolf, 1991).

Figure 8.10 shows the activity of serotonergic neurons, recorded by Trulson and Jacobs (1979). As you can see, these neurons, like the noradrenergic neurons studied by Aston-Jones and Bloom (1981), were most active during waking. Their firing rate declined during slow-wave sleep and became virtually zero during REM sleep. However, once the period of REM sleep ended, the neurons temporarily became very active again. (See **Figure 8.10.**)

FIGURE 8.9

Norepinephrine and the Sleep–Waking Cycle.   This graph shows the activity of noradrenergic neurons in the locus coeruleus of freely moving rats during various stages of sleep and waking.

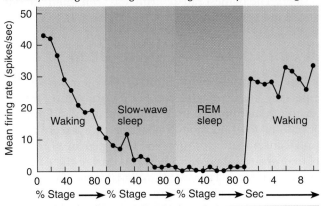

From Aston-Jones, G., and Bloom, F. E. *The Journal of Neuroscience*, 1981, *1*, 876–886. Copyright 1981, The Society for Neuroscience.

FIGURE 8.10

Serotonin and the Sleep–Waking Cycle   This graph shows the activity of serotonergic (5-HT-secreting) neurons in the dorsal raphe nuclei of freely moving cats during various stages of sleep and waking.

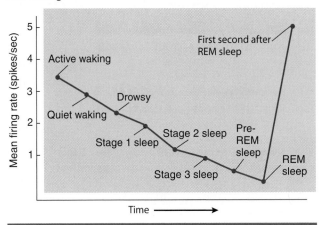

Adapted from Trulson, M. E., and Jacobs, B. L. *Brain Research*, 1979, *163*, 135–150. Redrawn with permission.

Histamine

The fourth neurotransmitter implicated in the control of wakefulness and arousal is histamine, a compound synthesized from histidine, an amino acid. You are undoubtedly aware that antihistamines, used to treat allergies, can cause drowsiness. They do so by blocking histamine receptors in the brain. More modern antihistamines cannot cross the blood–brain barrier, so they do not cause drowsiness.

The cell bodies of histaminergic neurons are located in the **tuberomammillary nucleus (TMN)** of the hypothalamus, located at the base of the brain just rostral to the mammillary bodies. The axons of these neurons project primarily to the cerebral cortex, thalamus, basal ganglia, basal forebrain, and hypothalamus. The projections to the cerebral cortex directly increase cortical activation and arousal, and projections to ACh neurons of the basal forebrain and dorsal pons do so indirectly, by increasing the release of acetylcholine in the cerebral cortex (Khateb et al., 1995; Brown, Stevens, and Haas, 2001). The activity of histaminergic neurons is high during waking but low during slow-wave sleep and REM sleep (Steininger et al., 1996). In addition, injections of drugs that prevent the synthesis of histamine or block histamine receptors decrease waking and increase sleep (Lin, Sakai, and Jouvet, 1998). Also, infusion of histamine into the basal forebrain region of rats causes an increase in waking and a decrease in non-REM sleep (Ramesh et al., 2004)

Orexin

As we saw in the section on sleep disorders, the cause of narcolepsy is degeneration of orexinergic neurons in humans and a hereditary absence of orexin-B receptors in dogs. The cell bodies of neurons that secrete orexin (as we saw, also called hypocretin) are located in the lateral hypothalamus. Although there are only about 7000 orexinergic neurons in the human brain, the axons of these neurons project to almost every part of the brain, including the cerebral cortex and all of the regions involved in arousal and wakefulness, including the locus coeruleus, raphe nuclei, tuberomammillary nucleus, and acetylcholinergic neurons in the dorsal pons and basal forebrain (Sakurai, 2007). Orexin has an excitatory effect in all of these regions.

tuberomammillary nucleus (TMN)
A nucleus in the ventral posterior hypothalamus, just rostral to the mammillary bodies; contains histaminergic neurons involved in cortical activation and behavioral arousal.

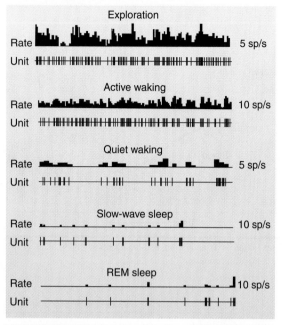

Reprinted from *Neuron, 46*, Mileykovskiy, B. Y., Kiyashchenko, L. I., and Siegel, J. M., Behavioral Correlates of Activity in Identified Hypocretin/ Orexin Neurons, 787–798, Copyright 2005, with permission from Elsevier.

Mileykovskiy, Kiyashchenko, and Siegel (2005) recorded the activity of single orexinergic neurons in unanesthetized rats and found that the neurons fired at a high rate during alert or active waking, and at a low rate during quiet waking, slow-wave sleep, and REM sleep. The highest rate of firing was seen when the rats were engaged in exploratory activity. (See *Figure 8.11*.)

Neural Control of Slow-Wave Sleep

When we are awake and alert, most of the neurons in our brain—especially those of the forebrain—are active, which enables us to pay attention to sensory information and process this information, to think about what we are perceiving, to retrieve and think about memories, and to engage in a variety of behaviors that we are called on to perform during the day. The level of brain activity is largely controlled by the five sets of arousal neurons described in the previous section. A high level of activity of these neurons keeps us awake, and a low level puts us to sleep.

But what controls the activity of the arousal neurons? What causes this activity to fall, thus putting us to sleep? The first hint at an answer to this question was suggested in the early 20th century by careful observations of a Viennese neurologist, Constantin von Economo, who noticed that patients afflicted by a new type of encephalitis that was sweeping through Europe and North America showed severe disturbance in sleep and waking (Triarhou, 2006). Most patients slept excessively, waking only to eat and drink. According to von Economo, these patients had brain damage at the junction of the brain stem and forebrain, at a location that would destroy the axons of the arousal neurons entering the forebrain. Some patients, however, showed just the opposite symptoms: They slept only a few hours each day. Although they were tired, they had difficulty falling asleep and usually awakened shortly thereafter. Von Economo reported that patients who displayed insomnia had damage to the region of the anterior hypothalamus. We now know that this region, usually referred to as the *preoptic area*, is the one most involved in control of sleep. The preoptic area contains neurons whose axons form inhibitory synaptic connections with the brain's arousal neurons. When our preoptic neurons (let's call them *sleep neurons*) become active, they suppress the activity of our arousal neurons, and we fall asleep (Saper, Scammell, and Lu, 2005).

The majority of the sleep neurons are located in the **ventrolateral preoptic area (vlPOA)**. Damage to vlPOA neurons suppresses sleep (Lu et al., 2000), and the activity of these neurons, measured by their levels of Fos protein, increases during sleep. Anatomical and histochemical studies indicate that the sleep neurons secrete the inhibitory neurotransmitter GABA, and that they send their axons to the five regions involved in arousal and wakefulness (Sherin et al., 1998; Gvilia et al., 2006; Suntsova et al., 2007). As we saw in the previous section, activity of neurons in these five regions causes cortical activation and behavioral arousal. Inhibition of these regions, then, is a necessary condition for sleep.

The sleep neurons in the vlPOA receive inhibitory inputs from some of the same regions they inhibit, including the tuberomammillary nucleus, raphe nuclei, and locus coeruleus (Chou et al., 2002). As Saper, Chou, and Scammell (2001) suggest, this mutual inhibition may provide the basis for establishing periods of sleep and waking. They note that reciprocal inhibition also characterizes an electronic circuit known as a *flip-flop*. A flip-flop can assume one of two states, usually referred to as on or off—or 0 or 1 in computer applications. Thus, either the sleep neurons

ventrolateral preoptic area (vlPOA) A group of GABAergic neurons in the preoptic area whose activity suppresses alertness and behavioral arousal and promotes sleep.

FIGURE 8.12

The Sleep/Waking Flip-Flop. According to Saper et al. (2001), the major sleep-promoting region (the vlPOA) and the major wakefulness-promoting regions (basal forebrain and pontine regions that contain acetylcholinergic neurons; the locus coeruleus, which contains noradrenergic neurons; the raphe nuclei, which contain serotonergic neurons; and the tuberomammillary nucleus of the hypothalamus, which contains histaminergic neurons) are reciprocally connected by inhibitory GABAergic neurons. (a) When the flip-flop is in the "wake" state, the arousal systems are active and the vlPOA is inhibited, and the animal is awake. (b) When the flip-flop is in the "sleep" state, the vlPOA is active and the arousal systems are inhibited, and the animal is asleep.

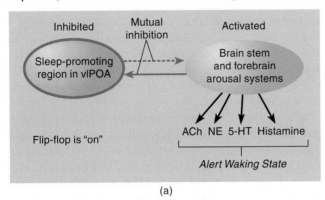

(a)

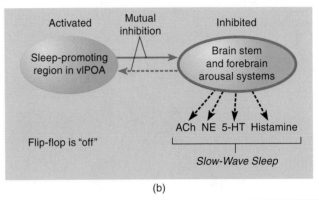

(b)

are active and inhibit the wakefulness neurons or the wakefulness neurons are active and inhibit the sleep neurons. Because these regions are mutually inhibitory, it is impossible for neurons in both sets of regions to be active at the same time. (See *Figure 8.12*.)

A flip-flop has an important advantage: When it switches from one state to the other, it does so quickly. Clearly, it is most advantageous to be either asleep or awake; a state that has some of the characteristics of both sleep and wakefulness would be maladaptive. However, there is one problem with flip-flops: They can be unstable. In fact, people with narcolepsy and animals with damage to the orexinergic system of neurons exhibit just this characteristic. They have great difficulty remaining awake when nothing interesting is happening, and they have trouble remaining asleep for an extended amount of time. (They also show intrusions of the characteristics of REM sleep at inappropriate time. I will discuss this phenomenon in the next section.)

Saper et al. (2001) suggest that an important function of orexinergic neurons is to help stabilize the sleep/waking flip-flop through their excitatory connections to the wakefulness neurons. Activity of this system of neurons tips the activity of the flip-flop toward the waking state, thus promoting wakefulness and inhibiting sleep. Perhaps your success at staying awake during a boring lecture depends on maintaining a high rate of firing of your orexinergic neurons, which would keep the flip-flop in the waking state. (See *Figure 8.13*.)

As we saw earlier in this chapter, adenosine is produced when neurons are metabolically active, and the accumulation of adenosine produces drowsiness and sleep. Porkka-Heiskanen, Strecker, and McCarley (2000) used microdialysis to measure adenosine levels in several regions of the brain. They found that the level of adenosine

FIGURE 8.13

Role of Orexinergic Neurons in Sleep. The schematic diagram shows the effect of activation of the orexinergic system of neurons of the lateral hypothalamus on the sleep/waking flip-flop. Motivation to remain awake or events that disturb sleep activate the orexinergic neurons.

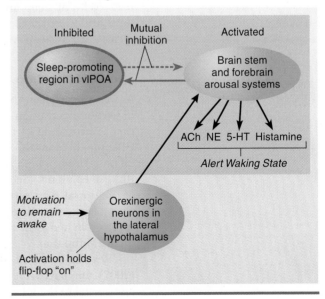

FIGURE 8.14

Adenosine, Time of Day, and Hunger. This figure shows the role of adenosine, time of day, and hunger and satiety signals on the sleep/waking flip-flop.

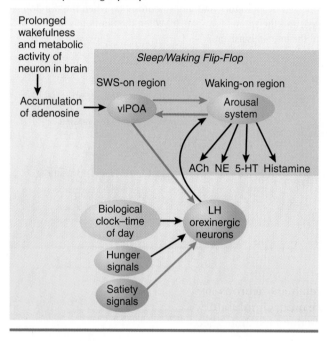

increased during wakefulness and slowly decreased during sleep, especially in the basal forebrain. Scammell et al. (2001) found that infusion of an adenosine agonist into the vlPOA activated neurons there, decreased the activity of histaminergic neurons of the tuberomammillary nucleus, and increased slow-wave sleep.

Seeing that orexinergic neurons help hold the sleep/waking flip-flop in the waking state, the obvious question to ask is what factors control the activity of orexinergic neurons? During the waking part of the day/night cycle, orexinergic neurons receive an excitatory signal from the biological clock that controls daily rhythms of sleep and waking. These neurons also receive signals from brain mechanisms that monitor the animal's nutritional state: Hunger-related signals activate orexinergic neurons, and satiety-related signals inhibit them. Thus, orexinergic neurons maintain arousal during the times that an animal should search for food. In fact, if normal mice (but not mice with a targeted mutation against orexin receptors) are given less food than they would normally eat, they stay awake longer each day (Yamanaka et al., 2003, Sakurai, 2007). Finally, orexinergic neurons receive inhibitory input from the vlPOA, which means that sleep signals that arise from the accumulation of adenosine can eventually overcome excitatory input to orexinergic neurons and sleep can occur. (See *Figure 8.14*.)

Neural Control of REM Sleep

As we saw earlier in this chapter, REM sleep consists of desynchronized EEG activity, muscular paralysis, rapid eye movements, and increased genital activity. The rate of cerebral metabolism during REM sleep is as high as it is during waking (Maquet et al., 1990), and were it not for the state of paralysis, the level of *physical* activity would also be high.

As we shall see, REM sleep is controlled by a flip-flop similar to the one that controls cycles of sleep and waking. The sleep/waking flip-flop determines when we wake and when we sleep, and once we fall asleep, the REM flip-flop controls our cycles of REM sleep and slow-wave sleep.

The REM Flip-Flop

As we saw earlier in this chapter, acetylcholinergic neurons play an important role in cerebral activation during alert wakefulness. Researchers have also found that they are involved in the neocortical activation that accompanies REM sleep. For example, El Mansari, Sakai, and Jouvet (1989) found that ACh neurons in the dorsal pons fire at a high rate during both REM sleep and active wakefulness or during REM sleep alone. (See *Figure 8.15*.) Such findings suggested that the ACh neurons of the dorsal pons served as the trigger mechanism that initiated a period of REM sleep. However, more recent research suggests that although ACh neurons are involved in neocortical activation that accompanies REM sleep, they are not part of the REM flip-flop.

Reviews by Lu et al. (2006); Fuller, Saper, and Lu (2007); and Luppi et al. (2007) summarize the evidence for the REM flip-flop. A region of the dorsal pons, just ventral to the locus coeruleus, contains REM-ON neurons. In rats, this region is

FIGURE 8.15

Firing Pattern of a REM-ON Cell.   The acetylcholinergic REM-ON cell is located in the dorsal pons. The figure shows (a) action potentials during 60-minute intervals during waking, slow-wave sleep, and REM sleep, and (b) the rate of firing just before and after the transition from slow-wave sleep to REM sleep. The increase in activity begins approximately 80 seconds before the onset of REM sleep.

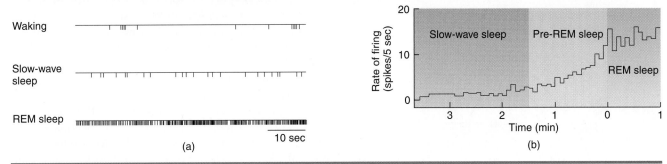

(a)

(b)

Adapted from El Mansari, M., Sakai, K., and Jouvet, M. *Experimental Brain Research*, 1989, 76, 519–529.

known as the **sublaterodorsal nucleus (SLD)**. A region of the dorsal midbrain, the **ventrolateral periaqueductal gray matter (vlPAG)** contains REM-OFF neurons. For simplicity, I will simply refer to the *REM-ON* and *REM-OFF* regions. The REM-ON and REM-OFF regions are interconnected by means of inhibitory GABAergic neurons. Stimulation of the REM-ON region with infusions of glutamate agonists elicits most of the elements of REM sleep, whereas inhibition of this region with GABA agonists disrupts REM sleep. In contrast, stimulation of the REM-OFF region suppresses REM sleep, whereas damage to this region or infusions of GABA agonists dramatically increases REM sleep. (See *Figure 8.16.*)

The mutual inhibition of these two regions means that they function like a flip-flop: Only one region can be active at any given time. During waking, the REM-OFF region receives excitatory input from the orexinergic neurons of the lateral hypothalamus, and this activation tips the REM flip-flop into the OFF state. Additional excitatory input to the REM-OFF region is received from two other sets of wakefulness neurons, the noradrenergic neurons of the locus coeruleus and the serotonergic neurons of the raphe nuclei.

When the sleep/waking flip-flop switches into the sleep phase, slow-wave sleep begins. The activity of the excitatory orexinergic, noradrenergic, and

sublaterodorsal nucleus (SLD) A region of the dorsal pons, just ventral to the locus coeruleus, that forms the REM-ON portion of the REM sleep flip-flop.

ventrolateral periaqueductal gray matter (vlPAG) A region of the dorsal midbrain that forms the REM-OFF portion of the REM sleep flip-flop.

FIGURE 8.16

The REM-Sleep Flip-Flop

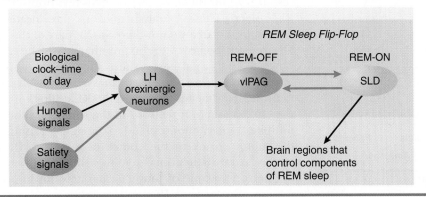

FIGURE 8.17

REM Sleep.   This schematic diagram shows the interaction between the sleep/waking flip-flop and the REM sleep flip-flop.

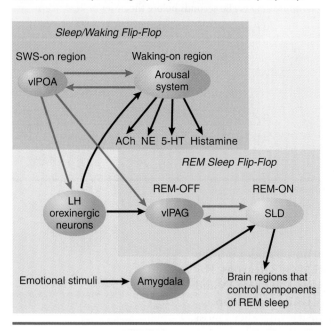

serotonergic inputs to the REM-OFF region begins to decrease. As a consequence, the excitatory input to the REM-OFF region is removed. The REM flip-flop tips to the ON state, and REM sleep begins. Presumably, an internal clock—perhaps located in the pons—controls the alternating periods of REM sleep and slow-wave sleep that follow. Figure 8.17 shows the control of the REM-sleep flip-flop by the sleep-waking flip-flop. (See *Figure 8.17.*)

We can see now why degeneration of orexinergic neurons causes narcolepsy. The daytime sleepiness and the fragmented sleep occur because without the influence of orexin, the sleep/waking flip-flop becomes unstable. The secretion of orexin in the REM-OFF region normally keeps the REM flip-flop in the OFF state. With the loss of orexinergic neurons, emotional episodes such as laughter or anger, which activate the amygdala, tip the REM flip-flop into the ON state, and the result is an attack of cataplexy. (See *Figure 8.17.*) In fact, a functional imaging study by Schwartz et al. (2008) found that when people with cataplexy watched humorous sequences of photographs, the hypothalamus was activated less, and the amygdala was activated more, than the same structures in control subjects. The investigators suggest that the loss of hypocretinergic neurons removed an inhibitory influence of the hypothalamus on the amygdala. The increased amygdala activity could account at least in part for the increased activity of REM-ON neurons that occurs even during waking in people with cataplexy. (See *Figure 8.18.*)

As we saw earlier, patients with REM sleep behavior disorder fail to become paralyzed during REM sleep and therefore act out their dreams. The same thing happens to cats when a lesion is placed in a particular region of the midbrain. Jouvet (1972) described this phenomenon:

FIGURE 8.18

Humor and Narcolepsy.   The graph shows the activation of the hypothalamus and amygdala in normal subjects and patients with narcolepsy watching neutral and humorous sequences of photos.

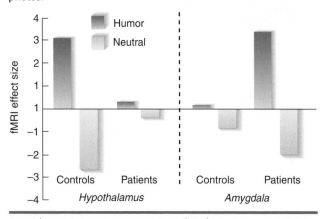

From Schwartz, S., Ponz, A., Poryazova, R., et al. *Brain*, 2008, *131*, 514–522. Reprinted by permission.

To a naive observer, the cat, which is standing, looks awake since it may attack unknown enemies, play with an absent mouse, or display flight behavior. There are orienting movements of the head or eyes toward imaginary stimuli, although the animal does not respond to visual or auditory stimuli. These extraordinary episodes . . . are a good argument that "dreaming" occurs during [REM sleep] in the cat. (Jouvet, 1972, pp. 236–237)

Jouvet's lesions destroyed a set of neurons that are responsible for the muscular paralysis that occurs during REM sleep. These "paralysis neurons" are located just ventral to the area we now know to be part of the REM-ON region. Some of the axons that leave this region travel to the spinal cord, where they excite inhibitory interneurons whose axons form synapses with motor neurons. This means that when the REM flip-flop tips to the ON state, motor neurons in the spinal cord become inhibited, and cannot respond to the signals arising from the motor cortex in the course of a dream. Damage to the "paralysis neurons" removes this inhibition, and the person (or one of Jouvet's cats) acts out his or her dreams. (See *Figure 8.19.*)

The fact that our brains contain an elaborate mechanism whose sole function is to keep us paralyzed while we dream—that is, to prevent us from acting out our dreams—suggests that the motor components of dreams are as important as the sensory components. Perhaps the practice our motor system gets during REM sleep helps us to improve our performance of behaviors we have learned that day. The inhibition of the motor neurons in the spinal cord prevents the movements being practiced from actually occurring, with the exception of a few harmless twitches of the hands and feet.

Little is known about the function of genital activity that occurs during REM sleep or about the neural mechanisms responsible for them. A study by Schmidt et al. (2000) found that lesions of the lateral preoptic area in rats suppressed penile erections during REM sleep but had no effect on erections during waking. Salas et al. (2007) found that penile erections could be triggered by electrical stimulation of acetylcholinergic neurons in the pons that become active during REM sleep. The investigators note that evidence suggests that these pontine neurons may be directly connected with neurons in the lateral preoptic area and thus may be responsible for the erections. (See *Figure 8.19*.)

FIGURE 8.19

Control of REM sleep. Components of REM sleep are controlled by the REM-ON region.

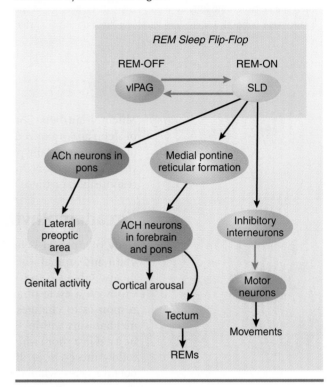

InterimSummary

Physiological Mechanisms of Sleep and Waking

The fact that the amount of sleep is regulated suggests that a sleep-promoting substance is produced during wakefulness. The sleeping pattern of the dolphin brain suggests that such a substance does not accumulate in the blood. Evidence suggests that adenosine, released when neurons are obliged to utilize the supply of glycogen stored in astrocytes, serves as the link between increased brain metabolism and the necessity of sleep.

Five systems of neurons appear to be important for alert, active wakefulness: the acetylcholinergic system of the dorsal pons and the basal forebrain, involved in cortical activation; the noradrenergic system of the locus coeruleus, involved in vigilance; the serotonergic system of the raphe nuclei, involved in activation of automatic behaviors such as locomotion; the histaminergic neurons of the tuberomammillary nucleus, involved in maintaining wakefulness; and the orexinergic system of the lateral hypothalamus, also involved in maintaining wakefulness.

Slow-wave sleep occurs when neurons in the ventrolateral preoptic area (vlPOA) become active. These neurons inhibit the systems of neurons that promote wakefulness. In turn, the vlPOA is inhibited by these same wakefulness-promoting regions, thus forming a kind of flip-flop that keeps us either awake or asleep. The accumulation of adenosine promotes sleep by activating the sleep-promoting neurons of the vlPOA, which inhibits the wakefulness-promoting regions. Activity of the orexinergic neurons of the lateral hypothalamus helps keep the flip-flop that controls sleep and waking in the "waking" state.

REM sleep is controlled by another flip-flop. The sublaterodorsal nucleus (SLD) serves as the REM-ON region, and the ventrolateral periaqueductal gray region (vlPAG) serves as the REM-OFF region. This flip-flop is controlled by the sleep/waking flip-flop; only when the sleep/waking flip-flop is in the "sleeping" state can the REM flip-flop switch to the "REM" state. The muscular paralysis that prevents our acting out our dreams is produced by connections between neurons adjacent to the SLD that excite inhibitory interneurons in the spinal cord. Penile erections during REM sleep (but not during waking) are abolished by lesions of the lateral preoptic area. Rapid eye movements are produced by indirect connections between the SLD and the tectum, through the medial pontine reticular formation and acetylcholinergic neurons in the pons.

Biological Clocks

Much of our behavior follows regular rhythms. For example, we saw that the stages of sleep are organized around a 90-minute cycle of REM and slow-wave sleep—and, of course, our daily pattern of sleep and waking follows a 24-hour cycle. In recent years investigators have learned much about the neural mechanisms that are responsible for these rhythms.

Circadian Rhythms and Zeitgebers

Daily rhythms in behavior and physiological processes are found throughout the plant and animal world. These cycles are generally called **circadian rhythms**. (*Circa* means "about," and *dies* means "day"; therefore, a circadian rhythm is one that varies on a cycle of approximately 24 hours.) Some of these rhythms are passive responses to changes in illumination. However, other rhythms are controlled by mechanisms within the organism—by "internal clocks." For example, if a rat is housed in a room where lights are on for 12 hours each day, its circadian rhythm will follow the cycle of illumination: The animal will sleep when the light is on and become active when the room is dark. If the lights are then turned on (or off) all day, the animal will continue to show rhythms of sleep and wakefulness. In the absence of external stimuli, the rhythm must be provided by some sort of internal clock. In fact, the internal clock tends to run a little slow. The cycle of the internal clock of most mammals tends to be approximately 25 hours.

In the natural environment, where day and night are defined by the rising and setting of the sun, the internal clock is reset each day so that the cycles take 24 hours. Light serves as a **zeitgeber** (German for "time giver"); it synchronizes the endogenous rhythm. Studies with many species of animals have shown that if they are maintained in constant darkness (or constant dim light), a brief period of bright light will reset their internal clock, advancing or retarding it, depending upon when the light flash occurs (Aschoff, 1979). For example, if an animal is exposed to bright light soon after dusk, the biological clock is set back to an earlier time—as if dusk had not yet arrived. On the other hand, if the light occurs late at night, the biological clock is set ahead to a later time—as if dawn had already come.

People, too, have circadian rhythms, but without the benefits of modern civilization we would probably go to sleep earlier and get up earlier than we do; we use artificial lights to delay our bedtime and window shades to extend our time for sleep. Under constant illumination our biological clocks will run free, gaining or losing time like a watch that runs too slow or too fast. Different people have different cycle lengths, but most people in that situation will begin to live a "day" that is approximately 25 hours long. This works out quite well, because the morning light, acting as a zeitgeber, simply resets the clock.

The Suprachiasmatic Nucleus

Researchers working independently in two laboratories (Moore and Eichler, 1972; Stephan and Zucker, 1972) discovered that the primary biological clock of the rat is located in the **suprachiasmatic nucleus (SCN)** of the hypothalamus; they found that

circadian rhythm (*sur **kay** dee un* or *sur ka **dee** un*) A daily rhythmical change in behavior or physiological process.

zeitgeber (*tsite gay ber*) A stimulus (usually the light of dawn) that resets the biological clock that is responsible for circadian rhythms.

suprachiasmatic nucleus (SCN) (*soo pra ky az **mat** ik*) A nucleus situated atop the optic chiasm. It contains a biological clock that is responsible for organizing many of the body's circadian rhythms.

lesions disrupted circadian rhythms of wheel running, drinking, and hormonal secretion. The SCN also provides the primary control over the timing of sleep cycles. Rats are nocturnal animals; they sleep during the day and forage and feed at night. Lesions of the SCN abolish this pattern; sleep occurs in bouts randomly dispersed throughout both day and night (Ibuka and Kawamura, 1975; Stephan and Nuñez, 1977). However, rats with SCN lesions still obtain the same amount of sleep that normal animals do. The lesions disrupt the circadian pattern but do not affect the total amount of sleep.

Anatomy and Connections

Figure 8.20 shows the suprachiasmatic nuclei in a cross section through the hypothalamus of a rat; they appear as two clusters of dark-staining neurons at the base of the brain, just above the optic chiasm. (See *Figure 8.20.*) The suprachiasmatic nuclei of the rat consist of approximately 8600 small neurons, tightly packed into a volume of 0.036 mm^3 (Moore, Speh, and Leak, 2002).

Because light is the primary zeitgeber for most mammals' activity cycles, we would expect that the SCN receives fibers from the visual system. Indeed, anatomical studies have revealed a direct projection of fibers from the retina to the SCN: the *retinohypothalamic pathway* (Hendrickson, Wagoner, and Cowan, 1972; Aronson et al., 1993). If you look carefully at Figure 8.20, you can see small dark spots within the optic chiasm, just ventral and medial to the base of the SCN; these are cell bodies of oligodendroglia that serve axons that enter the SCN and provide information from the retina. (See *Figure 8.20.*)

The photoreceptors in the retina that provide photic information to the SCN are neither rods nor cones—the cells that provide us with the information used for visual perception. Indeed, Freedman et al. (1999) found that targeted mutations against genes necessary for production of both rods and cones did not disrupt the synchronizing effects of light. However, when they removed the mice's eyes, these effects *were* disrupted. These results suggested that there is a special photoreceptor that provides information about the ambient level of light that synchronizes circadian rhythms. Provencio et al. (2000) found the photochemical responsible for this effect, which they named **melanopsin**.

Unlike the other retinal photopigments, which are found in rods and cones, melanopsin is present in ganglion cells—the neurons whose axons transmit information from the eyes to the rest of the brain. Melanopsin-containing ganglion cells are sensitive to light, and their axons terminate in the SCN and in a region of the tectum involved in the response of the pupils to light (Berson, Dunn, and Takao, 2002; Hattar et al., 2002). (See *Figure 8.21.*)

Evidence indicates that SCN controls cycles of sleep and waking by two means: direct neural connections and the secretion of chemicals that affect the activity of neurons in other regions of the brain. Researchers have found multisynaptic pathways from the SCN to the *subparaventricular zone (SPZ)*, located just dorsal to the SCN, to the *dorsomedial nucleus of the hypothalamus (DMH)* and then to regions involved in the control of sleep and waking, such as the vlPOA and the orexinergic neurons of the lateral hypothalamus. The projections to the vlPOA are inhibitory and thus inhibit sleep, whereas the projections to the orexinergic neurons are excitatory, and thus promote wakefulness (Saper, Scammell, and Lu, 2005). Of course, the activity of these connections varies across the day/night cycle. In

FIGURE 8.20

The SCN.   The figure shows the location and appearance of the suprachiasmatic nuclei in a rat. Cresyl violet stain was used to color the nuclei in this cross section of a rat brain.

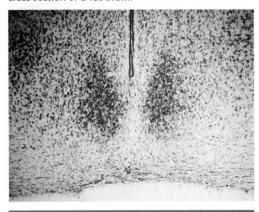

Courtesy of Geert DeVries, University of Massachusetts.

melanopsin (*mell a **nop** sin*) A photopigment present in ganglion cells in the retina whose axons transmit information to the SCN, the thalamus, and the olivary pretectal nuclei.

FIGURE 8.21

Melanopsin-Containing Ganglion Cells in the Retina.   The axons of the ganglion cells form the retinohypothalamic tract. These neurons detect the light of dawn that resets the biological clock in the SCN.

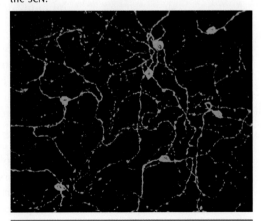

From Hattar, S., Liao, H.-W., Takao, et al. *Science*, 2002, *295*, 1065–1070. Copyright © 2002. Reprinted with permission from AAAS.

FIGURE 8.22

Control of Circadian Rhythms. The SCN controls circadian rhythms in sleep and waking by the SCN. During the day cycle, the DMH inhibits the vlPOA and excites the brain stem and forebrain arousal systems, thus stimulating wakefulness.

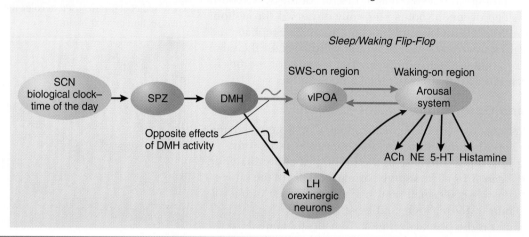

FIGURE 8.23

Circadian Rhythms in the SCN. The autoradiographs show cross sections through the brains of rats that had been injected with carbon 14–labeled 2-deoxyglucose during the day (*top*) and the night (*bottom*). The dark region at the base of the brain (*arrows*) indicates increased metabolic activity of the suprachiasmatic nuclei.

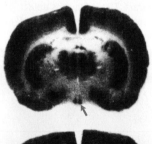

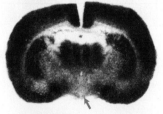

From Schwartz, W. J., and Gainer, H. *Science*, 1977, *197*, 1089–1091. Copyright © 1977 The American Association for the Advancement of Science. Reprinted with permission.

diurnal animals (such as ourselves), the activity of these connections is high during the day and low during the night. (See *Figure 8.22.*)

Although neurons of the SCN project to several parts of the brain, transplantation studies suggest that the SCN controls some functions by releasing chemical signals. Lehman et al. (1987) destroyed the SCN and then transplanted in their place a new set of suprachiasmatic nuclei obtained from donor animals. The grafts succeeded in reestablishing circadian rhythms, even though very few efferent connections were observed between the graft and the recipient's brain. Even more convincing evidence comes from a transplantation study by Silver et al. (1996). Silver and her colleagues first destroyed the SCN in a group of hamsters, abolishing their circadian rhythms. Then, a few weeks later, they removed SCN tissue from donor animals and placed it in very small semipermeable capsules, which they then implanted in the animals' third ventricles. Nutrients and other chemicals could pass through the walls of the capsules, keeping the SCN tissue alive, but the neurons inside the capsules were not able to establish synaptic connections with the surrounding tissue. Nevertheless, the transplants reestablished circadian rhythms in the recipient animals. Presumably, the chemicals secreted by cells in the SCN affect rhythms of sleep and waking by diffusing into the SPZ and binding with receptors on neurons located there.

The Nature of the Clock

All clocks must have a time base. Mechanical clocks use flywheels or pendulums; electronic clocks use quartz crystals. The SCN, too, must contain a physiological mechanism that parses time into units. After years of research, investigators are finally beginning to discover the nature of the biological clock in the SCN.

Several studies have demonstrated daily activity rhythms in the SCN, which indicates that the circadian clock is located there. A study by Schwartz and Gainer (1977) nicely demonstrated day–night fluctuations in the activity of the SCN. These investigators injected rats with radioactive 2-deoxyglucose (2-DG).

Schwartz and Gainer injected some rats with radioactive 2-DG during the day and injected others at night. The animals were then killed, and autoradiographs of cross sections through the brain were prepared. Figure 8.23 shows photographs of two of these cross sections. Note the evidence of radioactivity (and hence a high metabolic rate) in the SCN of the brain that was injected during the day (*top*). (See *Figure 8.23.*)

What causes SCN neurons to "tick"? For many years investigators have believed that circadian rhythms were produced by the production of a protein that, when it reached a certain level in the cell, inhibited its own production. As a result, the levels of the protein would begin to decline, which would remove the inhibition, starting the production cycle again. (See *Figure 8.24*.)

Just such a mechanism was discovered in *Drosophila melanogaster*, the common fruit fly. Subsequent research with mammals discovered a similar system (Shearman et al., 2000; Reppert and Weaver, 2001; Van Gelder et al., 2003; Yan and Silver, 2004). The system involves at least seven genes and their proteins and two interlocking feedback loops. When one of the proteins produced by the first loop reaches a sufficient level, it starts the second loop, which eventually inhibits the production of proteins in the first loop, and the cycle begins again. Thus, the intracellular ticking is regulated by the time it takes to produce and degrade a set of proteins.

It appears that the circadian clock in the human brain works the same way. Toh et al. (2001) found that a mutation on chromosome 2 of a gene for one of the proteins involved in these feedback loops (*per2*) is responsible for the **advanced sleep phase syndrome**. This syndrome causes a 4-hour advance in rhythms of sleep and temperature cycles. People with this syndrome fall asleep around 7:30 P.M. and awaken around 4:30 A.M. The mutation appears to change the relationship between the zeitgeber of morning light and the phase of the circadian clock that operates in the cells of the SCN. Ebisawa et al. (2001) found evidence that the opposite disorder, the **delayed sleep phase syndrome**, may be caused by mutations of the *per3* gene, found on chromosome 1. This syndrome consists of a 4-hour delay in sleep/waking rhythms. People with this disorder are typically unable to fall asleep before 2:00 A.M. and have great difficulty waking before midmorning.

Changes in Circadian Rhythms: Shift Work and Jet Lag

When people abruptly change their daily rhythms of activity, their internal circadian rhythms, controlled by the SCN, become desynchronized with those in the external environment. For example, if a person who normally works on the day

advanced sleep phase syndrome A 4-hour advance in rhythms of sleep and temperature cycles, apparently caused by a mutation of a gene (*per2*) involved in the rhythmicity of neurons of the SCN.

delayed sleep phase syndrome A 4-hour delay in rhythms of sleep and temperature cycles, possibly caused by a mutation of a gene (per3) involved in the rhythmicity of neurons of the SCN.

FIGURE 8.24

Circadian Rhythms in the SCN.   This schematic is a simplified explanation of the molecular control of the "ticking" of neurons of the SCN.

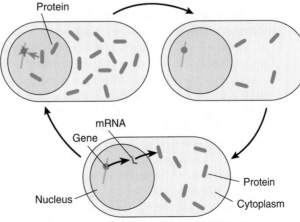

The protein enters the nucleus, suppressing the gene responsible for its production. No more messenger RNA is made.

The level of the protein falls, so the gene becomes active again.

The gene is active; messenger RNA leaves the the nucleus and causes the production of the protein

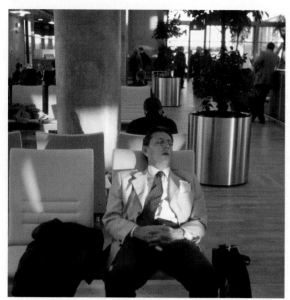

Researchers are beginning to understand the role of the suprachiasmatic nucleus and the pineal gland in phenomena such as jet lag.

shift begins working on a night shift or if someone travels east or west across several time zones, his or her SCN will signal the rest of the brain that it is time to sleep during the work shift (or the middle of the day, in the case of jet travel). This disparity between internal rhythms and the external environment results in sleep disturbances and mood changes and interferes with people's ability to function during waking hours. Problems such as ulcers, depression, and accidents related to sleepiness are more common in people whose work schedules regularly shift (Drake et al., 2004).

Jet lag is a temporary phenomenon; after several days people who have crossed several time zones find it easier to fall asleep at the appropriate time, and their daytime alertness improves. Shift work can present a more enduring problem when people are required to change shifts frequently. Obviously, the solution to jet lag and to the problems caused by shift work is to get the internal clock synchronized with the external environment as quickly as possible. The most obvious way to start is to try to provide strong zeitgebers at the appropriate time. If a person is exposed to bright light before the low point in the daily rhythm of body temperature (which occurs an hour or two before the person usually awakens), the person's circadian rhythm is delayed. If the exposure to bright light occurs after the low point, the circadian rhythm is advanced (Dijk et al., 1995). In fact, several studies have shown that exposure to bright lights at the appropriate time helps to ease the transition (Boulos et al., 1995). Similarly, people adapt to shift work more rapidly if artificial light is kept at a brighter level and if their bedroom is kept as dark as possible (Eastman et al., 1995).

The control of biological rhythms also involves another part of the brain: the **pineal gland** (Bartness et al., 1993). This structure sits on top of the midbrain, just in front of the cerebellum. The pineal gland secretes a hormone called **melatonin**, so named because it has the ability in certain animals (primarily fish, reptiles, and amphibians) to turn the skin temporarily dark. (The dark color is produced by a chemical known as *melanin*.) Neurons in the SCN make synaptic connections with neurons in the *paraventricular nucleus of the hypothalamus* (the PVN). The axons of these neurons travel all the way to the spinal cord, where they form synapses with preganglionic neurons of the sympathetic nervous system. The postganglionic neurons innervate the pineal gland and control the secretion of melatonin.

In response to input from the SCN, the pineal gland secretes melatonin during the night. This melatonin acts back on various structures in the brain (including the SCN, whose cells contain melatonin receptors) and controls various hormones, physiological processes, and behaviors. Studies have found that melatonin, acting on receptors in the SCN, can affect the sensitivity of SCN neurons to zeitgebers and can itself alter circadian rhythms (Gillette and McArthur, 1995; Starkey et al., 1995). Researchers do not yet understand exactly what role melatonin plays in the control of circadian rhythms, but they have already discovered practical applications. Melatonin secretion normally reaches its highest levels early in the night, at around bedtime. Investigators have found that the administration of melatonin at the appropriate time (in most cases, just before going to bed) significantly reduces the adverse effects of both jet lag and shifts in work schedules (Arendt et al., 1995; Deacon and Arendt, 1996). Bedtime melatonin has even helped to synchronize circadian rhythms and improve the sleep of blind people for whom light cannot serve as a zeitgeber (Skene, Lockley, and Arendt, 1999).

pineal gland (*py nee ul*) A gland attached to the dorsal tectum; produces melatonin and plays a role in circadian and seasonal rhythms.

melatonin (*mell a tone in*) A hormone secreted during the night by the pineal body; plays a role in circadian and seasonal rhythms.

InterimSummary

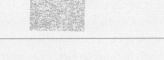

Biological Clocks

Our daily lives are characterized by cycles in physical activity, sleep, body temperature, secretion of hormones, and many other physiological changes. Circadian rhythms—those with a period of approximately 1 day—are controlled by biological clocks in the brain. The principal biological clock appears to be located in the suprachiasmatic nuclei of the hypothalamus; lesions of these nuclei disrupt most circadian rhythms, and the activity of neurons located there correlates with the day–night cycle. Light, detected by special cells in the retina that are not involved in visual perception, serves as a zeitgeber for most circadian rhythms. That is, the biological clocks tend to run a bit slow, with a period of approximately 25 hours. The presence of sunlight in the morning is detected by melanopsin-containing photoreceptors in the retina and conveyed to the SCN. The effect of the light is to reset the clock to the start of a new cycle.

"Ticking" of the neurons that constitute the biological clock in the SNC is accomplished by cycles of production and destruction of proteins. At least seven genes and their proteins and two interlocking feedback loops are involved in this process. Two human genetic disorders, advanced sleep phase syndrome and delayed sleep phase syndrome, are caused by a mutation of two of the genes responsible for circadian rhythms.

During the night the SCN signals the pineal gland to secrete melatonin, which appears to be involved in synchronizing circadian rhythms: The hormone can help people to adjust to the effects of shift work or jet lag and even synchronize the daily rhythms of blind people for whom light cannot serve as a zeitgeber.

Thought Question

Until recently (in terms of the evolution of our species), our ancestors tended to go to sleep when the sun set and wake up when it rose. Once our ancestors learned how to control fire, they undoubtedly stayed up somewhat later, sitting in front of a fire. But it was only with the development of cheap, effective lighting that many members of our species adopted the habit of staying up late and waking several hours after sunrise. Considering that our biological clock and the neural mechanisms it controls evolved long ago, do you think the changes in our daily rhythms impair any of our physical and intellectual abilities?

⠿ EPILOGUE   Functions of Dreams

Even though we are still not sure why REM sleep occurs, the elaborate neural circuitry involved with its control indicates that it must be important. Nature would probably not invent this circuitry if it did not do something useful. Michael's attacks of sleep paralysis, hypnagogic hallucinations, and cataplexy, described in the chapter prologue, occurred when two of the aspects of REM sleep (paralysis and dreaming) occurred at inappropriate times. Normally, the brain mechanisms responsible for these phenomena are inhibited during waking; in Michael's case, degeneration of orexinergic neurons caused instability in his sleep/waking flip-flop and permitted some of the phenomena of REM sleep to occur at inappropriate times.

As we saw, REM sleep appears to play a role in learning and brain development. But what about the subjective aspect of REM sleep dreaming? Is there some special purpose served by those vivid, story-like hallucinations we have while we sleep, or are dreams just irrelevant side effects of more important things going on in the brain?

Since ancient times, people have regarded dreams as important, using them to prophesy the future, decide whether to go to war, or determine the guilt or innocence of a person accused of a crime. In the twentieth century Sigmund Freud proposed a very influential theory about dreaming. He said that dreams arise out of inner conflicts between unconscious desires (primarily sexual ones) and prohibitions against acting out these desires, which we learn from society. According to Freud, although all dreams represent unfulfilled wishes, their contents are disguised. The *latent content* of the dream (from the Latin word for "hidden") is transformed into the *manifest content* (the actual story line or plot). Taken at face value, the manifest content is innocuous, but a knowledgeable psychoanalyst can recognize unconscious desires disguised as symbols in the dream. For example, climbing a set of stairs might represent sexual intercourse. The problem with Freud's theory is that it is not disprovable; even if it is wrong, a psychoanalyst can always provide a plausible interpretation of a dream that reveals hidden conflicts, disguised in obscure symbols.

Many sleep researchers—especially those who are interested in the biological aspects of dreaming—disagree with Freud and suggest alternative explanations. For example, Hobson (1988) suggests that the brain activation that occurs during REM sleep leads to hallucinations that we try to make sense of by creating a more- or less-plausible story. As you learned in this chapter, REM sleep is accompanied by rapid eye movements and cortical arousal. The visual system is especially active; so is the motor system—in fact, we have a mechanism that paralyzes and prevents the activity of the motor system from causing us to get out of bed and doing something that might harm us. (As we saw, people who suffer from REM without atonia actually *do* act out their dreams and sometimes injure themselves. On occasion they have even attacked their spouses while dreaming that they were fighting with someone.)

Research indicates that the two systems of the brain that are most active, the visual system and the motor system, account for most of the sensations that occur during dreams. Many dreams are silent, but almost all are full of visual images. In addition, many dreams contain sensations of movements, which are probably caused by feedback from the activity of the motor system. Very few dreamers report tactile sensations, smells, or tastes. Hobson, a wine lover, reported that although he has drunk wine in his dreams, he has never experienced any taste or smell. (He reported this fact rather wistfully; I suspect that he would have appreciated the opportunity to taste a fine wine without having to open one of his own bottles.) Why are these sensations absent? Is it because our "hidden desires" involve only sight and movement, or is it because the neural activation that occurs during REM sleep simply does not involve other systems to a very great extent? Hobson suggests the latter, and I agree with him.

Key Concepts

A PHYSIOLOGICAL AND BEHAVIORAL DESCRIPTION OF SLEEP

1. Sleep consists of slow-wave sleep, divided into four stages, and REM sleep. Dreaming occurs during REM sleep.

DISORDERS OF SLEEP

2. People sometimes suffer from such sleep disorders as insomnia, sleep apnea, narcolepsy, REM without atonia, bedwetting, sleepwalking, or night terrors. Three symptoms of narcolepsy (cataplexy, sleep paralysis, and hypnagogic hallucinations) can be understood as components of REM sleep occurring at inappropriate times. Narcolepsy is caused by a hereditary disorder that causes the degeneration of orexin-secreting neurons during adolescence.

WHY DO WE SLEEP?

3. Slow-wave sleep appears to permit the cerebral cortex to rest. REM sleep may be important in brain development, and it plays a role in formation of nondeclarative memories. Slow-wave sleep is involved in formation of declarative memories.

PHYSIOLOGICAL MECHANISMS OF SLEEP AND WAKING

4. Adenosine, a neuromodulator that is produced as a by-product of cerebral metabolism, appears to play a role in initiating sleep.

5. The brain stem contains an arousal mechanism with five major components: the acetylcholinergic system of the dorsolateral pons and basal forebrain; the noradrenergic system of the locus coeruleus; the serotonergic system of the raphe nuclei; the histaminergic system of the tuberomammillary nucleus of the hypothalamus; and the orexinergic system of the lateral hypothalamus. The ventrolateral preoptic area (vlPOA) appears to be necessary for sleep; its neurons inhibit the brain regions responsible for arousal.

6. Orexinergic neurons help stabilize the sleep/waking flip-flop, which consists of the vlPOA and the regions involved in arousal.

7. REM sleep is controlled by the REM sleep flip-flop, which consists of the SLD (the REM-ON region) and the vlPAG (the REM-OFF region) and their reciprocal, inhibitory, connections.

BIOLOGICAL CLOCKS

8. Circadian rhythms are largely under the control of a mechanism located in the suprachiasmatic nucleus. They are synchronized by the day–night light cycle, which is detected by a special category of photoreceptors in the retina. The ticking of the internal clock responsible for these rhythms appears to involve the production and degradation of proteins.

Suggested Readings

Hobson, J. A. *Dreaming: An Introduction to the Science of Sleep.* Oxford, England: Oxford University Press, 2004.

Jouvet, M. *The Paradox of Sleep: The Story of Dreaming.* Cambridge, MA: The MIT Press, 2001.

Kryger, M. H., Roth, T., and Dement, W. C. *Principles and Practice of Sleep Medicine,* 3rd ed. Philadelphia: Saunders, 2000.

Luppi, P.-H. *Sleep: circuits and function.* Boca Raton, FL: CRC Press, 2005.

Pace-Schott, E. F., Solms, M., Blagrove, M., and Harnad, S. *Sleep and Dreaming: Scientific Advances and Reconsiderations.* Cambridge, England: Cambridge University Press, 2003.

Vu, T. T., Desseilles, M., Petit, D., Mazza, S., Montplaisir, J., and Maquet, P. Neuroimaging in sleep medicine. *Sleep Medicine,* 2007, *8,* 350–373.

Additional Resources

Visit www.mypsychkit.com for additional review and practice of the material covered in this chapter. Within MyPsychKit, you can take practice tests and receive a customized study plan to help you review. Dozens of animations, tutorials, and Web links are also available. You can even review using the interactive electronic version of this textbook. You will need to register for MyPsychKit. See www.mypsychkit.com for complete details.

chapter 9 : Reproductive Behavior

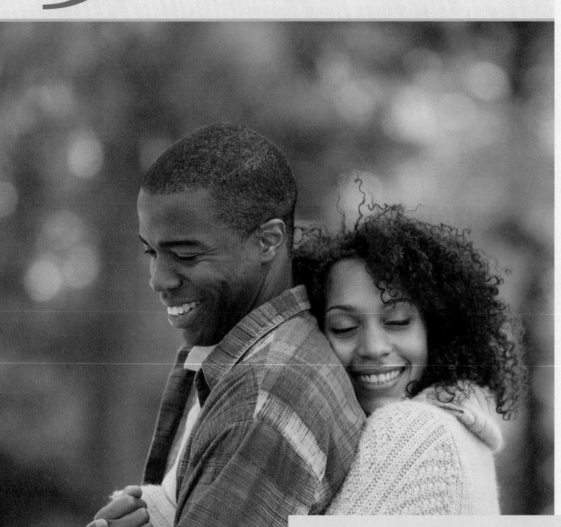

LEARNING OBJECTIVES

1. Describe mammalian sexual development and explain the factors that control it.

2. Describe the hormonal control of the female reproductive cycle and of male and female sexual behavior.

3. Describe the role of pheromones in reproductive physiology and sexual behavior.

4. Discuss the activational effects of gonadal hormones on the sexual behavior of women and men.

5. Discuss sexual orientation and the effects of prenatal androgenization of genetic females and the failure of androgenization of genetic males.

6. Discuss the neural control of male sexual behavior.

7. Discuss the neural control of female sexual behavior.

8. Describe the maternal behavior of rodents and discuss the hormonal and neural mechanisms that control maternal behavior and paternal behavior.

PROLOGUE   From Boy to Girl

The aftermath of a tragic surgical accident suggested that people's sexual identity and sexual orientation were not under the strong control of biological factors and that these characteristics could be shaped by the way a child was raised (Money and Ehrhardt, 1972). Identical twin boys were raised normally until 7 months of age, at which time one of the boys' penis was accidentally destroyed during circumcision. The cautery (a device that cuts tissue by means of electric current) was adjusted too high, and instead of removing the foreskin, the current burned off the entire penis. After a period of agonized indecision, the parents decided, on the advice of an expert in human sexuality, to raise the child as a girl. Bruce became Brenda.

Bruce's parents started dressing her in girl's clothing and treating her like a little girl. Surgeons removed the child's testes. Reports of this case stated that Brenda was a normal, happy girl, and many experts concluded that children's sexual identities were determined by the way that they were raised, not by their chromosomes or sex hormones. After all, Brenda's identical twin brother provided the perfect control. Many writers saw this case as a triumph of socialization over biology.

As you will see in the chapter epilogue, this conclusion was premature.

Reproductive behaviors constitute the most important category of social behaviors, because without them, most species would not survive. These behaviors—which include courting, mating, parental behavior, and most forms of aggressive behaviors—are the most striking categories of **sexually dimorphic behaviors**; that is, behaviors that differ in males and females (*di + morphous*, "two forms"). As you will see, hormones that are present both before and after birth play a very special role in the development and control of sexually dimorphic behaviors.

This chapter describes male and female sexual development and then discusses the neural and hormonal control of two sexually dimorphic behaviors that are most important to reproduction: sexual behavior and parental behavior.

Sexual Development

A person's chromosomal sex is determined at the time of fertilization. However, this event is merely the first in a series of steps that culminate in the development of a male or female. This section considers the major features of sexual development.

Production of Gametes and Fertilization

All cells of the human body (other than sperms or ova) contain twenty-three pairs of chromosomes. The genetic information that programs the development of a human is contained in the DNA that constitutes these chromosomes. We pride ourselves on our ability to miniaturize computer circuits on silicon chips, but that accomplishment looks primitive when we consider that the blueprint for a human being is too small to be seen by the naked eye.

The production of **gametes** (ova and sperms; *gamein* means "to marry") entails a special form of cell division. This process produces cells that contain one member of each of the twenty-three pairs of chromosomes. The development of a human begins at the time of fertilization, when a single sperm and ovum join, sharing their twenty-three single chromosomes to reconstitute the twenty-three pairs.

A person's genetic sex is determined at the time of fertilization of the ovum by the father's sperm. Twenty-two of the twenty-three pairs of chromosomes determine the organism's physical development independent of its sex. The last pair consists of two **sex chromosomes**, which determine whether the offspring will be a boy or a girl.

sexually dimorphic behavior A behavior that has different forms or that occurs with different probabilities or under different circumstances in males and females.

gamete (*gamm eet*) A mature reproductive cell; a sperm or ovum.

sex chromosome The X and Y chromosomes, which determine an organism's gender. Normally, XX individuals are female, and XY individuals are male.

Determination of Gender. The gender of the offspring depends on whether the sperm cell that fertilizes the ovum carries an X or a Y chromosome.

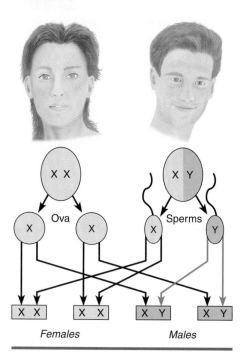

There are two types of sex chromosomes: X chromosomes and Y chromosomes. Females have two X chromosomes (XX); thus, all the ova that a woman produces will contain an X chromosome. Males have an X and a Y chromosome (XY). When a man's sex chromosomes divide, half the sperms contain an X chromosome and the other half contain a Y chromosome. A Y-bearing sperm produces an XY-fertilized ovum and therefore a male. An X-bearing sperm produces an XX-fertilized ovum and therefore a female. (See *Figure 9.1*.)

Development of the Sex Organs

Men and women differ in many ways: Their bodies are different, parts of their brains are different, and their reproductive behaviors are different. Are all these differences encoded on the tiny Y chromosome, the sole piece of genetic material that distinguishes males from females? The answer is no. The X chromosome and the twenty-two nonsex chromosomes found in the cells of both males and females contain all the information needed to develop the bodies of either sex. Exposure to sex hormones, both before and after birth, is responsible for our sexual dimorphism. What the Y chromosome does control is the development of the glands that produce the male sex hormones.

Gonads

There are three general categories of sex organs: the gonads, the internal sex organs, and the external genitalia. The **gonads**—testes or ovaries—are the first to develop. Gonads (from the Greek *gonos*, "procreation") have a dual function: They produce ova or sperms, and they secrete hormones. Through the sixth week of prenatal development, male and female fetuses are identical. Both sexes have a pair of identical undifferentiated gonads, which have the potential of developing into either testes or ovaries. The factor that controls their development appears to be a single gene on the Y chromosome called **Sry** (sex-determining region Y). This gene produces a protein that binds to the DNA of cells in the undifferentiated gonads and causes them to become testes. (Testes are also known as *testicles*, Latin for "little testes.") Believe it or not, the words "testis" and "testify" have the same root, meaning "witness." Legend has it that ancient Romans placed their right hand over their genitals while swearing that they would tell the truth in court. (Only men were permitted to testify.) If the Sry gene is not present, the undifferentiated gonads become ovaries (Sinclair et al., 1990; Smith, 1994; Koopman, 2001). In fact, a few cases of XX males have been reported. This anomaly can occur when the Sry gene becomes translocated from the Y chromosome to the X chromosome during production of the father's sperms (Warne and Zajac, 1998). (A test based on a molecular probe for Sry is used to ensure that the chromosomes of potential competitors for the women's Olympic events do not contain an Sry gene.)

Once the gonads have developed, a series of events is set into action that determines the individual's gender. These events are directed by hormones, which affect sexual development in two ways. During prenatal development these hormones have **organizational effects**, which influence the development of a person's sex organs and brain. These effects are permanent; once a particular path is followed in the course of development, there is no going back. The second role of sex hormones is their **activational effect**. These effects occur later in life, after the sex organs have developed. For example, hormones activate the production of sperms, make erection and ejaculation possible, and induce ovulation. Because the bodies of adult males and females have been organized differently, sex hormones will have different activational effects in the two sexes.

gonad (rhymes with *moan ad*) An ovary or testis.

Sry The gene on the Y chromosome whose product instructs the undifferentiated fetal gonads to develop into testes.

organizational effect (of hormone) The effect of a hormone on tissue differentiation and development.

activational effect (of hormone) The effect of a hormone that occurs in the fully developed organism; may depend on the organism's prior exposure to the organizational effects of hormones.

Internal Sex Organs

Early in embryonic development, the internal sex organs are *bisexual*; that is, all embryos contain the precursors for both female and male sex organs. However, during the third month of gestation, only one of these precursors develops; the other withers away. The precursor of the internal female sex organs, which develops into the *fimbriae* and *Fallopian tubes*, the *uterus*, and the *inner two-thirds of the vagina*, is called the **Müllerian system**. The precursor of the internal male sex organs, which develops into the *epididymis, vas deferens*, and *seminal vesicles*, is called the **Wolffian system**. (These systems were named after their discoverers, Müller and Wolff. See *Figure 9.2*.)

The gender of the internal sex organs of a fetus is determined by the presence or absence of hormones secreted by the testes. If these hormones are present, the Wolffian system develops. If they are not, the Müllerian system develops. The Müllerian (female) system needs no hormonal stimulus from the gonads to develop; it just normally does so. (Turner's syndrome, a disorder of sexual development that I will discuss later, provides the evidence for this assertion.) In contrast, the cells of the Wolffian (male) system do not develop unless they are stimulated to do so by a hormone. Thus, testes secrete two types of hormones. The first, a peptide hormone called **anti-Müllerian hormone**, does exactly what its name says: It prevents the Müllerian (female) system from developing. It therefore has a **defeminizing effect**. The second, a set of steroid hormones called **androgens**, stimulates the development of the Wolffian system. (This class of hormone is also aptly named: *Andros*

Müllerian system The embryonic precursors of the female internal sex organs.

Wolffian system The embryonic precursors of the male internal sex organs.

anti-Müllerian hormone A peptide secreted by the fetal testes that inhibits the development of the Müllerian system, which would otherwise become the female internal sex organs.

defeminizing effect An effect of a hormone present early in development that reduces or prevents the later development of anatomical or behavioral characteristics typical of females.

androgen (*an dro jen*) A male sex steroid hormone. Testosterone is the principal mammalian androgen.

FIGURE 9.2

Development of the Internal Sex Organs

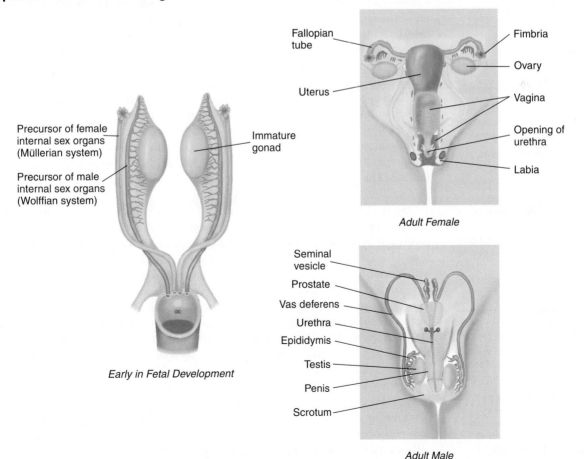

Precursor of female internal sex organs (Müllerian system)

Precursor of male internal sex organs (Wolffian system)

Immature gonad

Early in Fetal Development

Fallopian tube

Uterus

Fimbria

Ovary

Vagina

Opening of urethra

Labia

Adult Female

Seminal vesicle

Prostate

Vas deferens

Urethra

Epididymis

Testis

Penis

Scrotum

Adult Male

means "man," and *gennan* means "to produce.") Androgens have a **masculinizing effect**.

Two different androgens are responsible for masculinization. The first, **testosterone**, is secreted by the testes and gets its name from these glands. An enzyme converts some of the testosterone into another androgen, known as **dihydrotestosterone**.

As you will recall from Chapter 2, hormones exert their effects on target cells by stimulating the appropriate hormone receptor. Thus, the precursor of the male internal sex organs—the Wolffian system—contains androgen receptors that are coupled to cellular mechanisms that promote growth and division. When molecules of androgens bind with these receptors, the epididymis, vas deferens, and seminal vesicles develop and grow. In contrast, the cells of the Müllerian system contain receptors for anti-Müllerian hormone that *prevent* growth and division. Thus, the presence of anti-Müllerian hormone prevents the development of the female internal sex organs.

The fact that the internal sex organs of the human embryo are bisexual and could potentially develop as either male or female is dramatically illustrated by two genetic disorders: *androgen insensitivity syndrome* and *persistent Müllerian duct syndrome*. Some people are insensitive to androgens; they have **androgen insensitivity syndrome**, one of the more aptly named disorders (Money and Ehrhardt, 1972; MacLean, Warne, and Zajac, 1995). The cause of androgen insensitivity syndrome is a genetic mutation that prevents the formation of functioning androgen receptors. (The gene for the androgen receptor is located on the X chromosome.) The primitive gonads of a genetic male fetus with androgen insensitivity syndrome become testes and secrete both anti-Müllerian hormone and androgens. The lack of androgen receptors prevents the androgens from having a masculinizing effect; thus, the epididymis, vas deferens, seminal vesicles, and prostate fail to develop. However, the anti-Müllerian hormone still has its defeminizing effect, preventing the female internal sex organs from developing. The uterus, fimbriae, and Fallopian tubes fail to develop, and the vagina is shallow. The external genitalia are female, and at puberty the person develops a woman's body. Of course, lacking a uterus and ovaries, the person cannot have children.

The second genetic disorder, **persistent Müllerian duct syndrome**, has two causes: either a failure to produce anti-Müllerian hormone or the absence of receptors for this hormone (Warne and Zajac, 1998). When this syndrome occurs in genetic males, androgens have their masculinizing effect but defeminization does not occur. Thus, the person is born with *both* sets of internal sex organs, male and female. The presence of the additional female sex organs usually interferes with normal functioning of the male sex organs.

So far, I have been discussing only male sex hormones. What about prenatal sexual development in females? A chromosomal anomaly indicates that the hormones produced by female sex organs are not needed for development of the Müllerian system. This fact has led to the dictum "Nature's impulse is to create a female." People with **Turner's syndrome** have only one sex chromosome: an X chromosome. (Thus, instead of having XX cells, they have X0 cells—0 indicating a missing sex chromosome.) In most cases the existing X chromosome comes from the mother, which means that the cause of the disorder lies with a defective sperm (Knebelmann et al., 1991). Because a Y chromosome is not present, testes do not develop. In addition, because two X chromosomes are needed to produce ovaries, these glands are not produced either. But even though people with Turner's syndrome have no gonads at all, they develop into females, with normal female internal sex organs and external genitalia—which proves that fetuses do not need ovaries or the hormones they produce to develop as females. Of course, they must be given estrogen pills to induce puberty and sexual maturation—and they cannot bear children, because without ovaries they cannot produce ova.

masculinizing effect An effect of a hormone present early in development that promotes the later development of anatomical or behavioral characteristics typical of males.

testosterone (*tess **tahss** ter own*) The principal androgen found in males.

dihydrotestosterone (*dy hy dro tess **tahss** ter own*) An androgen, produced from testosterone through the action of an enzyme.

androgen insensitivity syndrome A condition caused by a congenital lack of functioning androgen receptors; in a person with XY sex chromosomes, causes the development of a female with testes but no internal sex organs.

persistent Müllerian duct syndrome A condition caused by a congenital lack of anti-Müllerian hormone or receptors for this hormone; in a male, causes development of both male and female internal sex organs.

Turner's syndrome The presence of only one sex chromosome (an X chromosome); characterized by lack of ovaries but otherwise normal female sex organs and genitalia.

External Genitalia

The external genitalia are the visible sex organs, including the penis and scrotum in males and the labia, clitoris, and outer part of the vagina in females. (See *Figure 9.3.*) As we just saw, the external genitalia do not need to be stimulated by female sex hormones to become female; they just naturally develop that way. In the presence of dihydrotestosterone the external genitalia will become male. Thus, the gender of a person's external genitalia is determined by the presence or absence of an androgen, which explains why people with Turner's syndrome have female external genitalia even though they lack ovaries. People with androgen insensitivity syndrome have female external genitalia too, because without androgen receptors their cells cannot respond to the androgens produced by their testes.

Figure 9.4 summarizes the factors that control the development of the gonads, internal sex organs, and genitalia. (See *Figure 9.4*.)

Sexual Maturation

The *primary* sex characteristics include the gonads, internal sex organs, and external genitalia. These organs are present at birth. The *secondary* sex characteristics, such as enlarged breasts and widened hips or a beard and deep voice, do not appear until puberty. Without seeing genitals, we must guess the sex of a prepubescent child from his or her haircut and clothing; the bodies of young boys and girls are rather similar. However, at puberty the gonads are stimulated to produce their hormones, and these hormones cause the person to mature sexually. The onset of puberty occurs when cells in the hypothalamus secrete

FIGURE 9.3

Development of the External Genitalia

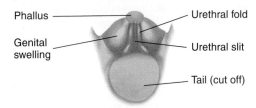

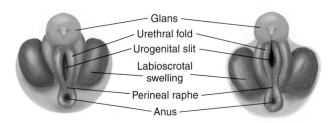

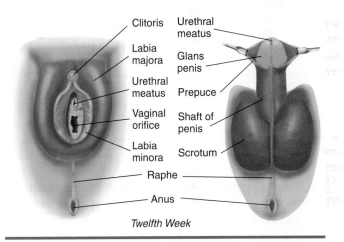

Adapted from Spaulding, M. H., in *Contributions to Embryology*, Vol. 13. Washington, DC: Carnegie Institute of Washington, 1921.

FIGURE 9.4

Hormonal Control of Development of the Internal Sex Organs

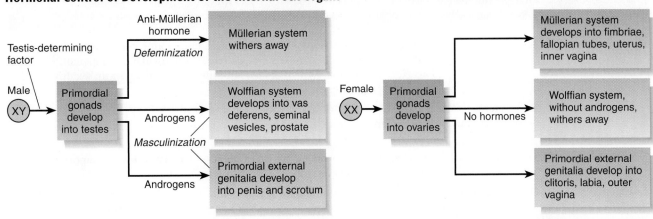

FIGURE 9.5

Sexual Maturation.   Puberty is initiated when the hypothalamus secretes gonadotropin-releasing hormones (GnRH), which stimulate the release of gonadotropic hormones by the anterior pituitary gland.

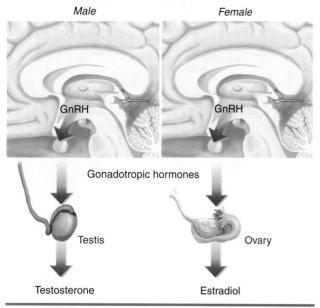

Male

Female

GnRH

GnRH

Gonadotropic hormones

Testis

Ovary

Testosterone

Estradiol

gonadotropin-releasing hormone
(*go nad oh* **trow** *pin*) A hypothalamic hormone that stimulates the anterior pituitary gland to secrete gonadotropic hormone.

gonadotropic hormone A hormone of the anterior pituitary gland that has a stimulating effect on cells of the gonads.

follicle-stimulating hormone (FSH)
The hormone of the anterior pituitary gland that causes development of an ovarian follicle and the maturation of an ovum.

gonadotropin-releasing hormones (GnRH), which stimulate the production and release of two **gonadotropic hormones** by the anterior pituitary gland. The gonadotropic ("gonad-turning") hormones stimulate the gonads to produce *their* hormones, which are ultimately responsible for sexual maturation. (See *Figure 9.5*.)

The two gonadotropic hormones are **follicle-stimulating hormone (FSH)** and **luteinizing hormone (LH)**, named for the effects they produce in the female (production of a *follicle* and its subsequent *luteinization*, to be described in the next section of this chapter). However, the same hormones are produced in the male, where they stimulate the testes to produce sperms and to secrete testosterone.

In response to the gonadotropic hormones (usually called *gonadotropins*), the gonads secrete steroid sex hormones. The ovaries produce **estradiol**, one of a class of hormones known as **estrogens**. As we saw, the testes produce testosterone, an androgen. Both types of glands also produce a small amount of the hormones of the other sex. The gonadal steroids affect many parts of the body. Both estradiol and androgens initiate closure of the growing portions of the bones and thus halt skeletal growth. In females, estradiol also causes breast development, growth of the lining of the uterus, changes in the deposition of body fat, and maturation of the female genitalia. In males, androgens stimulate growth of facial, axillary (underarm), and pubic hair; lower the voice; alter the hairline on the head (often causing baldness later in life); stimulate muscular development; and cause genital growth. This description leaves out two of the female secondary characteristics: axillary hair and pubic hair. These characteristics are produced not by estradiol but rather by androgens secreted by the cortex of the adrenal glands. Even a male who is castrated before puberty (whose testes are removed) will grow axillary and pubic hair, stimulated by his own adrenal androgens. A list of the principal sex hormones and examples of their effects are presented in Table 9.1. Note that some of these effects are discussed later in this chapter. (See *Table 9.1*.)

TABLE 9.1   Classification of Sex Steroid Hormones

Class	Principal Hormone in Humans (where produced)	Examples of Effects
Androgens	Testosterone (testes)	Development of Wolffian system; production of sperms; growth of facial, pubic, and axillary hair; muscular development; enlargement of larynx; inhibition of bone growth; sex drive in men (and women?)
	Dihydrotestosterone (produced from testosterone by action of an enzyme)	Maturation of male external genitalia
	Androstenedione (adrenal glands)	In women, growth of pubic and axillary hair; less important than testosterone and dihydrotestosterone in men
Estrogens	Estradiol (ovaries)	Maturation of female genitalia; growth of breasts; alterations in fat deposits; growth of uterine lining; inhibition of bone growth; sex drive in women (?)

TABLE 9.1   Classification of Sex Steroid Hormones *(continued)*

Class	Principal Hormone in Humans (where produced)	Examples of Effects
Gestagens	Progesterone (ovaries)	Maintenance of uterine lining
Hypothalamic hormones	Gonadotropin-releasing hormone (hypothalamus)	Secretion of gonadotropins
Gonadotropins	Follicle-stimulating hormone (anterior pituitary)	Development of ovarian follicle
	Luteinizing hormone (anterior pituitary)	Ovulation; development of corpus luteum
Other hormones	Prolactin (anterior pituitary)	Milk production; male refractory period (?)
	Oxytocin (posterior pituitary)	Milk ejection; orgasm; pair bonding (especially females); bonding with infants
	Vasopressin (posterior pituitary)	Pair bonding (especially males)

The bipotentiality of some of the secondary sex characteristics remains throughout life. If a man is treated with an estrogen (for example, to control an androgen-dependent tumor), he will grow breasts, and his facial hair will become finer and softer. However, his voice will remain low, because the enlargement of the larynx is permanent. Conversely, a woman who receives high levels of an androgen (usually from a tumor that secretes androgens) will grow a beard, and her voice will become lower.

luteinizing hormone (LH) (*lew tee a nize ing*) A hormone of the anterior pituitary gland that causes ovulation and development of the ovarian follicle into a corpus luteum.

estradiol (*ess tra dye ahl*) The principal estrogen of many mammals, including humans.

estrogen (*ess trow jen*) A class of sex hormones that cause maturation of the female genitalia, growth of breast tissue, and development of other physical features characteristic of females.

Interim Summary

Sexual Development

Gender is determined by the sex chromosomes: XX produces a female, and XY produces a male. Males are produced by the action of the *Sry* gene on the Y chromosome, which contains the code for the production of a protein that in turn causes the primitive gonads to become testes. The testes secrete two kinds of hormones that cause a male to develop. Testosterone and dihydrotestosterone (androgens) stimulate the development of the Wolffian system (masculinization), and anti-Müllerian hormone suppresses the development of the Müllerian system (defeminization). Androgen insensitivity syndrome results from a hereditary defect in androgen receptors, and persistent Müllerian duct syndrome results from a hereditary defect in production of anti-Müllerian hormone or its receptors.

By default the body is female ("Nature's impulse is to create a female"); only by the actions of testicular hormones does it become male. Masculinization and defeminization are referred to as *organizational* effects of hormones; *activational* effects occur after development is complete. A person with Turner's syndrome (X0) fails to develop gonads but nevertheless develops female internal sex organs and external genitalia. The external genitalia develop from common precursors. In the absence of gonadal hormones the precursors develop the female form; in the presence of androgens (primarily dihydrotestosterone, which derives from testosterone

through the action of an enzyme) they develop the male form (masculinization).

Sexual maturity occurs when the hypothalamus begins secreting gonadotropin-releasing hormone, which stimulates the secretion of follicle-stimulating hormone and luteinizing hormone by the anterior pituitary gland. These hormones stimulate the gonads to secrete their hormones, thus causing the genitals to mature and the body to develop the secondary sex characteristics (activational effects).

Thought Questions

1. Suppose that people could easily determine the sex of their child, say, by having one of the would-be parents take a drug before conceiving the baby. What would the consequences be?

2. With appropriate hormonal treatment, the uterus of a postmenopausal woman can be made ready for the implantation of another woman's ovum, fertilized in vitro, and she can become a mother. In fact, several women in their fifties and sixties have done so. What do you think about this procedure? Should decisions about using it be left to couples and their physicians, or does the rest of society (represented by their legislators) have an interest?

Hormonal Control of Sexual Behavior

We have seen that hormones are responsible for sexual dimorphism in the structure of the body and its organs. Hormones have organizational and activational effects on the internal sex organs, genitals, and secondary sex characteristics. Naturally, all of these effects influence a person's behavior. Simply having the physique and genitals of a man or a woman exerts a powerful effect. But hormones do more than give us masculine or feminine bodies; they also affect behavior by interacting directly with the nervous system. Androgens that are present during prenatal development affect the development of the nervous system. In addition, both male and female sex hormones have activational effects on the adult nervous system that influence both physiological processes and behavior. This section considers some of these hormonal effects.

Hormonal Control of Female Reproductive Cycles

menstrual cycle (*men* strew al) The female reproductive cycle of most primates, including humans; characterized by growth of the lining of the uterus, ovulation, development of a corpus luteum, and (if pregnancy does not occur) menstruation.

estrous cycle The female reproductive cycle of mammals other than primates.

ovarian follicle A cluster of epithelial cells surrounding an oocyte, which develops into an ovum.

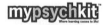

Animation 9.1
The Menstrual Cycle

corpus luteum (*lew* tee um) A cluster of cells that develops from the ovarian follicle after ovulation; secretes estradiol and progesterone.

progesterone (*pro jess* ter own) A steroid hormone produced by the ovary that maintains the endometrial lining of the uterus during the later part of the menstrual cycle and during pregnancy; along with estradiol it promotes receptivity in female mammals with estrous cycles.

The reproductive cycle of female primates is called a **menstrual cycle** (from *mensis*, meaning "month"). Females of other species of mammals also have reproductive cycles, called **estrous cycles**. *Estrus* means "gadfly"; when a female rat is in estrus, her hormonal condition goads her to act differently than she does at other times. (For that matter, it goads male rats to act differently too.) The primary feature that distinguishes menstrual cycles from estrous cycles is the monthly growth and loss of the lining of the uterus. The other features are approximately the same—except that the estrous cycle of rats takes 4 days. Also, the sexual behavior of female mammals with estrous cycles is linked with ovulation, whereas most female primates can mate at any time during their menstrual cycle.

Menstrual cycles and estrous cycles consist of a sequence of events that are controlled by hormonal secretions of the pituitary gland and ovaries. These glands interact, the secretions of one affecting those of the other. A cycle begins with the secretion of gonadotropins by the anterior pituitary gland. These hormones (especially FSH) stimulate the growth of **ovarian follicles**, small spheres of epithelial cells surrounding each ovum. Women normally produce one ovarian follicle each month; if two are produced and fertilized, dizygotic (fraternal) twins will develop. As ovarian follicles mature, they secrete estradiol, which causes the lining of the uterus to grow in preparation for implantation of the ovum, should it be fertilized by a sperm. Feedback from the increasing level of estradiol eventually triggers the release of a surge of LH by the anterior pituitary gland. (See *Figure 9.6* and *MyPsychKit 9.1, The Menstrual Cycle.*)

The LH surge causes *ovulation*: The ovarian follicle ruptures, releasing the ovum. Under the continued influence of LH, the ruptured ovarian follicle becomes a **corpus luteum** ("yellow body"), which produces estradiol and **progesterone**. (See *Figure 9.6.*) The latter hormone promotes pregnancy (*gestation*). It maintains the lining of the uterus, and it inhibits the ovaries from producing another follicle. Meanwhile, the ovum enters one of the Fallopian tubes and begins its progress toward the uterus. If it meets sperm cells during its travel down the Fallopian tube and becomes fertilized, it begins to divide, and several days later it attaches itself to the uterine wall.

If the ovum is not fertilized or if it is fertilized too late to develop sufficiently by the time it gets to the uterus, the corpus luteum will stop producing estradiol and progesterone, and then the lining of the walls of the uterus will slough off. At this point, menstruation will commence.

Hormonal Control of Sexual Behavior of Laboratory Animals

The interactions between sex hormones and the human brain are difficult to study. We must turn to two sources of information: experiments with animals and various developmental disorders in humans, which serve as nature's own "experiments." Let us first consider the evidence gathered from research with laboratory animals.

Males

Male sexual behavior is quite varied, although the essential features of *intromission* (entry of the penis into the female's vagina), *pelvic thrusting* (rhythmic movement of the hindquarters, causing genital friction), and *ejaculation* (discharge of semen) are characteristic of all male mammals. Humans, of course, have invented all kinds of copulatory and noncopulatory sexual behavior. For example, the pelvic movements leading to ejaculation may be performed by the woman, and sex play can lead to orgasm without intromission.

The sexual behavior of rats has been studied more than that of any other laboratory animal (Hull and Dominguez, 2007). When a male rat encounters a receptive female, he will spend some time nuzzling her and sniffing and licking her genitals, mount her, and engage in pelvic thrusting. He will mount her several times, achieving intromission on most of the mountings. After eight to fifteen intromissions approximately 1 minute apart (each lasting only about one-quarter of a second), the male will ejaculate.

After ejaculating, the male refrains from sexual activity for a period of time (minutes, in the rat). Most mammals will return to copulate several times, finally showing a longer pause, called a **refractory period**. (The term comes from the Latin *refringere*, "to break off.") An interesting phenomenon occurs in some mammals. If a male, after finally becoming "exhausted" by repeated copulation with the same female, is presented with a new female, he begins to respond quickly—often as fast as he did in his initial contact with the first female. Successive introductions of new females can keep up his performance for prolonged periods of time. This phenomenon is undoubtedly important in species in which a single male inseminates all the females in his harem. Species with approximately equal numbers of reproductively active males and females are less likely to act this way.

FIGURE 9.6

Neuroendocrine Control of the Menstrual Cycle

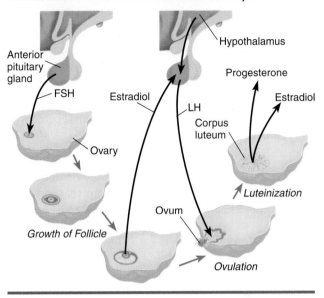

In one of the most unusual studies I have read about, Beamer, Bermant, and Clegg (1969) tested the ability of a ram (male sheep) to recognize ewes with which he had mated. A ram that is given a new ewe each time will quickly begin copulating and will ejaculate within 2 minutes. (In one study, a ram kept up this performance with twelve ewes. The experimenters finally got tired of shuffling sheep around; the ram was still ready to go.) Beamer and his colleagues tried to fool rams by putting trench coats and Halloween face masks on females with which the rams had mated. (No, I'm not making this up.) The males were not fooled by the disguise; they apparently recognized their former partners by their odor and were no longer interested in them.

The rejuvenating effect of a new female, also seen in roosters, is usually called the **Coolidge effect.** The following story is reputed to be true, but I cannot vouch for that. (If it is not true, it ought to be.) The late former U.S. president Calvin Coolidge and his wife were touring a farm when Mrs. Coolidge asked the farmer whether the continuous and vigorous sexual activity among the flock of hens was the work of just one rooster. The reply was yes. She smiled and said, "You might point that

refractory period (*ree frak to ree*) A period of time after a particular action (for example, an ejaculation by a male) during which that action cannot occur again.

Coolidge effect The restorative effect of introducing a new female sex partner to a male that has apparently become "exhausted" by sexual activity.

out to Mr. Coolidge." The president looked thoughtfully at the birds and then asked the farmer whether a different hen was involved each time. The answer, again, was yes. "You might point *that* out to Mrs. Coolidge," he said.

Sexual behavior of male rodents depends on testosterone, a fact that has long been recognized (Bermant and Davidson, 1974). If a male rat is castrated (that is, if his testes are removed), his sexual activity eventually ceases. However, the behavior can be reinstated by injections of testosterone. I will describe the neural basis of this activational effect later in this chapter.

Females

The mammalian female has been described as the passive participant in copulation. It is true that in some species the female's role during the act of copulation is merely to assume a posture that exposes her genitals to the male. This behavior is called the **lordosis** response (from the Greek *lordos*, meaning "bent backward"). The female will also move her tail away (if she has one) and stand rigidly enough to support the weight of the male. However, the behavior of a female rodent in *initiating* copulation is often very active. Certainly, if a male attempts to copulate with a nonestrous rodent, the female will either actively flee or rebuff him. But when the female is in a receptive state, she will often approach the male, nuzzle him, sniff his genitals, and show behaviors characteristic of her species. For example, a female rat will exhibit quick, short, hopping movements and rapid ear wiggling, which most male rats find irresistible (McClintock and Adler, 1978).

Sexual behavior of female rodents depends on the gonadal hormones present during estrus: estradiol and progesterone. In rats, estradiol increases about 40 hours before the female becomes receptive; just before receptivity occurs, the corpus luteum begins secreting large quantities of progesterone (Feder, 1981). Ovariectomized rats (rats whose ovaries have been removed) are not sexually receptive. Although sexual receptivity can be produced in ovariectomized rodents by administering large doses of estradiol alone, the most effective treatment duplicates the normal sequence of hormones: a small amount of estradiol, followed by progesterone. Progesterone alone is ineffective; thus, the estradiol "primes" its effectiveness. Priming with estradiol takes about 16–24 hours, after which an injection of progesterone produces receptive behaviors within an hour (Takahashi, 1990). The neural mechanisms that are responsible for these effects will be described later in this chapter.

The sequence of estradiol followed by progesterone has three effects on female rats: It increases their receptivity, their proceptivity, and their attractiveness. *Receptivity* refers to their ability and willingness to copulate—to accept the advances of a male by holding still and displaying lordosis when he attempts to mount her. *Proceptivity* refers to a female's eagerness to copulate, as shown by the fact that she seeks out a male and engages in behaviors that tend to arouse his sexual interest. *Attractiveness* refers to physiological and behavioral changes that affect the male. The male rat (along with many other male mammals) is most responsive to females who are in estrus ("in heat"). Males will ignore a female whose ovaries have been removed, but injections of estradiol and progesterone will restore her attractiveness (and also change her behavior toward the male). The stimuli that arouse a male rat's sexual interest include her odor and her behavior. In some species visible changes, such as the swollen sex skin in the genital region of a female monkey, also affect sex appeal.

Even though women do not show obvious physical changes during the fertile period of their menstrual cycle, some subtle changes do occur. Roberts et al. (2004) took photos of women's faces during fertile and non-fertile periods of their menstrual cycle and found that both men and women judged the photos taken during

lordosis A spinal sexual reflex seen in many four-legged female mammals; arching of the back in response to approach of a male or to touching the flanks, which elevates the hindquarters.

the fertile period were more attractive than those taken during a non-fertile period. (The women whose pictures were taken were not told the object of the study until afterward to prevent them from unknowingly changing their facial expressions in a way that might bias the results.)

Organizational Effects of Androgens on Behavior: Masculinization and Defeminization

The dictum "Nature's impulse is to create a female" applies to sexual behavior as well as to sex organs. That is, if a rodent's brain is *not* exposed to androgens during a critical period of development, the animal will engage in female sexual behavior as an adult (if it is then given estradiol and progesterone). Fortunately for experimenters, this critical time comes shortly after birth for rats and for several other species of rodents that are born in a rather immature condition. Thus, if a male rat is castrated immediately after birth, permitted to grow to adulthood, and then given injections of estradiol and progesterone, it will respond to the presence of another male by arching its back and presenting its hindquarters. In other words, it will act as if it were a female (Blaustein and Olster, 1989).

In contrast, if a rodent brain is exposed to androgens during development, two phenomena occur: behavioral defeminization and behavioral masculinization. *Behavioral defeminization* refers to the organizational effect of androgens that prevents the animal from displaying female sexual behavior in adulthood. As we shall see later, this effect is accomplished by suppressing the development of neural circuits controlling female sexual behavior. For example, if a female rodent is ovariectomized and given an injection of testosterone immediately after birth, she will *not* respond to a male rat when, as an adult, she is given injections of estradiol and progesterone. *Behavioral masculinization* refers to the organizational effect of androgens that enables animals to engage in male sexual behavior in adulthood. This effect is accomplished by stimulating the development of neural circuits controlling male sexual behavior. For example, if the female rodent in my previous example is given testosterone in adulthood rather than estradiol and progesterone, she will mount and attempt to copulate with a receptive female. (See Breedlove, 1992, and Carter, 1992, for references to specific studies.) (See *Figure 9.7*.)

Effects of Pheromones

Hormones transmit messages from one part of the body (the secreting gland) to another (the target tissue). Another class of chemicals, called **pheromones**, carries messages from one animal to another. Some of these chemicals, like hormones, affect reproductive behavior. Karlson and Luscher (1959) coined the term, from the Greek *pherein*, "to carry," and *horman*, "to excite." Pheromones are released by one animal and directly affect the physiology or behavior of another. In mammalian species most pheromones are detected by means of olfaction.

Pheromones can affect reproductive physiology or behavior. First, let us consider the effects on reproductive physiology. When groups of female mice are housed together, their estrous cycles slow down and eventually stop. This phenomenon is known as the **Lee-Boot effect** (van der Lee and Boot, 1955). If groups of females are exposed to the odor of a male (or of his urine), they begin cycling again,

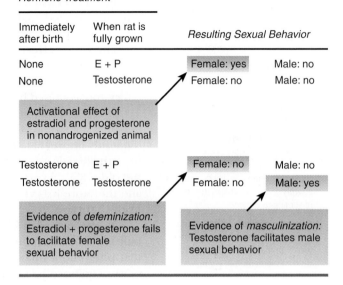

FIGURE 9.7

Organizational Effects of Testosterone.   Around the time of birth, testosterone masculinizes and defeminizes rodents' sexual behavior.

Hormone Treatment

Immediately after birth	When rat is fully grown	*Resulting Sexual Behavior*	
None	E + P	Female: yes	Male: no
None	Testosterone	Female: no	Male: no

Activational effect of estradiol and progesterone in nonandrogenized animal

Testosterone	E + P	Female: no	Male: no
Testosterone	Testosterone	Female: no	Male: yes

Evidence of *defeminization*: Estradiol + progesterone fails to facilitate female sexual behavior

Evidence of *masculinization*: Testosterone facilitates male sexual behavior

pheromone (*fair* oh moan) A chemical released by one animal that affects the behavior or physiology of another animal; usually smelled or tasted.

Lee-Boot effect The slowing and eventual cessation of estrous cycles in groups of female animals that are housed together; caused by a pheromone in the animals' urine; first observed in mice.

Whitten effect The synchronization of the menstrual or estrous cycles of a group of females, which occurs only in the presence of a pheromone in a male's urine.

Vandenbergh effect The earlier onset of puberty seen in female animals that are housed with males; caused by a pheromone in the male's urine; first observed in mice.

Bruce effect Termination of pregnancy caused by the odor of a pheromone in the urine of a male other than the one that impregnated the female; first identified in mice.

vomeronasal organ (VNO) (*voah mer oh nay zul*) A sensory organ that detects the presence of certain chemicals, especially when a liquid is actively sniffed; mediates the effects of some pheromones.

accessory olfactory bulb A neural structure located in the main olfactory bulb that receives information from the vomeronasal organ.

and their cycles tend to be synchronized. This phenomenon is known as the **Whitten effect** (Whitten, 1959). The **Vandenbergh effect** (Vandenbergh, Whitsett, and Lombardi, 1975) is the acceleration of the onset of puberty in a female rodent caused by the odor of a male. Both the Whitten effect and the Vandenbergh effect are caused by a group of compounds that are present only in the urine of intact adult males (Ma, Miao, and Novotny, 1999; Novotny et al., 1999); the urine of a juvenile or castrated male has no effect. Thus, the production of the pheromone requires the presence of testosterone.

The **Bruce effect** (Bruce, 1960a, 1960b) is a particularly interesting phenomenon: When a recently impregnated female mouse encounters a normal male mouse other than the one with which she mated, the pregnancy is very likely to fail. This effect, too, is caused by a substance secreted in the urine of intact males—but not of males that have been castrated. Thus, a male mouse that encounters a pregnant female is able to prevent the birth of infants carrying another male's genes and subsequently impregnate the female himself. This phenomenon is advantageous even from the female's point of view. The fact that the new male has managed to take over the old male's territory indicates that he is probably healthier and more vigorous, and therefore his genes will contribute to the formation of offspring that are more likely to survive.

As you learned in Chapter 7, detection of odors is accomplished by the olfactory bulbs, which constitute the primary olfactory system. However, some of the effects that pheromones have on reproductive cycles appear to be mediated by another sensory organ—the **vomeronasal organ (VNO)**—which consists of a small group of sensory receptors arranged around a pouch connected by a duct to the nasal passage. The vomeronasal organ, which is present in all orders of mammals except for cetaceans (whales and dolphins), projects to the **accessory olfactory bulb**, located immediately behind the olfactory bulb (Wysocki, 1979). (See *Figure 9.8*.)

Although the vomeronasal organ can respond to some airborne molecules, it is primarily sensitive to nonvolatile compounds found in urine or other substances (Brennan and Keverne, 2004). In fact, stimulation of a nerve that serves the nasal region of the hamster causes fluid to be pumped into the vomeronasal organ, which exposes the receptors to any substances that may be present (Meredith and O'Connell, 1979). This pump is activated whenever the animal encounters a novel stimulus (Meredith, 1994). Removal of the accessory olfactory bulb disrupts the Lee-Boot effect, the Whitten effect, the Vandenbergh effect, and the Bruce effect; thus, the vomeronasal system is essential for these phenomena (Halpern, 1987).

Besides having effects on reproductive physiology, some pheromones directly affect behavior. For example, pheromones present in the vaginal secretions of female hamsters stimulate sexual behavior in males. Males are attracted to the secretions of females, and they sniff and lick the female's genitals before copulating (Powers and Winans, 1975; Winans and Powers, 1977). In addition, the males of some species produce sex-attractant pheromones that affect the behavior of females. For example, a pheromone present in the saliva of boars (male pigs) elicits sexual behavior in sows (Dorries, Adkins, and Halpern, 1997). Some male pheromones that attract females are detected by the main olfactory system. For example, Mak et al. (2007) found that the odor of soiled bedding taken from the cage of a male mouse activated neurons in the main olfactory system and hippocampus. The odor even stimulated neurogenesis (production of new neurons); Mak and her colleagues found new neurons in the olfactory bulb and hippocampus. Moreover, bedding from

FIGURE 9.8

The Rodent Accessory Olfactory System

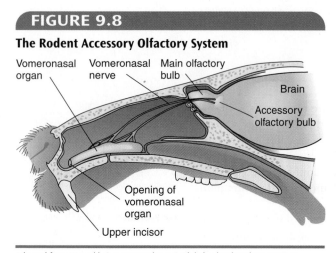

Adapted from Wysocki, C. J. *Neuroscience & Biobehavioral Reviews*, 1979, *3*, 301–341.

cages of dominant males stimulated neurogenesis more effectively than did bedding from subordinate males.

Stowers et al. (2002) found that a targeted mutation against a protein that is essential for the detection of pheromones by the vomeronasal organ abolishes a male mouse's ability to discriminate between males and females. As a result, male mice with this mutation attempted to copulate with both males and females. (See *MyPsychKit 9.2, Role of Pheromones in Intermale Aggression.*) Luo, Fee, and Katz (2003) recorded from single neurons in the accessory olfactory bulb in mice and found that specific neurons responded selectively to either males or females. (See *MyPsychKit 9.3, VNO Responses.*)

It appears that at least some pheromone-related phenomena occur in humans. McClintock (1971) studied the menstrual cycles of women attending an all-female college. She found that women who spent a large amount of time together tended to have synchronized cycles: Their menstrual periods began within a day or two of one another. In addition, women who regularly spent some time in the presence of men tended to have shorter cycles than those who rarely spent time with (smelled?) men.

Russell, Switz, and Thompson (1980) obtained direct evidence that pheromones can synchronize women's menstrual cycles. The investigators collected daily samples of a woman's underarm sweat. They dissolved the samples in alcohol and swabbed them on the upper lips of a group of women three times each week, in the order in which they were originally taken. The cycles of the women who received the extract (but not those of control subjects whose lips were swabbed with pure alcohol) began to synchronize with the cycle of the odor donor.

Several studies have found that two compounds present in human sweat have different effects in men and women. Singh and Bronstad (2001) had men smell T-shirts that had been worn by women for several days. The men reported that shirts worn by women during the fertile phase of their menstrual cycle smelled more pleasant and more sexy than those worn during the nonfertile phase. Jacob and McClintock (2000) found that the androgenic chemical *androstadienone* (*AND*) increases alertness and positive mood in women but decreased positive mood in men. Wyart et al. (2007) found that women who smelled AND showed higher levels of cortisol (an adrenal hormone involved in a variety of emotional behaviors) as well as reporting a more positive mood and an increase in sexual arousal. A functional imaging study by Savic et al. (2001) found that AND activated the preoptic area and ventromedial hypothalamus in women but not in men, whereas the estrogenic chemical *estratetraene* (*EST*) activated the paraventricular nucleus and dorsomedial hypothalamus in men but not in women.

Whether or not pheromones play a role in sexual attraction in humans, the familiar odor of a sex partner probably has a positive effect on sexual arousal—just like the sight of a sex partner or the sound of his or her voice. It is likely that men and women can learn to be attracted by their partners' characteristic odors, just as they can learn to be attracted by the sound of their voice. In an instance like this, the odors are serving simply as sensory cues, not as pheromones.

What sensory organ detects the presence of human pheromones? Although humans have a small vomeronasal organ located along the nasal septum (bridge of tissue between

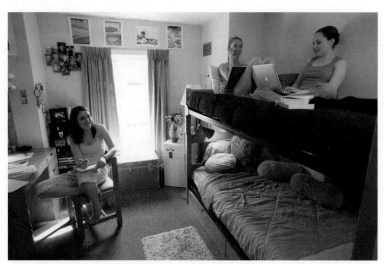

The presence of pheromone-related phenomena in humans was confirmed by the discovery that women who regularly spend time together tend to have synchronized menstrual cycles.

the nostrils) approximately 2 cm from the opening of the nostril (Garcia-Velasco and Mondragon, 1991), the human VNO appears to be a vestigial, nonfunctional, organ. The density of neurons in the VNO is very sparse, and investigators have not found any neural connections from this organ to the brain (Doty, 2001). Evidence clearly shows that human reproductive physiology is affected by pheromones, but it appears that these chemical signals are detected by the "standard" olfactory system—the receptor cells in the olfactory epithelium—and not by cells in the VNO.

Human Sexual Behavior

Human sexual behavior, like that of other mammals, is influenced by activational effects of gonadal hormones and, almost certainly, by organizational effects as well. If hormones have organizational effects on human sexual behavior, they must exert these effects by altering the development of the brain. Although there is good evidence that prenatal exposure to androgens affects development of the human brain, we cannot yet be certain that this exposure has long-lasting behavioral effects. The evidence pertaining to these issues is discussed later, in a section on sexual orientation.

Activational Effects of Sex Hormones in Women

As we saw, the sexual behavior of most female mammals other than higher primates is controlled by the ovarian hormones estradiol and progesterone. (In some species, such as cats and rabbits, only estradiol is necessary.) As Wallen (1990) pointed out, the ovarian hormones control not only the *willingness* (or even eagerness) of an estrous female to mate but also her *ability* to mate. That is, a male rat cannot copulate with a female rat that is not in estrus. Even if he would overpower her and mount her, her lordosis response would not occur, and he would be unable to achieve intromission. Thus, the evolutionary process seems to have selected animals that mate only at a time when the female is able to become pregnant. (The neural control of the lordosis response and the effects of ovarian hormones on it are described later in this chapter.)

In higher primates (including our own species), the ability to mate is not controlled by ovarian hormones. There are no physical barriers to sexual intercourse during any part of the menstrual cycle. If a woman or other female primate consents to sexual activity at any time (or is forced to submit by a male), intercourse can certainly take place.

Although ovarian hormones do not *control* women's sexual activity, they may still have an influence on their sexual interest. Early studies reported that fluctuations in the level of ovarian hormones had only a minor effect on women's sexual interest (Adams, Gold, and Burt, 1978; Morris et al., 1987). However, as Wallen (1990) notes, these studies have almost all involved married women who live with their husbands. In stable, monogamous relationships in which the partners are together on a daily basis, sexual activity can be instigated by either of them. Normally, a husband does not force his wife to have intercourse with him, but even if she is not interested in engaging in sexual activity at that moment, she may find that she wants to do so because of her affection for him. Thus, changes in sexual interest and arousability might not always be reflected in changes in sexual behavior.

A study by Van Goozen et al. (1997) supports this suggestion. The investigators found that the sexual activity initiated by men and women showed very different relations to the woman's menstrual cycle (and hence to her level of ovarian hormones). Men initiated sexual activity at about the same rate throughout the woman's cycle, whereas sexual activity initiated by women showed a distinct peak around the time of ovulation, when estradiol levels are highest. (See *Figure 9.9*.) Bullivant et al. (2004) found that women were more likely to initiate sexual activity and were more likely to engage in sexual fantasies just before and during the surge in luteinizing hormone that stimulates ovulation.

Activational Effects of Sex Hormones in Men

Although women and mammals with estrous cycles differ in their behavioral responsiveness to sex hormones, men resemble other mammals in their behavioral responsiveness to testosterone. With normal levels they can be potent and fertile; without testosterone sperm production ceases, and sooner or later, so does sexual potency. In a double-blind study, Bagatell et al. (1994) gave a placebo or a gonadotropin-releasing hormone (GnRH) antagonist to young male volunteers to temporarily suppress secretion of testicular androgens. Within 2 weeks, the subjects who received the GnRH antagonist reported a decrease in sexual interest, sexual fantasy, and intercourse. Men who received replacement doses of testosterone along with the antagonist did not show these changes.

The decline of sexual activity after castration is quite variable. As reported by Money and Ehrhardt (1972), some men lose potency immediately, whereas others show a slow, gradual decline over several years. Perhaps at least some of the variability is a function of prior experience; practice not only may "make perfect," but also may forestall a decline in function. Although there is no direct evidence with respect to this possibility in humans, Wallen and his colleagues (Wallen et al., 1991; Wallen, 2001) injected a GnRH antagonist in seven adult male rhesus monkeys that were part of a larger group. The injection suppressed testosterone secretion, and sexual behavior declined after 1 week. However, the decline was related to the animal's social rank and sexual experience: More sexually experienced, high-ranking males continued to copulate. In fact, the highest-ranking male continued to copulate and ejaculate at the same rate as before, even though his testosterone secretion was suppressed for almost 8 weeks. The mounting behavior of the lowest-ranking monkey completely ceased and did not resume until testosterone secretion recovered from the anti-GnRH treatment.

Testosterone not only affects sexual activity but also is affected by it—or even by thinking about it. A scientist stationed on a remote island (Anonymous, 1970) removed his beard with an electric shaver each day and weighed the clippings. Just before he left for visits to the mainland (and to the company of a female companion), his beard began growing faster. Because rate of beard growth is related to androgen levels, the effect indicates that his anticipation of sexual activity stimulated testosterone production. Confirming these results, Hellhammer, Hubert, and Schurmeyer (1985) found that watching an erotic film increased men's testosterone level.

Sexual Orientation

What controls a person's sexual orientation; that is, the gender of the preferred sex partner? Some investigators believe that sexual orientation is determined by childhood experiences, especially interactions between the child and parents. A large-scale study of several hundred male and female homosexuals reported by Bell, Weinberg, and Hammersmith (1981) attempted to assess the effects of these factors. The researchers found no evidence that homosexuals had been raised by domineering mothers or submissive fathers, as some clinicians had suggested. The best predictor of adult homosexuality was a self-report of homosexual feelings, which usually preceded homosexual activity by 3 years. The investigators concluded that their data did not support social explanations for homosexuality but were consistent with the possibility that homosexuality is at least partly biologically determined.

FIGURE 9.9

Sexual Activity of Heterosexual Couples.   This graph shows the distribution of sexual activity initiated by the man and by the woman.

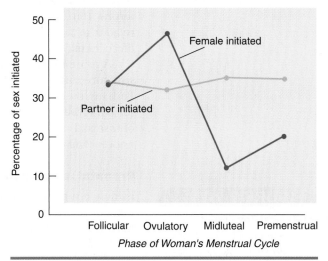

Adapted from Wallen, K. *Hormones and Behavior*, 2001, *40*, 339–357. After data from Van Goozen et al., 1997.

congenital adrenal hyperplasia (CAH) (*hy per play zha*) A condition characterized by hypersecretion of androgens by the adrenal cortex; in females, causes masculinization of the external genitalia.

If homosexuality does have a physiological cause, it certainly is not variations in the levels of sex hormones during adulthood. Many studies have examined the levels of sex steroids in male homosexuals (Meyer-Bahlburg, 1984), and the vast majority of them found these levels to be similar to those of heterosexuals. A few studies suggest that about 30 percent of female homosexuals have elevated levels of testosterone (but still lower than those found in men). Whether these differences are related to a biological cause of female homosexuality or whether differences in lifestyles may increase the secretion of testosterone is not yet known.

A more likely biological cause of homosexuality is a subtle difference in brain structure caused by differences in the amount of prenatal exposure to androgens. Perhaps, then, the brains of male homosexuals are neither masculinized nor defeminized, those of female homosexuals are masculinized and defeminized, and those of bisexuals are masculinized but not defeminized. Of course, these are *hypotheses*, not *conclusions*. They should be regarded as suggestions to guide future research.

Prenatal Androgenization of Genetic Females

Evidence suggests that prenatal androgens can affect human social behavior and sexual orientation, as well as anatomy. In a disorder known as **congenital adrenal hyperplasia (CAH)**, the adrenal glands secrete abnormal amounts of androgens. (*Hyperplasia* means "excessive formation.") The secretion of androgens begins prenatally; thus, the syndrome causes prenatal masculinization. Boys born with CAH develop normally; the extra androgen does not seem to have significant effects. However, a girl with CAH will be born with an enlarged clitoris, and her labia may be partly fused together. (As Figure 9.3 shows, the scrotum and labia develop from the same tissue in the fetus.) If masculinization of the genitals is pronounced, surgery is sometimes performed to correct them. In any event, once the syndrome is identified, the person will be given a synthetic hormone that suppresses the abnormal secretion of androgens.

As a group, females with CAH have an increased likelihood of becoming sexually attracted to other women; approximately one-third describe themselves as bisexual or homosexual (Cohen-Bendahan, van de Beek, and Berenbaum, 2005). Presumably, prenatal androgenization is responsible for this increased incidence of a masculinized sexual orientation. If the differences seen in sexual orientation *are* caused by effects of prenatal androgens on brain development, then we could reasonably conclude that exposure of the male brain to prenatal androgens plays a role in establishing a sexual orientation toward females, too. That is, sexual orientation in men is probably affected by masculinizing (and defeminizing) effects of androgens on the brain.

Children typically show sex differences in behaviors such as toy preferences (Alexander, 2003). Boys generally prefer toys that can be used actively, especially those that move or can be propelled by the child. Girls generally prefer toys that provide the opportunity for nurturance. Of course, it is an undeniable fact that both caregivers and peers encourage "sex-typical" toy choices. However, evidence suggests that biology may play a role in the nature of these choices. For example, even at 1 day of age, baby boys prefer to watch a moving mobile and baby girls prefer to look at a female face (Connellan et al., 2000). Alexander and Hines (2002) found that young vervet monkeys showed the same sexually dimorphic preferences in choice of toys that children do: Males chose to play with a car and a ball, whereas females preferred to play with a doll and a pot. (See *Figure 9.10*.)

Pasterski et al. (2005) found that girls with CAH were more likely to choose male toys than were their non-CAH sisters or female cousins. The girls' parents reported that they made a special effort to encourage their CAH daughters to play with "girls' toys" but that this encouragement appeared not to succeed. Thus, the girls' tendencies to make male toy choices did not seem to be a result of parental pressure.

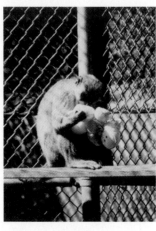
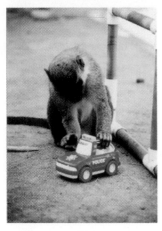

Failure of Androgenization of Genetic Males

As we saw, genetic males with androgen insensitivity syndrome develop as females, with female external genitalia—but also with testes and without uterus or fallopian tubes. If an individual with this syndrome is raised as a girl, all is well. Normally, the testes are removed because they often become cancerous, but if they are not, the body will mature into that of a woman at the time of puberty through the effects of the small amounts of estradiol produced by the testes. (If the testes are removed, the person will be given estradiol to accomplish the same result.) At adulthood the individual will function sexually as a woman, although surgical lengthening of the vagina may be necessary. Women with this syndrome report average sex drives, including normal frequency of orgasm in intercourse. Most marry and lead normal sex lives.

There are no reports of bisexuality or homosexuality (sexual orientation toward women) of XY women with androgen insensitivity syndrome. Thus, the lack of androgen receptors appears to prevent both the masculinizing and defeminizing effects of androgens on a person's sexual interest. Of course, it is also possible that rearing an XY child with androgen insensitivity syndrome as a girl plays a role in that person's sexual orientation.

Sexual Orientation and the Brain

The human brain is a sexually dimorphic organ. This fact has long been suspected, even before confirmation was received from anatomical studies and studies of regional cerebral metabolism using PET and functional MRI. For example, neurologists discovered that the two hemispheres of a woman's brain appear to share functions more than those of a man's brain do. If a man sustains a stroke that damages the left side of the brain, he is more likely to show impairments in language than will a woman with similar damage. Presumably, the woman's right hemisphere shares language functions with the left, so damage to one hemisphere is less devastating than it is in men. Also, men's brains are, on the average, somewhat larger—apparently because men's bodies are generally larger than those of women. In addition, the sizes of some specific regions of the telencephalon and diencephalon are different in males and females, and the shape of the corpus callosum may also be sexually dimorphic. (See Breedlove, 1994; Swaab, Gooren, and Hofman, 1995; and Goldstein et al., 2001, for specific references.)

Most investigators believe that the sexual dimorphism of the human brain is a result of differential exposure to androgens prenatally and during early postnatal life. Of course, additional changes could occur at the time of puberty, when another surge in androgens occurs. Sexual dimorphisms in the human brain could even be a result of differences in the social environments of males and females. We cannot manipulate the hormone levels of humans before and after birth as we can with laboratory animals, so it might be a long time before enough evidence is gathered to permit us to make definite conclusions.

Several studies have examined the brains of deceased heterosexual and homosexual men and heterosexual women. So far, these studies have found differences in the size of three different subregions of the brain (Swaab and Hofman, 1990; LeVay, 1991; Allen and Gorski, 1992). However, a follow-up study confirmed the existence of a sexually dimorphic nucleus in the hypothalamus but failed to find a relationship between its size and sexual orientation in men (Byne et al., 2001). At this point there is no good evidence for differences in brain structure that might account for differences in sexual orientation.

As we saw earlier, a functional imaging study by Savic et al. (2001) found that the brains of heterosexual men and women reacted differently to the odors of AND and EST, two chemicals that may serve as human pheromones. Savic, Berglund, and Lindström (2005) investigated the patterns of brain activation in heterosexual women and homosexual and heterosexual men in response to the odors of these chemicals. They found the same sex differences in the responses of heterosexual men and women that were seen in the earlier study. They also found that the response of homosexual men was similar to that of heterosexual women, which suggests that the response pattern was affected by the person's sexual orientation. People with an orientation to women (heterosexual men) showed brain activation in the paraventricular and dorsomedial nuclei of the hypothalamus when they smelled EST, whereas people with an orientation to men (heterosexual women and homosexual men) showed brain activation in the preoptic area and ventromedial hypothalamus when they smelled AND.

Studies by Blanchard and his colleagues (Blanchard, 2001) and by Bogaert (2006) suggest that another factor can influence sexual differentiation of the brain. These studies found that homosexual men tend to have more older brothers—but not older sisters or younger brothers or sisters—than heterosexual men. In contrast, the numbers of brothers or sisters (younger or older) of homosexual and heterosexual women did not differ, nor did the age of the mother or father or the interval between births. The presence of older brothers and sisters had no effect on women's sexual orientation. The data obtained by Blanchard and his colleagues suggest that the odds of a boy becoming homosexual increased by approximately 3.3 percent for each older brother. Assuming a 2 percent rate of homosexuality in boys without older brothers, the predicted rate would be 3.6 percent for a boy with two older brothers and 6.3 percent for one with four older brothers. Thus, the odds are still strongly against the incidence of homosexuality even in a family with several boys.

Why would the existence of older brothers increase the likelihood of a boy's becoming homosexual? The authors suggest that when mothers are exposed to several male fetuses, their immune system may become sensitized to proteins that only males possess. As a result, the response of the mother's immune system may affect the prenatal brain development of later male fetuses. Of course, most men who have several older brothers are heterosexual, so even if this hypothesis is correct, it appears that only some women become sensitized to a protein produced by their male fetuses. In addition, many homosexual men do not have older brothers, so the phenomenon discovered by Blanchard and his colleagues cannot be the sole cause of male homosexuality.

Heredity and Sexual Orientation

Another factor that may play a role in sexual orientation is heredity. Twin studies take advantage of the fact that identical twins have identical genes, whereas the genetic similarity between fraternal twins is, on the average, 50 percent. Bailey and Pillard (1991) studied pairs of male twins in which at least one member identified himself as homosexual. If both twins are homosexual, they are said to be *concordant* for this trait. If only one is homosexual, the twins are said to be *discordant*. Thus, if homosexuality has a genetic basis, the percentage of monozygotic twins who are concordant for homosexuality should be higher than that for dizygotic twins. This is exactly what Bailey and Pillard found: The concordance rate was 52 percent for identical twins and only 22 percent for fraternal twins—a difference of 30 percent. Other studies have shown differences of up to 60 percent (Gooren, 2006).

Genetic factors also appear to affect female homosexuality. Bailey et al. (1993) found that the concordance rate of female monozygotic twins for homosexuality was 48 percent, while that of dizygotic twins was 16 percent. Another study, by Pattatucci and Hamer (1995), found an increased incidence of homosexuality and bisexuality in sisters, daughters, nieces, and female cousins (through a paternal uncle) of homosexual women.

For several years, investigators have been puzzled by an apparent paradox. On average, male homosexuals have approximately 80 percent fewer children than male heterosexuals do (Bell and Weinberg, 1981). This reduced fecundity should

Hormonal Control of Sexual Behavior

exert strong selective pressure against any genes that predispose men to become homosexual. A study by Camperio-Ciani, Corna, and Capiluppi (2004) suggests a possible explanation. They found that the female maternal relatives (for example, maternal aunts and grandmothers) of male homosexuals had higher fecundity rates than female maternal relatives of male heterosexuals. No differences were found in the female *paternal* relatives of homosexuals and heterosexuals. Because men are likely to share an X chromosome with female maternal relatives but not with female paternal relatives, the investigators suggested that a gene or genes on the X chromosome that increase a male's likelihood of becoming homosexual also increase a female's fecundity.

To summarize, evidence suggests that two biological factors—prenatal hormonal exposure and heredity—may affect a person's sexual orientation. These research findings certainly contradict the suggestion that a person's sexual orientation is a moral issue. It appears that homosexuals are no more responsible for their sexual orientation than heterosexuals are. Morris et al. (2004) pointed out the unlikelihood of a person's sexual orientation being a simple matter of choice. It is difficult to imagine someone saying to himself, "Let's see, I'll have gym at school today, so I'll wear white socks and tennis shoes. Gosh, as long as I'm making decisions I guess I better be attracted to girls for the rest of my life, too." (Morris et al., 2004, p. 475). The question "Why does someone become homosexual?" will probably be answered when we find out why someone becomes *heterosexual*.

Interim Summary

Hormonal Control of Sexual Behavior

Sexual behaviors are controlled by the organizational and activational effects of hormones. The female reproductive cycle (menstrual cycle or estrous cycle) begins with the maturation of one or more ovarian follicles, which occurs in response to the secretion of FSH by the anterior pituitary gland. As the ovarian follicle matures, it secretes estradiol, which causes the lining of the uterus to develop. When estradiol reaches a critical level, it causes the pituitary gland to secrete a surge of LH, triggering ovulation. The empty ovarian follicle becomes a corpus luteum, under the continued influence of LH, and secretes estradiol and progesterone. If pregnancy does not occur, the corpus luteum dies and stops producing hormones, and menstruation begins.

The sexual behavior of males of all mammalian species appears to depend on the presence of androgens. The proceptivity, receptivity, and attractiveness of female mammals other than primates depend primarily on estradiol and progesterone. In particular, estradiol has a priming effect on the subsequent appearance of progesterone.

In most mammals, female sexual behavior is the norm, just as the female body and female sex organs are the norm. That is, unless prenatal androgens masculinize and defeminize the animal's brain, its sexual behavior will be feminine. Behavioral masculinization refers to the androgen-stimulated development of neural circuits that respond to testosterone in adulthood, producing male sexual behavior. Behavioral defeminization refers to the inhibitory effects of androgens on the development of neural circuits that respond to estradiol and progesterone in adulthood, producing female sexual behavior.

Pheromones can affect sexual physiology and behavior. Odorants present in the urine of female mice affect their estrous cycles, lengthening and eventually stopping them (the Lee-Boot effect). Odorants present in the urine of male mice abolish these effects and cause the females' cycles to become synchronized (the Whitten effect). (Phenomena similar to the Lee-Boot effect and the Whitten effect also occur in women.) Odorants can also accelerate the onset of puberty in females (the Vandenbergh effect). In addition, the odor of the urine from a male other than the one that impregnated a female mouse will cause her to abort (the Bruce effect). Most, but not all, of the effects of pheromones on reproductive physiology and behavior are mediated by the vomeronasal organ/accessory olfactory system.

Pheromones present in the underarm sweat of both men and women affect women's menstrual cycles, and substances present in male sweat improves women's mood. Because the human vomeronasal organ does not appear to have sensory functions, these effects must be mediated by the main olfactory bulb. The search for sex-attractant pheromones in humans has so far been fruitless, although we might well recognize our sex partners by their odors.

Testosterone has an activational effect on the sexual behavior of men, just as it does on the behavior of other male mammals. Although women do not require estradiol or progesterone to experience sexual interest or to engage in sexual behavior, estrogen appears to affect the quality and intensity of their sex drive.

Sexual orientation (that is, heterosexuality or homosexuality) may be influenced by prenatal exposure to androgens. Studies of prenatally androgenized girls suggest that organizational effects of androgens influence the development of sexual orientation; androgenization appears to enhance interest in activities and toys usually preferred by boys and to increase the likelihood of a sexual orientation toward women. If androgens cannot act (as they cannot in cases of androgen insensitivity syndrome), the person's anatomy and behavior are feminine. So far, evidence concerning specific brain structures and sexual orientation is inconclusive. The fact that male homosexuals tend to have more older brothers than male heterosex-uals do has led to the suggestion that a woman's immune system may become sensitized to a protein that is expressed only in male fetuses. Finally, twin studies suggest that heredity may play a role in sexual orientation in both men and women.

Thought Question

Whatever the relative roles played by biological and environmental factors may be, most investigators believe that a person's sexual orientation is not a matter of choice. Why do you think so many people consider sexual orientation to be a moral issue?

Neural Control of Sexual Behavior

The control of sexual behavior—at least in laboratory animals—involves different brain mechanisms in males and females. This section describes these mechanisms.

Males

Erection and ejaculation are controlled by circuits of neurons that reside in the spinal cord. However, brain mechanisms have both excitatory and inhibitory control of these circuits. The **medial preoptic area (MPA)**, located just rostral to the hypothalamus, is the forebrain region most critical for male sexual behavior. (As we will see later in this chapter, it is also critical for other sexually dimorphic behavior, including maternal behavior.) Electrical stimulation of this region elicits male copulatory behavior (Malsbury, 1971), and sexual activity increases the firing rate of single neurons in the MPA (Shimura, Yamamoto, and Shimokochi, 1994; Mas, 1995). In addition, the act of copulation increases the activity of the MPA (Oaknin et al., 1989; Robertson et al., 1991; Wood and Newman, 1993). Finally, destruction of the MPA abolishes male sexual behavior (Heimer and Larsson, 1966/1967).

The organizational effects of androgens are responsible for sexual dimorphisms in brain structure. Gorski et al. (1978) discovered a nucleus within the MPA of the rat that is three to seven times larger in males than in females. This area is called (appropriately enough) the **sexually dimorphic nucleus (SDN)** of the preoptic area. The size of this nucleus is controlled by the amount of androgens present during fetal development. According to Rhees, Shryne, and Gorski (1990a, 1990b), the critical period for masculinization of the SDN appears to start on the eighteenth day of gestation and end once the animals are 5 days old. (Normally, rats are born on the twenty-second day of gestation.) Lesions of the SDN decrease masculine sexual behavior (De Jonge et al., 1989).

Of course, the MPA does not stand alone. It receives chemosensory input from the vomeronasal organ through connections with the medial amygdala and the bed nucleus of the stria terminalis (BNST). The MPA also receives somatosensory information from the genitals, the central tegmental field of the midbrain, and the medial amygdala. (See *Figure 9.11*.)

Androgens exert their activational effects on neurons in the MPA and associated brain regions. If a male rodent is castrated in adulthood, its sexual behavior will cease. However, the behavior can be reinstated by implanting a small amount of testosterone directly into the MPA or in two regions whose axons project to the MPA: the central tegmental field and the medial amygdala (Sipos and Nyby, 1996; Coolen and Wood, 1999). Both of these regions contain a high concentration of androgen receptors in the male rat brain (Cottingham and Pfaff, 1986).

medial preoptic area (MPA) An area of cell bodies just rostral to the hypothalamus; plays an essential role in male sexual behavior.

sexually dimorphic nucleus (SDN) A nucleus in the preoptic area that is much larger in males than in females; first observed in rats; plays a role in male sexual behavior.

FIGURE 9.11

Brain Regions Involved in Sexual Behavior.   This schematic cross section through the rat brain shows the location of the medial preoptic area, the medial amygdala, and the bed nucleus of the stria terminalis.

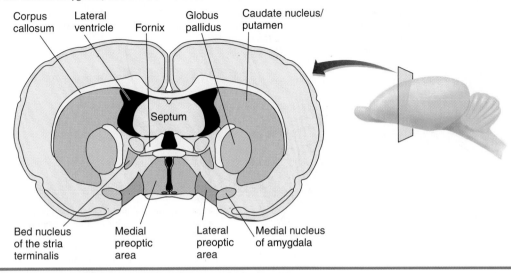

Adapted from Swanson, L. W. *Brain Maps: Structure of the Rat Brain.* New York: Elsevier, 1992.

The motor neurons that innervate the pelvic organs involved in copulation are located in the lumbar region of the spinal cord (Coolen et al., 2004). Anatomical tracing studies suggest that the most important connections between the MPA and the motor neurons of the spinal cord are accomplished through the **periaqueductal gray matter (PAG)** of the midbrain and the **nucleus paragigantocellularis (nPGi)** of the medulla (Marson and McKenna, 1992; Normandin and Murphy, 2008). The nPGi has inhibitory effects on spinal cord sexual reflexes, so one of the tasks of the pathway originating in the MPA is to suppress this inhibition. The MPA suppresses the nPGi directly through an inhibitory pathway and also does so indirectly by inhibiting the activity of the PAG, which normally excites the nPGi.

The inhibitory connections between neurons of the nPGi and those of the spinal cord motor neurons are serotonergic. As Marson and McKenna (1992) showed, application of serotonin (5-HT) to the spinal cord suppresses ejaculation. This connection may explain a well-known side effect of selective serotonin reuptake inhibitors (SSRIs). Men who take SSRIs as a treatment for depression often report that they have no trouble attaining an erection but have difficulty achieving an ejaculation. Presumably, the action of the drug as an agonist at serotonergic synapses in the spinal cord increases the inhibitory influence of nPGi neurons on spinal neurons responsible for ejaculation.

Figure 9.12 summarizes the evidence presented so far in this section. (See *Figure 9.12.*)

A functional imaging study by Holstege et al. (2003b) examined the pattern of brain activation during ejaculation in men that was elicited by the men's female partners by means of manual stimulation. Ejaculation was accompanied by neural activity in many brain regions, including the junction between the midbrain and the diencephalon, which includes the ventral tegmental area (probably involved in the pleasurable, reinforcing effects of orgasm), other midbrain regions, several thalamic nuclei, the lateral putamen (part of the basal ganglia), and the cerebellum. *Decreased* activity was seen in the amygdala and nearby entorhinal cortex. As we will see in Chapter 10, the amygdala is involved in defensive behavior and in negative emotions such as fear and anxiety. Decreased activation is also seen in this structure

periaqueductal gray matter (PAG) The region of the midbrain that surrounds the cerebral aqueduct; plays an essential role in various species-typical behaviors, including female sexual behavior.

nucleus paragigantocellularis (nPGi) A nucleus of the medulla that receives input from the medial preoptic area and contains neurons whose axons form synapses with motor neurons in the spinal cord that participate in sexual reflexes in males.

FIGURE 9.12

Male Sexual Behavior.   This schematic diagram shows a possible explanation of the interacting excitatory effects of pheromones, genital stimulation, and testosterone on male sexual behavior.

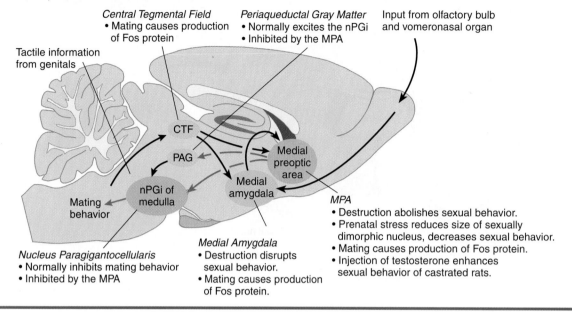

when people who are deeply in love see pictures of their loved one (Bartels and Zeki, 2000, 2004).

Females

Just as the MPA plays an essential role in male sex behavior, another region in the ventral forebrain plays a similar role in female sexual behavior: the **ventromedial nucleus of the hypothalamus (VMH)**. A female rat with bilateral lesions of the ventromedial nuclei will not display lordosis, even if she is treated with estradiol and progesterone. Conversely, electrical stimulation of the ventromedial nucleus facilitates female sexual behavior (Pfaff and Sakuma, 1979). (See *Figure 9.13.*)

The medial amygdala of males receives chemosensory information from the vomeronasal system and somatosensory information from the genitals, and it sends efferent axons to the medial preoptic area. These connections are found in females as well. In addition, neurons in the medial amygdala also send efferent axons to the VMH. In fact, copulation or mechanical stimulation of the genitals or flanks increases the production of Fos protein in both the medial amygdala and the VMH (Pfaus et al., 1993; Tetel, Getzinger, and Blaustein, 1993).

As we saw earlier, sexual behavior of female rats is activated by a priming dose of estradiol, followed by progesterone. The estrogen sets the stage, so to speak, and the progesterone stimulates the sexual behavior. Injections of these hormones directly into the VMH will stimulate sexual behavior even in females whose ovaries have been removed (Rubin and Barfield, 1980; Pleim and Barfield, 1988)—and if a chemical that blocks the production of progesterone receptors is injected into the VMH, the animal's sexual behavior is disrupted (Ogawa et al., 1994). Thus, estradiol and progesterone exert their effects on female sexual behavior by activating neurons in this nucleus.

The neurons of the ventromedial nucleus send axons to the periaqueductal gray matter. This region, too, has been implicated in female sexual behavior (Sakuma and Pfaff, 1979a, 1979b, 1980a, 1980b).

ventromedial nucleus of the hypothalamus (VMH) A large nucleus of the hypothalamus located near the walls of the third ventricle; plays an essential role in female sexual behavior.

The Ventromedial Nucleus of the Hypothalamus.   This schematic cross section through the rat brain shows the location of the ventromedial nucleus of the hypothalamus.

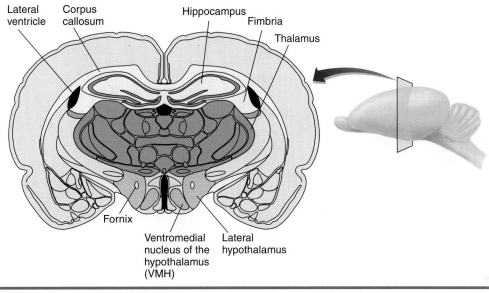

Adapted from Swanson, L. W. *Brain Maps: Structure of the Rat Brain.* New York: Elsevier, 1992.

Daniels, Miselis, and Flanagan-Cato (1999) injected a transneuronal retrograde tracer, pseudorabies virus, in the muscles responsible for the lordosis response in female rats. They found that the pathway innervating these muscles was as previous studies predicted: VMH→PAG→nPGi→motor neurons in the ventral horn of the lumbar region of the spinal cord.

Figure 9.14 summarizes the evidence I have presented so far in this section. (See *Figure 9.14.*)

A functional imaging study by Holstege et al. (2003a) investigated the neural activation that accompanies orgasm in women, elicited by manual clitoral stimulation supplied by the women's male partners. They observed activation in the junction between the midbrain and diencephalon, the lateral putamen, and the cerebellum, just as they observed in men (Holstege et al., 2003b). They also saw activation in the PAG—a critical region for copulatory behavior in female laboratory animals.

Formation of Pair Bonds

In approximately 5 percent of mammalian species, heterosexual couples form monogamous, long-lasting bonds. In humans, such bonds can be formed between members of homosexual couples as well. As naturalists and anthropologists have pointed out, monogamy is not always exclusive: In many species of animals, humans included, individuals sometimes cheat on their partners. In addition, some people display serial monogamy—intense relationships that last for a period of time, only to be replaced with similarly intense relationships with new partners. However, there is no doubt that pair bonding occurs in some species, including our own.

Several laboratories have investigated pair bonding in some closely related species of voles (small rodents that are often mistaken for mice). Prairie voles (*Microtus ochrogaster*) are monogamous; males and females form pair bonds after mating, and the fathers help to care for the pups. In the wild, most prairie voles whose mates die never take another partner (Getz and Carter, 1996). Meadow voles

FIGURE 9.14

Female Sexual Behavior.   This schematic diagram shows a possible explanation of the interacting excitatory effects of pheromones, genital stimulation, and estradiol and progesterone on female sexual behavior.

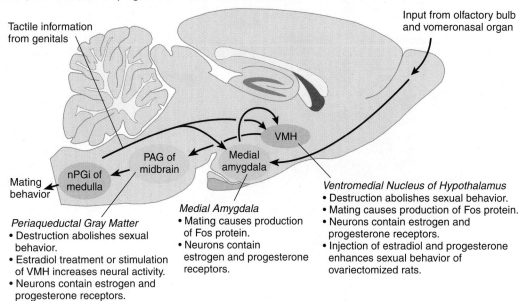

(*Microtus pennsylvanicus*) are promiscuous; after mating, the male leaves, and the mother cares for the pups by herself.

Several studies have revealed a relation between monogamy and the levels of two peptides in the brain: vasopressin and oxytocin. These compounds are both released as hormones by the posterior pituitary gland and as neurotransmitters by neurons in the brain. In males, vasopressin appears to play the more important role. Monogamous voles have a higher level of vasopressin receptors in the ventral forebrain than do polygamous voles (Insel, Wang, and Ferris, 1994). This difference appears to be responsible for the presence or absence of monogamy. Lim and Young (2004) found that mating induced the production of Fos protein in the ventral forebrain of male prairie voles, and that an injection into this region of a drug that blocks vasopressin receptors disrupted the formation of pair bonds. In female voles, oxytocin appears to play a major role in pair bonding. Mating stimulates the release of oxytocin, and injection of oxytocin into the cerebral ventricles facilitates pair bonding in female prairie voles (Williams et al., 1994). In contrast, a drug that blocks oxytocin receptors disrupts formation of pair bonds (Cho et al., 1999).

Many investigators believe that oxytocin and vasopressin may play a role in the formation of pair bonding in humans. For example, after intercourse, at a time when blood levels of oxytocin are increased, people report feelings of calmness and well-being, which are certainly compatible with the formation of bonds with one's partner. However, it is difficult to envision ways to perform definitive research on this topic. Experimenters can study the effects of these hormones or their antagonists on pair bonding in laboratory animals, but they certainly cannot do so with humans. Studies *have* found that oxytocin affects human social behaviors less momentous than pair bonding. For example, Rimmele et al. (2009) found that people who received an intranasal spray of oxytocin before looking at photos of faces were more likely to remember these faces later. The hormone had no effect on memory of photos of nonsocial stimuli such as houses, sculptures, or landscapes.

InterimSummary

Neural Control of Sexual Behavior

In laboratory animals, different brain mechanisms control male and female sexual behavior. The medial preoptic area is the forebrain region that is most critical for male sexual behavior. Stimulating this area produces copulatory behavior; destroying it permanently abolishes the behavior. The sexually dimorphic nucleus, located in the medial preoptic area, develops only if an animal is exposed to androgens early in life. A sexually dimorphic nucleus is found in humans as well. Destruction of the SDN (part of the MPA) in laboratory animals impairs mating behavior.

Neurons in the MPA contain androgen receptors. Copulatory activity causes an increase in the activity of neurons in this region. Implantation of testosterone directly into the MPA reinstates copulatory behavior that was previously abolished by castration in adulthood. Neurons in the MPA are part of a circuit that includes the periaqueductal gray matter, the nucleus paragigantocellularis of the medulla, and motor neurons controlling genital reflexes in the spinal cord. Connections of the nPGi with the spinal cord are inhibitory. Ejaculation in men is accompanied by increased behavior in the brain's reinforcement mechanisms, several thalamic nuclei, the lateral putamen, and the cerebellum. Activity of the amygdala decreases.

The most important forebrain region for female sexual behavior is the ventromedial nucleus of the hypothalamus (VMH). Its destruction abolishes copulatory behavior, and its stimulation facilitates this behavior. Both estradiol and progesterone exert their facilitating effects on female sexual behavior in this region, and studies have confirmed the existence of progesterone and estrogen receptors there. The priming effect of estradiol is caused by an increase in progesterone receptors in the VMH. Neurons that contain these receptors send axons to the periaqueductal gray matter (PAG) of the midbrain; these neurons, through their connections with the medullary reticular formation, control the particular responses that constitute female sexual behavior. Orgasm in women is accompanied by increased activity in regions similar to those activated during ejaculation in men, and in addition, in the periaqueductal gray matter.

Vasopressin and oxytocin, peptides that serve as hormones and as neurotransmitters in the brain, appear to facilitate pair bonding. Vasopressin plays the most important role in males, and oxytocin plays the most important role in females.

Parental Behavior

In most mammalian species, reproductive behavior takes place after the offspring are born as well as at the time they are conceived. This section examines the role of hormones in the initiation and maintenance of maternal behavior and the role of the neural circuits that are responsible for their expression. Most of the research has involved rodents; less is known about the neural and endocrine bases of maternal behavior in primates.

Although most research on the physiology of parental behavior has focused on maternal behavior, some researchers are now studying paternal behavior shown by the males of some species of rodents. It goes without saying that the human paternal behavior is very important for the offspring of our species, but the physiological basis of this behavior has not yet been studied.

Maternal Behavior of Rodents

The final test of the fitness of an animal's genes is the number of offspring that survive to a reproductive age. Just as the process of natural selection favors reproductively competent animals, it favors those that care adequately for their young, if their young in fact require care. Rat and mouse pups certainly do; they cannot survive without a mother to attend to their needs.

At the time of **parturition** (delivery of offspring), the female begins to groom and lick the area around her vagina. As a pup begins to emerge, she assists the uterine contractions by pulling the pup out with her teeth. She then eats the placenta and umbilical cord and cleans off the fetal membranes—a quite delicate operation.

parturition (*par tew ri shun*) The act of giving birth.

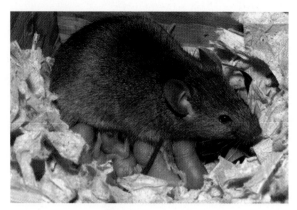

A mother mouse nurses her young pups.

(A newborn pup looks as though it is sealed in very thin plastic wrap.) After all the pups are born and cleaned up, the mother will probably nurse them. Milk is usually present in the mammary glands very near the time of birth.

Periodically, the mother licks the pups' anogenital region, stimulating reflexive urination and defecation. Friedman and Bruno (1976) have shown the utility of this mechanism. They noted that a lactating female rat produces approximately 48 grams (g) of milk on the tenth day of lactation. This milk contains approximately 35 milliliters (ml) of water. The experimenters injected some of the pups with tritiated (radioactive) water and later found radioactivity in the mother and in the littermates. They calculated that a lactating rat normally consumes 21 ml of water in the urine of her young, thus recycling approximately two-thirds of the water she gives to the pups in the form of milk. The water, traded back and forth between mother and young, serves as a vehicle for the nutrients—fats, protein, and sugar—contained in milk. Because each day the milk production of a lactating rat is approximately 14 percent of her body weight (for a human weighing 120 pounds, that would be around 2 gallons), the recycling is extremely useful, especially when the availability of water is a problem.

Hormonal Control of Maternal Behavior

As we saw earlier in this chapter, most sexually dimorphic behaviors are controlled by the organizational and activational effects of sex hormones. Maternal behavior is somewhat different in this respect. First, there is no evidence that organizational effects of hormones play a role; as we will see, under the proper conditions even males will take care of infants. (Obviously, males cannot provide infants with milk.) Second, although maternal behavior is affected by hormones, it is not *controlled* by them. Most virgin female rats will begin to retrieve and care for young pups after having infants placed with them for several days (Wiesner and Sheard, 1933). And once the rats are sensitized, they will thereafter take care of pups as soon as they encounter them; sensitization lasts for a lifetime.

Although pregnant female rats will not immediately care for foster pups that are given to them during pregnancy, they will do so as soon as their own pups are born. The hormones that influence a female rodent's responsiveness to her offspring are the ones that are present shortly before parturition. Figure 9.15 shows the levels of the three hormones that have been implicated in maternal behavior: progesterone, estradiol, and prolactin. Note that just before parturition the level of estradiol begins rising, then the level of progesterone falls dramatically, followed by a sharp increase in prolactin, the hormone produced by the anterior pituitary gland that is responsible for milk production. (See **Figure 9.15**.) If ovariectomized virgin female rats are given progesterone, estradiol, and prolactin in a pattern that duplicates this sequence, the time it takes to sensitize their maternal behavior is drastically reduced (Bridges et al., 1985).

FIGURE 9.15

Hormones in Pregnant Rats.   The graph shows blood levels of progesterone, estradiol, and prolactin in pregnant rats.

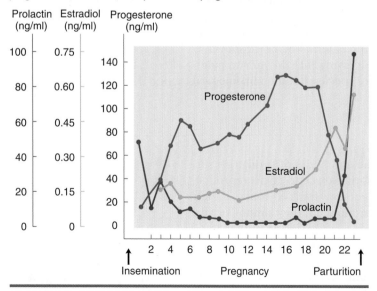

Adapted from Rosenblatt, J. S., Siegel, H. I., and Mayer, A. D. *Advances in the Study of Behavior,* 1979, *10,* 225–310.

As we saw in the previous section, pair bonding involves vasopressin and oxytocin. In at least some species, oxytocin also appears to be involved in formation of a bond between mother and offspring. In rats, the administration of oxytocin facilitates the establishment of maternal behavior (Insel, 1997). Van Leengoed, Kerker, and Swanson (1987) injected an oxytocin antagonist into the cerebral ventricles of rats as soon as they began giving birth. The experimenters removed the pups from the cage as soon as they were born. When the pups were given back to the mothers 40 minutes later, their mothers ignored them. Control rats given a placebo began caring for their pups as soon as the pups were returned to them.

Neural Control of Maternal Behavior

The medial preoptic area, the region of the forebrain that plays the most critical role in male sexual behavior, appears to play a similar role in maternal behavior. Numan (1974) found that lesions of the MPA disrupted both nest building and pup care. The mothers simply ignored their offspring. However, female sexual behavior was unaffected by these lesions. Del Cerro et al. (1995) found that the metabolic activity of the MPA, measured by 2-DG autoradiography increased immediately after parturition. They also found that virgin females whose maternal behavior had been sensitized by exposure to pups showed increased activity in the MPA. Thus, stimuli that facilitate pup care activate the MPA.

Numan and Numan (1997) found that neurons of the MPA that were activated by the performance of maternal behavior (as indicated by the production of Fos protein) sent their axons to two regions of the midbrain: the ventral tegmental area (VTA) and the retrorubral field. The retrorubral field of the midbrain sends axons to regions of the brain stem reticular formation that may be involved in the expression of maternal behavior. Cutting the connections of the MPA with the brain stem abolishes maternal behavior (Numan and Smith, 1984).

An fMRI study with rats (yes, they really put their little heads in a special fMRI scanner) found that regions of the brain are involved in reinforcement when the mothers are presented with their pups (Ferris et al., 2005). The same regions are activated by artificial reinforcers such as cocaine. However, cocaine activates this region only in virgin females; lactating females actually showed a reduction when their received injections of the drug. To a lactating female the presence of pups becomes extremely reinforcing, and the potency of other stimuli, which might distract her from providing maternal care, appears to become weaker. Perhaps, say the authors, oxytocin plays a role in this phenomenon.

An fMRI study—this time with humans—found that when mothers looked at pictures of their infants, brain regions involved in reinforcement and those that contain receptors for oxytocin and vasopressin showed increased activity. Regions involved with negative emotions, such as the amygdala, showed decreased activity (Bartels and Zeki, 2004). We already know that mothers (and fathers too, for that matter) form intense bonds with their infants, so it should not come as a surprise that regions involved with reinforcement should be activated by the sight of their faces.

Neural Control of Paternal Behavior

Newborn infants of most species of mammals are cared for by their mother, and it is, of course, their mother that feeds them. However, males of a few species of rodents share the task of infant care with the mothers, and the brains of these nurturing fathers show some interesting differences compared with those of nonpaternal fathers of other species.

You will recall that monogamous prairie voles form pair bonds with their mates and help to care for their offspring, while polygamous meadow voles leave the female after mating. As we saw, the release of vasopressin, elicited by mating, facilitates this process. The size of the MPA, which plays an essential role in maternal behavior, shows less sexual dimorphism in monogamous voles than in promiscuous voles (Shapiro et al., 1991).

Kirkpatrick, Kim, and Insel (1994) found that when male prairie voles were exposed to a pup, Fos production increased in the MPA (and also several other regions of the forebrain). In addition, lesions of the MPA produce severe deficits in paternal behavior of male rats and another species of monogamous voles (Rosenblatt, Hazelwood, and Poole, 1996; Sturgis and Bridges, 1997; Lee and Brown, 2007). Thus, the MPA appears to play a similar roles in parental behavior of both males and females.

Interim Summary

Parental Behavior

Many species must care for their offspring. Among most rodents this duty falls to the mother, which must build a nest, deliver her own pups, clean them, keep them warm, nurse them, and retrieve them if they are moved out of the nest. The mother must even induce her pups' urination and defecation, and the mother's ingestion of the urine recycles water, which is often a scarce commodity.

Exposure of virgin females to young pups stimulates maternal behavior within a few days. The stimuli that normally induce maternal behavior are those produced by the act of parturition and the hormones present around the end of pregnancy. Injections of progesterone, estradiol, and prolactin that duplicate the sequence that occurs during pregnancy facilitate maternal behavior. The hormones appear to act in the medial preoptic area (MPA). Oxytocin, which facilitates the formation of pair bonds in female rodents, is also involved in formation of a bond between mother and her pups.

An fMRI study with rats showed activation of brain mechanisms of reinforcement when the mothers were presented with their pups.

Women who look at pictures of their infants show increased activity in similar brain regions.

Paternal behavior is relatively rare in mammalian species, but research indicates that sexual dimorphism of the MPA is less pronounced in male voles of monogamous, but not promiscuous, species. Lesions of the MPA abolish paternal behavior of male rats.

Thought Questions

As you saw, both male sexual behavior and maternal behavior are disrupted by lesions of the medial preoptic area; thus, the MPA performs some functions necessary for both behaviors. Do you think that the functions are common to both categories of behavior, or do you think that different functions are involved? If you think the former possibility is true, what might these functions be? Can you think of any common features of male sexual behavior and maternal behavior?

⋮ EPILOGUE   From Boy to Girl and Back Again

Unfortunately, the case of Bruce/Brenda was not what it seemed to be (Diamond and Sigmundson, 1997). It turned out that although Brenda did not know she had been born as a boy, she was unhappy as a girl. As her twin brother said, "I recognized Brenda as my sister, [b]ut she never, ever acted the part. . . . When I say there was nothing feminine about Brenda, . . . I mean there was *nothing* feminine. She walked like a guy. Sat with her legs apart. She talked about guy things, didn't give a crap about cleaning house, getting married, wearing makeup. . . . She played with *my* toys: Tinkertoys, dump trucks. This toy sewing machine she got just sat" (Colapinto, 2000, p. 57).

Brenda's childhood was lonely and miserable. She had no real friends. She was teased by her classmates, who recognized that there was something different about her. Brenda tried, unsuccess-

fully, to convince the girls in her class to play games that boys played. One of her classmates asked the teacher, "How come Brenda stands *up* when she goes to the bathroom?" (Colapinto, 2000, p. 61) When Brenda was 7 years old, she daydreamed of herself as a man with a mustache, driving a sports car, yet, reports of her case described "the identical twin boy whose penis was cauterized at birth and who, now that his parents have opted for surgical reconstruction to make him appear female, has been sailing contentedly through childhood as a genuine girl" (Wolfe, 1975, quoted by Colapinto, 2000, p. 107).

In the summer of 1977 Brenda began taking estrogen pills to stimulate the changes that normally occur at puberty. The hormone caused her breasts to grow, which mortified her. She began to overeat so that her breasts would be hidden by fat; in fact, her

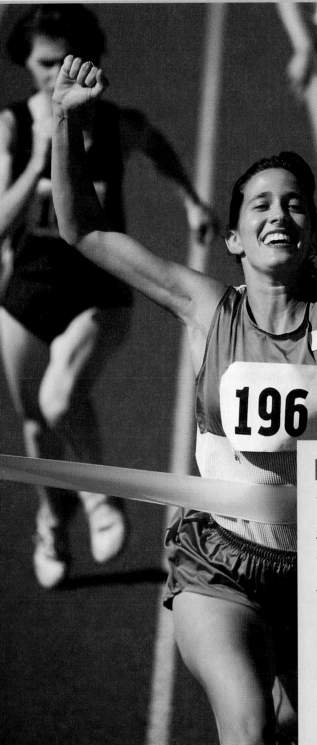

chapter 10 : ● Emotion

LEARNING OBJECTIVES

1. Discuss the behavioral, autonomic, and hormonal components of an emotional response and the role of the amygdala in controlling them.

2. Discuss the nature, functions, and neural control of aggressive behavior.

3. Discuss the role of the ventromedial prefrontal cortex in anger, aggression, and impulse control.

4. Discuss cross-cultural studies on the expression and comprehension of emotions.

5. Discuss the neural control of the recognition of emotional expression.

6. Discuss the neural control of emotional expression.

7. Discuss the James-Lange theory of feelings of emotion and evaluate relevant research.

PROLOGUE   Intellect and Emotion

Several years ago, while I was on a sabbatical leave, a colleague stopped by my office and asked whether I would like to see an interesting patient. The patient, a 72-year-old man, had suffered a massive stroke in his right hemisphere that had paralyzed the left side of his body.

Mr. V. was seated in a wheelchair equipped with a large tray on which his right arm was resting; his left arm was immobilized in a sling, to keep it out of the way. He greeted us politely, almost formally, articulating his words carefully with a slight Central European accent.

Mr. V. seemed intelligent, and this impression was confirmed when we gave him some of the subtests of the Wechsler Adult Intelligence Test. His verbal intelligence appeared to be in the upper 5 percent of the population. The fact that English was not his native language made his performance even more remarkable.

The most interesting aspect of Mr. V.'s behavior after his stroke was his lack of reaction to his symptoms. After we had finished with the testing, we asked him to tell us a little about himself and his lifestyle. What, for example, was his favorite pastime?

"I like to walk," he said. "I walk at least 2 hours each day around the city, but mostly I like to walk in the woods. I have maps of most of the national forests in the state on the walls of my study, and I mark all of the trails I've taken. I figure that in about 6 months I will have walked all of the trails that are short enough to do in a day."

"You're going to finish up those trails in the next 6 months?" asked Dr. W.

"Yes, and then I'll start over again!" he replied.

"Mr. V., are you having any trouble?" asked Dr. W.

"Trouble? What do you mean?"

"I mean physical difficulty."

"No." Mr. V. gave him a slightly puzzled look.

"Well, what are you sitting in?"

Mr. V. gave him a look that indicated he thought that the question was rather stupid–or perhaps insulting. "A wheelchair, of course," he answered.

"Why are you in a wheelchair?"

Now Mr. V. looked frankly exasperated; he obviously did not like to answer foolish questions. "Because my left leg is paralyzed!" he snapped.

Mr. V. clearly knew what his problem was, but he failed to understand its implications. He could verbally describe his disability, but he was unable to grasp its significance. Thus, he blandly accepted the fact that he was confined to a wheelchair. The implications of his disability did not affect him emotionally or figure into his plans.

The word *emotion* can mean several things. Most of the time, it refers to positive or negative feelings that are produced by particular situations. For example, being treated unfairly makes us angry, seeing someone suffer makes us sad, and being close to a loved one makes us feel happy. Emotions consist of patterns of physiological responses and species-typical behaviors. In humans these responses are accompanied by feelings. In fact, most of us use the word *emotion* to refer to the feelings, not to the behaviors. But it is behavior, and not private experience, that has consequences for survival and reproduction. Thus, the useful functions served by emotional behaviors are what guided the evolution of our brain. The feelings that accompany these behaviors came rather late in the game.

This chapter is divided into three major sections. The first considers the patterns of behavioral and physiological responses that constitute the negative emotions of fear and anger. It describes the nature of these response patterns, their neural and hormonal control, and the role of emotions in moral judgments and social behavior. The second section describes the communication of emotions—their expression and recognition. The third section examines the nature of the feelings that accompany emotions.

Emotions as Response Patterns

An emotional response consists of three types of components: behavioral, autonomic, and hormonal. The *behavioral* component consists of muscular movements that are appropriate to the situation that elicits them. For example, a dog defending its territory against an intruder first threatens the intruder by adopting an aggressive posture, growling, and showing its teeth. If the intruder does not leave, the defender runs toward the intruder and attacks. *Autonomic* responses facilitate the behaviors and provide quick mobilization of energy for vigorous movement. In this example the activity of the sympathetic branch of the autonomic nervous system increases while that of the parasympathetic branch decreases. As a consequence the dog's heart rate increases, and changes in the size of blood vessels shunt the circulation of blood away from the digestive organs toward the muscles. *Hormonal* responses reinforce the autonomic responses. The hormones secreted by the adrenal medulla—epinephrine and norepinephrine—further increase blood flow to the muscles and cause nutrients stored in the muscles to be converted into glucose. In addition, the adrenal cortex secretes steroid hormones, which also help to make glucose available to the muscles.

This section discusses research on the control of overt emotional behaviors and the autonomic and hormonal responses that accompany them. Special behaviors that serve to communicate emotional states to other animals, such as the threat gestures that precede an actual attack and the smiles and frowns used by humans, are discussed in the second section of the chapter. As you will see, negative emotions receive much more attention than positive ones. Most of the research on the physiology of emotions has been confined to fear and anger—emotions associated with situations in which we must defend ourselves or our loved ones. The physiology of behaviors associated with positive emotions—such as those associated with lovemaking, caring for one's offspring, or enjoying a good meal or a cool drink of water (or some other beverage)—is described in other chapters but not in the specific context of emotions. Chapter 16 discusses the consequences of situations that evoke negative emotions: stress.

Fear

As we just saw, emotional responses involve behavioral, autonomic, and hormonal components. These components are controlled by separate neural systems. The *integration* of the components of fear appears to be controlled by the amygdala.

Research with Laboratory Animals

The amygdala plays a special role in physiological and behavioral reactions to objects and situations that have biological significance, including those that warn of pain or other unpleasant consequences. Researchers in several different laboratories have shown that single neurons in various nuclei of the amygdala become active when emotionally relevant stimuli are presented. For example, these neurons are excited by such stimuli as the sight of a device that has been used to squirt either a bad-tasting solution or a sweet solution into the animal's mouth, the sound of another animal's vocalization, the sound of the opening of the laboratory door, the smell of smoke, or the sight of another animal's face (O'Keefe and Bouma, 1969; Jacobs and McGinty, 1972; Rolls, 1982; Leonard et al., 1985). As we saw in Chapter 9, the amygdala is involved in the effects of olfactory stimuli on reproductive physiology and behavior. This section describes research on the role of the amygdala in organizing emotional responses produced by aversive stimuli.

The amygdala (or more precisely, the *amygdaloid complex*) is located within the temporal lobes. It consists of several groups of nuclei, each with different inputs and outputs—and with different functions (Amaral et al., 1992; Pitkänen, Savander, and LeDoux, 1997; Stefanacci and Amaral, 2000). The amygdala has been subdivided into approximately twelve regions, each containing several subregions. However, we need concern ourselves with just three major regions: the *lateral nucleus*, the *basal nucleus*, and the *central nucleus*.

FIGURE 10.1

The Amygdala.   This much-simplified diagram of the major divisions and connections of the amygdala that play a role in emotions.

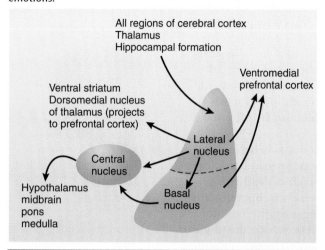

All regions of cerebral cortex
Thalamus
Hippocampal formation

Ventromedial prefrontal cortex

Ventral striatum
Dorsomedial nucleus of thalamus (projects to prefrontal cortex)

Lateral nucleus

Central nucleus

Hypothalamus midbrain pons medulla

Basal nucleus

lateral nucleus (LA) A nucleus of the amygdala that receives sensory information from the neocortex, thalamus, and hippocampus and sends projections to the basal, accessory basal, and central nucleus of the amygdala.

central nucleus (CE) The region of the amygdala that receives information from the basal, lateral, and accessory basal nuclei and sends projections to a wide variety of regions in the brain; involved in emotional responses.

conditioned emotional response A classically conditioned response that occurs when a neutral stimulus is followed by an aversive stimulus; usually includes autonomic, behavioral, and endocrine components such as changes in heart rate, freezing, and secretion of stress-related hormones.

The **lateral nucleus (LA)** receives information from all regions of the neocortex, including the ventromedial prefrontal cortex, thalamus, and hippocampal formation. The lateral nucleus sends information to the basal nucleus (B) and to other parts of the brain, including the ventral striatum (a region involved in the effects of reinforcing stimuli on learning) and the dorsomedial nucleus of the thalamus, whose projection region is the prefrontal cortex. The LA and B nuclei send information to the ventromedial prefrontal cortex and the **central nucleus (CE)**, which projects to regions of the hypothalamus, midbrain, pons, and medulla that are responsible for the expression of the various components of emotional responses. As we will see, activation of the central nucleus elicits a variety of emotional responses: behavioral, autonomic, and hormonal. (See *Figure 10.1*.)

The central nucleus of the amygdala is the single most important part of the brain for the expression of emotional responses provoked by aversive stimuli. When threatening stimuli are perceived, increases are seen in the neural activity of the central nucleus and the production of Fos protein there (Pascoe and Kapp, 1985; Campeau et al., 1991). Damage to the central nucleus (or to the nuclei that provide it with sensory information) reduces or abolishes a wide range of emotional behaviors and physiological responses. After the central nucleus has been destroyed, animals no longer show signs of fear when confronted with stimuli that have been paired with aversive events. They also act more tamely when handled by humans, their blood levels of stress hormones are lower, and they are less likely to develop ulcers or other forms of stress-induced illnesses (Coover, Murison, and Jellestad, 1992; Davis, 1992; LeDoux, 1992). Normal monkeys show signs of fear when they see a snake, but those with amygdala lesions do not (Amaral, 2003). In contrast, when the central amygdala is stimulated by means of electricity or by an injection of an excitatory amino acid, the animal shows physiological and behavioral signs of fear and agitation (Davis, 1992), and long-term stimulation of the central nucleus produces stress-induced illnesses such as gastric ulcers (Henke, 1982). These observations suggest that the autonomic and endocrine responses controlled by the central nucleus are among those responsible for the harmful effects of long-term stress, which are discussed in Chapter 16. Rather than describing the regions to which the amygdala projects and the responses these regions control, refer to Figure 10.2, which summarizes them. (See *Figure 10.2*.)

A few stimuli automatically activate the central nucleus of the amygdala and produce fear reactions—for example, loud unexpected noises, the approach of large animals, heights, or (for some species) specific sounds or odors. Even more important, however, is the ability to *learn* that a particular stimulus or situation is dangerous or threatening. Once the learning has taken place, that stimulus or situation will evoke fear; heart rate and blood pressure will increase, the muscles will become more tense, the adrenal glands will secrete epinephrine, and the animal will proceed cautiously, alert and ready to respond.

The most basic form of emotional learning is a **conditioned emotional response**, which is produced by a neutral stimulus that has been paired with an emotion-producing stimulus. The word *conditioned* refers to the process of *classical conditioning*, which is described in greater detail in Chapter 12. Briefly, classical conditioning occurs when a neutral stimulus is regularly followed by a stimulus that automatically evokes a response. For example, if a dog regularly hears a bell ring just before it receives some food that makes it salivate, the dog will begin salivating as soon as it hears the sound of the bell. (You probably already know that this phenomenon was discovered by Ivan Pavlov.)

Several laboratories have investigated the role of the amygdala in the development of classically conditioned emotional responses. For example, LeDoux and his colleagues have studied these responses in rats by pairing an auditory stimulus with a brief electrical shock delivered to the feet (reviewed by LeDoux, 2000). In their studies they presented an 800-Hz tone for 10 seconds, and then they delivered a brief (0.5-second) shock to the floor on which the animals were standing. (See *Figure 10.3*.) By itself the shock produces an *unconditional* emotional response: The animal jumps into the air, its heart rate and blood pressure increase, its breathing becomes more rapid, and its adrenal glands secrete catecholamines and steroid stress hormones. The experimenters presented several pairings of the two stimuli, which established classical conditioning.

The investigators tested conditioned emotional responses the next day by presenting the 800-Hz tone several times and measuring the animals' blood pressure and heart rate and observing their behavior. (This time, they did not present the shock.) Upon hearing the tone, the rats showed the same type of physiological responses as they had when they were shocked the previous day. In addition, they showed behavioral arrest—a species-typical defensive response called *freezing*. That is, the animals acted as if they were expecting to receive a shock.

Research indicates that the physical changes responsible for classical conditioning take place in the lateral nucleus of the amygdala (Paré, Quirk, and LeDoux, 2004). Neurons in the lateral nucleus communicate with neurons in the central nucleus, which in turn communicate with regions in the hypothalamus, midbrain, pons, and medulla that are responsible for the behavioral, autonomic, and hormonal components of a conditioned emotional response. Research on the details of the physical changes responsible for classical conditioning has provided some interesting information about the physiology of learning and memory. This research is discussed in greater detail in Chapter 12.

The amygdala appeared early in the evolution of the brain and is involved in responses vital to survival. However, under some conditions, emotional responses are inappropriate. As we will see later in this chapter, the **ventromedial prefrontal cortex (vmPFC)** plays an important role in controlling the expression of emotional responses. For example, the vmPFC is involved in the process of *extinction*. As we saw, when a neutral stimulus such as a tone is paired with an aversive stimulus such as a painful electrical shock, the tone begins to elicit the emotional response. That is, the tone becomes a *conditional stimulus (CS)* that elicits a *conditional response (CR).* However, if the CS (tone) is then presented repeatedly by itself, the CR (emotional response) eventually disappears—it becomes *extinguished*. After all, the value of a conditioned emotional response is that it prepares an animal to confront (or perhaps even avoid) an aversive stimulus. If the CS occurs repeatedly but the aversive

FIGURE 10.2

Amygdala Connections.   This schematic diagram shows some important brain regions that receive input from the central nucleus of the amygdala and the emotional responses controlled by these regions.

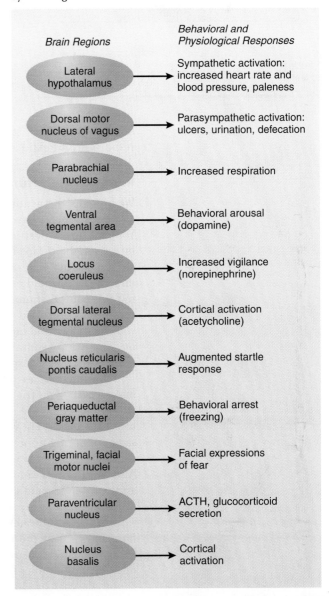

Brain Regions	Behavioral and Physiological Responses
Lateral hypothalamus	Sympathetic activation: increased heart rate and blood pressure, paleness
Dorsal motor nucleus of vagus	Parasympathetic activation: ulcers, urination, defecation
Parabrachial nucleus	Increased respiration
Ventral tegmental area	Behavioral arousal (dopamine)
Locus coeruleus	Increased vigilance (norepinephrine)
Dorsal lateral tegmental nucleus	Cortical activation (acetycholine)
Nucleus reticularis pontis caudalis	Augmented startle response
Periaqueductal gray matter	Behavioral arrest (freezing)
Trigeminal, facial motor nuclei	Facial expressions of fear
Paraventricular nucleus	ACTH, glucocorticoid secretion
Nucleus basalis	Cortical activation

Adapted from Davis, M., *Trends in Pharmacological Sciences*, 1992, *13*, 35–41.

ventromedial prefrontal cortex (vmPFC) The region of the prefrontal cortex at the base of the anterior frontal lobes, adjacent to the midline; plays an inhibitory role in the expression of emotions.

FIGURE 10.3

Conditioned Emotional Responses.   The diagram shows the procedure used to produce conditioned emotional responses.

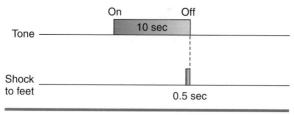

stimulus does not follow, then it is better for the emotional response—which itself is disruptive and unpleasant—to disappear.

Behavioral studies have shown that extinction is not the same as forgetting. Instead, the animal learns that the CS is no longer followed by an aversive stimulus, and as a result of this learning the expression of the CR is inhibited; the memory for the association between the CS and the aversive stimulus is not erased (Pavlov, 1927; Bouton and King, 1983; Quirk, 2002). This inhibition is supplied by the ventromedial prefrontal cortex. Evidence for this conclusion comes from several studies (Quirk, Garcia, and González-Lima, 2006). For example, lesions of the ventromedial prefrontal cortex impair extinction, stimulation of this region inhibits conditioned emotional responses, and extinction training activates neurons there.

Research with Humans

We humans also acquire conditioned emotional responses. Let's examine a specific (if somewhat contrived) example. Suppose you are helping a friend prepare a meal. You pick up an electric mixer to mix some batter for a cake. Before you can turn the mixer on, the device makes a sputtering noise and then gives you a painful electrical shock. Your first response would be a defensive reflex: You would let go of the mixer, which would end the shock. This response is *specific*; it is aimed at terminating the painful stimulus. In addition, the painful stimulus would elicit *nonspecific* responses controlled by your autonomic nervous system: Your eyes would dilate, your heart rate and blood pressure would increase, you would breathe faster, and so on. The painful stimulus would also trigger the secretion of some stress-related hormones, another nonspecific response.

Suppose that a while later you visit your friend again and once more agree to make a cake. Your friend tells you that the electric mixer is perfectly safe. It has been fixed. Just seeing the mixer and thinking of holding it again makes you a little nervous, but you accept your friend's assurance and pick it up. Just then, it makes the same sputtering noise that it did when it shocked you. What would your response be? Almost certainly, you would drop the mixer again, even if it did not give you a shock. Also, your pupils would dilate, your heart rate and blood pressure would increase, and your endocrine glands would secrete some stress-related hormones. In other words, the sputtering sound would trigger a conditioned emotional response.

Evidence indicates that the amygdala is involved in emotional responses in humans. One of the earliest studies observed the reactions of people who were being evaluated for surgical removal of parts of the brain to treat severe seizure disorders. These studies found that stimulation of parts of the brain (for example, the hypothalamus) produced autonomic responses that are often associated with fear and anxiety but that only when the amygdala was stimulated did people also report that they actually *felt* afraid (White, 1940; Halgren et al., 1978; Gloor et al., 1982).

Many studies have shown that lesions of the amygdala decrease people's emotional responses. For example, Bechara et al. (1995) and LaBar et al. (1995) found that people with lesions of the amygdala showed impaired acquisition of a conditioned emotional response, just as rats do.

Most human fears are probably acquired socially, not through first-hand experience with painful stimuli. For example, a child does not have to be attacked by a dog to develop a fear of dogs: He or she can do so by watching another person being attacked or (more often) see another person display signs of fear when encountering a dog. People can also acquire a conditioned fear response through instruction. A functional imaging study by Phelps et al. (2001) attached electrodes to subjects' wrists, and told them that they were going to watch blue and yellow squares that

FIGURE 10.4

Control of Extinction.   The graphs show that activation of the amygdala is related to the acquisition of a conditioned emotional response and that activation of the medial prefrontal cortex is related to the extinction of this response.

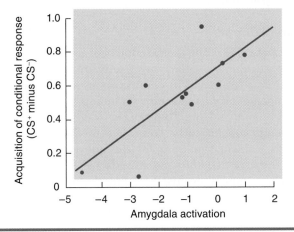
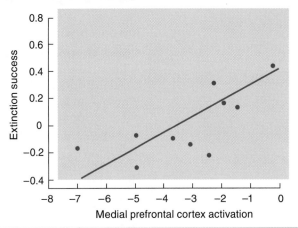

Data from a functional-imaging study by Phelps, E. A., Delgado, M. R., Nearing, K. U., and LeDoux, J. E. *Neuron*, 2004, *43*, 897–905.

would appear, one at a time, on a computer screen. One of the colors was the danger signal, warning that they would receive a shock, and the other was the safety signal. (The subjects did not actually receive a shock.) The instructions given by the experimenters was sufficient to evoke a fear response—and increased activation of the amygdala—when the danger signal appeared.

We saw that studies with laboratory animals indicate that the medial prefrontal cortex plays a critical role in extinction of a conditioned emotional response. The same is true for humans. Phelps et al. (2004) directly established a conditioned emotional response in human subjects (the blue/yellow square procedure) by administering actual shocks to the wrist, and then extinguished the response by presenting the squares alone, without any shocks. As Figure 10.4 shows, increased activity of the amygdala correlated with acquisition of a conditioned emotional response, and increased activity of the medial prefrontal cortex correlated with extinction of the conditioned response. (See *Figure 10.4*.)

As we saw in Chapter 7, Patient I. R., a woman who had sustained damage to the auditory association cortex, was unable to perceive or produce melodic or rhythmic aspects of music (Peretz et al., 2001). She could not even tell the difference between consonant (pleasant) and dissonant (unpleasant) music. However, she was still able to recognize the mood conveyed by music. (*MyPsychLab 7.4* contains recordings of dissonant music and consonant music that varies in emotional content—happy, sad, peaceful, and scary.) Gosselin et al. (2005) found that patients with damage to the amygdala showed the opposite symptoms: They had no trouble with musical perception but were unable to recognize scary music. They could still recognize happy and sad music. Thus, amygdala lesions impair recognition of a musical style that is normally associated with fear.

Anger, Aggression, and Impulse Control

Almost all species of animals engage in aggressive behaviors, which involve threatening gestures or actual attack directed toward another animal. Aggressive behaviors are species-typical; that is, the patterns of movements (for example, posturing, biting, striking, and hissing) are organized by neural circuits whose development is largely programmed by an animal's genes. Many aggressive behaviors are related to reproduction. For example, aggressive behaviors that gain access to mates, defend territory needed to attract mates or to provide a site for building a nest, or defend offspring against intruders can all be regarded as reproductive behaviors. Other aggressive behaviors are related to self-defense, such as that of an animal threatened by a predator or an intruder of the same species.

Research with Laboratory Animals

Neural Control of Aggressive Behavior   The neural control of aggressive behavior is hierarchical. That is, the particular muscular movements an animal makes in attacking or defending itself are programmed by neural circuits in the brain stem. Whether an animal attacks depends on many factors, including the nature of the eliciting stimuli in the environment and the animal's previous experience. The activity of the brain stem circuits appears to be controlled by the hypothalamus and the amygdala, which also influence many other species-typical behaviors— and, of course, the activity of the hypothalamus and amygdala is controlled by perceptual systems that detect environmental events, including the presence of other animals.

Role of Serotonin   An overwhelming amount of evidence suggests that the activity of serotonergic synapses inhibits aggression. In contrast, destruction of serotonergic axons in the forebrain facilitates aggressive behavior, presumably by removing an inhibitory effect (Vergnes et al., 1988).

A group of researchers has studied the relationship between serotonergic activity and aggressiveness in a free-ranging colony of rhesus monkeys (reviewed by Howell et al., 2007). The researchers assessed serotonergic activity by capturing the monkeys, removing a sample of cerebrospinal fluid, and analyzing it for 5-HIAA, a metabolite of serotonin (5-HT). When 5-HT is released, most of the neurotransmitter is taken back into the terminal buttons by means of reuptake, but some escapes and is broken down to 5-HIAA, which finds its way into the cerebrospinal fluid. Thus, high levels of 5-HIAA in the CSF indicates an elevated level of serotonergic activity. The investigators found that young male monkeys with the lowest levels of 5-HIAA showed a pattern of risk-taking behavior, including high levels of aggression directed toward animals that were older and much larger than themselves. They were much more likely to take dangerous unprovoked long leaps from tree to tree at a height of more than 7 m (27.6 ft). They were also more likely to pick fights that they could not possibly win. Of the preadolescent male monkeys that the investigators followed for 4 years, a large percentage of those with the lowest 5-HIAA levels died, while all of the monkeys with the highest levels survived. (See *Figure 10.5*.) Most of the monkeys that died were killed by other monkeys. In fact, the first monkey to be killed had the lowest level of 5-HIAA and was seen attacking two mature males the night before his death. Clearly, serotonin does not simply inhibit aggression; rather, it exerts a controlling influence on risky behavior, which includes aggression.

Genetic studies with other species confirm that serotonin has an inhibitory role in aggression. For example, selective breeding of rats and silver foxes has yielded animals that display tameness and friendly responses to humans. These animals show increased brain levels of serotonin and 5-HIAA (Popova, 2006).

Research with Humans

Human violence and aggression are serious social problems. Consider the following case histories:

FIGURE 10.5

Serotonin and Risk-Taking Behavior.   The graph shows the percentage of young male monkeys alive or dead as a function of 5-HIAA level in the CSF, measured 4 years previously.

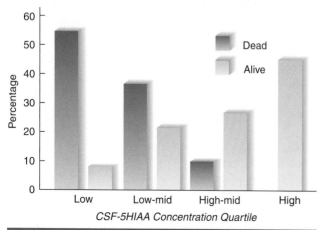

Adapted from Higley, J. D., Mehlman, P. T., Higley, S. B., Fernald, B., et al. *Archives of General Psychiatry*, 1996, 53, 537–543.

Born to an alcoholic teen mother who raised him with an abusive alcoholic stepfather, Steve was hyperactive, irritable, and disobedient as a toddler. . . . After dropping out of school at age 14, Steve spent his teen years fighting, stealing, taking drugs, and beating up girlfriends. . . . School counseling, a probation officer, and meetings with child protective service failed to forestall disaster: At 19, several weeks after his last interview with researchers, Steve visited a girlfriend who had recently dumped him, found her with another man, and shot him to death. The same day he tried to kill himself. Now he's serving a life sentence without parole. (Holden, 2000, p. 580)

By the time Joshua had reached the age of 2, . . . he would bolt out of the house and into traffic. He kicked and head-butted relatives and friends. He poked the family hamster with a pencil and tried to strangle it. He threw regular temper tantrums and would stage toy-throwing frenzies. "At one point he was hurting himself—banging his head against a wall, pinching himself, not to mention leaping off the refrigerator. . . . Showering Joshua with love . . . made little difference: By age 3, his behavior got him kicked out of his preschool. (Holden, 2000, p. 581)

Role of Serotonin   Several studies have found that serotonergic neurons play an inhibitory role in human aggression. For example, a depressed rate of serotonin release (indicated by low levels of 5-HIAA in the CSF) are associated with aggression and other forms of antisocial behavior, including assault, arson, murder, and child beating (Lidberg, Asberg, and Sundqvist-Stensman, 1984; Lidberg et al., 1985; Virkkunen et al., 1989).

If low levels of serotonin release contribute to aggression, perhaps drugs that act as serotonin agonists might help to reduce antisocial behavior. In fact, a study by Coccaro and Kavoussi (1997) found that fluoxetine (Prozac), a serotonin agonist, decreased irritability and aggressiveness, as measured by a psychological test. Joshua, the little boy described in the introduction to this subsection came under the care of a psychiatrist who prescribed monoaminergic agonists and began a course of behavior therapy that managed to stem Joshua's violent outbursts and risk-taking behaviors.

Functional imaging studies by Hariri and his colleagues (Hariri et al., 2002, 2005) found an association between differences in the genes responsible for production of serotonin transporters and the reaction of people's amygdala to the viewing of facial expressions of negative emotions. (Serotonin transporters play a role in regulating the amount of serotonin that remains in the synaptic cleft after it is released by the terminal button.) The serotonin transporter gene has two common alleles, one long and one short. People who carry at least one short allele are slightly more likely to show higher levels of anxiety or develop an affective disorder such as depression (Lesch and Mossner, 1998). Hariri and his colleagues had people perform a task that required them to look at faces expressing fear or anger. The investigators found that the right amygdala of people carrying the short form of the serotonin transporter gene showed a higher rate of activity during this task. (See ***Figure 10.6.***) Rhodes et al. (2007) used a PET scanner to measure levels of the serotonin transporter—and hence lower levels of serotonin—in the brains of human subjects. They found that people with higher levels of the transporter in the amygdala showed less activation of the amygdala when the people looked at emotional faces. A possible explanation for the influence of the alleles on the reactivity of the amygdala to emotional stimuli is described in Chapter 16.

Role of the Ventromedial Prefrontal Cortex   Many investigators believe that impulsive violence is a consequence of faulty emotional regulation. For most of us, frustrations may elicit an urge to respond emotionally, but we usually manage to calm ourselves and suppress these urges. As we shall see, the ventromedial prefrontal cortex plays an important role in

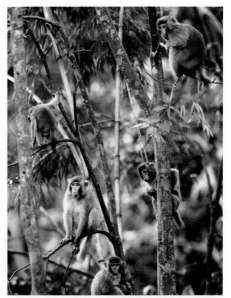

Study of free-ranging colonies of rhesus monkeys has provided important information about the role of serotonin in risk-taking behavior and aggression.

FIGURE 10.6

The Serotonin Transporter Gene and Amygdala Reactivity.   The graph shows the relative activity of the right amygdala of people with the short and long alleles of the serotonin transporter (5-HTT) gene, measured by fMRI, while the people looked at photographs of angry or fearful faces.

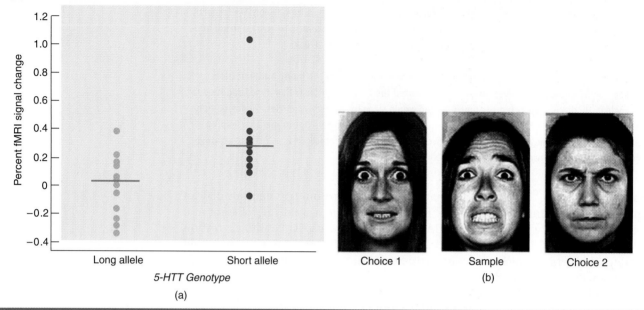

Long allele   Short allele
5-HTT Genotype
(a)

Choice 1   Sample   Choice 2
(b)

Adapted from Hariri, A. R., Mattay, V. S., Tessitore, A., Kolachana, B., et al. *Science*, 2002, *297*, 400–403.

regulating our responses to such situations. The analysis of social situations involves much more than sensory analysis; it involves experiences and memories, inferences and judgments. In fact, the skills involved include some of the most complex ones we possess. These skills are not localized in any one part of the cerebral cortex, although research does suggest that the right hemisphere is more important than the left. But the ventromedial prefrontal cortex—which includes the medial *orbitofrontal cortex* and the *subgenual anterior cingulate cortex*—plays a special role.

The ventromedial prefrontal cortex (vmPFC) is located just where its name suggests. (See *Figure 10.7.*) The vmPFC receives direct inputs from the dorsomedial thalamus, temporal cortex, ventral tegmental area, olfactory system, and amygdala. Its outputs go to several brain regions, including the cingulate cortex, hippocampal formation, temporal cortex, lateral hypothalamus, and amygdala. Finally, it communicates with other regions of the frontal cortex. Thus, its inputs provide it with information about what is happening in the environment and what plans are being made by the rest of the frontal lobes, and its outputs permit it to affect a variety of behaviors and physiological responses, including emotional responses organized by the amygdala.

The fact that the ventromedial prefrontal cortex plays an important role in control of emotional behavior is shown by the effects of damage to this region.

The first—and most famous—case comes from the mid-1800s. Phineas Gage, the foreman of a railway construction crew, was using a steel rod to ram a charge of blasting powder into a hole drilled in solid rock. Suddenly, the charge exploded and sent the rod into his cheek, through his brain, and out the top of his head. (See *Figure 10.8.*) He survived, but he was a different man. Before his injury he was serious, industrious, and energetic. Afterward, he became childish, irresponsible, and thoughtless of others. His outbursts of temper led some people to remark that it looked as if Dr. Jekyll had become Mr. Hyde. He was unable to make or carry out plans, and his actions appeared to be capricious and whimsical. His accident had largely destroyed the orbitofrontal cortex (Damasio et al., 1994).

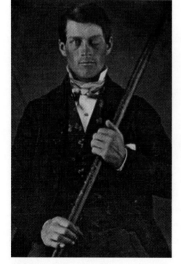

Phineas Gage

People whose ventromedial prefrontal cortex has been damaged by disease or accident are still able to accurately assess the significance of particular situations but only in a *theoretical* sense.

FIGURE 10.7

The Location of the Ventromedial Prefrontal Cortex

Eslinger and Damasio (1985) found that a patient with bilateral damage of the ventromedial prefrontal cortex (produced by a benign tumor, which was successfully removed) displayed excellent social judgment. When he was given hypothetical situations that required him to make decisions about what the people involved should do—situations involving moral, ethical, or practical dilemmas—he always gave sensible answers and justified them with carefully reasoned logic. However, his own life was a different matter. He frittered away his life's savings on investments that his family and friends pointed out were bound to fail. He lost one job after another because of his irresponsibility. He became unable to distinguish between trivial decisions and important ones, spending hours trying to decide where to have dinner but failing to use good judgment in situations that concerned his occupation and family life. (His wife finally left him and sued for divorce.) As the authors noted, "He had learned and used normal patterns of social behavior before his brain lesion, and although he could recall such patterns when he was questioned about their applicability, *real-life situations failed to evoke them*" (p. 1737). Evidence suggests that the vmPFC serves as an interface between brain mechanisms involved in automatic emotional responses (both learned and unlearned) and those involved in the control of complex behaviors. This role includes the using our emotional reactions to guide our behavior and in controlling the occurrence of emotional reactions in various social situations.

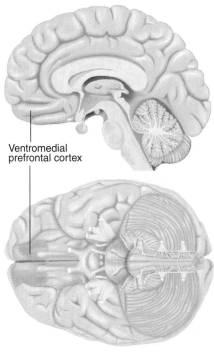

Ventromedial
prefrontal cortex

Damage to the vmPFC causes serious and often debilitating impairments of behavioral control and decision making. These impairments appear to be a consequence of emotional dysregulation. Anderson et al. (2006) obtained ratings of emotional behaviors of patients with ventromedial prefrontal lesions—such as frustration tolerance, emotional instability, anxiety, and irritability—from the patients' relatives. They also obtained ratings of the patients' real-world competencies, such as judgment, planning, social inappropriateness, and financial and occupational status, from both relatives and clinicians. They found a significant correlation between emotional dysfunction and impairments in real-world competencies. There was no relation between these impairments and the patients' cognitive abilities, which strongly suggests that emotional problems, and not problems in cognition, lie at the base of the real-world difficulties exhibited by people with vmPFC damage.

Evidence suggests that emotional reactions guide moral judgments as well as decisions involving personal risks and rewards and that the prefrontal cortex plays a role in these judgments as well. Consider the following moral dilemma (Thomson, 1986): You see a runaway trolley with five people aboard hurtling down a track leading to a cliff. Without your intervention these people will soon die. However, you are standing near a switch that will shunt the trolley off to another track, where the vehicle will stop safely. But a worker is standing on that track, and he will be killed if you throw the switch to save the five helpless passengers. Should you stand by and watch the trolley go off the cliff, or should you save them—and kill the man on the track?

Most people conclude that the better choice would be to throw the switch; saving five people justifies the sacrifice of one man. This decision is based on conscious, logical application of a rule that it is better to kill one person than five people—but consider a variation of this dilemma. As before, the trolley is hurtling toward doom, but there is no switch at hand to shunt it to another track. Instead, you are standing on a bridge over the track. An obese man is standing there too, and if you give him a push, his body will fall on the track and stop the trolley. (You are too small to stop the trolley, so you cannot save the five people by sacrificing yourself.) What should you do?

FIGURE 10.8

Phineas Gage's Accident. As shown in this image, in the accident the steel rod entered his left cheek and exited through the top of his head.

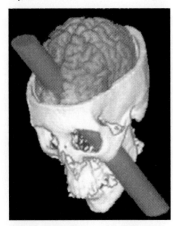

From Damasio, H., Grabowski, T., Frank, R., Galaburda, A. M., and Damasio, A. R. *Science*, 1994, *264*, 1102–1105. Copyright © 1994. Reprinted with permission from AAAS.

Most people feel repugnant at the thought of pushing the man off the bridge and balk at the idea of doing so, even though the result would be the same as the first dilemma: one person lost, five people saved. Whether we kill someone by sending a trolley his way or by pushing him off a bridge into the path of an oncoming trolley, he dies when the trolley strikes him. But somehow, imagining yourself pushing a person's body and causing his death seems more emotionally wrenching than throwing a switch that changes the course of a runaway trolley. Thus, moral judgments appear to be guided by emotional reactions and are not simply the products of rational, logical decision-making processes.

In a functional imaging study, Greene et al. (2001) presented people with the moral dilemmas such as the one just described and found that thinking about them activated several brain regions involved in emotional reactions, including the vmPFC. Making innocuous decisions, such as whether to take a bus or train to some destination, did not activate these regions. Perhaps, then, our reluctance to push someone to his death is guided by the unpleasant emotional reaction we feel when we contemplate this action.

Considering whether to throw a switch to save four lives evokes a much smaller emotional reaction than considering whether to shove someone on the tracks to accomplish the same goal. Indeed, considering the second dilemma, and not the first, strongly activates the vmPFC. Therefore, we might expect that people with vmPFC damage might be more willing to chose to push the man onto the track in the second dilemma. In fact, that is exactly what they do: They demonstrate *utilitarian* moral judgment. Koenigs et al. (2007) presented nonmoral, impersonal moral, and personal moral scenarios to patients with vmPFC lesions, patients with brain damage not including this region, and normal controls. For example, the switch-throwing scenario we just considered is an impersonal moral dilemma, and the person-pushing dilemma is a personal moral dilemma. The following examples are some of the scenarios that the investigators of the present study presented to their subjects.

Brownies (Nonmoral scenario)

You have decided to make a batch of brownies for yourself. You open your recipe book and find a recipe for brownies. The recipe calls for a cup of chopped walnuts. You don't like walnuts, but you do like macadamia nuts. As it happens, you have both kinds of nuts available to you.

Would you substitute macadamia nuts for walnuts in order to avoid eating walnuts?

Speedboat (Impersonal moral scenario)

While on vacation on a remote island, you are fishing from a seaside dock. You observe a group of tourists board a small boat and set sail for a nearby island. Soon after their departure you hear over the radio that there is a violent storm brewing, a storm that is sure to intercept them. The only way that you can ensure their safety is to warn them by borrowing a nearby speedboat. The speedboat belongs to a miserly tycoon who would not take kindly to your borrowing his property.

Would you borrow the speedboat in order to warn the tourists about the storm?

Lifeboat (Personal moral scenario)

You are on a cruise ship when there is a fire on board, and the ship has to be abandoned. The lifeboats are carrying many more people than they were designed to carry. The lifeboat you're in is sitting dangerously low in the water—a few inches lower and it will sink. The seas start to get rough, and the boat begins to fill with water. If nothing is done, it will sink before the rescue boats arrive and everyone on board will die. However, there is an injured person who will not survive in any case. If you throw that person overboard, the boat will stay afloat and the remaining passengers will be saved.

Would you throw this person overboard in order to save the lives of the remaining passengers?

Figure 10.9 shows the proportion of the subjects from each of the three groups who endorsed a decision to act in high-conflict personal moral dilemmas, such as the lifeboat scenario. As you can see, the patients with vmPFC lesions were much more likely to say "yes" to the question posed at the end of the scenarios. (See *Figure 10.9*.)

It might seem that I have been getting away from the topic of this section: anger and aggression. However, recall that many investigators believe that impulsive violence is a consequence of faulty emotional regulation. The amygdala plays an important role in provoking anger and violent emotional reactions, and the prefrontal cortex plays an important role in suppressing such behavior by making us see its negative consequences. As we saw earlier, antisocial behavior may be associated with decreased volume of the prefrontal cortex; thus, activation of the prefrontal cortex may reflect its role in inhibiting aggressive behavior. Raine et al. (1998) found evidence of decreased prefrontal activity and increased subcortical activity (including the amygdala) in the brains of convicted murderers. These changes were primarily seen in impulsive, emotional murderers. The prefrontal activity of cold-blooded, calculating, predatory murderers—whose crimes were not accompanied by anger and rage—was closer to normal. Presumably, increased activation of the amygdala reflected an increased tendency for display of negative emotions, and the decreased activation of the prefrontal cortex reflected a decreased ability to inhibit the activity of the amygdala and thus control the people's emotions. Raine et al. (2002) found that people with antisocial personality disorder showed an 11 percent reduction in volume of the gray matter of the prefrontal cortex.

Earlier in this chapter we saw that decreased activity of serotonergic neurons is associated with aggression, violence, and risk taking. As we saw in this subsection, decreased activity of the prefrontal cortex is also associated with antisocial behavior. These two facts appear to be linked. The prefrontal cortex receives a major projection of serotonergic axons. Research indicates that serotonergic input to the prefrontal cortex activates this region. A functional imaging study by New et al. (2004) measured regional brain activity of people with histories of impulsive aggression before and after 12 weeks of treatment with a specific serotonin reuptake inhibitor. They found that the drug increased the activity of the prefrontal cortex and reduced aggressiveness.

FIGURE 10.9

Moral Decisions and the vmPFC.   The graph shows the percentage of people with lesions of the ventromedial prefrontal cortex and normal controls who endorse decisions of nonmoral, impersonal moral, and personal moral scenarios like the ones listed in the box.

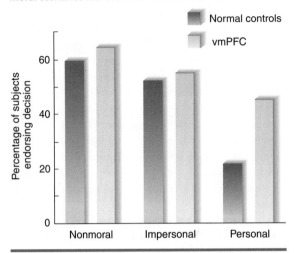

Data from Koenigs, M., Young, L., Adolphs, R., Tranel, D. et al., *Nature*, 2007, *446*, 908–911.

InterimSummary

Emotions as Response Patterns

The word *emotion* refers to behaviors, physiological responses, and feelings. This section has discussed emotional response patterns, which consist of behaviors that deal with particular situations and physiological responses (both autonomic and hormonal) that support the behaviors. The amygdala organizes behavioral, autonomic, and hormonal responses to a variety of situations, including those that produce fear, anger, or disgust. It receives inputs from the olfactory system, the association cortex of the temporal lobe, the frontal cortex, and the rest of the limbic system. Its outputs go to the frontal cortex, hypothalamus, hippocampal formation, and brain stem nuclei that control autonomic functions and some species-typical behaviors. Electrical recordings of single neurons in the amygdala indicate that some of them respond when the animal perceives particular stimuli with emotional significance. Stimulation of the amygdala leads to emotional responses, and its destruction disrupts them. Pairing of neutral stimuli with those that elicit emotional responses results in classically conditioned emotional responses. Learning of these responses takes place primarily in the amygdala. Extinction of conditioned emotional responses involves inhibitory control of amygdala activity by the ventromedial prefrontal cortex.

Studies of people with amygdala lesions and functional imaging studies with humans indicate that the amygdala is involved in emotional reactions in our species, too. However, many of our conditioned emotional responses are acquired by observing the responses of other people or even through verbal instruction.

Aggressive behaviors are species-typical and serve useful functions most of the time. These behaviors are organized by circuits in the brain stem, which are modulated by the amygdala and hypothalamus. The activity of serotonergic neurons appears to inhibit risk-taking behaviors, including aggression. Destruction of serotonergic axons in the forebrain enhances aggression, and administration of drugs that facilitate serotonergic transmission reduces it. Low CSF levels of 5-HIAA (a metabolite of serotonin) are correlated with increased risk-taking and aggressive behavior in monkeys and humans.

The ventromedial prefrontal cortex plays an important role in emotional reactions. This region communicates with the dorsomedial thalamus, temporal cortex, ventral tegmental area, olfactory system, amygdala, cingulate cortex, lateral hypothalamus, and other regions of the frontal cortex. People with lesions of the vmPFC show impulsive behavior and often display outbursts of inappropriate anger. Their lack of an emotional response in a situation that has important consequences for them often leads to poor decision making.

Evidence suggests that the prefrontal cortex is involved in making moral judgments. When people make judgments that involve conflicts between utilitarian judgments (one person dies but five people live) and personal moral judgments (are you willing to push a man to his death?), the ventromedial prefrontal cortex is activated. Activation of one part of this region, the anterior cingulate cortex, is involved in weighing emotional and rational factors and coming to a decision about what action to take. People with damage to the vmPFC display utilitarian moral judgments. The release of serotonin in the prefrontal cortex activates this region, and some investigators believe that the serotonergic input to this region is responsible for the ability of serotonin to inhibit aggression and risky behavior.

Thought Questions

1. Phobias can be seen as dramatic examples of conditioned emotional responses. These responses can even be contagious; we can acquire them without direct experience with an aversive stimulus. For example, a child who sees a parent show signs of fright in the presence of a dog may also develop a fear reaction to the dog. Do you think that some prejudices might be learned in this way, too?

2. From the point of view of evolution, aggressive behavior and a tendency to establish dominance have useful functions. In particular, they increase the likelihood that only the most healthy and vigorous animals will reproduce. Can you think of examples of good and bad effects of these tendencies among members of our own species?

Communication of Emotions

The previous section described emotions as organized responses (behavioral, autonomic, and hormonal) that prepare an animal to deal with existing situations in the environment, such as events that pose a threat to the organism. For our earliest premammalian ancestors that is undoubtedly all there was to emotions. But over time other responses, with new functions, evolved. Many species of animals (including our own) communicate their emotions to others by means of postural changes, facial expressions, and nonverbal sounds (such as sighs, moans, and growls). These expressions serve useful social functions; they tell other individuals how we feel and—more to the point—what we are likely to do. For example, they warn a rival that we are angry or tell friends that we are sad and would like some comfort and reassurance. They can also indicate that a danger might be present or that something interesting seems to be happening. This section examines such expression and communication of emotions.

Facial Expression of Emotions: Innate Responses

Charles Darwin (1872/1965) suggested that human expressions of emotion have evolved from similar expressions in other animals. He said that emotional expressions are innate, unlearned responses consisting of a complex set of movements, principally of the facial muscles. Thus, a person's sneer and a wolf's snarl are biologically determined response patterns, both controlled by innate brain mechanisms, just as coughing and sneezing are. (Of course, people can sneer and wolves can snarl for quite different reasons.) Some of these movements resemble the behaviors themselves and may have evolved from them. For example, a snarl shows one's teeth and can be seen as an anticipation of biting.

Darwin obtained evidence for his conclusion that emotional expressions were innate by observing his own children and by corresponding with people living in various isolated cultures around the world. He reasoned that if people all over the world, no matter how isolated, show the same facial expressions of emotion, then these expressions must be inherited instead of learned. The logical argument goes like this: When groups of people are isolated for many years, they develop different languages. Thus, we can say that the words people use are arbitrary; there is no biological basis for using particular words to represent particular concepts. However, if facial expressions are inherited, then they should take approximately the same form in people from all cultures, despite their isolation from one another. Darwin did, indeed, find that people in different cultures used the same patterns of movement of facial muscles to express a particular emotional state.

Research by Ekman and his colleagues (Ekman and Friesen, 1971; Ekman, 1980) tends to confirm Darwin's hypothesis that facial expression of emotion uses an innate, species-typical repertoire of movements of facial muscles (Darwin, 1872/1965). For example, Ekman and Friesen (1971) studied the ability of members of an isolated tribe in New Guinea to recognize facial expressions of emotion produced by Westerners. They had no trouble doing so and themselves produced facial expressions that Westerners readily recognized. Figure 10.10 shows four photographs taken from videotapes of a man from this tribe reacting to stories designed to evoke facial expressions of happiness, sadness, anger, and disgust. I am sure that you will have no trouble recognizing which is which. (See *Figure 10.10*.)

Because the same facial expressions were used by people who had not previously been exposed to each other, Ekman and Friesen concluded that the expressions were unlearned behavior patterns. In contrast, different cultures use different words to express particular concepts; production of these words does not involve innate responses but must be learned.

Other researchers have compared the facial expressions of blind and normally sighted people. They reasoned that if the facial expressions of the two groups are similar, then the expressions are natural for our species and do not require learning by imitation. In fact, the facial expressions of young blind and sighted children are very similar (Woodworth and Schlosberg, 1954; Izard, 1971). In addition, a study of the emotional expressions of people competing (and winning or losing) athletic events in the 2004 Paralympic Games found no differences between the expressions

FIGURE 10.10

Facial Expressions in a New Guinea Tribesman   The tribesman made faces when told stories: (a) "Your friend has come and you are happy." (b) "Your child had died." (c) "You are angry and about to fight." (d) "You see a dead pig that has been lying there a long time."

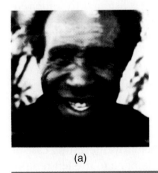 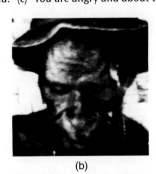 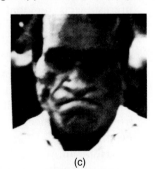 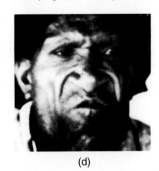

(a)   (b)   (c)   (d)

From Ekman, P., *The Face of Man: Expressions of Universal Emotions in a New Guinea Village.* New York: Garland STPM Press, 1980. Reprinted with permission.

of congenitally blind, noncongenitally blind, and sighted athletes (Matsumoto and Willingham, 2009). Thus, both the cross-cultural studies and the investigations of blind people confirm the naturalness of these facial expressions of emotion.

Neural Basis of the Communication of Emotions: Recognition

Effective communication is a two-way process. That is, the ability to display one's emotional state by changes in expression is useful only if other people are able to recognize them. In fact, Kraut and Johnston (1979) unobtrusively observed people in circumstances that would be likely to make them happy. They found that happy situations (such as making a strike while bowling, seeing the home team score, or experiencing a beautiful day) produced only small signs of happiness when the people were alone. However, when the people were interacting socially with other people, they were much more likely to smile. For example, bowlers who made a strike usually did not smile when the ball hit the pins, but when they turned around to face their companions, they often smiled. Jones, Collins, and Hong (1991) found that even 10-month-old children showed this tendency. (No, I'm not suggesting that infants have been observed while bowling.)

Recognition of another person's facial expression of emotions is generally automatic, rapid, and accurate. Tracy and Robbins (2008) found that observers quickly recognized brief expressions of a variety of emotions. If they were given more time to think about the expression they had seen, they showed very little improvement.

People can express emotions through their body language, as well as through muscular movements of their face (de Gelder, 2006). For example, a clenched fist might accompany an angry facial expression, and a fearful person may run away. The sight of photographs of bodies posed in gestures of fear activates the amygdala, just as the sight of fearful faces does (Hadjikhani and de Gelder, 2003). Meeren, van Heijnsbergen, and de Gelder (2005) prepared computer-modified photographs of people showing facial expressions of emotions that were either congruent with the person's body posture (for example, a facial expression of fear and a body posture of fear) or incongruent (for example, a facial expression of anger and a body posture of fear). The investigators asked people to identify the *facial* expressions shown in the photos and found that the ratings were faster and more accurate when the facial and body expressions were congruent. In other words, when we look at other people's faces, our perception of their emotion is affected by their body posture as well as by their facial expression.

Laterality of Emotional Recognition

We recognize other people's feelings by means of vision and audition—seeing their facial expressions and hearing their tone of voice and choice of words. Many studies have found that the right hemisphere plays a more important role than the left hemisphere in comprehension of emotion. For example, George et al. (1996) measured subjects' regional cerebral blood flow while the subjects listened to some sentences and identified their emotional content. In one condition the subjects listened to the meaning of the words and said whether they described a situation in which someone would be happy, sad, angry, or neutral. In another condition they judged the emotional state from the tone of the voice. The investigators found that comprehension of emotion from word meaning increased the activity of the prefrontal cortex bilaterally, the left more than the right. Comprehension of emotion from tone of voice increased the activity of only the right prefrontal cortex. (See *Figure 10.11.*)

Heilman, Watson, and Bowers (1983) recorded a particularly interesting case of a man with a disorder called *pure word deafness*, caused by damage to the left temporal cortex. (This syndrome is described in Chapter 13). The man could not compre-

FIGURE 10.11

Perception of Emotions.   The PET scans indicate brain regions activated by listening to emotions expressed by tone of voice (green) or by meanings of words (red).

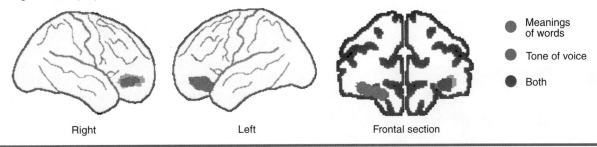

Right   Left   Frontal section

- Meanings of words
- Tone of voice
- Both

From George, M. S., Parekh, P. I., Rosinsky, N., Ketter, T. A., et al. *Archives of Neurology*, 1996, *53*, 665–670.

hend the meaning of speech but had no difficulty identifying the emotion being expressed by its intonation. This case, like the functional imaging study by George et al. (1996), indicates that comprehension of words and recognition of tone of voice are independent functions.

Role of the Amygdala

As we saw in the previous section, the amygdala plays a special role in emotional responses. It plays a role in emotional recognition as well. For example, several studies have found that lesions of the amygdala (the result of degenerative diseases or surgery for severe seizure disorders) impair people's ability to recognize facial expressions of emotion, especially expressions of fear (Adolphs et al., 1994, 1995; Young et al., 1995; Calder et al., 1996). In addition, functional imaging studies (Morris et al., 1996; Whalen et al., 1998) have found large increases in the activity of the amygdala when people view photographs of faces expressing fear but only small increases (or even decreases) when they look at photographs of happy faces. However, amygdala lesions do not appear to affect people's ability to recognize emotions in tone of voice (Anderson and Phelps, 1998; Adolphs and Tranel, 1999).

Krolak-Salmon et al. (2004) recorded electrical potentials from the amygdala and visual association cortex through electrodes that had been implanted in people who were being evaluated for neurosurgery to alleviate a seizure disorder. They presented the people with photographs of faces showing neutral expressions or expressions of fear, happiness, or disgust. The found that fearful faces produced the largest response and that the amygdala showed activity before the visual cortex did. The rapid response suggests that visual information that the amygdala receives directly from the subcortical visual system (which conducts information very rapidly) permits it to recognize facial expressions of fear.

Role of Imitation in Recognition of Emotional Expressions

Adolphs et al. (2000) discovered a possible link between somatosensation and emotional recognition. They compiled computerized information about the locations of brain damage in 108 patients with localized brain lesions and correlated this information with the patients' ability to recognize and identify facial expressions of emotions. They found that the most severe damage to this ability was caused by damage to the somatosensory cortex of the right hemisphere. (See *Figure 10.12*.) They suggest that when we see a facial expression of an emotion, we unconsciously imagine ourselves making that expression. Often, we do more than imagine making the expressions—we actually imitate what we see. Adolphs et al. suggest that the somatosensory representation of what it feels like to make the perceived expression provides cues we use to recognize the emotion being expressed in the face we are

FIGURE 10.12

Brain Damage and Recognition of Facial Expressions of Emotion. In this computer-generated representation, the colored areas outline the site of the lesions in a group of patients. Good performance in recognition of facial expressions of emotion is shown in shades of blue; poor performance is shown in red and yellow.

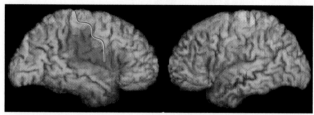

Right hemisphere   Left hemisphere

From Adolphs, R., Damasio, H., Tranel, D., Cooper, G., and Damasio, A. R. *The Journal of Neuroscience*, 2000, 20, 2683–2690. Copyright © 2000 by the Society for Neuroscience. Reprinted with permission.

viewing. In support of this hypothesis, Adolphs and his colleagues report that the ability of patients with right hemisphere lesions to recognize facial expressions of emotions is correlated with their ability to perceive somatosensory stimuli. That is, patients with somatosensory impairments (caused by right-hemisphere lesions) also had impairments in recognition of emotions.

Hussey and Safford (2009) review a considerable amount of evidence that supports this hypothesis (the so-called *simulationist* hypothesis). For example, neuroimaging studies have shown that brain regions that are activated when particular emotional expressions are observed are also activated when these expressions are imitated. In addition, a study by Pitcher et al. (2008) used transcranial magnetic stimulation to disrupt the normal activity of brain regions involved in visual perception of faces or perception of somatosensory feedback from one's own face. They found that disruption of *either* region impaired people's ability to recognize facial expressions of emotion. Finally, a study by Oberman, Winkielman, and Ramachandran (2007) had people hold a pen between their teeth, which interfered with smiling. When they did so, they had difficulty recognizing facial expressions of happiness, but not expressions of disgust, fear, and sadness, which involve the upper part of the face more than smiling does.

Neural Basis of the Communication of Emotions: Expression

Facial expressions of emotion are automatic and involuntary (although, as we saw, they can be modified by display rules). It is not easy to produce a realistic facial expression of emotion when we do not really feel that way. In fact, Ekman and Davidson have confirmed an early observation by a nineteenth-century neurologist, Guillaume-Benjamin Duchenne de Boulogne, that genuinely happy smiles, as opposed to false smiles or social smiles people make when they greet someone else, involve contraction of a muscle near the eyes, the lateral part of the orbicularis oculi—now sometimes referred to as Duchenne's muscle (Ekman, 1992; Ekman and Davidson, 1993). As Duchenne put it, "The first [zygomatic major muscle] obeys the will but the second [orbicularis oculi] is only put in play by the sweet emotions of the soul; the . . . fake joy, the deceitful laugh, cannot provoke the contraction of this latter muscle" (Duchenne, 1862/1990, p. 72). (See *Figure 10.13*.) The difficulty actors have in voluntarily producing a convincing facial expression of emotion is one of the reasons that led Constantin Stanislavsky to develop his system of *method acting*, in which actors attempt to imagine themselves in a situation that would lead to the desired emotion. Once the emotion is evoked, the facial expressions follow naturally (Stanislavsky, 1936).

This observation is confirmed by two neurological disorders with complementary symptoms (Hopf, Mueller-Forell, and Hopf, 1992; Topper, Kosinski, and Mull, 1995; Urban et al., 1998; Michel et al., 2008). The first, **volitional facial paresis**, is caused by damage to the face region of the primary motor cortex or to the fibers connecting this region with the motor nucleus of the facial nerve, which controls the muscles responsible for movement of the facial muscles. (*Paresis*, from the Greek "to let go," refers to a partial paralysis.) The interesting thing about volitional facial paresis is that the patient cannot voluntarily move the facial muscles but will express

volitional facial paresis Difficulty in moving the facial muscles voluntarily; caused by damage to the face region of the primary motor cortex or its subcortical connections.

emotional facial paresis Lack of movement of facial muscles in response to emotions in people who have no difficulty moving these muscles voluntarily; caused by damage to the insular prefrontal cortex, subcortical white matter of the frontal lobe, or parts of the thalamus.

a genuine emotion with those muscles. For example, Figure 10.14(a) shows a woman trying to pull her lips apart and show her teeth. Because of the lesion in the face region of her right primary motor cortex, she could not move the left side of her face. However, when she laughed (Figure 10.14b), both sides of her face moved normally. (See *Figure 10.14a* and *10.14b*.)

In contrast, **emotional facial paresis** is caused by damage to the insular region of the prefrontal cortex, to the white matter of the frontal lobe, or to parts of the thalamus. This system joins the system responsible for voluntary movements of the facial muscles in the medulla or caudal pons. People with this disorder can move their face muscles voluntarily but do not express emotions on the affected side of the face. Figure 10.14(c) shows a man pulling his lips apart to show his teeth, which he had no trouble doing. Figure 10.14(d) shows him smiling; as you can see, only the left side of his mouth is raised. He had a stroke that damaged the white matter of the left frontal lobe. (See *Figure 10.14c* and *10.14d*.) These two syndromes clearly indicate that different brain mechanisms are responsible for voluntary movements of the facial muscles and automatic, involuntary expression of emotions involving the same muscles.

As we saw in the previous subsection, the right hemisphere plays a more significant role in recognizing emotions in the voice or facial expressions of other people—especially negative emotions. The same hemispheric specialization appears to be true for expressing emotions. When people show emotions with their facial muscles, the left side of the face usually makes a more intense expression. For example, Sackeim and Gur (1978) cut photographs of people who were expressing emotions into right and left halves, prepared mirror images of each of them, and pasted them together, producing so-called *chimerical faces* (from the mythical Chimera, a fire-breathing monster, part goat, part

FIGURE 10.13

An Artificial Smile.   The photograph shows Dr. Duchenne electrically stimulating muscles in the face of a volunteer, causing contraction of muscles around the mouth that become active during a smile. As Duchenne discovered, however, a true smile also involves muscles around the eyes.

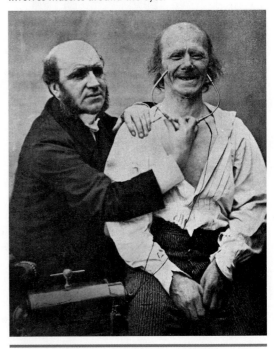

© Hulton-Deutsch Collection/Corbis

FIGURE 10.14

Emotional and Volitional Paresis.   This figure shows examples of emotional and volitional paresis: (a) A woman with volitional facial paresis caused by a right hemisphere lesion tries to pull her lips apart and show her teeth. Only the right side of her face responds. (b) The same woman shows a genuine smile. (c) A man with emotional facial paresis caused by a left-hemisphere lesion shows his teeth. (d) The same man is smiling. Only the left side of his face responds.

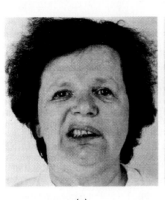 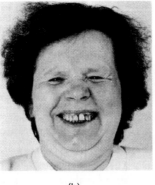 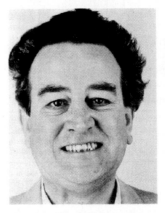 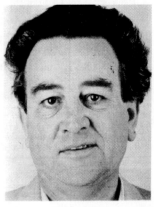

(a)   (b)   (c)   (d)

From Hopf, H. C., Mueller-Forell, W., and Hopf, N. J., *Neurology*, 1992, *42*, 1918–1923.

FIGURE 10.15

Chimerical Faces.   The figure shows (a) the original photo, (b) a composite of the right side of the man's face, and (c) a composite of the left side of the man's face.

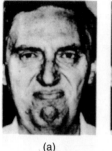 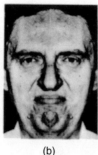 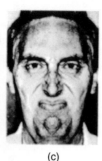

(a)   (b)   (c)

Reprinted from *Neuropsychologia, 16*, H. A. Sackeim and R. C. Gur, Lateral Asymmetry in Intensity of Emotional Expression, 473–481, Copyright 1978, with permission from Elsevier.

lion, and part serpent). They found that the left halves were more expressive than the right ones. (See *Figure 10.15*.) Because motor control is contralateral, the results suggest that the right hemisphere is more expressive than the left.

Moscovitch and Olds (1982) made more natural observations of people in restaurants and parks and found that the left side of their faces appeared to make stronger expressions of emotions. They confirmed these results in the laboratory by analyzing videotapes of people telling sad or humorous stories. A review of the literature by Borod et al. (1998) found forty-eight other studies that obtained similar results.

Left hemisphere lesions do not usually impair vocal expressions of emotion. For example, people with Wernicke's aphasia (described in Chapter 13) usually modulate their voice according to mood, even though the words they say make no sense. In contrast, right-hemisphere lesions do impair expression of emotion, both facially and by tone of voice.

We saw in the previous subsection that the amygdala is involved in the recognition of facial expression of emotions. Research indicates that it is *not* involved in emotional *expression*.

Anderson and Phelps (2000) reported the case of S. P., a 54-year-old woman whose right amygdala was removed to treat a serious seizure disorder. Because of a preexisting lesion of the left amygdala, the surgery resulted in a bilateral amygdalectomy. After the surgery, S. P. lost the ability to recognize facial expressions of fear, but she had no difficulty recognizing individual faces, and she could easily identify male and female faces and accurately judge their ages. What is particularly interesting is that the amygdala lesions did not impair S. P.'s ability to produce her own facial expressions of fear. She had no difficulty accurately expressing fear, anger, happiness, sadness, disgust, and surprise. By the way, when she saw a photograph of herself showing fear, she could not tell what emotion her face had been expressing.

InterimSummary

Communication of Emotions

We (and members of other species) communicate our emotions primarily through facial gestures. Darwin believed that such expressions of emotion were innate—that these muscular movements were inherited behavioral patterns. Ekman and his colleagues performed cross-cultural studies with members of an isolated tribe in New Guinea. Their results supported Darwin's hypothesis. We also receive information about people's emotions from their body posture or movement.

Recognition of other people's emotional expressions involves the right hemisphere more than the left. Functional imaging indicates that when people judge the emotions of voices, the right hemisphere is activated more than the left. In addition, some people with

pure word deafness, caused by damage to the left hemisphere, cannot recognize words but can still recognize the emotions portrayed by tone of voice. The amygdala plays a role in recognition of facial expressions of fearfulness; lesions of the amygdala disrupt this ability, and functional imaging studies show increased activity of the amygdala while the subject is engaging in this task. The ability to judge emotions by a person's tone of voice is not affected.

The amygdala receives more primitive visual information from subcortical regions of the brain, and this information is used in making judgments about fearful expressions. There is a natural tendency to imitate the emotional expressions of other people. Feedback from this activity, which is transmitted to the somatosensory cortex, appears to help us to comprehend the emotional intentions of other people.

Facial expression of emotions (and other stereotypical behaviors such as laughing and crying) are almost impossible to simulate. For example, only a genuine smile of pleasure causes the contraction of the lateral part of the orbicularis oculi (Duchenne's muscle). Genuine expressions of emotion are controlled by special neural circuits.

The best evidence for this assertion comes from the complementary syndromes of emotional and volitional facial paresis. People with emotional facial paresis can move their facial muscles voluntarily but not in response to an emotion, whereas people with volitional facial paresis show the opposite symptoms. In addition, the left halves of people's faces tend to be more expressive than the right halves.

Feelings of Emotions

So far, we have examined two aspects of emotions: the organization of patterns of responses that deal with the situation that provokes the emotion and the communication of emotional states with other members of the species. The final aspect of emotion to be examined in this chapter is the subjective component: feelings of emotion.

The James-Lange Theory

William James (1842–1910), an American psychologist, and Carl Lange (1834–1900), a Danish physiologist, independently suggested similar explanations for emotion, which most people refer to collectively as the **James-Lange theory** (James, 1884; Lange, 1887). Basically, the theory states that emotion-producing situations elicit an appropriate set of physiological responses, such as trembling, sweating, and increased heart rate. The situations also elicit behaviors, such as clenching of the fists or fighting. The brain receives sensory feedback from the muscles and from the organs that produce these responses, and it is this feedback that constitutes our feeling of emotion.

James-Lange theory A theory of emotion that suggests that behaviors and physiological responses are directly elicited by situations and that feelings of emotions are produced by feedback from these behaviors and responses.

James says that our own emotional feelings are based on what we find ourselves doing and on the sensory feedback we receive from the activity of our muscles and internal organs. Thus, when we find ourselves trembling and feel queasy, we experience fear. Where feelings of emotions are concerned, we are self-observers. Thus, the two aspects of emotions reported in the first two sections of this chapter (patterns of emotional responses and expressions of emotions) give rise to the third: feelings. (See *Figure 10.16*.)

James's description of the process of emotion might strike you as being at odds with your own experience. Many people think that they experience emotions directly, internally. They consider the outward manifestations of emotions to be secondary events. But have you ever found yourself in an unpleasant confrontation with someone else and discovered that you were trembling, even though you did not think that you were so bothered by the encounter? Or did you ever find yourself blushing in response to some public remark that was made about you? Or did you ever find tears coming to your eyes while you watched a film that you did not think was affecting you? What would you conclude about your emotional states in situations like these? Would you ignore the evidence from your own physiological reactions?

James's theory is difficult to verify experimentally because it attempts to explain *feelings* of emotion, not the causes of emotional responses, and feelings are private events. Some anecdotal evidence supports the theory. For example, Sweet (1966)

FIGURE 10.16

The James-Lange Theory of Emotion. This schematic diagram indicates that an event in the environment triggers behavioral, autonomic, and endocrine responses. Feedback from these responses produces feelings of emotions.

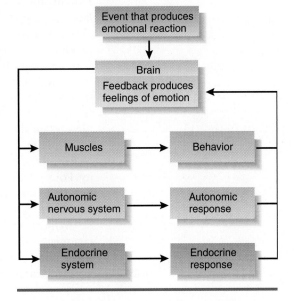

reported the case of a man in whom some sympathetic nerves were severed on one side of the body to treat a cardiovascular disorder. The man—a music lover—reported that the shivering sensation he felt while listening to music now occurred only on the unoperated side of his body. He still enjoyed listening to music, but the surgery altered his emotional reaction.

In one of the few tests of James's theory, Hohman (1966) collected data from people with spinal cord damage. He asked these people about the intensity of their emotional feelings. If feedback is important, one would expect that emotional feelings would be less intense if the injury were high (that is, close to the brain) than if it were low, because a high spinal cord injury would make the person become insensitive to a larger part of the body. In fact, this result is precisely what Hohman found: The higher the injury, the less intense the feeling was. As one of Hohman's subjects said:

> I sit around and build things up in my mind, and I worry a lot, but it's not much but the power of thought. I was at home alone in bed one day and dropped a cigarette where I couldn't reach it. I finally managed to scrounge around and put it out. I could have burned up right there, but the funny thing is, I didn't get all shook up about it. I just didn't feel afraid at all, like you would suppose. (Hohman, 1966, p. 150)

Another subject showed that angry behavior (an emotional response) does not appear to depend on *feelings* of emotion. Instead, the behavior is evoked by the situation (and by the person's evaluation of it) even if the spinal cord damage has reduced the intensity of the person's emotional feelings.

> Now, I don't get a feeling of physical animation, it's sort of cold anger. Sometimes I act angry when I see some injustice. I yell and cuss and raise hell, because if you don't do it sometimes, I've learned people will take advantage of you, but it doesn't have the heat to it that it used to. It's a mental kind of anger. (Hohman, 1966, p. 151)

Feedback from Simulated Emotions

James stressed the importance of two aspects of emotional responses: emotional behaviors and autonomic responses. As we saw earlier in this chapter, a particular set of muscles—those of the face—helps us to communicate our emotional state to other people. Several experiments suggest that feedback from the contraction of facial muscles can affect people's moods and even alter the activity of the autonomic nervous system.

Ekman and his colleagues (Ekman, Levenson, and Friesen, 1983; Levenson, Ekman, and Friesen, 1990) asked subjects to move particular facial muscles to simulate the emotional expressions of fear, anger, surprise, disgust, sadness, and happiness. They did not tell the subjects what emotion they were trying to make them produce, but only what movements they should make. For example, to simulate fear, they told the subjects, "Raise your brows. While holding them raised, pull your brows together. Now raise your upper eyelids and tighten the lower eyelids. Now stretch your lips horizontally." (These movements produce a facial expression of fear.) While the subjects made the expressions, the investigators monitored several physiological responses controlled by the autonomic nervous system.

The simulated expressions *did* alter the activity of the autonomic nervous system. In fact, different facial expressions produced somewhat different patterns of activity. For example, anger increased heart rate and skin temperature, fear increased heart rate but decreased skin temperature, and happiness decreased heart rate without affecting skin temperature.

Why should a particular pattern of movements of the facial muscles cause changes in mood or in the activity of the autonomic nervous system? Perhaps the connection is a result of experience; in other words, perhaps the occurrence of particular facial movements along with changes in the autonomic nervous system leads to classical conditioning, so that feedback from the facial movements becomes capable of eliciting the autonomic response—and a change in perceived emotion. Or perhaps the connection is innate. As we saw earlier, the adaptive value of emotional expressions is that they communicate feelings and intentions to others. The research presented earlier in this chapter on the role of the somatosensory cortex in recognition of emotions suggests that one of the ways we communicate feelings is through unconscious imitation.

A functional imaging study by Damasio et al. (2000) asked people to recall and try to re-experience past episodes from their lives that evoked feelings of sadness, happiness, anger, and fear. The investigators found that recalling these emotions activated the subjects' somatosensory cortex and upper brain stem nuclei involved in control of internal organs and detection of sensations received from them. These responses are certainly compatible with James's theory. As Damasio et al. put it,

> [Emotions are part of a neural mechanism] based on structures that regulate the organism's current state by executing specific actions via the musculoskeletal system, ranging from facial and postural expressions to complex behaviors, and by producing chemical and neural responses aimed at the internal milieu, viscera and telencephalic neural circuits. The consequences of such responses are represented in both subcortical regulatory structures . . . and in cerebral cortex . . . , and those representations constitute a critical aspect of the neural basis of feelings. (p. 1049)

I suspect that if James were still alive, he would approve of these words.

The tendency to imitate the expressions of other people appears to be innate. Field et al. (1982) had adults make facial expressions in front of infants. The infants' own facial expressions were videotaped and were subsequently rated by people who did not know what expressions the adults were displaying. Field and her colleagues found that even newborn babies (with an average age of 36 hours) tended to imitate the expressions they saw. Clearly, the effect occurs too early in life to be a result of learning. Figure 10.17 shows three photographs of the adult expressions and the expressions they elicited in a baby. Can you look at them yourself without changing your own expression, at least a little? (See *Figure 10.17*.)

Perhaps imitation provides one of the channels by which organisms communicate their emotions—and evoke feelings of empathy. For example, if we see someone looking sad, we tend to assume a sad expression ourselves. The feedback from our own expression helps to put us in the other person's place and makes us more likely to respond with solace or assistance. And perhaps one of the reasons we derive pleasure from making someone else smile is that their smile makes *us* smile and feel happy.

FIGURE 10.17

Imitation in an Infant.   The photographs show happy, sad, and surprised faces posed by an adult and the responses made by the infant.

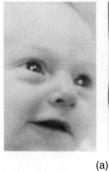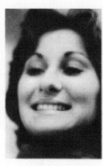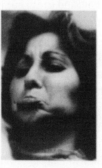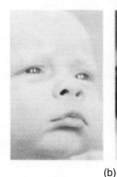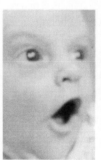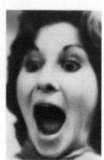

(a)   (b)   (c)

Photographs courtesy of Tiffany Field, Fielding Graduate University.

InterimSummary

Feelings of Emotions

From the earliest times people recognized that emotions were accompanied by feelings that seemed to come from inside the body, which probably provided the impetus for developing physiological theories of emotion. James and Lange suggested that emotions were primarily responses to situations. Feedback from the physiological and behavioral reactions to emotion-producing situations gave rise to the feelings of emotion; thus, feelings are the *results*, not the *causes*, of emotional reactions. Hohman's study of people with spinal cord damage supported the James-Lange theory; people who could no

longer feel the reactions from most of their body reported that they no longer experienced intense emotional states.

Ekman and his colleagues have shown that even simulating an emotional expression causes changes in the activity of the autonomic nervous system. Perhaps feedback from these changes explains why an emotion can be "contagious": We see someone smile with pleasure, we ourselves imitate the smile, and the internal feedback makes us feel at least somewhat happier.

⋮ EPILOGUE   Mr. V. Revisited

After our visit to Mr. V. (described in the chapter prologue), we were discussing the case. A student asked why Mr. V. talked about continuing his walking schedule when he obviously knew that he couldn't walk. Did he think that he would recover soon?

"No, that's not it," said Dr. W. "He *knows* what his problem is, but he doesn't really *understand* it. The people at the rehab center are having trouble with him because he keeps trying to go outside for a walk. The first time, he managed to wheel his chair to the top of the stairs, but someone caught him just in time. Now they have a chain across the door frame of his room so that he can't get into the hall without an attendant.

"Mr. V.'s problem is not that he can't verbally recognize what's going on; it's that he just can't grasp its significance. The right hemisphere is specialized in seeing many things at once: in seeing all the parts of a geometric shape and grasping its form or in seeing all the elements of a situation and understanding what they mean. That's what's wrong. He can tell you about his paralyzed leg, about the fact that he is in a wheelchair, and so on, but he can't put these facts together and realize that his days of walking are over.

"As you could see, Mr. V. can still express emotions." We all smiled at the thought of the contemptuous look on Mr. V.'s face. "But the right hemisphere is especially important in assessing the significance of a situation and making conclusions that lead to our being happy or sad or whatever. People with certain right-hemisphere lesions are not bothered at all by their conditions. They can *tell* you about their problems, so I guess they verbally understand it, but their problems just don't affect them emotionally."

He turned to me. "Neil, do you remember Mr. P.?" I nodded. "Mr. P. had a left-hemisphere lesion. He had a severe aphasia and

could hardly say a word. We showed him a picture of some objects and asked him to try to name them. He looked at them and started crying. Although he couldn't talk, he knew that he had a serious problem and that things would never be the same for him. His right hemisphere was still working. It could assess the situation and give rise to feelings of sadness and despair."

Dr. W. suggested that the right hemisphere's special role in emotional processes is related to its ability to deal with perception and evaluation of patterns of stimuli that occur simultaneously. His suggestion is plausible, but we still do not know enough about hemispheric differences to be sure that it is correct. In any event, many studies have shown that the right hemisphere does play a special role in evaluating the emotional significance of a situation. I described some of these studies in the chapter, but let's look at a few more examples. Bear and Fedio (1977) reported that people with seizures that primarily involve the left hemisphere tend to have thought disorders, whereas those with right-hemisphere seizures tend to have emotional disorders. Mesulam (1985) reported that people with damage to the right temporal lobe (but not the left temporal lobe) are likely to lose their sensitivity to social cues. Obviously, this observation is meaningful only for patients who were sensitive to social cues before the brain damage; if someone is socially insensitive *before* having a stroke, we can hardly blame the behavior on brain damage. In particular, people with right temporal lobe lesions tend to show bad manners. They talk when they feel like it and do not yield the floor to someone else who has something to say; they simply ignore the social cues that polite people observe and follow. They also adopt a familiar conversational style with people to whom they would normally be deferential (for example, the physician who is treating them).

Perhaps my favorite example of possible hemispheric specialization is hypnosis. Sackeim (1982) reported that when people are hypnotized, the left side of their body is more responsive to hypnotic suggestion than the right side is. Because the left side of the body is controlled by the right hemisphere, this observation indicates that the right hemisphere may be more susceptible to hypnotic suggestion. In addition, Sackeim, Paulus, and Weiman (1979) found that students who are easily hypnotized tend to sit on the right side of the classroom. In this position they see most of the front of the room (including the teacher) with their right hemispheres, so perhaps their choice represents a preference for right-hemisphere involvement in watching another person.

One of the reasons I enjoy writing these epilogues is that I can permit myself to be more speculative than I am in the text of the chapter itself. Why might the right hemisphere be more involved in hypnosis? One explanation of hypnosis that I find appealing is that it derives from our ability to get emotionally involved in a story—to get wrapped up in what is happening to the characters in a film or a novel (Barber, 1975). When we become involved in a story, we experience genuine feelings of emotion: happiness, sadness, fear, or anger. We laugh, cry, and show the same sorts of physiological changes that we would if the story were really happening to us. Similarly, according to Barber, we become involved in the "story" that the hypnotist is creating for us, and we suspend our disbelief and act it out. According to this explanation, hypnosis is related to our susceptibility to social situations and to our ability to empathize with others. In fact, people with the ability to produce vivid mental images, a high capacity for becoming involved in imaginative activities, and a rich, vivid imagination are those who are most likely to be susceptible to hypnosis (Kihlstrom, 1985).

As we saw in this chapter, the right hemisphere appears to play a special role in assessing social situations and appreciating their emotional significance. If Barber's explanation of hypnosis is correct, then we can see why the right hemisphere might play a special role in hypnosis, too. Perhaps researchers interested in hypnosis will begin studying patients with right- or left-hemisphere damage, and neuropsychologists already studying these people will start investigating hypnosis and its possible relation to social and emotional variables and either confirm or disprove these speculations.

Key Concepts

EMOTIONS AS RESPONSE PATTERNS

1. Emotional responses consist of three components: behavioral, autonomic, and hormonal.

2. The amygdala plays a central role in coordinating all three components in response to threatening or aversive stimuli. In particular, the lateral nucleus is involved in acquisition of conditioned emotional responses.

3. Species-typical aggressive behaviors are controlled by neural circuits in the brain stem, which are modulated by the circuits in the hypothalamus and the amygdala.

4. The ventromedial prefrontal cortex plays a special role in the inhibitory control of emotional responses and in the evaluation of situations that involve moral judgments.

COMMUNICATION OF EMOTIONS

5. Facial expressions of emotions appear to be species-typical responses, even in humans.

6. Recognition of facial expressions of emotions may involve imitation, which gives rise to feedback from the somatosensory cortex.

7. The amygdala is involved in visual recognition of facial expressions of emotion but not in their production.

8. Difficulty in faking true expressions of emotion and the existence of emotional and volitional facial paresis indicate that special neural circuits are involved in expressions of emotion.

9. Expression and recognition of emotions is largely accomplished by neural mechanisms located in the right hemisphere.

FEELINGS OF EMOTION

10. The James-Lange theory suggests that we experience our own emotions through feedback from the expression of the physiological and behavioral components. Evidence from people with spinal cord injuries supports this theory.

Suggested Readings

Damasio, A. R. *Looking for Spinoza: Joy, Sorrow, and the Feeling Brain.* New York: Harcourt, 2003.

Goldman, A. I., and Sripada, C. S. Simulationist models of face-based emotion recognition. *Cognition*, 2005, *94*, 193–213.

Lane, R. D., and Nadel, L. (eds.). *Cognitive Neuroscience of Emotion.* New York: Oxford University Press, 2000.

LeDoux, J. E. Emotional circuits in the brain. *Annual Review of Neuroscience*, 2000, *23*, 155–184.

Moll, J., Zahn, R., de Oliveira-Souza, R., Krueger, F., and Grafman, J. The neural basis of human moral cognition. *Nature Reviews: Neuroscience*, 2005, *6*, 799–809.

Nelson, R. J., and Trainor, B. C. Neural mechanisms of aggression. *Nature Reviews: Neuroscience*, 2007, *8*, 536–546.

Pessoa, L. On the relationship between emotion and cognition. *Nature Reviews: Neuroscience*, 2008, *9*, 148–158.

Popova, N. K. From genes to aggressive behavior: The role of serotonergic system. *BioEssays*, 2006, *28*, 495–503.

Stoff, D. M., and Susman, E. J. (eds.) *Developmental Psychobiology of Aggression.* New York: Cambridge University Press, 2005.

Additional Resources

Visit www.mypsychkit.com for additional review and practice of the material covered in this chapter. Within MyPsychKit, you can take practice tests and receive a customized study plan to help you review. Dozens of animations, tutorials, and Web links are also available. You can even review using the interactive electronic version of this textbook. You will need to register for MyPsychKit. See www.mypsychkit.com for complete details.

chapter 11 : Ingestive Behavior

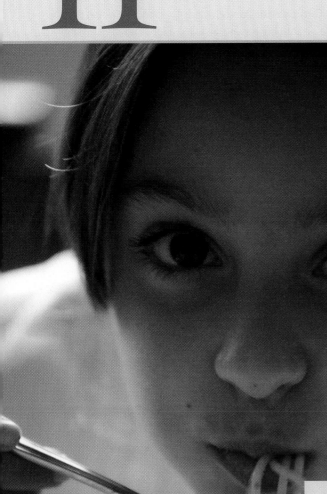

LEARNING OBJECTIVES

1. Explain the characteristics of a regulatory mechanism.
2. Describe the fluid compartments of the body.
3. Explain the control of osmometric thirst and volumetric thirst and the role of angiotensin.
4. Describe characteristics of the two nutrient reservoirs and the absorptive and fasting phases of metabolism.
5. Discuss the signals from the environment, the stomach, and the metabolism that begin a meal.
6. Discuss the long-term and short-term factors that stop a meal.
7. Describe research on the role of the brain stem and hypothalamus in hunger and satiety.
8. Discuss the social and physiological factors that contribute to obesity.
9. Discuss surgical, behavioral, and pharmacological treatments for obesity.
10. Discuss the physiological factors that may contribute to anorexia nervosa and bulimia nervosa.

Out of Control

Carrie was a frail little baby. She nursed poorly, apparently because she was so weak. For several years she was underweight. Her motor development and cognitive development were much slower than normal, she often seemed to have trouble breathing, and her hands and feet were especially small. Finally, her appetite seemed to improve. She began gaining weight and soon surpassed other children of her age. Previously, she was passive and well behaved, but she became difficult and demanding. She also showed compulsive behavior—picking at her skin, collecting and lining up objects, and protesting violently when her parents tried to put things away.

The worst problem, though, was her appetite. She ate everything she could and never seemed satisfied. At first her parents were so pleased to see her finally gaining weight that they gave her food whenever she asked for it. But after a while it was clear that she was becoming obese. A specialist diagnosed her condition and told her parents that they would have to strictly limit Carrie's food intake. Because of her weak muscles and low metabolic rate, she needed only 1200 calories per day to maintain a normal weight. But Carrie was constantly looking for food. She would raid the refrigerator until her parents installed a lock on it and on the cabinets where they put food. They had to be careful of how they disposed of leftover food, vegetable peels, or meat trimmings because Carrie would raid the garbage can and eat them.

When Carrie went to school, she began gaining weight once more. She would quickly eat everything on her tray and would then eat everything her classmates did not finish. If anyone dropped food on the floor near her, she would pick that up and eat it too. Because of Carrie's special needs, the school appointed an aide to monitor her food intake to be sure that she ate only the low-calorie meal that she was served.

As the French physiologist Claude Bernard (1813–1878) said, "The constancy of the internal milieu is a necessary condition for a free life." This famous quotation says succinctly what organisms must do to be able to exist in environments that are hostile to the living cells that compose them (that is, to live a "free life"): They must provide a barrier between their cells and the external environment—in the case of mammals this barrier consists of skin and mucous membrane. Within the barrier they must regulate the nature of the internal fluid that bathes the cells.

The physiological characteristics of the cells that constitute our bodies evolved long ago, when these cells floated freely in the ocean. In essence, what the evolutionary process has accomplished is the ability to make our own seawater for bathing our cells, to add to this seawater the oxygen and nutrients that our cells need, and to remove from it waste products that would otherwise poison them. To perform these functions, we have digestive, respiratory, circulatory, and excretory systems. We also have the behaviors necessary for finding and ingesting food and water.

Regulation of the fluid that bathes our cells is part of a process called **homeostasis** ("similar standing"). This chapter discusses the means by which we mammals achieve homeostatic control of the vital characteristics of our extracellular fluid through our **ingestive behavior**: intake of food, water, and minerals such as sodium. First, we will examine the general nature of regulatory mechanisms; then we will consider drinking and eating and the neural mechanisms that are responsible for these behaviors. Finally, we will look at some research on the eating disorders.

homeostasis (*home ee oh **stay** sis*) The process by which the body's substances and characteristics (such as temperature and glucose level) are maintained at their optimal level.

ingestive behavior (*in **jess** tiv*) Eating or drinking.

system variable A variable that is controlled by a regulatory mechanism; for example, temperature in a heating system.

Physiological Regulatory Mechanisms

A physiological regulatory mechanism is one that maintains the constancy of some internal characteristic of the organism in the face of external variability; for example, keeping body temperature constant despite changes in the ambient temperature. A regulatory mechanism contains four essential features: the **system variable** (the characteristic to be regulated), a **set point** (the optimal value of the system variable), a **detector** that monitors the value of the system variable, and a **correctional mechanism** that restores the system variable to the set point.

An example of a regulatory system is a room whose temperature is regulated by a thermostatically controlled heater. The system variable is the air temperature of the room, and the detector for this variable is a thermostat. This device can be adjusted so that contacts of a switch will be closed when the temperature falls below a preset value (the set point). Closure of the contacts turns on the correctional mechanism—the coils of the heater. (See *Figure 11.1*.) If the room cools below the set point of the thermostat, the thermostat turns the heater on, and the heater warms the room. The rise in room temperature causes the thermostat to turn the heater off. Because the activity of the correctional mechanism (heat production) feeds back to the thermostat and causes it to turn the heater off, this process is called **negative feedback**. Negative feedback is an essential characteristic of all regulatory systems.

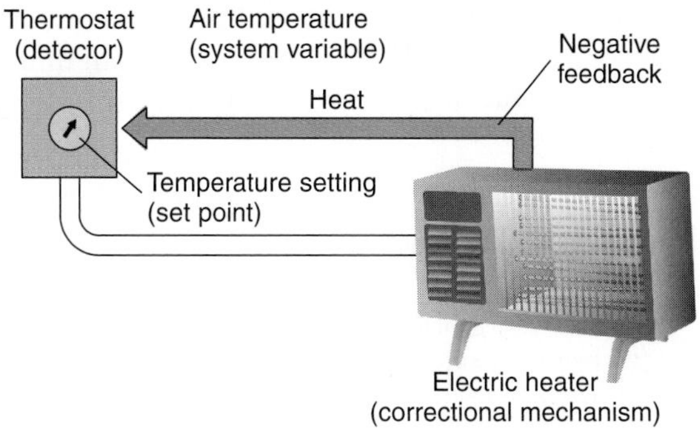

This chapter considers regulatory systems that involve ingestive behaviors: drinking and eating. These behaviors are correctional mechanisms that replenish the body's depleted stores of water or nutrients. Because of the delay between ingestion and replenishment of the depleted stores, ingestive behaviors are controlled by **satiety mechanisms** as well as by detectors that monitor the system variables. Satiety mechanisms are required because of the physiology of our digestive system. For example, suppose you spend some time in a hot, dry environment and lose body water. The loss of water causes internal detectors to initiate the correctional mechanism: drinking. You quickly drink a glass or two of water and then stop. What stops your ingestive behavior? The water is still in your digestive system, not yet in the fluid surrounding your cells, where it is needed. Therefore, although drinking was initiated by detectors that measure your body's need for water, *it was stopped by other means*. There must be a satiety mechanism that says, in effect, "Stop—this water, when absorbed by the digestive system into the blood, will eventually replenish the body's need." Satiety mechanisms monitor the activity of the correctional mechanism (in this case, drinking), not the system variables themselves. When a sufficient amount of drinking occurs, the satiety mechanisms stop further drinking *in anticipation* of the replenishment that will occur later. (See *Figure 11.2*.)

FIGURE 11.1

An Example of a Regulatory System

Thermostat (detector)   Air temperature (system variable)   Negative feedback   Heat   Temperature setting (set point)   Electric heater (correctional mechanism)

set point The optimal value of the system variable in a regulatory mechanism.

detector In a regulatory process, a mechanism that signals when the system variable deviates from its set point.

correctional mechanism In a regulatory process, the mechanism that is capable of changing the value of the system variable.

negative feedback A process whereby the effect produced by an action serves to diminish or terminate that action; a characteristic of regulatory systems.

satiety mechanism A brain mechanism that causes cessation of hunger or thirst, produced by adequate and available supplies of nutrients or water.

FIGURE 11.2

An Outline of the System That Controls Drinking

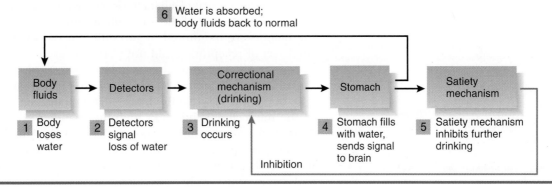

intracellular fluid The fluid contained within cells.

extracellular fluid All body fluids outside cells: interstitial fluid, blood plasma, and cerebrospinal fluid.

intravascular fluid The fluid found within the blood vessels.

interstitial fluid The fluid that bathes the cells, filling the space between the cells of the body (the "interstices").

isotonic Equal in osmotic pressure to the contents of a cell. A cell placed in an isotonic solution neither gains nor loses water.

hypertonic The characteristic of a solution that contains enough solute that it will draw water out of a cell placed in it, through the process of osmosis.

hypotonic The characteristic of a solution that contains so little solute that a cell placed in it will absorb water, through the process of osmosis.

hypovolemia (*hy poh voh **lee** mee a*) Reduction in the volume of the intravascular fluid.

Drinking

To maintain our internal milieu at its optimal state, we have to drink some water from time to time. This section describes the control of this form of ingestive behavior.

Some Facts About Fluid Balance

Before you can understand the physiological control of drinking, you must know something about the fluid compartments of the body and their relationships with each other. The body contains four major fluid compartments: one compartment of intracellular fluid and three compartments of extracellular fluid. Approximately two-thirds of the body's water is contained in the **intracellular fluid**, the fluid portion of the cytoplasm of cells. The rest is **extracellular fluid**, which includes the **intravascular fluid** (the blood plasma), the cerebrospinal fluid, and the **interstitial fluid**. *Interstitial* means "standing between"; indeed, the interstitial fluid stands between our cells—it is the "seawater" that bathes them. For the purposes of this chapter, we will ignore the cerebrospinal fluid and concentrate on the other three compartments. (See *Figure 11.3*.)

Two of the fluid compartments of the body must be kept within precise limits: the intracellular fluid and the intravascular fluid. The intracellular fluid is controlled by the concentration of solutes in the interstitial fluid. (*Solutes* are the substances dissolved in a solution.) Normally, the interstitial fluid is **isotonic** (from *isos*, "equal," and *tonos*, "tension") with the intracellular fluid. That is, the concentration of solutes in the cells and in the interstitial fluid that bathes them is balanced, so that water does not tend to move into or out of the cells. If the interstitial fluid loses water (becomes more concentrated, or **hypertonic**), water will be pulled out of the cells. On the other hand, if the interstitial fluid gains water (becomes more dilute, or **hypotonic**), water will move into the cells. Either condition endangers cells; a loss of water deprives them of the ability to perform many chemical reactions, and a gain of water can cause their membranes to rupture. Therefore, the concentration of the interstitial fluid must be closely regulated. (See *Figure 11.4*.)

The volume of the blood plasma must be closely regulated because of the mechanics of the operation of the heart. If the blood volume falls too low, the heart can no longer pump the blood effectively; if the volume is not restored, heart failure will result. This condition is called **hypovolemia**, literally "low volume of the blood" (*-emia* comes from the Greek *haima*, "blood"). The vascular system of the body can make some adjustments for loss of blood volume by contracting the muscles in smaller veins and arteries, thereby presenting a smaller space for the blood to fill, but this correctional mechanism has definite limits.

The two important characteristics of the body fluids—the solute concentration of the intracellular fluid and the volume of the blood—are monitored by two different sets of receptors. A single set of receptors would not work because it is possible for one of these fluid compartments to be changed without affecting the other. For example, a loss of blood obviously reduces the volume of the intravascular fluid, but it has no effect on the volume of the intracellular fluid. On the other hand, a salty meal will increase the solute concentration of the interstitial fluid, drawing water out of the cells, but it will not cause hypovolemia. Thus, the body needs two sets of receptors, one measuring blood volume and another measuring cell volume.

FIGURE 11.3

The Relative Size of the Body's Fluid Compartments

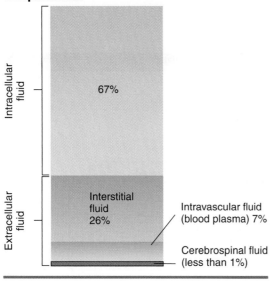

Intracellular fluid

67%

Extracellular fluid

Interstitial fluid 26%

Intravascular fluid (blood plasma) 7%

Cerebrospinal fluid (less than 1%)

FIGURE 11.4

Solute Concentration.   The figure shows the effects of differences in solute concentration on the movement of water molecules.

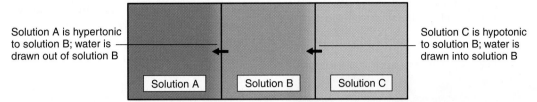

Solution A is hypertonic to solution B; water is drawn out of solution B

Solution C is hypotonic to solution B; water is drawn into solution B

Solution A   Solution B   Solution C

Two Types of Thirst

As we just saw, for our bodies to function properly, the volume of two fluid compartments—intracellular and intravascular—must be regulated. Most of the time, we ingest more water and sodium than we need, and the kidneys excrete the excess. However, if the levels of water or sodium fall too low, correctional mechanisms—drinking water or ingesting sodium—are activated. Everyone is familiar with the sensation of thirst, which occurs when we need to ingest water. However, a salt appetite is much more rare because it is difficult for people *not* to get enough sodium in their diet, even if they do not put extra salt on their food. Nevertheless, the mechanisms to increase sodium intake exist, even though they are seldom called upon in members of our species.

Because loss of water from either the intracellular or intravascular fluid compartments stimulates drinking, researchers have adopted the terms *osmometric thirst* and *volumetric thirst* to describe them. The term *volumetric* is clear; it refers to the metering (measuring) of the volume of the blood plasma. The term *osmometric* requires more explanation, which will be provided in the next section. The term *thirst* means different things in different circumstances. Its original definition referred to a sensation that people say they have when they are dehydrated. Here I use it in a descriptive sense. Because we do not know how other animals feel, *thirst* simply means a tendency to seek water and to ingest it.

Osmometric Thirst

Osmometric thirst occurs when the solute concentration of the interstitial fluid increases. This increase draws water out of the cells, and they shrink in volume. The term *osmometric* refers to the fact that the detectors are actually responding to (metering) changes in the concentration of the interstitial fluid that surrounds them. *Osmosis* is the movement of water through a semipermeable membrane from a region of low solute concentration to one of high solute concentration.

The existence of neurons that respond to changes in the solute concentration of the interstitial fluid was first hypothesized by Verney (1947). Verney suggested that these detectors, which he called **osmoreceptors**, were neurons whose firing rate was affected by their level of hydration. That is, if the interstitial fluid surrounding them became more concentrated, they would lose water through osmosis. The shrinkage would cause them to alter their firing rate, which would send signals to other parts of the brain. (See *Figure 11.5*.)

When we eat a salty meal, we incur a pure osmometric thirst. The salt is absorbed from the digestive system

osmometric thirst Thirst produced by an increase in the osmotic pressure of the interstitial fluid relative to the intracellular fluid, thus producing cellular dehydration.

osmoreceptor A neuron that detects changes in the solute concentration of the interstitial fluid that surrounds it.

FIGURE 11.5

An Osmoreceptor.   The figure shows a hypothetical explanation of the workings of an osmoreceptor.

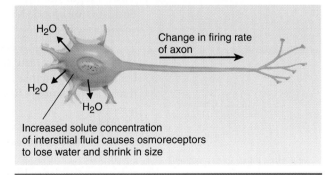

H_2O

Change in firing rate of axon

H_2O

H_2O

Increased solute concentration of interstitial fluid causes osmoreceptors to lose water and shrink in size

FIGURE 11.6

Osmometric Thirst in Humans. Functional MRI scans show brain activation produced by osmometric thirst: (a) Activation in the anterior cingulate cortex and hypothalamus, corresponding to a sensation of thirst; (b) Activation in the AV3V, the location of the brain's osmoreceptors.

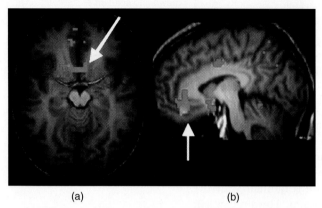

(a)   (b)

From Egan, G., Silk, T., Zamarripa, F., et al. *Proceedings of the National Academy of Science, USA*, 2004, *100*, 15241–15246. Reprinted with permission.

into the blood plasma; hence, the blood plasma becomes hypertonic. This condition draws water from the interstitial fluid, which makes this compartment become hypertonic too and thus causes water to leave the cells. As the blood plasma increases in volume, the kidneys begin excreting large amounts of both sodium and water. Eventually, the excess sodium is excreted, along with the water that was taken from the interstitial and intracellular fluid. The net result is a loss of water from the cells. *At no time does the volume of the blood plasma fall.*

Most researchers now believe that osmoreceptors responsible for osmometric thirst are located in the region of the anterior hypothalamus that borders the anteroventral tip of the third ventricle (the *AV3V*). Buggy et al. (1979) found that injections of hypertonic saline directly into this region produced drinking.

A functional imaging study by Egan et al. (2003) found that the human AV3V also appears to contain osmoreceptors. The investigators administered intravenous injections of hypertonic saline to normal subjects while their brain were being scanned. They observed strong activation of several brain regions, including the AV3V and the anterior cingulate cortex. When the subjects were permitted to drink water, they did so and almost immediately reported that their thirst had been satisfied. Simultaneously, the activity in the anterior cingulate cortex returned to baseline values. However, the activity in the AV3V remained high. These results suggest that the activity of the anterior cingulate cortex reflected the subjects' thirst, which was immediately relieved by a drink of water. (As we saw in Chapter 7, activity of this region is related to people's perception of the unpleasantness of painful stimuli.) In contrast, the continued activity in the AV3V reflected the fact that the blood plasma was still hypertonic. After all, it takes around 20 minutes for a drink of water to be absorbed into the general circulation. As we saw in the discussion of Figure 11.2, satiety is an anticipatory mechanism, triggered by the act of drinking. The fall in the activity of the anterior cingulate cortex appears to reflect the activation of this satiety mechanism. (See *Figure 11.6.*)

Volumetric Thirst

Volumetric thirst occurs when the volume of the blood plasma—the intravascular volume—decreases. As we saw earlier, when we lose water through evaporation, we lose it from all three fluid compartments: intracellular, interstitial, and intravascular. Thus, evaporation produces both volumetric thirst and osmometric thirst. In addition, loss of blood, vomiting, and diarrhea all cause loss of blood volume (hypovolemia) without depleting the intracellular fluid.

Loss of blood causes pure volumetric thirst. From the earliest recorded history, reports of battles note that the wounded survivors called out for water. In addition, because hypovolemia involves a loss of sodium as well as water (that is, the sodium that was contained in the isotonic fluid that was lost), volumetric thirst leads to a salt appetite.

What detectors are responsible for initiating volumetric thirst and a salt appetite? There are two sets of receptors that accomplish this dual function: one set in the kidneys, which controls the production of angiotensin, and one set in the heart and large blood vessels (atrial baroreceptors).

volumetric thirst Thirst produced by hypovolemia.

The Role of Angiotensin   The kidneys contain cells that are able to detect decreases in the flow of blood to the kidneys. The usual cause of a reduced flow of blood is a loss of blood volume; thus, these cells detect the presence of hypovolemia. When the flow of blood to the kidneys decreases, these cells secrete an enzyme called **renin**. Renin enters the blood, where it catalyzes the conversion of a protein called *angiotensinogen* into a hormone called **angiotensin**. In fact, there are two forms of angiotensin. Angiotensinogen becomes angiotensin I, which is quickly converted by an enzyme to angiotensin II. The active form is angiotensin II, which I shall abbreviate as *AII*.

AII has several physiological effects: It stimulates the secretion of hormones by the posterior pituitary gland and the adrenal cortex that cause the kidneys to conserve water and sodium, and it increases blood pressure by causing muscles in the small arteries to contract. In addition, AII has two behavioral effects: It initiates both drinking and a salt appetite. Therefore, a reduction in the flow of blood to the kidneys causes water and sodium to be retained by the body, helps to compensate for their loss by reducing the size of the blood vessels, and encourages the animal to find and ingest both water and salt. (See *Figure 11.7.*)

FIGURE 11.7

Detection of Hypovolemia by the Kidney and the Renin–Angiotensin System

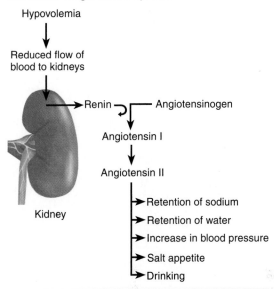

Little Billy started eating salt. He had always liked plenty of salt on his food, but his craving finally got out of hand. His mother noticed that a carton of salt lasted only a few days, and one afternoon she caught Billy in the kitchen with the container of salt on the counter next to him, eating something out of his hand. It was salt, pure salt! She grabbed his hand and shook the salt out of it into the sink and then put the container on a shelf where Billy couldn't reach it. Billy started crying and said, "Mommy, don't take it away—I need that!"

The next morning she heard a crash in the kitchen and found Billy on the floor, an overturned chair next to him. Clearly, he was trying to get at the salt. "What's wrong with you?" she cried. Billy sobbed and said, "Please, Mommy, I need some salt! I need it!" Bewildered but moved by his distress, she reached down the container and poured some salt in his hand, which he ate eagerly.

After consulting with the family physician, Billy's parents decided to have him admitted to the hospital, where his bizarre craving could be investigated. Although Billy cried piteously that he needed salt, the hospital staff made sure that he received no more than a child normally needs. He tried several times to leave his room, presumably to try to find some salt, but he was brought back, and the door to his room was finally locked. Unfortunately, before definitive testing could be begun, Billy died.

The diagnosis of Billy's craving came too late to help him. A disease process had caused his adrenal glands to stop secreting aldosterone, a steroid hormone that stimulates the kidneys to retain sodium. Without this hormone, excessive amounts of sodium are excreted by the kidneys, which causes the volume of the blood to fall. In Billy's case the fall in blood volume that occurred when his access to salt was blocked led to a fatal loss of blood pressure. This unhappy story occurred several decades ago, and we can hope that physicians today would recognize an intense salt craving as a cardinal symptom of adrenal insufficiency.

renin (*ree nin*) A hormone secreted by the kidneys that causes the conversion of angiotensinogen in the blood into angiotensin.

angiotensin (*ann gee oh ten sin*) A peptide hormone that constricts blood vessels, causes the retention of sodium and water, and produces thirst and a salt appetite.

subfornical organ (SFO) A small organ located in the confluence of the lateral ventricles, attached to the underside of the fornix; contains neurons that detect the presence of angiotensin in the blood and excite neural circuits that initiate drinking.

median preoptic nucleus A small nucleus situated around the front of the anterior commissure; plays a role in thirst stimulated by angiotensin.

Angiotensin acts on neurons found in one of the organs of the brain located outside the blood–brain barrier, the **subfornical organ (SFO)** (Phillips and Felix, 1976; Simpson, Epstein, and Camardo, 1978). This structure gets its name from its location, just below the commissure of the ventral fornix. Neurons in the SFO send their axons to the **median preoptic nucleus** (not to be confused with

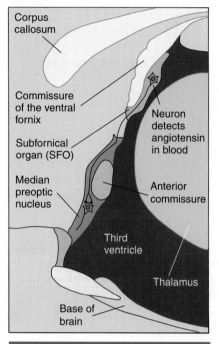

FIGURE 11.8

The Subfornical Organ. This sagittal section of the rat diencephalon shows the location of the subfornical organ and its connection with the median preoptic nucleus.

Corpus callosum

Commissure of the ventral fornix

Subfornical organ (SFO)

Median preoptic nucleus

Neuron detects angiotensin in blood

Anterior commissure

Third ventricle

Thalamus

Base of brain

the *medial* preoptic nucleus), a small nucleus wrapped around the front of the anterior commissure, a fiber bundle that connects the amygdala and anterior temporal lobe. Neurons in the median preoptic nucleus then communicate with the motor systems involved in drinking. (See *Figure 11.8.*)

Atrial Baroreceptors   The second set of receptors for volumetric thirst lies within the heart. Physiologists had long known that the *atria* of the heart (the parts that receive blood from the veins) contain sensory neurons that detect stretch. (The term *baro-* comes from the Greek *baros,* "heavy," and refers to weight or pressure.) The atria are passively filled with blood being returned from the body by the veins. The more blood in the veins, the fuller the atria become just before each contraction of the heart. Thus, when the volume of the blood plasma falls, the atria become less full, and the stretch receptors within them will detect this change.

Fitzsimons and Moore-Gillon (1980) showed that information from these receptors can stimulate thirst. They operated on dogs and placed a small balloon in the inferior vena cava, the vein that brings blood from most of the body (excluding the head and arms) to the heart. When the balloon was inflated, it reduced the flow of blood to the heart and thus lowered the amount of blood that entered the right atrium. Within 30 minutes the dogs began to drink. Quillen, Keil, and Reid (1990) confirmed these results. They also found that when the nerves connecting the atrial baroreceptors with the brain were cut, animals drank much less water when the blood flow to their heart was temporarily reduced.

InterimSummary

Physiological Regulatory Mechanisms and Drinking

A regulatory system contains four features: a system variable (the variable that is regulated), a set point (the optimal value of the system variable), a detector to measure the system variable, and a correctional mechanism to change it. Physiological regulatory systems, such as control of body fluids and nutrients, require a satiety mechanism to anticipate the effects of the correctional mechanism, because the changes brought about by eating and drinking occur only after a considerable period of time.

The body contains three major fluid compartments: intracellular, interstitial, and intravascular. Sodium and water can easily pass between the intravascular fluid and the interstitial fluid, but sodium cannot penetrate the cell membrane. The solute concentration of the interstitial fluid must be closely regulated. If it becomes hypertonic, cells lose water; if it becomes hypotonic, they gain water. The volume of the intravascular fluid (blood plasma) must also be kept within bounds.

Osmometric thirst occurs when the interstitial fluid becomes hypertonic, drawing water out of cells. This event, which can be caused by evaporation of water from the body or by ingestion of a salty meal, is detected by osmoreceptors in the region of the anteroventral third ventricle (AV3V). Activation of these osmoreceptors stimulates drinking. Osmometric thirst activates the human AV3V, and the anterior cingulate cortex may be involved in sensations of thirst.

Volumetric thirst occurs along with osmometric thirst when the body loses fluid through evaporation. Pure volumetric thirst is caused by blood loss, vomiting, and diarrhea. One stimulus for volumetric thirst is provided by a fall in blood flow to the kidneys. This event triggers the secretion of renin, which converts plasma angiotensinogen to angiotensin I. Angiotensin I is subsequently converted to its active form, angiotensin II, which acts on neurons in the SFO and stimulates thirst. The hormone also increases blood pressure and stimulates the secretion of pituitary and adrenal hormones that inhibit the secretion of water and sodium by the kidneys and induce a sodium appetite. (Sodium is needed to help restore the plasma volume.) Volumetric drinking can also be stimulated by a set of baroreceptors in the atria of the heart that detect decreased blood volume and send this information to the brain.

Thought Questions

How do we know that we are thirsty? What does thirst feel like? It cannot simply be a dry mouth or throat, because a real thirst is not quenched by taking a small sip of water, which moistens the mouth and throat as well as a big drink does.

Eating: Some Facts About Metabolism

Clearly, eating is one of the most important things we do, and it can also be one of the most pleasurable. Much of what an animal learns to do is motivated by the constant struggle to obtain food; therefore, the need to ingest undoubtedly shaped the evolutionary development of our own species. After having read the first part of this chapter, in which you saw that the signals that cause thirst are well understood, you might be surprised to learn that researchers are only now discovering what the system variables for hunger are. Control of ingestive behavior is even more complicated than the control of drinking and sodium intake. We can achieve water balance by the intake of two ingredients: water and sodium chloride. When we eat, we must obtain adequate amounts of carbohydrates, fats, amino acids, vitamins, and minerals other than sodium. Therefore, our food-ingestive behaviors are more complex, as are the physiological mechanisms that control them.

To stay alive, our cells must be supplied with fuel and oxygen. Obviously, fuel comes from the digestive tract, and its presence there is a result of eating. However, the digestive tract is sometimes empty; in fact, most of us wake up in the morning in that condition, so there has to be a reservoir that stores nutrients to keep the cells of the body nourished when the gut is empty. Indeed, there are two reservoirs: one short term and the other long term. The short-term reservoir stores carbohydrates, and the long-term reservoir stores fats.

The short-term reservoir is located in the cells of the liver and the muscles, and it is filled with a complex, insoluble carbohydrate called **glycogen**. For simplicity I will consider only one of these locations: the liver. Cells in the liver convert glucose (a simple, soluble carbohydrate) into glycogen and store the glycogen. They are stimulated to do so by the presence of **insulin**, a peptide hormone produced by the pancreas. Thus, when glucose and insulin are present in the blood, some of the glucose is used as a fuel, and some of it is stored as glycogen. Later, when all of the food has been absorbed from the digestive tract, the level of glucose in the blood begins to fall.

The fall in glucose is detected by cells in the pancreas and in the brain. The pancreas responds by stopping its secretion of insulin and starting to secrete a different peptide hormone: **glucagon**. The effect of glucagon is opposite that of insulin: It stimulates the conversion of glycogen into glucose. (Unfortunately, the terms *glucose, glycogen,* and *glucagon* are similar enough that it is easy to confuse them. Even worse, you will soon encounter another one: *glycerol.*) (See **Figure 11.9.**) Thus, the liver soaks up excess glucose and stores it as glycogen when plenty of glucose is available, and it releases glucose from its reservoir when the digestive tract becomes empty and the level of glucose in the blood begins to fall.

The carbohydrate reservoir in the liver is reserved primarily for the central nervous system. When you wake in the morning, your brain is being fed by your liver, which is in the process of converting glycogen to glucose and releasing it into the blood. The glucose reaches the CNS, where it is absorbed and metabolized by the neurons and the glia. This process can continue for a few hours, until all of the carbohydrate reservoir in the liver is used up. (The average liver holds approximately 300 calories of carbohydrate.) Usually, we eat some food before this reservoir gets depleted, which permits us to refill it. But if we do not eat, the CNS has to start living on the products of the long-term reservoir.

Our long-term reservoir consists of adipose tissue (fat tissue). This reservoir is filled with fats, or, more precisely, with **triglycerides**. Triglycerides are complex molecules that contain **glycerol** (a soluble carbohydrate, also called *glycerine*) combined with three **fatty acids** (stearic acid, oleic acid, and

glycogen (*gly ko jen*) A polysaccharide often referred to as *animal starch;* stored in liver and muscle; constitutes the short-term store of nutrients.

insulin A pancreatic hormone that facilitates entry of glucose and amino acids into the cell, conversion of glucose into glycogen, and transport of fats into adipose tissue.

glucagon (*gloo ka gahn*) A pancreatic hormone that promotes the conversion of liver glycogen into glucose.

triglyceride (*try gliss er ide*) The form of fat storage in adipose cells; consists of a molecule of glycerol joined with three fatty acids.

glycerol (*gliss er all*) A substance (also called glycerine) derived from the breakdown of triglycerides, along with fatty acids; can be converted by the liver into glucose.

fatty acid A substance derived from the breakdown of triglycerides, along with glycerol; can be metabolized by most cells of the body except for the brain.

FIGURE 11.9

Effects of Insulin and Glucagon on Glucose and Glycogen

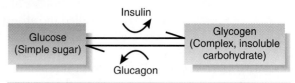

palmitic acid). Adipose tissue is found beneath the skin and in various locations in the abdominal cavity. It consists of cells that are capable of absorbing nutrients from the blood, converting them to triglycerides, and storing them. These cells can expand enormously in size; in fact, the primary physical difference between an obese person and a person of normal weight is the size of their fat cells, which is determined by the amount of triglycerides that these cells contain.

The long-term fat reservoir is obviously what keeps us alive when we are fasting. As we begin to use the contents of our short-term carbohydrate reservoir, fat cells start converting triglycerides into fuels that the cells can use and releasing these fuels into the bloodstream. As we just saw, when we wake in the morning with an empty digestive tract, our brain (in fact, all of the central nervous system) is living on glucose released by the liver. But what about the other cells of the body? They are living on fatty acids, sparing the glucose for the brain. As you will recall from Chapter 3, the sympathetic nervous system is primarily involved in the breakdown and utilization of stored nutrients. When the digestive system is empty, there is an increase in the activity of the sympathetic axons that innervate adipose tissue, the pancreas, and the adrenal medulla. All three effects (direct neural stimulation, secretion of glucagon, and secretion of catecholamines) cause triglycerides in the long-term fat reservoir to be broken down into glycerol and fatty acids. The fatty acids can be directly metabolized by cells in all of the body *except the brain*, which needs glucose. That leaves glycerol. The liver takes up glycerol and converts it to glucose. That glucose, too, is available to the brain.

You may be asking why the cells of the rest of the body treat the brain so kindly, letting it consume almost all the glucose that the liver releases from its carbohydrate reservoir and constructs from glycerol. The answer is simple: Insulin has several other functions besides causing glucose to be converted to glycogen. One of these functions is controlling the entry of glucose into cells. To be taken into a cell, glucose must be transported there by *glucose transporters*—protein molecules that are situated in the membrane and are similar to those responsible for the reuptake of transmitter substances. Glucose transporters contain insulin receptors, which control their activity; only when insulin binds with these receptors can glucose be transported into the cell. However, the cells of the nervous system are an exception to this rule. Their glucose transporters do not contain insulin receptors; thus, these cells can absorb glucose *even when insulin is not present.*

Figure 11.10 reviews what I have said so far about the metabolism that takes place while the digestive tract is empty, which physiologists refer to as the **fasting phase** of metabolism. A fall in the blood glucose level causes the pancreas to stop secreting insulin and to start secreting glucagon. The absence of insulin means that most of the cells of the body can no longer use glucose; thus, all the glucose present in the blood is reserved for the central nervous system. The presence of glucagon and the absence of insulin instructs the liver to start drawing on the short-term carbohydrate reservoir—to start converting its glycogen into glucose. The presence of glucagon and the absence of insulin, along with increased activity of the sympathetic nervous system, also instruct fat cells to start drawing on the long-term fat reservoir—to start breaking down triglycerides into fatty acids and glycerol. Most of the body lives on the fatty acids, and the glycerol, which is converted into glucose by the liver, gets used by the brain. If fasting is prolonged, proteins (especially protein found in muscle) will be broken down to amino acids, which can be metabolized by all of the body except the central nervous system. (See *Figure 11.10* and *MyPsychKit 11.1, Metabolism* .)

The phase of metabolism that occurs when food is present in the digestive tract is called the **absorptive phase**. Now that you understand the fasting phase, this one is simple. Suppose that we eat a balanced meal of carbohydrates, proteins, and fats. The carbohydrates are broken down into glucose, and the proteins are broken down into amino acids. The fats basically remain as fats. Let us consider each of these three nutrients.

fasting phase The phase of metabolism during which nutrients are not available from the digestive system; glucose, amino acids, and fatty acids are derived from glycogen, protein, and adipose tissue during this phase.

absorptive phase The phase of metabolism during which nutrients are absorbed from the digestive system; glucose and amino acids constitute the principal source of energy for cells during this phase, and excess nutrients are stored in adipose tissue in the form of triglycerides.

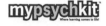

Animation 11.1
Metabolism

FIGURE 11.10

Metabolic Pathways During the Fasting Phase and Absorptive Phase of Metabolism

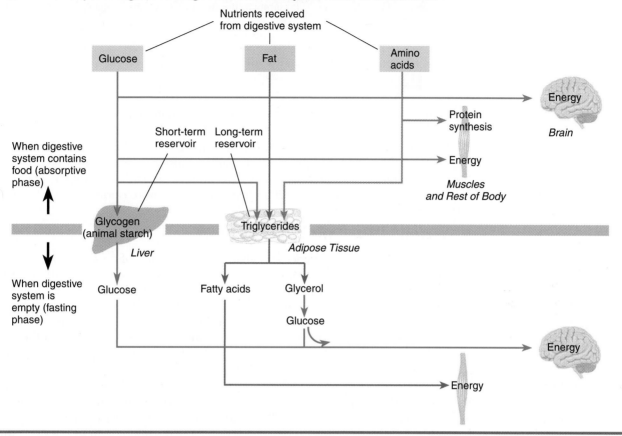

1. As we start absorbing the nutrients, the level of glucose in the blood rises. This rise is detected by cells in the brain, which causes the activity of the sympathetic nervous system to decrease and the activity of the parasympathetic nervous system to increase. This change tells the pancreas to stop secreting glucagon and to begin secreting insulin. The insulin permits all the cells of the body to use glucose as a fuel. Extra glucose is converted into glycogen, which fills the short-term carbohydrate reservoir. If some glucose is left over, it is converted into fat and absorbed by fat cells.
2. A small proportion of the amino acids received from the digestive tract are used as building blocks to construct proteins and peptides; the rest are converted to fats and stored in adipose tissue.
3. Fats are not used at this time; they are simply stored in adipose tissue. (See *Figure 11.10.*)

InterimSummary

Eating: Some Facts About Metabolism

Metabolism consists of two phases. During the absorptive phase we receive glucose, amino acids, and fats from the intestines. The blood level of insulin is high, which permits all cells to metabolize glucose. In addition, the liver and the muscles convert glucose to glycogen, which replenishes the short-term reservoir. Excess carbohydrates and amino acids are converted to fats, and fats are placed into the long-term reservoir in the adipose tissue.

During the fasting phase the activity of the parasympathetic nervous system falls, and the activity of the sympathetic nervous system increases. In response, the level of insulin falls, and the levels of glucagon and the adrenal catecholamines rise. These events cause liver glycogen to be converted to glucose and triglycerides to be broken down into glycerol and fatty acids. In the absence of insulin, only the central nervous system can use the glucose that is available in the blood; the rest of the body lives on fatty acids. Glycerol is converted to glucose by the liver, and the glucose is metabolized by the brain.

What Starts a Meal?

Regulation of body weight requires a balance between food intake and energy expenditure. If we ingest more calories than we burn, we will gain weight. Assuming that our energy expenditure is constant, we need two mechanisms to maintain a relatively constant body weight. One mechanism must increase our motivation to eat if our long-term nutrient reservoir is becoming depleted, and another mechanism must restrain our food intake if we begin to take in more calories than we need.

Signals from the Environment

The environment of our ancestors shaped the evolution of these regulatory mechanisms. In the past, starvation was a much greater threat to survival than overeating was. In fact, a tendency to overeat in times of plenty provided a reserve that could be drawn upon if food became scarce again—which it often did. A feast-or-famine environment favored the evolution of mechanisms that were quick to detect losses from the long-term reservoir and provide a strong signal to seek and eat food. Natural selection for mechanisms that detected weight gain and suppressed overeating was much less significant.

The answer to the question posed by the title of this section, "What starts a meal?" is not simple. Most people, if they were asked why they eat, would say that they do so because they get hungry. By that they probably mean that something happens inside their body that provides a sensation that makes them want to eat. But if this is true, just what is happening inside our bodies? The factors that motivate us to eat when food is readily available are very different from those that motivate us when food is scarce. When food is plentiful, we tend to eat when our stomach and upper intestine are empty. This emptiness provides a hunger signal—a message to our brain that indicates that we should begin to eat. The time it takes for food to leave our stomach would seem to encourage the establishment of a pattern of eating three meals a day. In addition, our ancestors undoubtedly found it most practical to prepare food for a group of people and have everyone eat at the same time. Most modern-day work schedules follow this routine as well.

Although an empty stomach is an important signal, many factors start a meal, including the sight of a plate of food, the smell of food cooking in the kitchen, the presence of other people sitting around the table, or the words "It's time to eat!" I am writing this in the late afternoon. I am anticipating a tasty meal this evening and look forward to eating it. I don't feel particularly hungry, but I like good food and expect to enjoy my dinner. My short-term and long-term nutrient reservoirs are well stocked, so my motivation to eat will not be based upon a physiological need for nourishment.

Signals from the Stomach

As we just saw, an empty stomach and upper intestine provide an important signal to the brain that it is time to start thinking about finding something to eat. Recently, researchers discovered one of the ways this signal may be communicated to the brain. The gastrointestinal system (especially the stomach) releases a peptide hormone called **ghrelin** (Kojima et al., 1999). The name *ghrelin* is a contraction

ghrelin (*grell in*) A peptide hormone released by the stomach that increases eating; also produced by neurons in the brain.

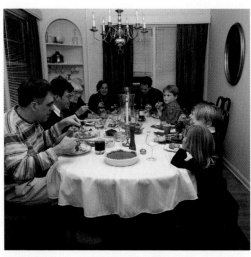

Social factors, and not just physiological ones, affect when and how much we eat.

of *GH releasin*, which reflects the fact that this peptide is involved in controlling the release of growth hormone, usually abbreviated as *GH*. Researchers have discovered that blood levels of this peptide increase with fasting and are reduced after a meal. In humans, blood levels of ghrelin increase shortly before each meal, which suggests that this peptide is involved in the initiation of a meal. (See *Figure 11.11*.) Ghrelin is a potent stimulator of food intake, and it even stimulates thoughts about food. Schmid et al. (2005) found that a single intravenous injection of ghrelin not only enhanced appetite in normal subjects, it also elicited vivid images of foods that the subjects liked to eat. Subcutaneous injection or infusion of ghrelin into the cerebral ventricles of laboratory animals causes weight gain by increasing food intake and decreasing the metabolism of fats (Tschöp, Smiley, and Heiman, 2000; Ariyasu et al., 2001; Bagnasco et al., 2003).

What controls ghrelin secretion? Secretion of this hormone is suppressed when an animal eats or when an experimenter infuses food into the animal's stomach. Injections of nutrients into the blood do *not* suppress ghrelin secretion, so the release of the hormone is controlled by the contents of the digestive system and not by the availability of nutrients in the blood (Schaller et al., 2003). In fact, the entry of food into the upper part of the small intestine—the **duodenum**—suppresses ghrelin secretion (Overduin et al., 2004). Thus, although the stomach secretes ghrelin, the secretion of this hormone appears to be controlled by receptors present in the upper part of the small intestine, not in the stomach itself. (If you're interested, the original Greek name for the duodenum was *dodekadaktulon*, or "twelve fingers long." More precisely, the duodenum is twelve finger *widths* long.)

Although ghrelin is an important short-term hunger signal, it clearly cannot be the only one. For example, people with successful gastric bypass surgery have almost negligible levels of ghrelin in the blood. Although they eat less and lose weight, they certainly do not stop eating. In addition, mice with a targeted mutation against the ghrelin gene or the ghrelin receptor have normal food intake and body weight (Sun, Ahmed, and Smith, 2003; Sun et al., 2004). However, Zigman et al. (2005) found that this mutation protected mice from overeating and gaining weight when fed a tasty high-fat diet that induces obesity in normal mice. Thus, alternative mechanisms can stimulate feeding which, given the vital importance of food, is not surprising. In fact, one of the factors that complicates research on ingestive behavior is the presence of redundant systems.

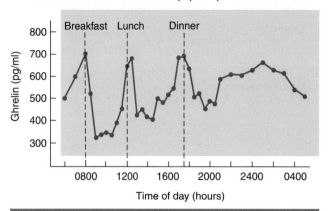

FIGURE 11.11

Levels of Ghrelin in Human Blood Plasma. The graph shows that a rise in the level of this peptide preceded each meal.

Adapted from Cummings, D. E., Purnell, J. Q., Frayo, R. S., et al. *Diabetes*, 2001, *50*, 1714–1719.

Metabolic Signals

Most of the time, we begin a meal a few hours after the previous meal, so our nutrient reservoirs are seldom in serious need of replenishment. But if we skip several meals, we get hungrier and hungrier, presumably because of physiological signals indicating that we have been withdrawing nutrients from our long-term reservoir. What happens to the level of nutrients in our body as time passes after a meal? As you learned earlier in this chapter, during the absorptive phase of metabolism we live on food that is being absorbed from the digestive tract. After that we start drawing on our nutrient reservoirs: The brain lives on glucose, and the rest of the body lives on fatty acids. Although the metabolic needs of the cells of the body are being met, we are taking fuel out of our long-term reservoir—making withdrawals rather than deposits. Clearly, this is the time to start thinking about our next meal.

A fall in blood glucose level (a condition known as *hypoglycemia*) is a potent stimulus for hunger. Hypoglycemia can be produced experimentally by giving an animal a large injection of insulin, which causes cells in the liver, muscles, and adipose

duodenum (*doo oh dee num*) The first portion of the small intestine, attached directly to the stomach.

glucoprivation A dramatic fall in the level of glucose available to cells; can be caused by a fall in the blood level of glucose or by drugs that inhibit glucose metabolism.

lipoprivation A dramatic fall in the level of fatty acids available to cells; usually caused by drugs that inhibit fatty acid metabolism.

hepatic portal vein The vein that transports blood from the digestive system to the liver.

tissue to take up glucose and store it away. We can also deprive cells of glucose by injecting an animal with a drug that interferes with the metabolism of glucose. Both of these treatments cause **glucoprivation**; that is, they deprive cells of glucose and glucoprivation, whatever its cause, stimulates eating. Hunger can also be produced by causing **lipoprivation**—depriving cells of lipids. More precisely, they are deprived of the ability to metabolize fatty acids through an injection of a drug that interferes with this process.

What is the nature of the detectors that monitor the level of metabolic fuels, and where are these detectors located? The evidence that has been gathered so far indicates that there are two sets of detectors: one set located in the brain and the other set located in the liver.

Let's first review the evidence for the detectors in the liver. A study by Novin, VanderWeele, and Rezek (1973) suggested that receptors in the liver can stimulate glucoprivic hunger; when these neurons are deprived of nutrients, they cause eating. The investigators infused 2-DG into the **hepatic portal vein**. This vein brings blood from the intestines to the liver; thus, an injection of a drug into this vein (an *intraportal* infusion) delivers it directly to the liver. (See *Figure 11.12.*) The investigators found that when they infused a drug that interferes with glucose metabolism into the hepatic portal vein, the animals immediately started eating. When the investigators cut the vagus nerve, which connects the liver with the brain, the infusions no longer stimulated eating. Thus, the brain receives the hunger signal through the vagus nerve.

Now let's look at some of the evidence that indicates that the brain has its own nutrient detectors. Because the brain can use only glucose, it would make sense that these detectors respond to glucoprivation—and, indeed, they do. Ritter, Dinh, and Zhang (2000) found that injections of a drug that interferes with glucose metabolism into the medulla induced eating. The role of the medulla in control of food intake and metabolism is discussed later in this chapter.

Liproprivic hunger appears to be stimulated by receptors in the liver. Ritter and Taylor (1990) induced liproprivic hunger and found that cutting the vagus nerve abolished this hunger. Thus, the liver appears to contain receptors that detect low availability of glucose or fatty acids (glucoprivation or lipoprivation) and send this information to the brain through the vagus nerve (Friedman, Horn, and Ji, 2005).

To summarize: The brain contains detectors that monitor the availability of glucose (its only fuel) inside the blood–brain barrier, and the liver contains detectors the monitor the availability of nutrients (glucose and fatty acids) outside the blood–brain barrier. (See *Figure 11.13.*)

FIGURE 11.12

The Hepatic Portal Blood Supply. The liver receives water, minerals, and nutrients from the digestive system through this blood supply.

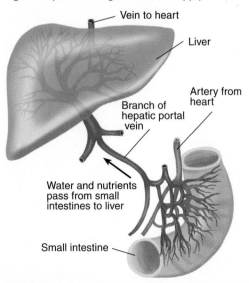

Vein to heart

Liver

Artery from heart

Branch of hepatic portal vein

Water and nutrients pass from small intestines to liver

Small intestine

FIGURE 11.13

Nutrient Receptors. The figure shows the probable location of nutrient receptors responsible for hunger signals.

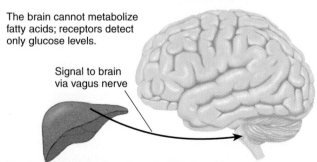

The brain cannot metabolize fatty acids; receptors detect only glucose levels.

Signal to brain via vagus nerve

The liver can metabolize glucose and fatty acids; receptors detect levels of both nutrients.

InterimSummary

What Starts a Meal?

Many stimuli, environmental and physiological, can initiate a meal. Natural selection has endowed us with strong mechanisms to encourage eating but weaker ones to prevent overeating and weight gain. Stimuli associated with eating—such as clocks indicating lunchtime or dinnertime, the smell or sight of food, or an empty stomach—increase appetite. Ghrelin, a peptide hormone released by the stomach when it and the upper intestine are empty, is a potent stimulator of food intake.

Studies with inhibitors of the metabolism of glucose and fatty acids indicate that low levels of both of these nutrients are involved in hunger; that is, animals will eat in response to both glucoprivation and lipoprivation. These signals are normally present only after several meals have been missed. Receptors in the liver detect both glucoprivation and lipoprivation and transmit this information to the brain through sensory axons of the vagus nerve. Glucoprivic eating can also be stimulated by interfering with glucose metabolism in the medulla; thus, the brain stem contains its own glucose-sensitive detectors.

What Stops a Meal?

There are two primary sources of satiety signals—the signals that stop a meal. Short-term satiety signals come from the immediate effects of eating a particular meal, which begin long before the food is digested. To search for these signals, we will follow the pathway traveled by ingested food: the stomach, the small intestine, and the liver. Each of these locations can potentially provide a signal to the brain that indicates that food has been ingested and is progressing on the way toward absorption. Long-term satiety signals arise in the adipose tissue, which contains the long-term nutrient reservoir. These signals do not control the beginning and end of a particular meal, but they do, in the long run, control the intake of calories by modulating the sensitivity of brain mechanisms to the hunger and satiety signals that they receive.

Gastric Factors

The stomach apparently contains receptors that can detect the presence of nutrients. Deutsch and Gonzalez (1980) found that when they removed food from the stomach of a rat that had just eaten all it wanted, the animal would immediately eat just enough food to replace what had been removed—even if the experimenters replaced the food with a nonnutritive saline solution. Obviously, the rats did not do so simply by measuring the volume of the food in their stomachs, because they were not fooled by the infusion of a saline solution. Of course, this study indicates only that the stomach contains nutrient receptors; it does not prove that there are not detectors in the intestines as well.

Intestinal Factors

Indeed, the intestines do contain nutrient detectors. Studies with rats have shown that afferent axons arising from the duodenum are sensitive to the presence of glucose, amino acids, and fatty acids (Ritter, Brener, and Yox, 1992). In fact, some of the chemoreceptors found in the duodenum are also found in the tongue. These axons may transmit a satiety signal to the brain.

Feinle, Grundy, and Read (1997) had people swallow an inflatable bag attached to the end of a thin, flexible tube. When the stomach and duodenum were empty, the subjects reported that they simply felt bloated when the bag was inflated, filling

FIGURE 11.14

Effects of PYY on Hunger.   The graph shows the amount of food (in kilocalories) eaten at a buffet meal 30 minutes after people received a 90-minute intravenous infusion of saline or PYY. Data points from each subject are connected by straight lines.

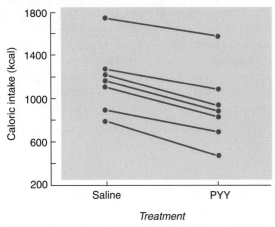

Data from Batterham, R. L., ffytche, D. H., Rosenthal, J. M., et al. *Nature*, 2007, *450*, 106–109.

the stomach. However, when fats or carbohydrates were infused into the duodenum while the bag was being inflated, the people reported sensations of fullness like those experienced after eating a meal. Thus, stomach and intestinal satiety factors can interact. That's not surprising, given the fact that by the time we finish a normal meal, our stomachs are full and a small quantity of nutrients has been received by the duodenum.

After food reaches the stomach, it is mixed with hydrochloric acid and pepsin, an enzyme that breaks proteins into their constituent amino acids. As digestion proceeds, food is gradually introduced from the stomach into the duodenum. There, the food is mixed with bile and pancreatic enzymes, which continue the digestive process. The duodenum controls the rate of stomach emptying by secreting a peptide hormone called **cholecystokinin (CCK)**. This hormone receives its name from the fact that it causes the gallbladder (cholecyst) to contract, injecting bile into the duodenum. (Bile breaks fats down into small particles so that they can be absorbed from the intestines.) CCK is secreted in response to the presence of fats, which are detected by receptors in the walls of the duodenum. In addition to stimulating contraction of the gallbladder, CCK causes the pylorus to constrict and inhibits gastric contractions, thus keeping the stomach from giving the duodenum more food.

Obviously, the blood level of CCK is related to the amount of nutrients (particularly fats) that the duodenum receives from the stomach. Thus, this hormone could potentially provide a satiety signal to the brain, telling it that the duodenum was receiving food from the stomach. Many studies have indeed found that injections of CCK suppress eating (Gibbs, Young, and Smith, 1973; Smith, Gibbs, and Kulkosky, 1982). CCK does not act directly on the brain; instead, it acts on receptors located in the junction between the stomach and the duodenum (Moran et al., 1989).

Investigators have discovered another chemical produced by cells in the gastrointestinal tract that serves as an additional satiety signal. This chemical, **peptide YY$_{3-36}$** (let's just call it **PYY**) is released after a meal in amounts proportional to the calories that were just ingested (Pedersen-Bjergaard et al., 1996). Only nutrients caused PYY to be secreted; a large drink of water had no effect. Injections of PYY significantly decreased the size of meals eaten by members of several species, including rats and humans (Batterham et al., 2002, 2007). (See *Figure 11.14.*)

Liver Factors

Satiety produced by gastric factors and duodenal factors is anticipatory; that is, these factors predict that the food in the digestive system will, when absorbed, eventually restore the system variables that cause hunger. Not until nutrients are absorbed from the intestines can they be used to nourish the cells of the body and replenish the body's nutrient reservoirs. The last stage of satiety appears to occur in the liver, which is the first organ to learn that food is finally being received from the intestines.

Evidence that nutrient detectors in the liver play a role in satiety comes from several sources. For example, Tordoff and Friedman (1988) infused small amounts of two nutrients, glucose and fructose, into the hepatic portal vein. The amounts they used were similar to those that are produced when a meal is being digested. The infusions "fooled" the liver; both nutrients reduced the amount of food that the rats ate. Fructose cannot cross the blood–brain barrier and is metabolized very poorly by cells in the rest of the body, but it can readily be metabolized by the liver. Therefore,

cholecystokinin (CCK) (*coal i sis toe ky nin*) A hormone secreted by the duodenum that regulates gastric motility and causes the gallbladder (cholecyst) to contract; appears to provide a satiety signal transmitted to the brain through the vagus nerve.

peptide YY$_{3-36}$ (PYY) A peptide released by the gastrointestinal system after a meal in amounts proportional to the size of the meal.

the signal from this nutrient must have originated in the liver. These results strongly suggest that when the liver receives nutrients from the intestines, it sends a signal to the brain that produces satiety. More accurately, the signal *continues* the satiety that was already started by signals arising from the stomach and upper intestine.

Insulin

As you will recall, the absorptive phase of metabolism is accompanied by an increased level of insulin in the blood. Insulin permits organs other than the brain to metabolize glucose, and it promotes the entry of nutrients into fat cells where they are converted into triglycerides. You will also recall that cells in the brain do not need insulin to metabolize glucose. Nevertheless, the brain contains insulin receptors (Unger et al., 1989). What purpose do these insulin receptors serve? The answer is that they appear to detect insulin present in the blood, which tells the brain that the body is probably in the absorptive phase of metabolism. Thus, insulin may serve as a satiety signal.

Insulin is a peptide and would not normally be admitted to the brain. However, a transport mechanism delivers it through the blood–brain barrier, and it reaches neurons in the hypothalamus that are involved in regulation of hunger and satiety. Infusion of insulin into the third ventricle inhibits eating and causes a loss of body weight (Woods et al., 1979). In addition, Brüning et al. (2000) prepared a mutation in mice that blocked the synthesis of insulin receptors in the brain without affecting their production elsewhere in the body. The mice became obese, especially when they were fed a tasty, high-fat diet, which would be expected if one of the factors that promotes satiety was absent.

FIGURE 11.15

Effects of Force Feeding.   After rats were fed an excess of their normal food intake, their subsequent food intake fell during the period of force feeding and recovered only when their body weight returned to normal.

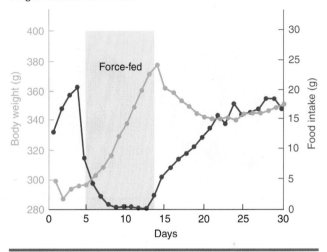

Adapted from Wilson, B. E., Meyer, G. E., Cleveland, J. C., and Weigle, D. S. *American Journal of Physiology*, 1990, *259*, R1148–R1155.

Long-Term Satiety: Signals from Adipose Tissue

So far, I have discussed short-term satiety factors—those arising from a single meal, but in most people, body weight appears to be regulated over a long-term basis. If an animal is force-fed so that it becomes fatter than normal, it will reduce its food intake once it is permitted to choose how much to eat (Wilson et al., 1990). (See *Figure 11.15*.) Similar studies have shown that an animal will adjust its food intake appropriately if it is given a high-calorie or low-calorie diet—and if an animal is put on a diet that reduces its body weight, short-term satiety factors become much less effective (Cabanac and Lafrance, 1991). Thus, signals arising from the long-term nutrient reservoir may alter the sensitivity of the brain to hunger signals or short-term satiety signals.

What exactly is the system variable that permits the body weight of most organisms to remain relatively stable? It seems highly unlikely that body *weight* itself is regulated; this variable would have to be measured by detectors in the soles of our feet or (for those of us who are sedentary) in the skin of our buttocks. What is more likely is that some variable related to body fat is regulated. The basic difference between obese and nonobese people is the amount of fat stored in their adipose tissue. Perhaps fat tissue provides a signal to the brain that indicates how much of it there is.

The discovery of a long-term satiety signal from fat tissue came after years of study with a strain of genetically obese mice. The **ob mouse** (as this strain is called)

ob mouse A strain of mice whose obesity and low metabolic rate are caused by a mutation that prevents the production of leptin.

FIGURE 11.16

Effects of Leptin on Obesity in Mice.   The ob (obese) strain mouse on the left is untreated; the one on the right received daily injections of leptin.

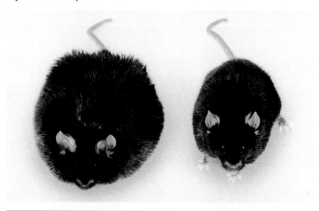

Photo courtesy of Dr. J. Sholtis, The Rockefeller University. Copyright © 1995 Amgen, Inc.

has a low metabolism, overeats, and gets exceedingly fat. It also develops diabetes in adulthood, just as many obese people do. Researchers in several laboratories reported the discovery of the cause of the obesity (Campfield et al., 1995; Halaas et al., 1995; Pelleymounter et al., 1995). A particular gene, called OB, normally produces a peptide that has been given the name **leptin** (from the Greek word *leptos,* "thin"). Leptin is normally secreted by well-nourished fat cells. Because of a genetic mutation, the fat cells of ob mice are unable to produce leptin.

Leptin has profound effects on metabolism and eating, acting as an antiobesity hormone. If ob mice are given daily injections of leptin, their metabolic rate increases, their body temperature rises, they become more active, and they eat less. As a result, their weight returns to normal. Figure 11.16 shows a picture of an untreated ob mouse and an ob mouse that has received injections of leptin. (See *Figure 11.16.*)

InterimSummary

What Stops a Meal?

Short-term satiety signals control the size of a meal. These signals include feedback from gastric factors that are activated by the entry of food into the stomach, from intestinal factors that are activated by the passage of food from the stomach into the duodenum, and from liver factors that are activated by the presence of newly digested nutrients in the blood carried by the hepatic portal artery.

The signals from the stomach include information about the volume and chemical nature of the food it contains. Another satiety signal from the intestine is provided by CCK, which is secreted by the duodenum when it receives food from the stomach. PYY, a peptide secreted after a meal by the intestines, also acts as a satiety signal. Another satiety signal comes from the liver, which detects nutrients being received from the intestines through the hepatic portal vein. Finally, moderately high levels of insulin in the blood, associated with the absorptive phase of metabolism, provide a satiety signal to the brain.

Signals arising from fat tissue affect food intake on a long-term basis, apparently by modulating the effectiveness of short-term hunger and satiety signals. Force-feeding facilitates satiety, and starvation inhibits it. Studies of the ob mouse led to the discovery of leptin, a peptide hormone secreted by well-nourished adipose tissue that increases an animal's metabolic rate and decreases food intake.

Thought Questions

1. Do you find hunger unpleasant? I find that when I'm looking forward to a meal I particularly like, I don't mind being hungry, knowing that I'll enjoy the meal that much more—but then, I've never gone without eating for several days.

2. The drive-reduction hypothesis of motivation and reinforcement says that drives are aversive and satiety is pleasurable. Clearly, *satisfying* hunger is pleasurable, but what about *satiety*? Which do you prefer, eating a meal while you are hungry or feeling full afterward?

Brain Mechanisms

Although hunger and satiety signals originate in the digestive system and in the body's nutrient reservoirs, the target of these signals is the brain. This section looks at some of the research on the brain mechanisms that control food intake and metabolism.

leptin A hormone secreted by adipose tissue; decreases food intake and increases metabolic rate, primarily by inhibiting NPY-secreting neurons in the arcuate nucleus.

Brain Stem

Ingestive behaviors are phylogenetically ancient; obviously, all our ancestors ate and drank or died. Therefore, we should expect that the basic ingestive behaviors of chewing and swallowing are programmed by phylogenetically ancient brain circuits. Indeed, studies have shown that these behaviors can be performed by decerebrate rats, whose brains were transected between the diencephalon and the midbrain (Norgren and Grill, 1982; Flynn and Grill, 1983; Grill and Kaplan, 1990). **Decerebration** disconnects the motor neurons of the brain stem and spinal cord from the neural circuits of the cerebral hemispheres (such as the cerebral cortex and basal ganglia) that normally control them. The only behaviors that decerebrate animals can display are those that are directly controlled by neural circuits located within the brain stem. (See *Figure 11.17*.)

Decerebrate rats cannot approach and eat food; the experimenters must place food, in liquid form, into their mouths. Decerebrate rats can distinguish between different tastes; they drink and swallow sweet or slightly salty liquids and spit out bitter ones. They even respond to hunger and satiety signals. They drink more sucrose after having been deprived of food for 24 hours, and they drink less of it if some sucrose is first injected directly into their stomachs. They also eat in response to glucoprivation. These studies indicate that the brain stem contains neural circuits that can detect hunger and satiety signals and control at least some aspects of food intake.

Two regions of the medulla, the *area postrema* and the *nucleus of the solitary tract* (henceforth referred to as the AP/NST), receive taste information from the tongue and a variety of sensory information from the internal organs, including signals from detectors in the stomach, duodenum, and liver. In addition, this region contains a set of detectors that are sensitive to the brain's own fuel: glucose. All this information is transmitted to regions of the forebrain that are more directly involved in control of eating and metabolism. Evidence indicates that events that produce hunger increase the activity of neurons in the AP/NST. In addition, lesions of this region abolish both glucoprivic and lipoprivic feeding (Ritter and Taylor, 1990; Ritter, Dinh, and Friedman, 1994).

Hypothalamus

Discoveries made in the 1940s and 1950s focused the attention of researchers interested in ingestive behavior on two regions of the hypothalamus: the lateral area and the ventromedial area. For many years investigators believed that these two regions controlled hunger and satiety, respectively; one was the accelerator, and the other was the brake. The basic findings were these: After the lateral hypothalamus was destroyed, animals stopped eating or drinking (Anand and Brobeck, 1951; Teitelbaum and Stellar, 1954). Electrical stimulation of the same region would produce eating, drinking, or both behaviors. Conversely, lesions of the ventromedial hypothalamus produced overeating that led to gross obesity, whereas electrical stimulation suppressed eating (Hetherington and Ranson, 1942).

Role in Hunger

Research in the last decade has discovered several peptides produced by neurons in the hypothalamus that play a special role in the control of feeding and metabolism (Arora and Anubhuti, 2006). Two of these peptides, **melanin-concentrating hormone (MCH)** and **orexin**, produced by neurons in the lateral hypothalamus, stimulate hunger and decrease metabolic rate, thus increasing and preserving the body's energy stores.

Decerebration. The operation disconnects the forebrain from the hindbrain so that the muscles involved in ingestive behavior are controlled solely by hindbrain mechanisms.

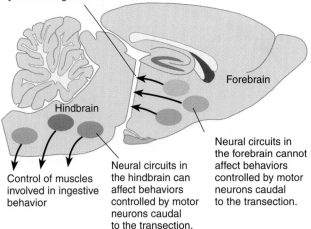

Decerebration is accomplished by transecting the brain stem.

Forebrain

Hindbrain

Control of muscles involved in ingestive behavior

Neural circuits in the hindbrain can affect behaviors controlled by motor neurons caudal to the transection.

Neural circuits in the forebrain cannot affect behaviors controlled by motor neurons caudal to the transection.

decerebration A surgical procedure that severs the brain stem, disconnecting the hindbrain from the forebrain.

melanin-concentrating hormone (MCH) One of two peptide neurotransmitters found in a system of lateral hypothalamic neurons that stimulate appetite and reduce metabolic rate.

orexin One of two peptide neurotransmitters found in a system of lateral hypothalamic neurons that stimulate appetite and reduce metabolic rate. Also called hypocretin.

FIGURE 11.18

Feeding Circuits in the Brain.   This schematic diagram shows connections of the MCH neurons and orexin neurons of the lateral hypothalamus.

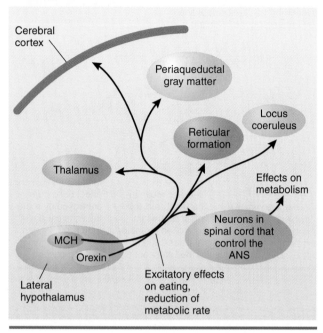

Melanin-concentrating hormone received its name from its role in regulating changes in skin pigmentation in fish and other nonmammalian vertebrates (Kawauchi et al., 1983). In mammals it serves as a neurotransmitter. Orexin (from the Greek word *orexis*, "desire, appetite") was discovered by Sakurai et al. (1998). (This peptide is also known as *hypocretin*.) As we saw in Chapter 8, degeneration of neurons that secrete orexin is responsible for narcolepsy. Evidence reviewed there indicates that it plays a role in keeping the brain's sleep–waking switch in the "waking" position.

Researchers refer to MCH and orexin as *orexigens*, "appetite-inducing chemicals." Injections of either of these peptides into the lateral ventricles or various regions of the brain induce eating. If rats are deprived of food, production of MCH and orexin in the lateral hypothalamus increases (Qu et al., 1996; Sakurai et al., 1998; Dube, Kalra, and Kalra, 1999). Of these two orexigenic hypothalamic peptides, MCH appears to play the more important role in stimulating feeding. Mice with a targeted mutation against the MCH gene eat less than normal mice and are consequently underweight (Shimada et al., 1998), and genetically engineered mice with increased production of MCH in the hypothalamus overeat and gain weight (Ludwig et al., 2001).

The axons of MCH and orexin neurons travel to a variety of brain structures that are known to be involved in motivation and movement, including the neocortex, periaqueductal gray matter, reticular formation, thalamus, and locus coeruleus. These neurons also have connections with neurons in the spinal cord that control the autonomic nervous system, which explains how they can affect the body's metabolic rate (Sawchenko, 1998; Nambu et al., 1999). These connections are shown in ***Figure 11.18***.

As we saw earlier, hunger signals caused by an empty stomach or by glucoprivation or lipoprivation arise from detectors in the abdominal cavity and brain stem. How do these signals activate the MCH and orexin neurons of the lateral hypothalamus? Part of the pathway involves a system of neurons that secrete a neurotransmitter called **neuropeptide Y (NPY)**, an extremely potent stimulator of food intake (Clark et al., 1984). Infusion of NPY into the hypothalamus produces ravenous, almost frantic eating.

The cell bodies of most of the neurons that secrete NPY are found in the **arcuate nucleus**, located in the hypothalamus at the base of the third ventricle. The arcuate nucleus also contains neurosecretory cells whose hormones control the secretions of the anterior pituitary gland. (Refer to ***Figure 11.19***.) Neurons that secrete NPY are affected by hunger and satiety signals; Sahu, Kalra, and Kalra (1988) found that hypothalamic levels of NPY are increased by food deprivation and lowered by eating. Glucose-sensitive neurons in the medulla also activate NPY neurons. Sindelar et al. (2004) found that in normal mice, glucoprivation caused an increase in NPY production. They also found that mice with a targeted mutation against the gene for NPY showed a feeding deficit in response to glucoprivation.

As we saw earlier, ghrelin, released by the stomach, provides a potent hunger signal to the brain. Shuto et al. (2002) found that rats with a genetic alteration that prevents ghrelin receptors from being produced in the hypothalamus ate less and gained weight more slowly than normal rats did. Evidence indicates the that ghrelin receptors that stimulate eating are located on NPY neurons (Willesen, Kristensen, and Romer, 1999; Nakazato et al., 2001; Van den Top et al., 2004). Thus, two im-

neuropeptide Y (NPY) A peptide neurotransmitter found in a system of neurons of the arcuate nucleus that stimulate feeding, insulin and glucocorticoid secretion, decrease the breakdown of triglycerides, and decrease body temperature.

arcuate nucleus A nucleus in the base of the hypothalamus that controls secretions of the anterior pituitary gland; contains NPY-secreting neurons involved in feeding and control of metabolism.

portant hunger signals—glucoprivation and ghrelin—activate the orexigenic NPY neurons.

Through what neural circuits does NPY exert its effects on eating and metabolic functions? NPY neurons of the arcuate nucleus send a projection directly to the MCH and orexin neurons in the lateral hypothalamus that stimulate eating (Broberger et al., 1998; Elias et al., 1998a). In addition, NPY neurons send a projection of axons to the **paraventricular nucleus (PVN)**—a region of the hypothalamus where infusions of NPY affect metabolic functions (Bai et al., 1985).

The terminals of hypothalamic NPY neurons release another orexigenic peptide in addition to neuropeptide Y: **agouti-related peptide**, otherwise known as **AGRP** (Hahn et al., 1998). AGRP, like NPY, is a potent and extremely long-lasting orexigen. Infusion of a very small amount of this peptide into the third ventricle of rats produces an increase in food intake that lasts for 6 days (Lu et al., 2001).

I should briefly mention one other category of orexigenic compounds: the endocannabinoids. (See Di Marzo and Matias, 2005, for a review of the evidence cited in this paragraph.) One of the effects of the THC contained in marijuana is an increase in appetite—especially for highly palatable foods. The endocannabinoids, whose actions are mimicked by THC, stimulate eating, apparently by increasing the release of MCH and orexin. (As you will recall from Chapter 4, cannabinoid receptors are found on terminal buttons, where they regulate the release of other neurotransmitters.) Levels of endocannabinoids are highest during fasting and lowest during feeding. A genetic mutation that disrupts the production of the enzyme that destroys the endocannabinoids after they have been released, causes overweight and obesity. Cannabinoid agonists have been used to increase the appetite of cancer patients, and cannabinoid antagonists have been used as an aid to weight reduction. (I will discuss this use later in this chapter, in the section on obesity.)

In summary, activity of MCH and orexin neurons of the lateral hypothalamus increases food intake and decreases metabolic rate. These neurons are activated by NPY/AGRP-secreting neurons of the arcuate nucleus, which also project to the paraventricular nucleus, which plays a role in control of insulin secretion and metabolism. The endocannabinoids stimulate appetite by increasing the release of MCH and orexin. (See *Figure 11.19*.)

Role in Satiety

As we saw earlier in this chapter, leptin, a hormone secreted by well-fed adipose tissue, suppresses eating and raises the animal's metabolic rate. The interactions of this long-term satiety signal with neural circuits involved in hunger are now being discovered. Leptin produces its behavioral and metabolic effects by binding with receptors in the brain—in particular, on neurons that secrete the orexigenic peptides NPY and AGRP.

Activation of leptin receptors found on NPY/AGRP-secreting neurons in the arcuate nucleus has an inhibitory effect on these neurons (Glaum et al., 1996; Jobst, Enriori, and Cowley, 2004). Because NPY/AGRP neurons normally activate orexin and MCH neurons, the presence of leptin in the arcuate nucleus decreases the release of these orexigens.

paraventricular nucleus (PVN) A nucleus of the hypothalamus located adjacent to the dorsal third ventricle; contains neurons involved in control of the autonomic nervous system and the posterior pituitary gland.

agouti-related protein (AGRP) A neuropeptide that acts as an antagonist at MC-4 receptors and increases eating.

FIGURE 11.19

Action of Hunger Signals on Feeding Circuits in the Brain. The diagram shows connections of the NPY neurons of the arcuate nucleus.

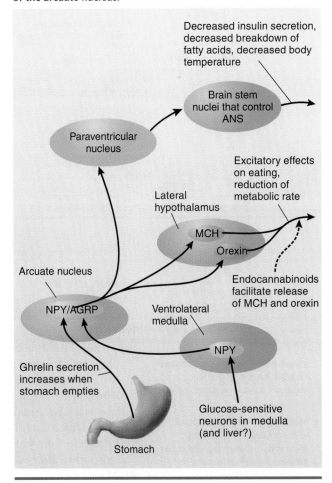

FIGURE 11.20

Action of Satiety Signals on Hypothalamic Neurons Involved in Control of Hunger and Satiety

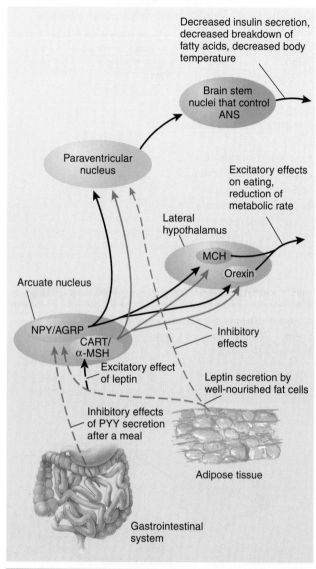

The arcuate nucleus contains two other systems of peptide-secreting neurons, both of which serve as *anorexigens* ("appetite-suppressing chemicals"). Douglass, McKinzie, and Couceyro (1995) discovered a peptide that is now called **CART** (for *cocaine- and amphetamine-regulated transcript*). When cocaine or amphetamine is administered to an animal, levels of this peptide increase, which may have something to do with the fact that these drugs suppress appetite. CART neurons appear to play an important role in satiety. If animals are deprived of food, levels of CART decrease. Injections of CART into their cerebral ventricles inhibit feeding, including the feeding stimulated by NPY, while infusion of a CART antibody increases feeding (Kristensen et al., 1998).

CART neurons are located in the arcuate nucleus and send their axons to a variety of locations (Koylu et al., 1998). In the context of the present topic, the most important connections are probably those with the paraventricular nucleus and those with the MCH and orexin neurons of the lateral hypothalamus. CART neurons increase metabolic rate through their connections with the paraventricular nucleus and appear to suppress eating by inhibiting MCH and orexin neurons. CART neurons contain leptin receptors that have an *excitatory* effect; thus, CART-secreting neurons appear to be responsible for at least part of the satiating effect of leptin (Elias et al., 1998b).

A second anorexigen, **α-melanocyte-stimulating hormone (α-MSH)**, is also released by CART neurons. This peptide is an agonist of the **melanocortin-4 receptor (MC-4R)**; it binds with the receptor and inhibits feeding. You will recall that NPY neurons also release AGRP, which stimulates eating. Both α-MSH and AGRP bind with the MC-4R. However, whereas AGRP binds with MC4 receptors and causes feeding (as we saw in the previous subsection), α-MSH binds with MC4 receptors and *inhibits* eating. CART/α-MSH neurons are activated by leptin, and NPY/AGRP neurons are inhibited by leptin. (See Elmquist, Elias, and Saper, 1999, and Wynne, Stanley, and McGowan, 2005, for specific references.) So leptin stimulates the release of the anorexigens CART and α-MSH and inhibits the release of the orexigens NPY and AGRP.

Earlier in this chapter, I mentioned an anorexigenic peptide, PYY, which is produced by cells in the gastrointestinal tract in amounts proportional to the calories that were just ingested. PYY binds with an inhibitory autoreceptor found on NPY/AGRP neurons in the arcuate nucleus of the hypothalamus. When PYY binds with this receptor, it suppresses the release of NPY and AGRP and suppresses food intake (Batterham et al., 2002).

In summary, leptin appears to exert at least some of its satiating effects by binding with receptors on neurons in the arcuate nucleus. Leptin inhibits NPY/AGRP neurons, which suppresses the feeding that these peptides stimulate and prevents the decrease in metabolic rate that they provoke. Leptin activates CART/α-MSH neurons, which then inhibit MCH and orexin neurons in the lateral hypothalamus and prevent their stimulatory effect on appetite. PYY, released by the gastrointestinal tract just after a meal, inhibits orexigenic NPY/AGRP neurons. (See *Figure 11.20*.)

CART Cocaine- and amphetamine-regulated transcript; a peptide neurotransmitter found in a system of neurons of the arcuate nucleus that inhibit feeding.

α-melanocyte-stimulating hormone (α-MSH) A neuropeptide that acts as an agonist at MC-4 receptors and inhibits eating.

melanocortin-4 receptor (MC-4R) A receptor found in the brain that binds with α-MSH and agouti-related protein; plays a role in control of appetite.

InterimSummary

Brain Mechanisms

The brain stem contains neural circuits that are able to control acceptance or rejection of sweet or bitter foods and can even be modulated by satiation or physiological hunger signals, such as a decrease in glucose metabolism or the presence of food in the digestive system. The area postrema and nucleus of the solitary tract and (AP/NST) receive signals from the tongue, stomach, small intestine, and liver and send the information on to many regions of the forebrain. These signals interact and help to control food intake. Lesions of the AP/NST disrupt both glucoprivic and lipoprivic eating.

The lateral hypothalamus contains two sets of neurons whose activity increases eating and decreases metabolic rate. These neurons secrete the peptides orexin and MCH (melanin-concentrating hormone). Food deprivation increases the level of these peptides, and mice with a targeted mutation against MCH undereat. The axons of these neurons project to regions of the brain involved in motivation, movement, and metabolism.

The release of neuropeptide Y in the lateral hypothalamus induces ravenous eating, an effect that is produced by excitatory connections of NPY-secreting neurons with the orexin and MCH neurons. NPY neurons in the hypothalamus receive input from glucose-sensitive neurons in the medulla. They are also activated by high blood levels of ghrelin. When NPY is infused in the paraventricular

nucleus, it decreases metabolic rate. Levels of NPY increase when an animal is deprived of food and fall again when the animal eats. NPY neurons also release a peptide called AGRP. This peptide serves as an antagonist at MC4 receptors and, like NPY, stimulates eating. Endocannabinoids, whose action is mimicked by THC, the active ingredient in marijuana, also stimulate eating, apparently by increasing the release of MCH and orexin.

Leptin, the long-term satiety hormone secreted by well-stocked adipose tissue, desensitizes the brain to hunger signals. It binds with receptors in the arcuate nucleus of the hypothalamus, where it inhibits NPY-secreting neurons, increasing metabolic rate and suppressing eating. The arcuate nucleus also contains neurons that secrete CART (cocaine- and amphetamine-regulated transcript), a peptide that suppresses eating. These neurons, which are *activated* by leptin, have inhibitory connections with MCH and orexin neurons in the lateral hypothalamus. CART neurons also secrete a peptide called α-MSH, which serves as an agonist at MC4 receptors and further inhibits eating. Ghrelin, which activates NPY/AGRP neurons and stimulates hunger, also inhibits CART/α-MSH neurons and suppresses the satiating effect of the peptides secreted by these neurons. The anorexigenic peptide, PYY, which is released by the gastrointestinal system, inhibits NPY neurons.

Obesity

Obesity is a widespread problem that can have serious medical consequences. In the United States, approximately 67 percent of men and 62 percent of women are overweight, defined as a body mass index (BMI) of over 25. In the past 20 years, the incidence of obesity, defined as a BMI of over 30, has doubled in the population as a whole, and has tripled for adolescents. Obesity is also increasing in developing countries as household incomes rise. For example, over a 10-year period, the incidence of obesity in young urban children in China increased by a factor of eight (Ogden, Carroll, and Flegal, 2003; Zorrilla et al., 2006). The known health hazards of obesity include cardiovascular disease, diabetes, stroke, arthritis, and some forms of cancer. One hundred years ago, type 2 diabetes was almost never seen in people before the age of 40. However, because of the increased incidence of obesity in children, this disorder is seen even in 10-year-old children. (See *Figure 11.21*.)

Possible Causes

What causes obesity? As we will see, genetic differences— and their effects on development of the endocrine

FIGURE 11.21

Obesity and Type 2 Diabetes.   The maps show the prevalence of obesity and type 2 ("adult onset") diabetes in the United States.

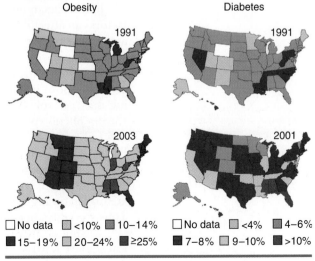

Based on data from the Centers for Disease Control and Prevention.

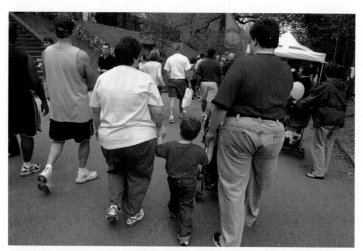

A greatly increased incidence of obesity has become a serious health problem, especially in industrialized societies. Presumably, the increase is a result of changes in lifestyle, including the ready availability of inexpensive high-calorie food.

system and brain mechanisms that control food intake and metabolism—appear to be responsible for the overwhelming majority of cases of extreme obesity. But as we just saw, the problem of obesity has been growing over recent years. Clearly, changes in the gene pool cannot account for this increase; instead, we must look to environmental causes that have produced changes in people's behavior.

Body weight is the result of the difference between two factors: calories consumed and energy expended. If we consume more calories than we expend as heat and work, we gain weight. If we expend more than we consume, we lose weight. In modern industrialized societies, inexpensive, convenient, good-tasting, high-fat food is readily available, which promotes an increase in intake. Fast-food restaurants are close at hand, parking is convenient (or even unnecessary at restaurants with drive-up windows), and the size of the portions they serve has increased in recent years. People eat out more often than they used to, and most often they do so at inexpensive fast-food restaurants.

Of course, fast-food restaurants are not the only environmental factor responsible for the increased incidence of obesity. Snack foods are available in convenience stores and vending machines, and even school cafeterias make high-calorie, high-fat foods and sweetened beverages available to their young students. In fact, school administrators often welcome the installation of vending machines because of the income they provide. As Bray, Nielsen, and Popkin (2004) point out, intake of high-fructose corn syrup, which is found in many prepared foods, including soft drinks, fruit drinks, flavored yogurts, and baked goods, may contribute to obesity. Fructose, unlike glucose, does not stimulate insulin secretion or enhance leptin production, so this form of sugar is less likely to activate the brain's satiety mechanisms. A 1994–1996 survey reported that the average daily consumption of fructose for an American over 2 years of age is approximately 318 kcal. Almost certainly, this figure is larger today (Nielsen, Siega-Riz, and Popkin, 2002).

Another modern trend that contributes to the obesity epidemic involves changes in people's expenditure of energy. The proportion of people employed in jobs that require a high level of physical activity has decreased considerably, which means that on the average we need less food than we did previously.

Just as cars differ in their fuel efficiency, so do living organisms, and hereditary factors can affect the level of efficiency. For example, farmers have bred cattle, pigs, and chickens for their efficiency in converting feed into muscle tissue, and researchers have done the same with rats (Pomp and Nielsen, 1999). People differ in this form of efficiency too. Those with an efficient metabolism have calories left over to deposit in the long-term nutrient reservoir; thus, they have difficulty keeping this reservoir from growing. Researchers have referred to this condition as a "thrifty phenotype." In contrast, people with an inefficient metabolism (a "spendthrift phenotype") can eat large meals without getting fat. A fuel-efficient automobile is desirable, but a fuel-efficient body runs the risk of becoming obese—at least in an environment where food is cheap and plentiful. Twin studies have found strong genetic effects on the amount of weight that people gain or lose when they are placed on high- or low-calorie diets (Bouchard et al., 1990; Hainer et al., 2001). Thus, heredity appears to affect people's metabolic efficiency.

The importance of heredity in metabolic efficiency is supported by epidemiological studies. Ravussin et al. (1994) studied two groups of Pima Indians, who live in the southwestern United States and northwestern Mexico. Members of the two groups appear to have the same genetic background; they speak the same language and have common historical traditions. The two groups separated 700–1000 years ago and now live under very different environmental conditions. The Pima Indians in the southwestern United States eat a high-fat American diet and weigh an average of 90 kg (198 lb), men and women combined. In contrast, the lifestyle of the Mexican Pimas is probably similar to that of their ancestors. They spend long hours working at subsistence farming and eat a low-fat diet—and weigh an average of 64 kg (141 lb). The cholesterol level of the American Pimas is much higher than that of the Mexican Pimas, and the American Pimas' rate of diabetes is more than five times higher. These findings show that genes that promote an efficient metabolism are of benefit to people who must work hard for their calories but that these same genes turn into a liability when people live in an environment where the physical demands are low and high-calorie food is cheap and plentiful.

As we saw earlier, study of the ob mouse led to the discovery of leptin, the hormone secreted by well-nourished adipose tissue. So far, researchers have found several cases of familial obesity caused by the absence of leptin produced by the mutation of the gene responsible for its production or the production of the leptin receptor (Farooqi and O'Rahilly, 2005). Treatment of leptin-deficient people with injections of leptin has dramatic effects on the people's body weights. (See *Figure 11.22.*) Unfortunately, leptin has no effect on people who lack leptin receptors. In any case, mutations of the genes for leptin or leptin receptors are very rare, so they do not explain the vast majority of cases of obesity. With the exception of these rare cases, leptin has not proved to provide a useful treatment for obesity. Indeed, obese people already have elevated blood levels of leptin, and additional leptin has no effect on their food intake or body weight. In other words, obese people show *leptin resistance.*

As we saw earlier in this chapter, the MC4 receptor plays a role in the control of eating and metabolism. Several groups of researchers have found families with severe obesity caused by mutations of the MC4 receptor gene (Farooqi and O'Rahilly, 2005). It appears that mutation of the MC4 receptor is the most common simple genetic cause of severe obesity. Approximately 4 percent of such people have a mutation of the gene for these receptors.

Research suggests that a chemical known as **uncoupling protein (UCP)** may play an important role in determining a person's metabolic efficiency. This protein is

uncoupling protein (UCP) A mitochondrial protein that facilitates the conversion of nutrients into heat.

FIGURE 11.22

Hereditary Leptin Deficiency. The photographs show three patients with hereditary leptin deficiency before (a) and after (b) treatment with leptin for 18 months. The faces of the patients are obscured for privacy. Two normal-weight nurses are shown for comparison purposes.

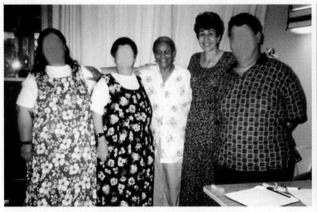 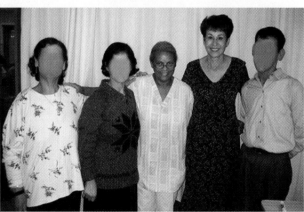

(a)   (b)

From Licinio, J., Caglayan, S., Ozata, M., et al. *Proceedings of the National Academy of Science, USA*, 2004, *101*, 4531–4536.

found in mitochondria and may be one of the factors that determine the rate at which the body burns off calories. Three different uncoupling proteins exist. One of them, UCP3, is found in muscles, and this form probably plays the most important role in metabolic efficiency. Several metabolic signals—including leptin—increase the production of UCP3, thus increasing metabolic rate and burning off calories (Scarpace et al., 2000). Schrauwen et al. (1999) found that levels of UCP3 in Pima Indians were negatively correlated with body mass index and positively correlated with metabolic rate. In other words, those Pima Indians who had high levels of UCP3 had spendthrift phenotypes that helped to protect them from developing obesity.

Treatment

Obesity is extremely difficult to treat; the enormous financial success of diet books, health spas, and weight reduction programs attests to the trouble people have in losing weight. More precisely, many programs help people to lose weight initially, but then the weight is quickly regained. Kramer et al. (1989) reported that 4 to 5 years after participating in a 15-week behavioral weight-loss program, fewer than 3 percent of the participants managed to maintain the weight loss they had achieved during the program.

Whatever the cause of obesity, the metabolic fact of life is this: If calories in exceed calories out, then body fat will increase. Because it is difficult to increase the "calories out" side of the equation enough to bring an obese person's weight back to normal, most treatments for obesity attempt to reduce the "calories in." The extraordinary difficulty that obese people have in reducing caloric intake for a sustained period of time (that is, for the rest of their lives) has led to the development of some extraordinary means. In this section I shall describe some surgical, pharmacological, and behavioral methods that have been devised to make obese people eat less.

Surgeons have become involved in trying to help obese people lose weight. The procedures they have developed (called *bariatric surgery*, from the Greek *barys*, "heavy," and *iatrikos*, "medical") are designed to reduce the amount of food that can be eaten during a meal or interfere with absorption of calories from the intestines. Bariatric surgery has been aimed at the stomach, the small intestine, or both.

The most effective form of bariatric surgery is a special form of gastric bypass called the *Roux-en-Y gastric bypass*, or *RYGB*. This procedure produces a small pouch in the upper end of the stomach. The jejunum (the second part of the small intestine, immediately "downstream" from the duodenum) is cut, and the upper end is attached to the stomach pouch. The effect is to produce a small stomach whose contents enter the jejunum, bypassing the duodenum. Digestive enzymes that are secreted into the duodenum pass through the upper intestine and meet up with the meal that has just been received from the stomach pouch. (See *Figure 11.23*.)

The RYGB procedure appears to work well, although it often causes an iron and vitamin B$_{12}$ deficiency. Brolin (2002) reported that the average postsurgical loss of excessive weight of obese patients was 65 to 75 percent, or about 35 percent of their initial weight. Even patients who sustained smaller weight losses showed improved health, including reductions in hypertension and diabetes. A meta-analysis of 147 studies by Maggard et al. (2005) reported an average weight loss of 43.5 kg (approximately 95 lb) 1 year after RYGB surgery and 41.5

FIGURE 11.23

Roux-en-Y Gastric Bypass (RYGB) Surgery. This procedure almost totally suppresses the secretion of ghrelin.

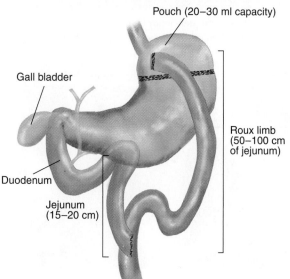

Pouch (20–30 ml capacity)

Gall bladder

Roux limb (50–100 cm of jejunum)

Duodenum

Jejunum (15–20 cm)

kg after 3 years. Unfortunately, a recent study of 16,155 patients in the United States who underwent bariatric surgery found a higher rate of mortality than had previously been reported (Flum et al., 2005). The 30-day, 90-day, and 1-year mortality rates were 2.0 percent, 2.8 percent, and 4.6 percent, respectively. Men were more likely than women to die, and the mortality rate increased with age. The mortality rate was also higher for patients of surgeons with less-than-average experience performing the procedures. Clearly, the decision to undergo bariatric surgery should not be taken lightly.

One important reason for the success of the RYGB procedure appears to be that it disrupts the secretion of ghrelin, either by disrupting communication between the upper intestine and the stomach or by damaging afferent axons in the vagus nerve. The procedure also increases blood levels of PYY (Chan et al., 2006; Reinehr et al., 2007). Both of these changes should decrease food intake: A decrease in ghrelin should reduce hunger, and an increase in PYY should increase satiety. A plausible explanation for the decreased secretion of ghrelin could be disruption of communication between the upper intestine and the stomach—as you will recall, although ghrelin is secreted by the stomach, the upper intestine controls this secretion. Presumably, because the surgery decreases the speed at which food moves through the small intestine, more PYY is secreted.

A less-drastic form of therapy for obesity—exercise—has significant benefits. As mentioned earlier, decreased physical activity is an important cause of the increased number of overweight people. Exercise burns off calories, of course, but it also appears to have beneficial effects on metabolic rate. Bunyard et al. (1998) found that when middle-aged men participated in an aerobic exercise program for 6 months, their body fat decreased and their daily energy requirement increased—by 5 percent for obese men and by 8 percent for lean men. (Remember, a less-efficient metabolism means that it is easier to avoid gaining weight.) Gurin et al. (1999) found that an exercise program helped obese children to lose fat and had the additional benefit of increasing bone density. Hill et al. (2003) calculated that an increased energy expenditure through exercise of only 100 kcal per day could prevent weight gain in most people. The effort would require only a small change in behavior—about 14 minutes of walking each day.

Another type of therapy for obesity—drug treatment—shows some promise. There are three possible ways in which drugs could help people lose weight: reduce the amount of food they eat, prevent some of the food they eat from being digested, and increase their metabolic rate (that is, provide them with a "spendthrift phenotype").

Some serotonergic agonists suppress eating. A review by Bray (1992) concluded that these drugs can be of benefit in weight-loss programs. However, one of the drugs most commonly used for this purpose, fenfluramine, was found to have hazardous side effects, including pulmonary hypertension and damage to the valves of the heart, so the drug was withdrawn from the market in the United States (Blundell and Halford, 1998). Fenfluramine acts by stimulating the release of 5-HT. Fortunately, another drug, sibutramine, has similar therapeutic effects and has not yet been associated with serious side effects.

Another drug, orlistat, interferes with the absorption of fats by the small intestine. As a result, some of the fat in the person's diet passes through the digestive system and is excreted with the feces. Possible side effects include a deficiency of fat-soluble vitamins and leaking of undigested fat from the anus. A double-blind, placebo-controlled study by Hill et al. (1999) found that orlistat helped people maintain weight loss they had achieved by participating in a conventional weight-loss program. People who received the placebo were much more likely to regain the weight they had lost.

As mentioned earlier, the fact that marijuana often elicits a craving for highly palatable foods led to the discovery that the endocannabinoids have an orexigenic effect. The drug rimonabant, which blocks CB1 cannabinoid receptors, was found to suppress appetite. Two large phase III clinical trials of rimonabant, with a total of 5580 patients, were carried out in North America and Europe. The results showed a significant weight loss, lower blood levels of triglycerides and insulin, increased blood levels of HDL ("good" cholesterol), and minimal adverse side effects (Di Marzo and Matias, 2005). Rimonabant is currently approved for the treatment of obesity in 42 countries, but the U.S. Food and Drug Administration has not yet approved it (Isoldi and Arrone, 2008). As we will see in Chapter 16, rimonabant has also been shown to help people stop smoking, which suggests that craving for nicotine also involves the release of endocannabinoids in the brain.

As we have seen, appetite can be stimulated by activation of NPY, MCH, orexin, and ghrelin receptors, and it can be suppressed by the activation of leptin, CCK, CART, and MC4 receptors. Most of these orexigenic and anorexigenic chemicals also affect metabolism: Orexigenic chemicals tend to decrease metabolic rate, and anorexigenic chemicals tend to increase it. In addition, uncoupling protein causes nutrients to be "burned"—converted into heat instead of adipose tissue. Do these discoveries hold any promise for the treatment of obesity? Is there any possibility that researchers will find drugs that will stimulate or block these receptors, thus decreasing people's appetite and increasing the rate at which they burn rather than store their calories? Drug companies certainly hope so, and they are working hard on developing medications that will do so, because they know that there will be a very large number of people willing to pay for them. If we learn more about the physiology of hunger signals, satiety signals, and the reinforcement provided by eating, we may be able to develop safe and effective drugs that attenuate the signals that encourage us to eat and strengthen those that encourage us to stop eating.

Interim Summary

Obesity

Obesity presents serious health problems. As we saw earlier, natural selection has given us strong hunger mechanisms and weaker mechanisms of long-term satiety. Obesity is strongly affected by heredity. Some people have inherited a thrifty metabolism, which makes it difficult for them to lose weight. A high percentage of Pima Indians who live in the United States and consume a high-fat diet become obese and, as a consequence, develop diabetes. In contrast, Mexican Pima Indians, who work hard at subsistence farming and eat a low-fat diet, remain thin and have a low incidence of obesity.

Obesity in humans is related to a hereditary absence of leptin or leptin receptors only in a few families. In general, obese people have very high levels of leptin in their blood. However, they show resistance to the effects of this peptide, apparently because the transport of leptin through the blood–brain barrier is reduced. The most significant simple genetic cause of severe obesity is mutation of the MC4 receptor, which responds to the orexigen AGRP and the anorexigen α-MSH. Genetic variations in uncoupling protein, which controls the conversion of nutrients into heat by the mitochondria, may also be involved in people's metabolic efficiency.

Researchers have tried many behavioral, surgical, and pharmacological treatments for obesity, but no panacea has yet been found. The RYGB procedure, a special form of gastric bypass operation, is the most successful form of bariatric surgery. The effectiveness of this operation is probably due primarily to its suppression of ghrelin secretion and stimulation of PYY secretion. The best hope for the future probably comes from drugs. One drug, rimonabant, blocks cannabinoid receptors and suppresses appetite. At present many pharmaceutical companies are trying to apply the results of the discoveries of orexigens and anorexigens described in this chapter to the development of antiobesity drugs.

This section and the previous one introduced several neuropeptides and peripheral peptides that play a role in control of eating and metabolism. Table 11.1 summarizes information about these compounds. (See *Table 11.1*.)

Thought Question
One of the last prejudices that people admit to publicly is a dislike of fat people. Is this fair, given that genetic differences in metabolism are such an important cause of obesity?

TABLE 11.1 Neuropeptides and Peripheral Peptides Involved in Control of Food Intake and Metabolism

NEUROPEPTIDES

Name	Location of Cell Bodies	Location of Terminals	Interaction with Other Peptides	Physiological or Behavioral Effects
Melanin-concentrating hormone (MCH)	Lateral hypothalamus	Neocortex, periaqueductal gray matter, reticular formation, thalamus, locus coeruleus, neurons in spinal cord that control the sympathetic nervous system	Activated by NPY/AGRP; inhibited by leptin and CART/α-MSH	Eating, decreased metabolic rate
Orexin	Lateral hypothalamus	Similar to those of MCH neurons	Activated by NPY/AGRP; inhibited by leptin and CART/α-MSH	Eating, decreased metabolic rate
Neuropeptide Y (NPY)	Arcuate nucleus of hypothalamus	Paraventricular nucleus, MCH and orexin neurons of the lateral hypothalamus	Activated by ghrelin; inhibited by leptin	Eating, decreased metabolic rate
Agouti-related protein (AGRP)	Arcuate nucleus of hypothalamus (colocalized with NPY)	Same regions as NPY neurons	Inhibited by leptin	Eating, decreased metabolic rate; acts as antagonist at MC4 receptors
Cocaine- and amphetamine-regulated transcript (CART)	Arcuate nucleus of hypothalamus	Paraventricular nucleus, lateral hypothalamus, periaqueductal gray matter, neurons in spinal cord that control the sympathetic nervous system	Activated by leptin	Suppression of eating, increased metabolic rate
α-melanocyte stimulating hormone (α-MSH)	Arcuate nucleus of hypothalamus (colocalized with CART)	Same regions as CART neurons	Activated by leptin	Suppression of eating, increased metabolic rate; acts as agonist at MC4 receptors

PERIPHERAL PEPTIDES

Name	Where Produced	Site of Actions	Physiological or Behavioral Effects
Leptin	Fat tissue	Inhibits NPY/AGRP neurons; excites CART/α-MSH neurons	Suppression of eating, increased metabolic rate
Insulin	Pancreas	Similar to leptin	Similar to leptin
Ghrelin	Gastrointestinal system	Activates NPY/AGRP neurons	Eating
Cholecystokinin (CCK)	Duodenum	Neurons in pylorus	Suppression of eating
Peptide YY_{3-36} (PYY)	Gastrointestinal system	Inhibits NPY/AGRP neurons	Suppression of eating

Anorexia Nervosa/Bulimia Nervosa

anorexia nervosa   A disorder that most frequently afflicts young women; exaggerated concern with overweight that leads to excessive dieting and often compulsive exercising; can lead to starvation.

bulimia nervosa   Bouts of excessive hunger and eating, often followed by forced vomiting or purging with laxatives; sometimes seen in people with anorexia nervosa.

Most people, if they have an eating problem, tend to overeat. However, some people, especially adolescent women, have the opposite problem: They eat too little, even to the point of starvation. This disorder is called **anorexia nervosa**. Another eating disorder, **bulimia nervosa**, is characterized by a loss of control of food intake. (The term *bulimia* comes from the Greek *bous*, "ox," and *limos*, "hunger.") People with bulimia nervosa periodically gorge themselves with food, especially dessert or snack food and especially in the afternoon or evening. These binges are usually followed by self-induced vomiting or the use of laxatives, along with feelings of depression and guilt. Episodes of bulimia are seen in some patients with anorexia nervosa. The incidence of anorexia nervosa is estimated at 0.5 to 2 percent; that of bulimia nervosa at 1 to 3 percent. Women are ten to twenty times more likely than men to develop anorexia nervosa and approximately ten times more likely to develop bulimia nervosa. (See Klein and Walsh, 2004.)

Possible Causes

The literal meaning of the word *anorexia* suggests a loss of appetite, but people with this disorder are usually interested in—even preoccupied with—food. They may enjoy preparing meals for others to consume, collect recipes, and even hoard food that they do not eat. Although anorexics might not be oblivious to the effects of food, they express an intense fear of becoming obese, which continues even if they become dangerously thin. Many exercise by cycling, running, or almost constant walking and pacing.

Anorexia is a serious disorder. Five to 10 percent die of complications of the disease or of suicide. Many anorexics suffer from osteoporosis, and bone fractures are common. When the weight loss becomes severe enough, anorexic women cease menstruating.

Many researchers and clinicians have concluded that anorexia nervosa and bulimia nervosa are symptoms of an underlying mental disorder. However, evidence suggests just the opposite: that the symptoms of eating disorders are actually symptoms of starvation. A famous study carried out at the University of Minnesota by Keyes and his colleagues (Keyes et al., 1950) recruited thirty-six physically and psychologically healthy young men to observe the effects of semistarvation. For 6 months, the men ate approximately 50 percent of what they had been eating previously, and as a result lost approximately 25 percent of their original body weight. As the volunteers lost weight, they began displaying disturbing symptoms, including preoccupation with food and eating, ritualistic eating, erratic mood, impaired cognitive performance, and physiological changes such as decreased body temperature. They began hoarding food and non-food objects and were unable to explain (even to themselves) why they bothered to accumulate objects that they had no use for. At first, they were gregarious, but as time when on they became withdrawn and isolated. They lost interest in sex, and many even "welcomed the freedom from sexual tensions and frustrations normally present in young adult men" (Keyes et al., 1950, p. 840).

The obsessions with food and weight loss and the compulsive rituals that people with anorexia nervosa develop suggest a possible linkage with obsessive-compulsive disorder (described in greater detail in Chapter 15). However, the fact that these obsessions and compulsions were seen in the subjects of the Minnesota study—

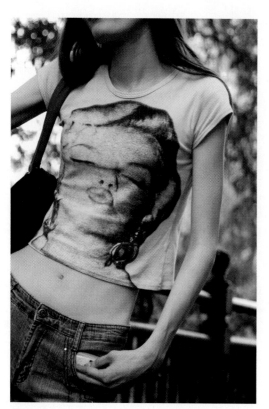

Anorexia nervosa most often occurs in young women.

none of whom showed these symptoms previously—suggests that they are effects rather than causes of the eating disorder.

Both anorexia and semistarvation include symptoms such as mood swings, depression, and insomnia. Even hair loss is seen in both conditions. The suicide rate in patients with anorexia is higher than that of the rest of the population (Pompili et al., 2004). None of the volunteers in the Minnesota study committed suicide, but one cut off three of his fingers. This volunteer said, "I have been more depressed than ever in my life. . . . I thought that there was only one thing that would pull me out of the doldrums, that is release from [the experiment]. I decided to get rid of some fingers. . . . It was premeditated (Keyes et al., 1950, pp. 894–895).

Although binge eating is a symptom of anorexia, eating very slowly is, too. Patients with anorexia tend to dawdle over a meal, and so did the volunteers in the Minnesota study. "Toward the end of starvation some of the men would dawdle for almost two hours over a meal which previously they would have consumed in a matter of minutes" (Keyes et al., p. 833).

As we saw, excessive exercising is a prominent symptom of anorexia (Zandian et al., 2007). In fact, Manley, O'Brien, and Samuels (2008) found that many fitness instructors recognize that some of their clients may have an eating disorder and expressed concern about ethical or liability issues about permitting such clients to participate in their classes or facilities.

Studies with animals suggest that the increased activity may actually be a result of the fasting. When rats are allowed access to food for 1 hour each day, they will spend more and more time running in a wheel if one is available and will lose weight and eventually die of emaciation (Smith, 1989). Nergårdh et al. (2007) placed rats in individual cages. Some of the cages were equipped with running wheels so that their running activity levels could be measured. After adaptation to the cages, the animals were given access to food once a day for varying amounts of time between 1 and 24 hours (no food restriction). The rats in cages with running wheels that received food on restricted schedules began to spend more time running. In fact, the rats with the most restrictive feeding schedules ran the most. Clearly, the increased running was counterproductive, because these animals lost much more weight than the animals housed in cages without running wheels. (See *Figure 11.24*.)

One explanation for the increased activity of rats on a semistarvation diet is that it reflects an innate tendency to seek food when it becomes scarce. Normally, rats would expend their activity by exploring the environment and searching for food, but because of their confinement, the tendency to explore results only in futile wheel running. Another possible explanation is the low body temperature that accompanies a semistarvation diet. (In fact, patients with anorexia complain that they feel cold.) The increased activity may simply reflect an attempt to keep warm. Whichever explanation is correct, the fact that starving rats increase their activity suggests that the excessive activity of anorexic patients may be a symptom of starvation, and not simply a weight-loss strategy.

Blood levels of NPY are elevated in patients with anorexia. As we saw earlier in this chapter, NPY normally stimulates eating. Nergårdh et al. (2007) found that intracerebroventricular infusions of NPY further increased the time spent running in rats on a restricted feeding schedule. Normally, NPY stimulates eating (as it did in rats with unlimited access to food), but under conditions of starvation, it stimulates wheel-running activity instead.

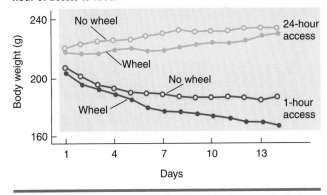

FIGURE 11.24

Activity, Food Restriction, and Weight Loss. The graph shows changes in body weight of rats permitted 1-hour or 24-hour access to food each day. Rats with access to a running wheel spent time running and lost weight, especially those with only 1 hour of access to food.

Data from Nergårdh, R., Ammar, A., Brodin, U., et al. *Psychoneuroendocrinology*, 2007, *32*, 493–502.

By now, you are probably wondering why anorexia gets started in the first place. Even if the symptoms of anorexia are largely those of starvation, what begins the behavior that leads to starvation? The simple answer is that we still do not know. One possibility is a genetic predisposition for this behavior. There is good evidence, primarily from twin studies, that hereditary factors play an important role in the development of anorexia nervosa (Russell and Treasure, 1989; Walters and Kendler, 1995; Kortegaard et al., 2001). In fact, between 58 and 76 percent of the variability in the occurrence of anorexia nervosa appears to be under control of genetic factors (Klein and Walsh, 2004). In addition, the incidence of anorexia nervosa is higher in girls who were born prematurely or who had sustained birth trauma during complicated deliveries (Cnattingius et al., 1999), which suggests that biological factors independent of heredity may play a role. Perhaps some young women (and a small number of young men) go on a diet to bring their body weight closer to what they perceive as ideal. Once they get set on this course and begin losing weight, physiological and endocrinological changes bring about the symptoms of starvation just outlined, and the vicious circle begins.

The fact that anorexia nervosa is seen primarily in young women has prompted both biological and social explanations. Most psychologists favor the latter, concluding that the emphasis that most modern industrialized societies places on slimness—especially in women—is responsible for this disorder. Another possible cause could be the changes in hormones that accompany puberty. Whatever the cause, young men and women differ in their response to even a short period of fasting. Södersten, Bergh, and Zandian (2006) had high school students visit their laboratory at noon one day, where they were given all the food that wanted to eat for lunch. Seven days later, they returned to the laboratory again. This time they had been fasting since lunch on the previous day. The men ate more food than they had the first time. However, the women actually ate *less* than they had before. (See *Figure 11.25.*) Apparently, women have difficulty compensating for a period of food deprivation by eating more food. As the authors note, "dieting may be dangerous in women and in particular in those who are physically active and therefore need to eat more food, [such as] athletes" (p. 575).

Treatment

Anorexia is very difficult to treat successfully. Cognitive behavior therapy, considered by many clinicians to be the most effective approach, has a success rate of less

FIGURE 11.25

Reactions of Young Men and Women to Fasting.   The graphs show food intake and eating rate of young men and women during a buffet lunch after a 24-hour period of fasting or after a period during which they ate meals at their normal times.

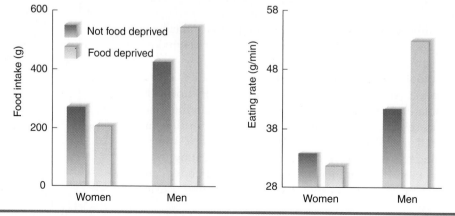

Data from Södersten, P., Bergh, C., and Zandian, M. *Hormones and Behavior*, 2006, *50*, 572–578.

than 50 percent and a relapse rate of 22 percent during a 1-year treatment period (Pike et al., 2003). A meta-analysis by Steinhausen (2002) indicates that the success rate in treating anorexia has not improved in the last 50 years. As Ben-Tovim (2003) notes, "Much of the literature on the treatment and outcome of eating disorders lacks methodological robustness and ignores basic epidemiological principles. The absence of authoritative evidence for treatment effectiveness makes it increasingly hard to protect resource intensive treatments in anorexia and bulimia nervosa, and existing theories of the causation of the disorders are too non-specific to generate effective programs of prevention. New models are urgently required" (p. 65).

Researchers have tried to treat anorexia nervosa with many drugs that increase appetite in laboratory animals or in people without eating disorders—for example, antipsychotic medications, drugs that stimulate adrenergic α_2 receptors, L-DOPA, and THC (the active ingredient in marijuana). Unfortunately, none of these drugs has been shown to be helpful (Mitchell, 1989). In any event the fact that anorexics are usually obsessed with food (and show high levels of neuropeptide Y and ghrelin) suggests that the disorder is not caused by the absence of hunger. Researchers have had better luck with bulimia nervosa; several studies suggest that serotonin agonists such as fluoxetine may aid in the treatment of this disorder (Advokat and Kutlesic, 1995; Kaye et al., 2001). However, fluoxetine does not help anorexic patients (Attia et al., 1998).

Bergh, Södersten, and their colleagues (Zandian et al., 2007; Court, Bergh, and Södersten, 2008) have devised a novel and apparently effective treatment protocol for anorexia. The patients are taught to eat faster by placing a plate of food on an electronic scale attached to a computer that displays the time course of their actual and ideal intake. After the meal, the patients are kept in a warm room, which reduces their anxiety and their activity level. A study with rats in cages with running wheels (Hillebrand et al., 2005) put the animals on a restricted feeding schedule and observed the symptoms described earlier: hyperactivity, reduced food intake, severe body weight loss, and decreased body temperature. If a warm metal plate was placed in the cage, the rats with restricted access to food spent less time running in the activity wheel and more time on the warm plate. Rats that had unrestricted access to food ignored the presence of the warm plate.

Anorexia nervosa and bulimia nervosa are serious conditions; understanding their causes is more than an academic matter. We can hope that research on the biological and social control of feeding and metabolism and the causes of compulsive behaviors will help us to understand this puzzling and dangerous disorder.

InterimSummary

Anorexia Nervosa/Bulimia Nervosa

Anorexia nervosa is a serious—even life-threatening—disorder. Although anorexic patients avoid eating, they are often preoccupied with food. Bulimia nervosa consists of periodic binging and purging and a low body weight. Anorexia nervosa has a strong hereditary component and is seen primarily in young women.

Some researchers believe that the symptoms of anorexia—preoccupation with food and eating, ritualistic eating, erratic mood, excessive exercising, impaired cognitive performance, and physiological changes such as decreased body temperature—are symptoms of starvation, and not the underlying causes of anorexia. A study carried out over 50 years ago found that several months of semistarvation caused similar symptoms to emerge in previously healthy people. If

rats are allowed access to food for a limited time each day, they will spend much time in a running wheel if one is available, and will consequently eat less and lose weight. This response may reflect increased exploratory behavior that, in the natural environment, might result in the discovery of food. It may also reflect an attempt to increase body temperature, which is lowered by fasting. A study with normal adolescents found that instead of eating more after a 24-hour fast, women actually ate less, which suggests that they have difficulty compensating for a period of food deprivation. Perhaps a period of dieting causes some young women to begin a vicious circle that leads to starvation and its ensuing symptoms. A therapeutic protocol based on findings such as these has shown promise in helping anorexic patients overcome the disorder. Researchers have tried to treat anorexia with drugs that increase appetite, but none has been found to be helpful. However, fluoxetine, a serotonin agonist used to treat depression, may help to suppress episodes of bulimia.

Thought Questions

Undoubtedly, anorexia has both environmental and physiological causes. After reading the last section of this chapter, what do you think is the cause of the sex difference in the incidence of this disorder (that is, the fact that almost all anorexics are female)? Is it caused entirely by social factors (such as the emphasis on thinness in our society), or do you think that biological factors also play a role?

EPILOGUE An Insatiable Appetite

As we saw in the chapter prologue, it was clear from birth that Carrie suffered from some kind of medical condition. She was a frail baby, had difficulty nursing, and exhibited several physical abnormalities, including a narrow forehead, almond-shaped eyes, mild strabismus (crossed eyes), a thin upper lip, small hands and feet, and a downturned mouth. Then, in early childhood she began overeating and became obese. Other behaviors changed; she had temper tantrums; she engaged in compulsive behaviors, including picking at her skin; and she was moderately mentally retarded.

The cause of Carrie's condition is genetic (Wattendorf and Muenke, 2005; Bittel and Butler, 2005). The defective genes are found on chromosome 15 and appear to be involved in production of proteins that are critical to normal development and functioning of the brain—especially the hypothalamus. Overeating appears to be caused by a deficiency in brain mechanisms of satiety rather than an increase in hunger. Normally, when people eat a meal, the rate of intake is initially high, but as satiety mechanisms begin to exert their control, eating slows down and eventually stops. However, Lindgren et al. (2000) found that although people with Prader-Willi syndrome began eating a meal at a slower rate than did obese or lean control subjects, they continued to eat for a much longer time, and their rate of eating stayed constant or even speeded up. Eating appeared to provide an inadequate satiety signal.

Ghrelin levels are abnormally high in people with Prader-Willi syndrome, which suggests that the overeating might be caused by increased hunger. However, a study by Tan et al. (2004) found that suppressing ghrelin secretion with injections of somatostatin, a peptide secreted by the pancreas, had no effect on appetite.

We do not yet know the cause of the impaired satiety mechanisms. Levels of leptin are high in people with Prader-Willi syndrome, just as they are in other obese people, and their leptin receptors appear to be normal. In addition, NPY and AGRP production appears to be normal (Bittel and Butler, 2005). Further study of people with Prader-Willi syndrome may help us learn more about the brain mechanisms that control ingestive behavior.

Key Concepts

PHYSIOLOGICAL REGULATORY MECHANISMS

1. Regulatory systems include four essential features: a system variable, a set point, a detector, and a correctional mechanism. Because of the time it takes for substances to be absorbed from the digestive system, eating and drinking behaviors are also controlled by satiety mechanisms.

DRINKING

2. The body's water is located in the intracellular and extracellular compartments; the latter consists of the interstitial fluid and the blood plasma.

3. Normal loss of water depletes both major compartments and produces both osmometric and volumetric thirst.

4. Osmometric thirst is detected by neurons in the anteroventral hypothalamus; volumetric thirst is detected by the kidney, which secretes an enzyme that produces angiotensin, and by baroreceptors in the atria of the heart, which communicate directly with the brain.

EATING: SOME FACTS ABOUT METABOLISM

5. The body has two nutrient reservoirs: a short-term reservoir containing glycogen (a carbohydrate) and a long-term reservoir containing fats.

6. Metabolism is divided into the absorptive and fasting phases, controlled primarily by the hormones insulin and glucagon.

WHAT STARTS A MEAL?

7. Hunger is affected by social and environmental factors, such as time of day and the presence of other people.

8. The most important physiological signal for hunger occurs when receptors located in the liver and the brain signal a low availability of nutrients.

WHAT STOPS A MEAL?

9. Satiety is controlled by receptors in several locations. Nutrient receptors in the stomach send signals to the brain. The release of CCK and PYY by the digestive system decreases food intake. Receptors in the small intestines and in the liver detect the presence of nutrients of a meal that is being digested and absorbed into the body.

BRAIN MECHANISMS

10. Neural mechanisms in the brain stem are able to control acceptance or rejection of food, even when they are isolated from the forebrain.

11. The hypothalamus in involved in the control of eating. Neurons in the lateral hypothalamus that secrete MCH or orexin increase appetite and decrease metabolic rate. These neurons are, in turn, activated by neurons that secrete neuropeptide Y and AGRP. Ghrelin, secreted by the stomach, activates NPY/AGRP neurons and stimulates hunger.

12. Well-fed adipose tissue releases a hormone, leptin, that suppresses eating by binding with leptin receptors on neuropeptide-Y–secreting neurons in the paraventricular nucleus of the hypothalamus, inhibiting them. Leptin also inhibits lateral hypothalamic neurons that secrete MCH and orexin, and it stimulates CART- and α-MSH–secreting neurons, whose activity inhibits eating.

OBESITY

13. An important cause of obesity is an efficient metabolism, which may have a genetic basis. Uncoupling protein may be involved in determining the efficiency of a person's metabolism.

14. Drugs that interact with the MCH, orexin, NPY, CART, or MC-4 receptors or alter the activity of uncoupling protein may be helpful in treating obesity.

ANOREXIA NERVOSA/BULIMIA NERVOSA

15. Anorexia nervosa is a serious eating disorder characterized by a drastic reduction in food intake and weight loss that is seen primarily in young women. Bulimia nervosa is characterized by periodic binges of overeating that are usually followed by vomiting or purging.

16. Recent research suggests that the symptoms of anorexia are actually those that accompany starvation. In susceptible individuals, a period of voluntary starvation may elicit these symptoms and begin a vicious circle.

17. An apparently successful treatment based on this analysis teaches patients with anorexia to eat more quickly and reduces hyperactivity by keeping them in a warm room after meals to reduce their anxiety and activity level.

Suggested Readings

Arora, S., and Anubhuti. Role of neuropeptides in appetite regulation and obesity—A review. *Neuropeptides*, 2006, *40*, 375–401.

Aylwin, S., and Al-Zaman, Y. Emerging concepts in the medical and surgical treatment of obesity. *Frontiers in Hormone Research*, 2008, *36*, 229–259.

Barsh, G. S., and Schwartz, M. W. Genetic approaches to studying energy balance: Perception and integration. *Nature Reviews: Genetics*, 2002, *3*, 589–600.

Crookes, P. F. Surgical treatment of morbid obesity. *Annual Review of Medicine*, 2006, *57*, 243–264.

de Castro, J. M. The control of eating behavior in free-living humans. In *Neurobiology of Food and Fluid Intake*, 2nd ed., edited by E. Stricker and S. Woods. New York: Kluwer Academic/Plenum Publishers, 2004.

Johnson, A. K. The sensory psychobiology of thirst and salt appetite. *Medicine and Science in Sports and Exercise*, 2007, *39*, 1388–1400.

Kreipe, R. E., and Mou, S. M. Eating disorders in adolescents and young adults. *Obstetrics and Gynecology Clinics of North America*, 2000, *27*, 101–124.

Rolls, E. T. Sensory processing in the brain related to the control of food intake. *Proceedings of the Nutrition Society*, 2007, *66*, 96–112.

Woods, S. C., Lutz, T. A., Geary, N., and Langhans, W. Pancreatic signals controlling food intake: Insulin, glucagon and amylin. *Philosophical Transactions of the Royal Society B*, 2006, *361*, 1219–1235.

Additional Resources

Visit www.mypsychkit.com for additional review and practice of the material covered in this chapter. Within MyPsychKit, you can take practice tests and receive a customized study plan to help you review. Dozens of animations, tutorials, and Web links are also available. You can even review using the interactive electronic version of this textbook. You will need to register for MyPsychKit. See www.mypsychkit.com for complete details.

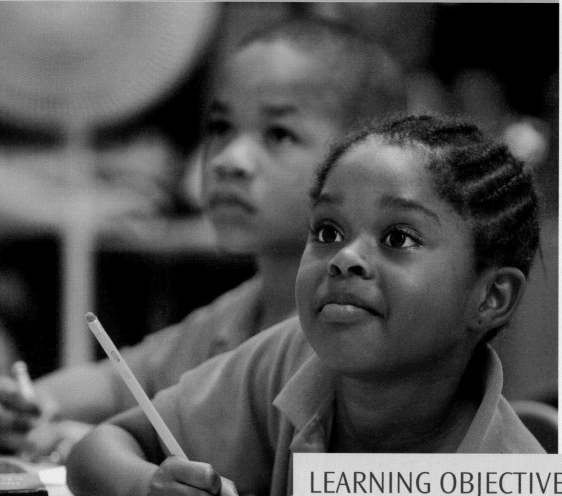

chapter 12: Learning and Memory

LEARNING OBJECTIVES

1. Describe each of four basic forms of learning: perceptual learning, stimulus–response learning, motor learning, and relational learning.

2. Describe the anatomy of the hippocampus, describe the establishment of long-term potentiation, and discuss the role of NMDA receptors in this phenomenon.

3. Discuss research on the physiological basis of synaptic plasticity during long-term potentiation and long-term depression.

4. Describe research on the role of the inferior temporal cortex in visual perceptual learning.

5. Discuss the physiology of the classically conditioned emotional response to aversive stimuli.

6. Describe the role of the basal ganglia in instrumental conditioning.

7. Describe the role of dopamine in reinforcing brain stimulation and discuss the effects of administering dopamine antagonists and agonists.

8. Describe the nature of human anterograde amnesia and explain what it suggests about the organization of learning.

9. Describe the role of the hippocampus in relational learning, including episodic and spatial learning, and discuss the function of hippocampal place cells.

Patient H. M. had a relatively pure amnesia. His intellectual ability and his immediate verbal memory was apparently normal. He could repeat seven numbers forward and five numbers backward, and he could carry on conversations, rephrase sentences, and perform mental arithmetic. He was unable to remember events that occurred during several years preceding his brain surgery, but he could recall older memories very well. He showed no personality change after the operation, and he was generally polite and good-natured.

However, after his surgery, H. M. was unable to learn anything new. He could not identify by name people he had met since the operation (performed in 1953, when he was 27 years old). His family moved to a new house after his operation, and he never learned how to get around in the new neighborhood. (After his parent's death, he lived in a nursing home, where he could be cared for.) He was aware of his disorder and often said something like this:

> Every day is alone in itself, whatever enjoyment I've had, and whatever sorrow I've had. . . . Right now, I'm wondering. Have I done or said anything amiss? You see, at this moment everything looks clear to me, but what happened just before? That's what worries me. It's like waking from a dream; I just don't remember. (Milner, 1970, p. 37)

H. M. was capable of remembering a small amount of verbal information as long as he was not distracted; constant rehearsal could keep information in his immediate memory for a long time. However, rehearsal did not appear to have any long-term effects; if he was distracted for a moment, he would completely forget whatever he had been rehearsing. He worked very well at repetitive tasks. Indeed, because he so quickly forgot what previously happened, he did not easily become bored. He could endlessly reread the same magazine or laugh at the same jokes, finding them fresh and new each time. His time was typically spent solving crossword puzzles and watching television.

On December 2, 2008, H. M., whom we now know as Henry Molaison, died at the age of 82.

Experiences change us; encounters with our environment alter our behavior by modifying our nervous system. As many investigators have said, an understanding of the physiology of memory is the ultimate challenge to neuroscience research. The brain is complex, and so are learning and remembering. However, despite the difficulties, the long years of work finally seem to be paying off. New approaches and new methods have evolved from old ones, and real progress has been made in understanding the anatomy and physiology of learning and remembering.

The Nature of Learning

Learning refers to the process by which experiences change our nervous system and hence our behavior. We refer to these changes as *memories*. Although it is convenient to describe memories as if they were notes placed in filing cabinets, this is certainly not the way experiences are reflected within the brain. Experiences are not "stored"; rather, they change the way we perceive, perform, think, and plan. They do so by physically changing the structure of the nervous system, altering neural circuits that participate in perceiving, performing, thinking, and planning.

Learning can take at least four basic forms: perceptual learning, stimulus–response learning, motor learning, and relational learning. **Perceptual learning** is the ability to learn to recognize stimuli that have been perceived before. The primary function of this type of learning is the ability to identify and categorize objects (including other members of our own species) and situations. Unless we have learned to recognize something, we cannot learn how we should behave with respect to it; we will not profit from our experiences with it, and profiting from experience is what learning is all about.

perceptual learning Learning to recognize a particular stimulus.

stimulus–response learning
Learning to automatically make a particular response in the presence of a particular stimulus; includes classical and instrumental conditioning.

classical conditioning A learning procedure; when a stimulus that initially produces no particular response is followed several times by an **unconditional stimulus** that produces a defensive or appetitive response (the **unconditional response**), the first stimulus (now called a **conditional stimulus**) itself evokes the response (now called a **conditional response**).

Each of our sensory systems is capable of perceptual learning. We can learn to recognize objects by their visual appearance, the sounds they make, how they feel, or how they smell. We can recognize people by the shape of their faces, the movements they make when they walk, or the sound of their voices. When we hear people talk, we can recognize the words they are saying and, perhaps, their emotional state. As we shall see, perceptual learning appears to be accomplished primarily by changes in the sensory association cortex. That is, learning to recognize complex visual stimuli involves changes in the visual association cortex, learning to recognize complex auditory stimuli involves changes in the auditory association cortex, etc.

Stimulus–response learning is the ability to learn to perform a particular behavior when a particular stimulus is present. Thus, it involves the establishment of connections between circuits involved in perception and those involved in movement. The behavior could be an automatic response such as a defensive reflex, or it could be a complicated sequence of movements. Stimulus–response learning includes two major categories of learning that psychologists have studied extensively: *classical conditioning* and *instrumental conditioning*.

Classical conditioning is a form of learning in which an unimportant stimulus acquires the properties of an important one. It involves an *association between two stimuli*. A stimulus that previously had little effect on behavior becomes able to evoke a reflexive, species-typical behavior. For example, a defensive eyeblink response can be conditioned to a tone. If we direct a brief puff of air toward a rabbit's eye, the eye will automatically blink. The response is called an **unconditional response (UR)** because it occurs unconditionally, without any special training. The stimulus that produces it (the puff of air) is called an **unconditional stimulus (US)**. Now we begin the training. We present a series of brief 1000-Hz tones, each followed 500 ms later by a puff of air. After several trials the rabbit's eye begins to close even before the puff of air occurs. Classical conditioning has occurred; the **conditional stimulus (CS**—the 1000-Hz tone) now elicits the **conditional response (CR**—the eye blink). (See *Figure 12.1*.)

When classical conditioning takes place, what kinds of changes occur in the brain? Figure 12.1 shows a simplified neural circuit that could account for this type of learning. For the sake of simplicity we will assume that the US (the puff of air) is detected by a single neuron in the somatosensory system and that the CS (the 1000-Hz tone) is detected by a single neuron in the auditory system. We will also assume that the response—the eyeblink—is controlled by a single neuron in the motor system. Of course, learning actually involves many thousands of neurons—sensory neurons, interneurons, and motor neurons—but the basic principle of synaptic change can be represented by this simple figure. (See *Figure 12.1*.)

Let's see how this circuit works. If we present a 1000-Hz tone, we find that the animal makes no reaction because the synapse connecting the tone-sensitive neuron with the neuron in the motor system is weak. That is, when an action potential reaches the terminal button of synapse T (tone), the excitatory postsynaptic potential (EPSP) that it produces in the dendrite of the motor neuron is too small to make that neuron fire. However, if we present a puff of air to the eye, the eye blinks. This reaction occurs because nature has provided the animal with a strong synapse between the somatosensory neuron and the motor neuron that causes a blink (synapse P, for "puff"). To establish classical conditioning, we first present the 1000-Hz tone and then quickly follow it with a puff of air. After we repeat these pairs of stimuli several times, we find that we can dispense with the air puff; the 1000-Hz tone produces the blink all by itself.

FIGURE 12.1

A Simple Neural Model of Classical Conditioning.
When the 1000-Hz tone is presented just before the puff of air to the eye, synapse T is strengthened.

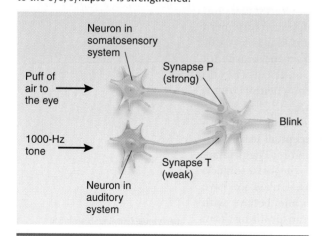

Neuron in somatosensory system

Puff of air to the eye

Synapse P (strong)

Blink

1000-Hz tone

Synapse T (weak)

Neuron in auditory system

Over 50 years ago, Donald Hebb proposed a rule that might explain how neurons are changed by experience in a way that would cause changes in behavior (Hebb, 1949). The **Hebb rule** says that if a synapse repeatedly becomes active at about the same time that the postsynaptic neuron fires, changes will take place in the structure or chemistry of the synapse that will strengthen it. How would the Hebb rule apply to our circuit? If the 1000-Hz tone is presented first, then weak synapse T (for "tone") becomes active. If the puff is presented immediately afterward, then strong synapse P becomes active and makes the motor neuron fire. The act of firing then strengthens any synapse with the motor neuron *that has just been active.* Of course, this means synapse T. After several pairings of the two stimuli and after several increments of strengthening, synapse T becomes strong enough to cause the motor neuron to fire by itself. Learning has occurred. (See *Figure 12.1*.)

When Hebb formulated his rule, he was unable to determine whether it was true or false. Now, finally, enough progress has been made in laboratory techniques that the strength of individual synapses can be determined, and investigators are studying the physiological bases of learning. We will see the results of some of these approaches in the next section of this chapter.

The second major class of stimulus–response learning is **instrumental conditioning** (also called *operant conditioning*). Whereas classical conditioning involves automatic, species-typical responses, instrumental conditioning involves behaviors that have been learned—and whereas classical conditioning involves an association between two stimuli, instrumental conditioning involves an *association between a response and a stimulus.* Instrumental conditioning is a more flexible form of learning: It permits an organism to adjust its behavior according to the consequences of that behavior. That is, when a behavior is followed by favorable consequences, the behavior tends to occur more frequently; when it is followed by unfavorable consequences, it tends to occur less frequently. Collectively, "favorable consequences" are referred to as **reinforcing stimuli**, and "unfavorable consequences" are referred to as **punishing stimuli**. For example, a response that enables a hungry organism to find food will be reinforced, and a response that causes pain will be punished. (Psychologists often refer to these terms as *reinforcers* and *punishers*.)

Let's consider the process of reinforcement. Briefly stated, reinforcement causes changes in an animal's nervous system that increase the likelihood that a particular stimulus will elicit a particular response. For example, when a hungry rat is first put in an operant chamber (a "Skinner box"), it is not very likely to press the lever mounted on a wall. However, if it does press the lever and if it receives a piece of food immediately afterward, the likelihood of its making another response increases. Put another way, reinforcement causes the sight of the lever to serve as the stimulus that elicits the lever-pressing response. It is not accurate to say simply that a particular behavior becomes more frequent. If no lever is present, a rat that has learned to press one will not wave its paw around in the air. The *sight of a lever* is needed to produce the response. Thus, the process of reinforcement strengthens a connection between neural circuits involved in perception (the sight of the lever) and those involved in movement (the act of lever pressing). As we will see later in this chapter, the brain contains reinforcement mechanisms that control this process. (See *Figure 12.2*.)

The third major category of learning, **motor learning**, is actually a component of stimulus–response learning. For simplicity's sake we can think of perceptual learning as the establishment of changes within the sensory systems of the brain, stimulus–response learning as the establishment of connections between sensory systems and motor systems, and motor learning as the establishment of changes within motor systems—but, in fact, motor learning cannot occur without sensory guidance from the environment. For example, most skilled movements involve interactions with objects: bicycles, pinball machines, tennis racquets, knitting needles, and so on. Even skilled movements that we make by ourselves, such as solitary dance steps, involve feedback from the joints, muscles, vestibular apparatus, eyes,

Hebb rule The hypothesis proposed by Donald Hebb that the cellular basis of learning involves strengthening of a synapse that is repeatedly active when the postsynaptic neuron fires.

instrumental conditioning A learning procedure whereby the effects of a particular behavior in a particular situation increase (reinforce) or decrease (punish) the probability of the behavior; also called *operant conditioning*.

reinforcing stimulus An appetitive stimulus that follows a particular behavior and thus makes the behavior become more frequent.

punishing stimulus An aversive stimulus that follows a particular behavior and thus makes the behavior become less frequent.

motor learning Learning to make a new response.

FIGURE 12.2

A Simple Neural Model of Instrumental Conditioning

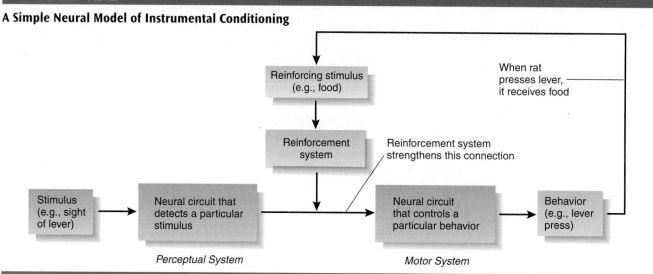

and contact between the feet and the floor. Motor learning differs from other forms of learning primarily in the degree to which new forms of behavior are learned; the more novel the behavior, the more the neural circuits in the motor systems of the brain must be modified. (See *Figure 12.3*.)

A particular learning situation can involve varying amounts of all three types of learning described so far: perceptual, stimulus–response, and motor. For example, if we teach an animal to make a new response whenever we present a stimulus it has never seen before, it must learn to recognize the stimulus (perceptual learning) and make the response (motor learning), and a connection must be established between these two new memories (stimulus–response learning). If we teach it to make a response it has already learned whenever we present a new stimulus, only perceptual learning and stimulus–response learning will take place.

The three forms of learning described so far consist primarily of changes in one sensory system, between one sensory system and the motor system, or in the motor system, but obviously, learning is usually more complex than that. The fourth form of learning, **relational learning**, involves learning the *relationships* among individual stimuli. For example, consider what we must learn to become familiar with the contents of a room. First, we must learn to recognize each of the objects. In addition, we must learn the relative locations of the objects with respect to each other. As a result, when we find ourselves located in a particular place in the room, our perceptions of these objects and their locations relative to us tell us exactly where we are.

FIGURE 12.3

An Overview of Perceptual, Stimulus–Response (S-R), and Motor Learning

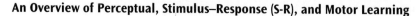
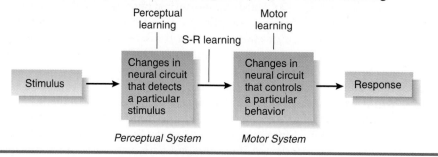

relational learning Learning the relationships among individual stimuli.

Other types of relational learning are even more complex. *Episodic learning*—remembering sequences of events (episodes) that we witness—requires us to keep track of and remember not only individual events but also the order in which they occur. As we will see in the last section of this chapter, a special system that involves the hippocampus and associated structures appears to perform coordinating functions required for many types of learning that go beyond simple perceptual, stimulus–response, or motor learning.

InterimSummary

The Nature of Learning

Learning produces changes in the way we perceive, act, think, and feel. It does so by producing changes in the nervous system in the circuits responsible for perception, in those responsible for the control of movement, and in connections between the two.

Perceptual learning consists primarily of changes in perceptual systems that make it possible for us to recognize stimuli so that we can respond to them appropriately. Stimulus–response learning consists of connections between perceptual and motor systems. The most important forms are classical and instrumental conditioning. Classical conditioning occurs when a neutral stimulus is followed by an unconditional stimulus (US) that naturally elicits an unconditional response (UR). After this pairing, the neutral stimulus becomes a conditional stimulus (CS); it now elicits the response by itself, which we refer to as the conditional response (CR).

Instrumental conditioning occurs when a response is followed by a reinforcing stimulus, such as a drink of water for a thirsty animal. The reinforcing stimulus increases the likelihood that the other stim-uli that were present when the response was made will evoke the response. Both forms of stimulus–response learning may occur as a result of strengthened synaptic connections, as described by the Hebb rule.

Motor learning, although it may primarily involve changes within neural circuits that control movement, is guided by sensory stimuli; thus, it is actually a form of stimulus–response learning. Relational learning, the most complex form of learning, includes the abilities to recognize objects through more than one sensory modality, to recognize the relative location of objects in the environment, and to remember the sequence in which events occurred during particular episodes.

Thought Questions

Can you think of specific examples of each of the categories of learning described in this section? Can you think of some examples that include more than one category?

Synaptic Plasticity: Long-Term Potentiation and Long-Term Depression

On theoretical considerations alone, it would appear that learning must involve synaptic plasticity: changes in the structure or biochemistry of synapses that alter their effects on postsynaptic neurons. Recent years have seen an explosion of research on this topic, largely stimulated by the development of methods that permit researchers to observe structural and biochemical changes in microscopically small structures: the presynaptic and postsynaptic components of synapses.

Induction of Long-Term Potentiation

Electrical stimulation of circuits within the hippocampal formation can lead to long-term synaptic changes that seem to be among those responsible for learning. Lømo (1966) discovered that intense electrical stimulation of axons leading from the entorhinal cortex to the dentate gyrus caused a long-term increase in the magnitude of excitatory postsynaptic potentials in the postsynaptic neurons; this increase has come to be called **long-term potentiation (LTP)**. (The word *potentiate* means "to strengthen, to make more potent.")

First, let's review some anatomy. The **hippocampal formation** is a specialized region of the limbic cortex located in the temporal lobe. (Its location in a human

long-term potentiation (LTP) A long-term increase in the excitability of a neuron to a particular synaptic input caused by repeated high-frequency activity of that input.

hippocampal formation A forebrain structure of the temporal lobe, constituting an important part of the limbic system; includes the hippocampus proper (Ammon's horn), dentate gyrus, and subiculum.

brain is shown in Figure 3.14.) Because the hippocampal formation is folded in one dimension and then curved in another, it has a complex, three-dimensional shape. Therefore, it is difficult to show what it looks like with a diagram on a two-dimensional sheet of paper. Fortunately, the structure of the hippocampal formation is orderly; a slice taken anywhere perpendicular to its curving long axis contains the same set of circuits.

Figure 12.4 shows a slice of the hippocampal formation, illustrating a typical procedure for producing long-term potentiation. The primary input to the hippocampal formation comes from the *entorhinal cortex.* The axons of neurons in the entorhinal cortex pass through the *perforant path* and form synapses with the granule cells of the *dentate gyrus.* A stimulating electrode is placed in the perforant path, and a recording electrode is placed in the dentate gyrus, near the granule cells. (See *Figure 12.4.*) First, a single pulse of electrical stimulation is delivered to the perforant path, and then the resulting population EPSP is recorded in the dentate gyrus. The **population EPSP** is an extracellular measurement of the excitatory postsynaptic potentials (EPSP) produced by the synapses of the perforant path axons with the dentate granule cells. The size of the first population EPSP indicates the strength of the synaptic connections before long-term potentiation has taken place. Long-term potentiation can be induced by stimulating the axons in the perforant path with a burst of approximately 100 pulses of electrical stimulation, delivered within a few seconds. Evidence that long-term potentiation has occurred is obtained by periodically delivering single pulses to the perforant path and recording the response in the dentate gyrus. If the response is greater than it was before the burst of pulses was delivered, long-term potentiation has occurred. (See *Figure 12.5.*)

Long-term potentiation can be produced in other regions of the hippocampal formation and in many other places in the brain. It can last for several months (Bliss and Lømo, 1973). It can be produced in isolated slices of the hippocampal formation as well as in the brains of living animals, which allows researchers to stimulate and record from individual neurons and to analyze biochemical changes. The brain

population EPSP An evoked potential that represents the EPSPs of a population of neurons.

FIGURE 12.4

The Hippocampal Formation and Long-Term Potentiation.   This schematic diagram shows the connections of the components of the hippocampal formation and the procedure for producing long-term potentiation.

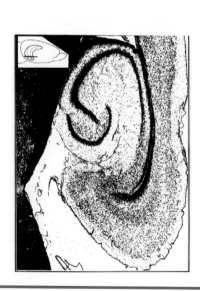
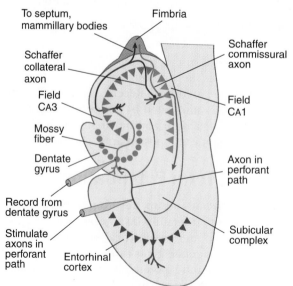

Photograph from Swanson, L. W., Köhler, C., and Björklund, A., in *Handbook of Chemical Neuroanatomy. Vol. 5: Integrated Systems of the CNS, Part I.* Amsterdam: Elsevier Science Publishers, 1987. Reprinted with permission.

FIGURE 12.5

Long-Term Potentiation.   Population EPSPs were recorded from the dentate gyrus before and after electrical stimulation that led to long-term potentiation.

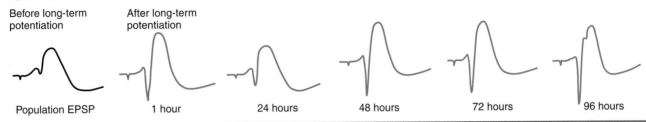

Before long-term potentiation

After long-term potentiation

Population EPSP

1 hour

24 hours

48 hours

72 hours

96 hours

From Berger, T. W. *Science*, 1984, *224*, 627–630. Copyright © 1984. Reprinted with permission from AAAS.

is removed from the skull, the hippocampal complex is dissected, and slices are placed in a temperature-controlled chamber filled with liquid that resembles interstitial fluid. Under optimal conditions a slice remains alive for up to 40 hours.

Many experiments have demonstrated that long-term potentiation in hippocampal slices can follow the Hebb rule. That is, when weak and strong synapses to a single neuron are stimulated at approximately the same time, the weak synapse becomes strengthened. This phenomenon is called **associative long-term potentiation**, because it is produced by the association (in time) between the activity of the two sets of synapses. (See *Figure 12.6*.)

Role of NMDA Receptors

Nonassociative long-term potentiation requires some sort of additive effect. That is, a series of pulses delivered at a high rate all in one burst will produce long-term potentiation, but the same number of pulses given at a slow rate will not. The reason for this phenomenon is now clear. Experiments have shown that synaptic strengthening occurs when molecules of the neurotransmitter bind with postsynaptic receptors located in a dendritic spine that is already depolarized. Kelso, Ganong, and Brown (1986) found that if they used a microelectrode to artificially depolarize neurons in field CA1 and then stimulated the axons that formed synapses with this neuron, the synapses became stronger; that is, they produced a stronger postsynaptic potential in the dendritic spine. However, if the stimulation of the synapses and the depolarization of the neuron occurred at different times, no effect was seen; thus, the release of the neurotransmitter and depolarization of the postsynaptic membrane had to occur at the same time. (See *Figure 12.7*.)

Experiments such as the ones just described indicate that long-term potentiation requires two events: activation of synapses and depolarization of the postsynaptic neuron. The explanation for this phenomenon, at least in some parts of the brain, lies in the characteristics of a very special type of glutamate receptor. The **NMDA receptor** has some unusual properties. It is found in the hippocampal formation, especially in field CA1. It gets its name from a drug that specifically activates it: *N*-methyl-D-aspartate. The NMDA receptor controls a calcium ion channel. However, this channel is normally blocked by a magnesium ion (Mg^{2+}), which prevents calcium ions from entering the cell even when the receptor is stimulated by glutamate. However, if the postsynaptic membrane is depolarized, the Mg^{2+} is ejected from the ion channel, and the channel is free to admit Ca^{2+} ions. Thus, calcium ions enter the cells through the channels controlled by NMDA receptors only when glutamate is present

FIGURE 12.6

Associative Long-Term Potentiation.   If the weak stimulus and strong stimulus are applied at the same time, the synapses activated by the weak stimulus will be strengthened.

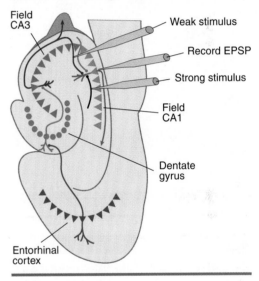

Field CA3

Weak stimulus

Record EPSP

Strong stimulus

Field CA1

Dentate gyrus

Entorhinal cortex

associative long-term potentiation
A long-term potentiation in which concurrent stimulation of weak and strong synapses to a given neuron strengthens the weak ones.

NMDA receptor A specialized ionotropic glutamate receptor that controls a calcium channel that is normally blocked by Mg^{2+} ions; involved in long-term potentiation.

and when the postsynaptic membrane is depolarized. This means that the ion channel controlled by the NMDA receptor is a neurotransmitter- *and* voltage-dependent ion channel. (See *Figure 12.8* and *MyPsychKit 12.1, The NMDA Receptor.*)

Cell biologists have discovered that the calcium ion is used by many cells as a second messenger that activates various enzymes and triggers biochemical processes. The entry of calcium ions through the ion channels controlled by NMDA receptors is an essential step in long-term potentiation (Lynch et al., 1984). **AP5** (2-amino-5-phosphonopentanoate), a drug that blocks NMDA receptors, prevents calcium ions from entering the dendritic spines and thus blocks the establishment of LTP (Brown et al., 1989). These results indicate that the activation of NMDA receptors is necessary for the first step in the process events that establishes LTP: the entry of calcium ions into dendritic spines.

In Chapter 2 you learned that only axons are capable of producing action potentials. Actually, they can also occur in dendrites of some types of pyramidal cells, including those in field CA1 of the hippocampal formation. The threshold of excitation for **dendritic spikes** (as these action potentials are called) is rather high. As far as we know, they occur only when an action potential is triggered in the axon of the pyramidal cell. The backwash of depolarization across the cell body triggers a dendritic spike, which is propagated up the trunk of the dendrite. This means that whenever the axon of a pyramidal cell fires, all of its dendritic spines become depolarized for a brief time.

I think that considering what you already know about associative long-term potentiation, you can anticipate the role that NMDA receptors play in this phenomenon. If weak synapses are active by themselves, nothing happens,

---

FIGURE 12.7

Long-Term Potentiation.   Synaptic strengthening occurs when synapses are active while the membrane of the postsynaptic cell is depolarized.

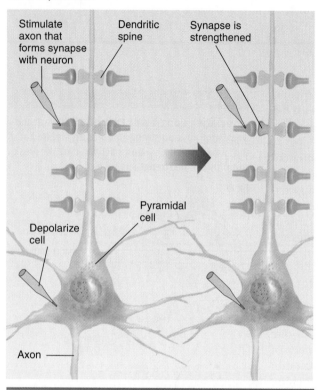

FIGURE 12.8

The NMDA Receptor   The NMDA receptor is a neurotransmitter- and voltage-dependent ion channel. (a) When the postsynaptic membrane is at the resting potential, Mg^{2+} blocks the ion channel, preventing Ca^{2+} from entering. (b) When the membrane is depolarized, the magnesium ion is evicted. Thus, the attachment of glutamate to the binding site causes the ion channel to open, allowing calcium ions to enter the dendritic spine.

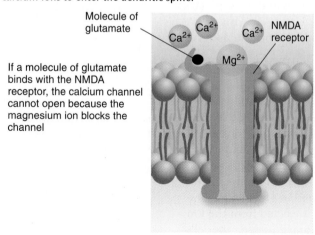

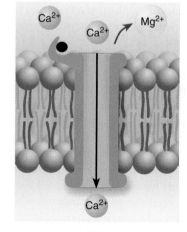

(a)

(b)

because the membrane of the dendritic spine does not depolarize sufficiently for the calcium channels controlled by the NMDA receptors to open. (Remember that for these channels to open, the postsynaptic membrane must first depolarize and displace the Mg^{2+} ions that normally block them.) However, if the activity of strong synapses located elsewhere on the postsynaptic cell has caused the cell to fire, then a dendritic spike will depolarize the postsynaptic membrane enough for calcium to enter the ion channels controlled by the NMDA receptors. Thus, the special properties of NMDA receptors account not only for the existence of long-term potentiation but also for its associative nature. (See *Figure 12.9* and *MyPsychKit 12.2, Associative LTP.*)

mypsychkit

Animation 12.2
Associative LTP

Mechanisms of Synaptic Plasticity

What is responsible for the increases in synaptic strength that occur during long-term potentiation? Dendritic spines on CA1 pyramidal cells contain two types of glutamate receptors: NMDA receptors and **AMPA receptors**. Research indicates that strengthening of an individual synapse appears to be accomplished by insertion of additional AMPA receptors into the postsynaptic membrane of the dendritic spine. AMPA receptors control sodium channels; thus, when they are activated by glutamate, they produce EPSPs in the membrane of the dendritic spine. Therefore, with more AMPA receptors present, the release of glutamate by the terminal button causes a larger excitatory postsynaptic potential. In other words, the synapse becomes stronger.

Where do these new AMPA receptors come from? Shi et al. (1999) used a harmless virus to insert a gene for a subunit of the AMPA receptor into rat hippocampal

AP5 2-amino-5-phosphonopentanoate; a drug that blocks NMDA receptors.

dendritic spike An action potential that occurs in the dendrite of some types of pyramidal cells.

AMPA receptor An ionotropic glutamate receptor that controls a sodium channel; when open, it produces EPSPs.

FIGURE 12.9

Associative Long-Term Potentiation.   If the activity of strong synapses is sufficient to trigger an action potential in the neuron, the dendritic spike will depolarize the membrane of dendritic spines, priming NMDA receptors so that any weak synapses active at that time will become strengthened.

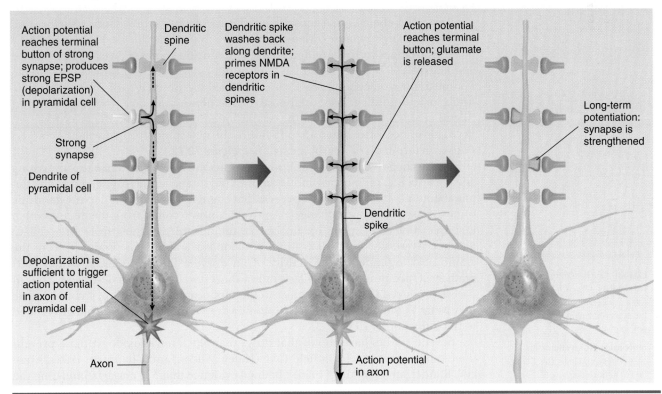

FIGURE 12.10

Role of AMPA Receptors in Long-Term Potentiation.
Two-photon laser scanning microscopy of the CA1 region of living hippocampal slices shows delivery of AMPA receptors into dendritic spines after long-term potentiation. The AMPA receptors were tagged with a fluorescent dye molecule. The arrows labeled *a* and *b* point to dendritic spines that became filled with AMPA receptors after the induction of long-term potentiation.

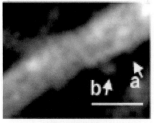 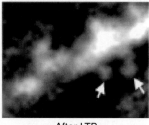

Before LTP   After LTP

From Shi, S.-H., Hayashi, Y., Petralia, R. S., et al. *Science*, 1999, *284*, 1811–1816. Copyright © 1999. Reprinted with permission from AAAS.

CaM-KII Type II calcium-calmodulin kinase, an enzyme that must be activated by calcium; may play a role in the establishment of long-term potentiation.

nitric oxide (NO) synthase An enzyme responsible for the production of nitric oxide.

neurons maintained in a tissue culture. The AMPA receptors produced by the gene had a fluorescent dye molecule attached to them, which permitted the investigators to use a special microscope to see the exact location of AMPA receptors in dendritic spines of CA1 neurons. The investigators induced LTP by stimulating axons that form synapses with these dendrites. Before LTP was induced, they saw AMPA receptors clustered at the base of the dendritic spines. Fifteen minutes after the induction of LTP, the AMPA receptors flooded into the spines and moved to their tips—the location of the postsynaptic membrane. This movement of AMPA receptors did not occur when AP5, the drug that blocks NMDA receptors, was added to the culture medium. (See *Figure 12.10*.)

How does the entry of calcium ions into the dendritic spine cause AMPA receptors to move into the postsynaptic membrane? This process appears to involve several enzymes, including **CaM-KII** (type II calcium-calmodulin kinase), an enzyme found in dendritic spines. CaM-KII is a *calcium-dependent* enzyme, which is inactive until a calcium ion binds with it and activates it. Many studies have shown that CaM-KII plays a critical role in long-term potentiation. For example, Silva et al. (1992) produced a targeted mutation against the gene responsible for the production of CaM-KII in mice. The mice had no obvious neuroanatomical defects, and the responses of their NMDA receptors were normal. However, the investigators were unable to produce LTP in field CA1 of hippocampal slices taken from these animals. Lledo et al. (1995) found that injection of activated CaM-KII directly into CA1 pyramidal cells mimicked the effects of LTP: It strengthened synaptic transmission in those cells. Shen and Meyer (1999) found that after LTP was induced, CaM-KII molecules became concentrated in the postsynaptic densities of dendritic spines, where the postsynaptic receptors are located.

Two other changes that accompany LTP are alteration of synaptic structure and production of new synapses. Many studies have found that the establishment of LTP includes changes in the size and shape of dendritic spines. For example, Bourne and Harris (2007) suggest that LTP causes the enlargement of thin spines into fatter, mushroom-shaped spines. Figure 12.11 shows the variety of shapes that dendritic spines and their associated postsynaptic density can take. (See *Figure 12.11*.) Nägerl et al. (2007) found that the establishment of LTP caused the growth of new dendritic spines. After about 15 to 19 hours, the new spines formed synaptic connections with terminals of nearby axons. (See *Figure 12.12*.)

Researchers believe that LTP may also involve *presynaptic* changes in existing synapses, such as an increase in the amount of glutamate that is released by the terminal button—but how could a process that begins postsynaptically, in the dendritic spines, cause presynaptic changes? A possible answer comes from the discovery that a simple molecule, nitric oxide, can communicate messages from one cell to another. As we saw in Chapter 4, nitric oxide is a soluble gas produced from the amino acid arginine by the activity of an enzyme known as **nitric oxide (NO) synthase**. Once produced, NO lasts only a short time before it is destroyed. Thus, if it were produced in dendritic spines in the hippocampal formation, it could diffuse only as far as the nearby terminal buttons, where it might produce changes related to the induction of LTP.

Several studies have shown that drugs that block nitric oxide synthase prevent the establishment of LTP in field CA1 (Haley, Wilcox, and Chapman, 1992). Arancio, Kandel, and Hawkins (1995) obtained evidence that NO acts by stimulating the production of cyclic GMP, a second messenger, in presynaptic terminals. Although there is good evidence that NO is one of the signals the dendritic spine uses to communicate with the terminal button, most investigators believe that there must be other signals as well. After all, alterations in synapses require coordinated changes in both presynaptic and postsynaptic elements.

For several years after its discovery, researchers believed that LTP involved a single process. Since then it has become clear that LTP consists of several stages. According to Raymond (2007), there are actually three types of LTP. The first type, LTP1, involves almost immediate changes in synaptic strength caused by insertion of AMPA receptors. This form of LTP lasts for an hour or two. The second type, LTP2, involves local protein synthesis. Dendrites contain molecules of RNA that can be translated into proteins. These RNAs include codes for various enzymes, components of receptors, and structural proteins (Martin and Zukin, 2006). The most durable type of long-term potentiation, LTP3, involved production of molecules of RNA in the nucleus that are then transported to the dendrites where protein synthesis takes place. The long-lasting form of LTP also requires the presence of dopamine, which stimulates D1 receptors present on the dendrites. The importance of dopamine in the establishment of long-term memories is discussed later in this chapter.

Figure 12.13 summarizes the biochemistry discussed in this subsection. I suspect that you might feel overwhelmed by all the new terms introduced here, and I hope that the figure will help to clarify things. The evidence we have seen so far indicates that activation of a terminal button releases glutamate, which binds with NMDA receptors in the postsynaptic membrane of the dendritic spine. If this membrane was depolarized by a dendritic spike, then calcium ions will enter through channels controlled by the NMDA receptors and activate

FIGURE 12.11

Dendritic Spines in Field CA1.   According to Bourne and Harris (2007), long-term potentiation may convert thin spines into mushroom-shaped spines. (a) In this colorized photomicrograph, dendrite shafts are yellow, spine necks are blue, spine heads are green, and presynaptic terminals are orange. (b) This three-dimensional reconstruction of a portion of a dendrite (yellow) shows the variation I size and shape of postsynaptic densities (red).

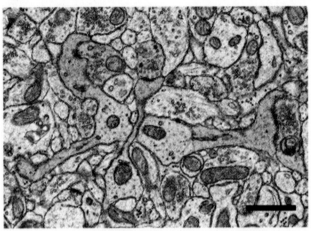

(a)

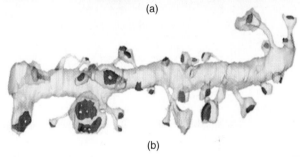

(b)

Reprinted from *Current Opinion in Neurobiology, 17*, Bourne, J., and Harris, K. M., Do Thin Spines Learn to be Mushroom Spines that Remember?, 381–386, Copyright 2007, with permission from Elsevier.

FIGURE 12.12

Growth of Dendritic Spines After Long-Term Potentiation.   Two-photon microscopic images show a segment of a dendrite of a CA1 pyramidal neuron before and after electrical stimulation that established long-term potentiation. Numbers in each box indicate the time before or after the stimulation.

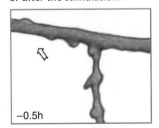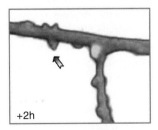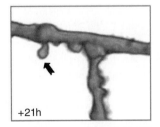

−0.5h   +2h   +21h

From Nägerl, U. V., Köstinger, G., Anderson, J. C., et al. *Journal of Neuroscience*, 2007, *27*, 8149–8156. Reprinted with permission.

FIGURE 12.13

Chemistry of Long-term Potentiation. These chemical reactions appear to be triggered by the entry of an adequate amount of calcium into the dendritic spine.

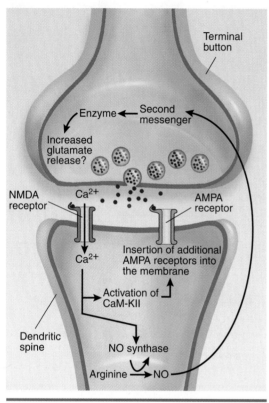

CaM-KII, a calcium-dependent protein kinase. Activated CaM-KII travels to the postsynaptic density of dendritic spines, where it causes the insertion of AMPA receptors into the postsynaptic density. In addition, LTP initiates rapid changes in synaptic structure and the production of new synapses. (See *Figure 12.13.*) The entry of calcium also activates a calcium-dependent NO synthase, and the newly produced NO then presumably diffuses out of the dendritic spine, back to the terminal button. There, it may trigger unknown chemical reactions that increase the release of glutamate. (See *Figure 12.13.*) Finally, long-lasting LTP (LTP2 and LTP3) requires the presence of dopamine and local and remote synthesis of new proteins that stabilize the changes made in the structure of the potentiated synapse. (See *MyPsychKit 12.3, Chemistry of LTP*.)

Long-Term Depression

I mentioned earlier that low-frequency stimulation of the synaptic inputs to a cell can *decrease* rather than increase their strength. This phenomenon, known as **long-term depression (LTD)**, also plays a role in learning. Apparently, neural circuits that contain memories are established by strengthening some synapses and weakening others. As we saw earlier, LTP occurs when synaptic inputs are activated at the same time that the postsynaptic membrane is strongly depolarized. (Refer to *Figure 12.7.*) In contrast, LTD occurs when the synaptic inputs are activated when the postsynaptic membrane is either weakly depolarized or hyperpolarized (Debanne, Gähwiler, and Thompson, 1994; Thiels et al., 1996).

As we saw, the early form of LTP involves an increase in the number of AMPA receptors in the postsynaptic membrane of dendritic spines. LTD appears to involve the opposite: a *decrease* in the number of AMPA receptors in these spines (Carroll et al., 1999). Just as AMPA receptors are inserted into dendritic spines during LTP, they are removed from the spines in vesicles during LTD (Lüscher et al., 1999).

InterimSummary

Synaptic Plasticity: Long-Term Potentiation and Long-Term Depression

The study of long-term potentiation in the hippocampal formation has suggested a mechanism that might be responsible for at least some of the synaptic changes that occur during learning. A circuit of neurons passes from the entorhinal cortex through the hippocampal formation. High-frequency stimulation of the axons in this circuit strengthens synapses; it leads to an increase in the size of the EPSPs in the dendritic spines of the postsynaptic neurons. Associative long-term potentiation can also occur, in which weak synapses are strengthened by the action of strong ones. In fact, the only requirement for LTP is that the postsynaptic membrane be depolarized at the same time that the synapses are active.

In field CA1, in the dentate gyrus, and in several other parts of

the brain, NMDA receptors play a special role in LTP. These receptors, sensitive to glutamate, control calcium channels but can open them only if the membrane is already depolarized. Thus, the combination of membrane depolarization (for example, from a dendritic spike produced by the activity of strong synapses) and activation of an NMDA receptor causes the entry of calcium ions. The increase in calcium activates several calcium-dependent enzymes, including CaM-KII. CaM-KII causes the insertion of AMPA receptors into the membrane of the dendritic spine, increasing their sensitivity to glutamate released by the terminal button. This change is accompanied by structural alterations in the shape of the dendritic spine and the growth of new spines, which establish new synapses. LTP may also involve presynaptic changes, through the activation of NO synthase, an enzyme responsible for the production of nitric oxide. This soluble gas may diffuse into nearby terminal buttons, where it facilitates the release of glutamate. Long-lasting forms of LTP (LTP2 and LTP3) require protein synthesis and the presence of dopamine. Long-term depression occurs when a synapse is activated at the time that the postsynaptic membrane is hyperpolarized or only slightly depolarized.

Thought Questions

The brain is the most complex organ in the body, and it is also the most malleable. Every experience leaves at least a small trace, in the form of altered synapses. When we tell someone something or participate in an encounter that the other person will remember, we are (literally) changing connections in the person's brain. How many synapses change each day? What prevents individual memories from becoming confused?

Perceptual Learning

Learning enables us to adapt to our environment and to respond to changes in it. In particular, learning provides us with the ability to perform an appropriate behavior in an appropriate situation. Situations can be as simple as the sound of a buzzer or as complex as the social interactions of a group of people. The first part of learning involves learning to perceive particular stimuli. In the interest of brevity, I will discuss only visual learning in this section. The same general principles are found in the results of research on learning to recognize stimuli by means of other sensory modalities. Furthermore, Chapter 13 discusses the role of learning in the acquisition and use of language.

Perceptual learning involves learning to *recognize* things, not *what to do* when they are present. (Learning what to do is discussed in the next three sections of this chapter.) Perceptual learning can involve learning to recognize entirely new stimuli, or it can involve learning to recognize changes or variations in familiar stimuli. For example, if a friend gets a new hairstyle or replaces glasses with contact lenses, our visual memory of that person changes. We also learn that particular stimuli are found in particular locations or contexts or in the presence of other stimuli. We can even learn and remember particular *episodes*: sequences of events taking place at a particular time and place. The more complex forms of perceptual learning will be discussed in the last section of this chapter, which is devoted to relational learning.

As we saw in Chapter 6, the primary visual cortex receives information from the lateral geniculate nucleus of the thalamus. After the first level of analysis the information is sent to the extrastriate cortex, which surrounds the primary visual cortex (striate cortex). After analyzing particular attributes of the visual scene, such as form, color, and movement, subregions of the extrastriate cortex send the results of their analysis to the next level of the visual association cortex, which is divided into two "streams." The *ventral stream*, which is involved with object recognition, continues ventrally into the inferior temporal cortex. The *dorsal stream*, which is involved with perception of the location of objects, continues dorsally into the posterior parietal cortex. As some investigators have said, the ventral stream is involved with the *what* of visual perception; the dorsal stream is involved with the *where*. (See *Figure 12.14*.)

Many studies have shown that lesions that damage the inferior temporal cortex—part of the ventral stream—disrupt the ability to discriminate between different visual stimuli. These lesions impair the ability to perceive (and thus to learn to recognize) particular kinds of visual information. As we saw in Chapter 6, people with damage to the inferior temporal cortex

long-term depression (LTD) A long-term decrease in the excitability of a neuron to a particular synaptic input caused by stimulation of the terminal button while the postsynaptic membrane is hyperpolarized or only slightly depolarized.

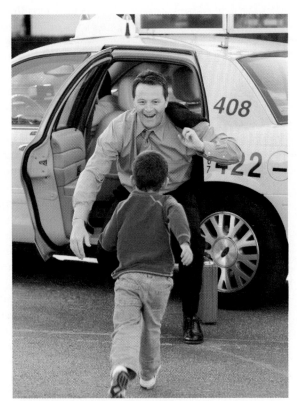

Learning to recognize another person's face is an important form of perceptual learning.

FIGURE 12.14

The Major Divisions of the Visual Cortex of the Rhesus Monkey. The arrows indicate the primary direction of the flow of information in the dorsal and ventral streams.

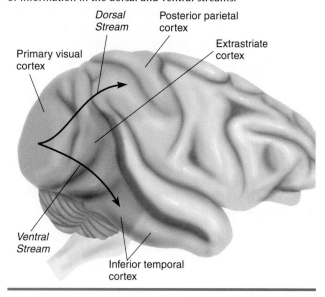

FIGURE 12.15

Evidence of Retrieval of Visual Memories of Movement. The bars represent the level of activation, measured by fMRI, of MT/MST, regions of the visual association cortex that respond to movement. Subjects looked at photographs of static scenes or scenes that implied motion similar to the ones shown here.

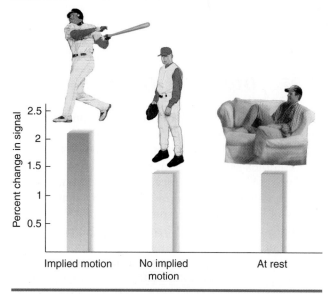

Adapted from Kourtzi, A., and Kanwisher, N. *Journal of Cognitive Neuroscience,* 2000, *12,* 48–55.

may have excellent vision but be unable to recognize familiar, everyday objects such as scissors, clothespins, or light bulbs—and faces of friends and relatives.

Perceptual learning clearly involves changes in synaptic connections in the visual association cortex that establish new neural circuits—changes such as the ones described in the previous section of this chapter. At a later time, when the same stimulus is seen again and the same pattern of activity is transmitted to the cortex, these circuits become active again. This activity constitutes the recognition of the stimulus—the readout of the visual memory, so to speak. For example, Yang and Maunsell (2004) trained monkeys to detect small differences in visual stimuli whose images were projected onto a specific region of the retina. After the training was complete, the monkeys were able to detect differences much smaller than those they could detect when the training first started. However, they were unable to detect these differences when the patterns were projected onto other regions of the retina. Recordings of single neurons in the visual association cortex showed that the response properties of neurons that received information from the "trained" region of the retina—but not from other regions—had become sensitive to small differences in the stimuli. Clearly, neural circuits in that region alone had been modified by the training.

Let's look at some evidence from studies with humans that supports the conclusion that activation of neural circuits in sensory association cortex constitutes the "readout" of a perceptual memory. Many years ago, Penfield and Perot (1963) discovered that when they stimulated the visual and auditory association cortex as patients were undergoing seizure surgery, the patients reported memories of images or sounds—for example, images of a familiar street or the sound of the patient's mother's voice. (Seizure surgery is performed under a local anesthetic so that the surgeons can test the effects of brain stimulation on the patient's cognitive abilities to be sure that they do not remove brain tissue that performs vital functions.)

Damage to regions of the brain involved in visual perception not only impair the ability to recognize visual stimuli but also disrupt people's memory of the visual properties of familiar stimuli. For example, Vandenbulcke et al. (2006) found that Patient J. A., who had sustained damage to the right fusiform gyrus, performed poorly on tasks that required her to draw or describe visual features of various animals, fruits, vegetables, tools, vehicles, or pieces of furniture. Her other cognitive abilities, including the ability to describe nonvisual attributes of objects, were normal. In addition, an fMRI study found that when normal control subjects were asked to perform the visual tasks that she performed poorly, activation was seen in the region of their brains that corresponded to J. A.'s lesion.

Kourtzi and Kanwisher (2000) found that specific kinds of visual information can activate very specific regions of visual association cortex. As we saw in Chapter 6, a region of the visual association cortex, MT/MST, plays an essential role in perception of movement. The investigators presented subjects with photographs that implied motion—for example, an athlete getting ready to throw a ball. They found that photographs like these, but not photographs of people remaining still, activated area MT/MST. Obviously, the photographs did not move, but presumably, the subjects' memories contained information about movements they had previously seen. (See *Figure 12.15.*)

A functional-imaging study by Goldberg, Perfetti, and Schneider (2006) asked people questions that involved visual, auditory, tactile, and gustatory information. They found that answering the questions activated the regions of association cortex involved in perception of the relevant sensory information. For example, questions about flavor activated the gustatory cortex, questions about tactile information activated the somatosensory cortex, and questions about visual and auditory information activated the visual and auditory association cortex.

Interim Summary

Perceptual Learning

Perceptual learning occurs as a result of changes in synaptic connections within the sensory association cortex. Damage to the inferior temporal cortex—the highest level of the ventral stream of the visual association cortex—disrupts visual perceptual learning. Functional imaging studies with humans have shown that retrieval of memories of pictures, sounds, movements, or spatial locations activate the appropriate regions of sensory association cortex.

Thought Questions

1. How many perceptual memories does your brain hold? How many images, sounds, and odors can you recognize, and how many objects and surfaces can you recognize by touch? Is there any way we could estimate these quantities?

2. Can you think of times that you saw something that you needed to remember and did so by keeping in mind a response you would need to make rather than an image of the stimulus you just perceived?

Classical Conditioning

Neuroscientists have studied the anatomy and physiology of classical conditioning using many models, such as the gill withdrawal reflex in *Aplysia* (a marine invertebrate) and the eyeblink reflex in the rabbit (Lavond, Kim, and Thompson, 1993; Bailey and Kandel, 2008). I have chosen to describe a simple mammalian model of classical conditioning—the conditioned emotional response—to illustrate the results of such investigations.

The amygdala is part of an important system involved in a particular form of stimulus–response (S-R) learning: classically conditioned emotional responses. An aversive stimulus such as a painful foot shock produces a variety of behavioral, autonomic, and hormonal responses: freezing, increased blood pressure, secretion of adrenal stress hormones, and so on. A classically conditioned emotional response is established by pairing a neutral stimulus (such as a tone of a particular frequency) with an aversive stimulus (such as a brief foot shock). As we saw in Chapter 10, after these stimuli are paired, the tone becomes a CS; when it is presented by itself, it elicits the same type of responses as the unconditional stimulus does.

A conditioned emotional response can occur in the absence of the auditory cortex (LeDoux, Sakaguchi, and Reis , 1984); therefore, I will confine my discussion to the subcortical components of this process. Information about the CS (the tone) reaches the lateral nucleus of the amygdala. This nucleus also receives information about the US (the foot shock) from the somatosensory system. Thus, these two sources of information converge in the lateral nucleus, which means that synaptic changes responsible for learning could take place in this location.

A hypothetical neural circuit is shown in Figure 12.16. The lateral nucleus of the amygdala contains neurons whose axons project to the central nucleus. Terminal buttons from neurons that transmit auditory and somatosensory information to the lateral nucleus form synapses with dendritic spines on these neurons. When a rat encounters a painful stimulus, somatosensory input activates strong synapses in the lateral nucleus. As a result, the neurons in this nucleus begin firing, which activates neurons in the central nucleus, evoking an unlearned (unconditional) emotional response. If a tone is paired with the painful stimulus, the weak synapses in the lateral amygdala that respond to the sound of the tone are strengthened through the action of the Hebb rule. (See *Figure 12.16*.)

This hypothesis has a considerable amount of support. Lesions of the lateral nucleus of the amygdala disrupt conditioned emotional responses that involve a simple auditory stimulus as a CS and a shock to the feet as a US (Kapp et al., 1979; Nader et al., 2001). Thus, the synaptic changes responsible for this learning may take place within this circuit.

Quirk, Repa, and LeDoux (1995) found evidence for synaptic changes in the lateral nucleus of the amygdala. They recorded the activity of neurons in this nucleus in freely moving rats before, during, and after pairing of a tone with a foot shock. Within a few trials the neurons became more responsive to the tone, and many neurons that had not previously responded to the tone began doing so. When they repeatedly presented the tone *without* the foot shock, the response extinguished and the rate of firing of the neurons in the lateral nucleus returned to baseline levels. (See *Figure 12.17*.)

Wilensky, Schafe, and LeDoux (1999) temporarily inactivated the lateral amygdala by infusing muscimol, a drug that activates inhibitory GABA receptors and hence suppresses neural firing. They found that if the lateral amygdala was inactivated during training, when the CS and US pairing were taking place, the animals did not acquire a conditioned emotional response.

The evidence from many studies indicates that the changes in the lateral amygdala responsible for acquisition of a conditioned emotional response involve LTP. LTP in many parts of the brain—including the amygdala—is accomplished through the activation of NMDA

FIGURE 12.16

Conditioned Emotional Responses. The figure shows the probable location of the changes in synaptic strength produced by the classically conditioned emotional response that results from pairing a tone with a foot shock.

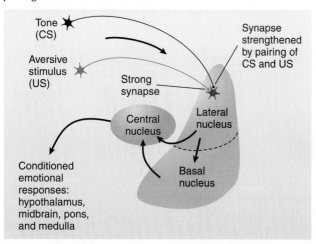

receptors. Rodrigues, Schafe, and LeDoux (2001) used a drug that blocks a subunit of the NMDA receptor. The investigators found that infusion of this drug into the lateral amygdala prevented the acquisition of a conditioned emotional response.

Rumpel et al. (2005) used a harmless virus to insert a gene for a fluorescent dye coupled to the AMPA receptor into the lateral amygdala of rats. They paired a tone with a shock and established a conditioned emotional response. They found that the learning experience caused AMPA receptors to be driven into dendritic spines of synapses that provide auditory input to lateral amygdala neurons. The investigators also inserted a defective gene that prevented AMPA receptors from being driven into the dendritic spines. As a result, conditioning did not take place. In fact, infusion of a wide variety of drugs into the lateral amygdala that prevent long-term potentiation in this nucleus disrupt acquisition of a conditioned emotional response (Rodrigues, Schafe, and LeDoux, 2004; Schafe et al., 2005; Schafe, Doyère, and LeDoux, 2005). The results of these studies support the conclusion that LTP in the lateral amygdala, mediated by NMDA receptors, plays a critical role in the establishment of conditioned emotional responses.

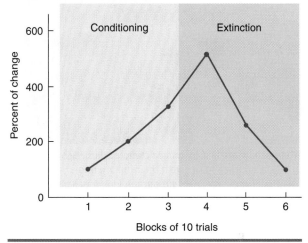

FIGURE 12.17

Classical Conditioning in the Lateral Amygdala.   The graph shows the change in rate of firing of neurons in the lateral amygdala in response to the tone, relative to baseline levels.

Adapted from Quirk, G. J., Repa, J. C., and LeDoux, J. E. *Neuron*, 1995, *15*, 1029–1039.

InterimSummary

Classical Conditioning

You have already encountered the conditioned emotional response in Chapter 10. When an auditory stimulus (CS) is paired with a foot shock (US), the two types of information converge in the lateral nucleus of the amygdala. This nucleus is connected, directly and via the basal nucleus and accessory basal nucleus, with the central nucleus, which is connected with brain regions that control various components of the emotional response. Lesions anywhere in this circuit disrupt the response.

Damage to the lateral nucleus of the amygdala or inhibition of neural activity there disrupts the establishment of conditioned emotional responses. Recordings of single neurons in this nucleus indicate that classical conditioning changes the response of neurons to the CS. The mechanism of synaptic plasticity in this system appears to be NMDA-mediated long-term potentiation. When a tone is paired with a foot shock, neurons in the lateral amygdala become more sensitive to auditory stimuli. Infusion of drugs that block NMDA receptors into the lateral nucleus blocks the establishment of conditioned emotional responses, and the insertion of AMPA receptors into synapses in the lateral nucleus is seen as a result of pairing a tone with a foot shock.

Instrumental Conditioning

Instrumental (operant) conditioning is the means by which we (and other animals) profit from experience. If, in a particular situation, we make a response that has favorable outcomes, we will tend to make the response again. This section first describes the neural pathways involved in instrumental conditioning and then discusses the neural basis of reinforcement.

Role of the Basal Ganglia

As we saw earlier in this chapter, instrumental conditioning entails the strengthening of connections between neural circuits that detect a particular stimulus and

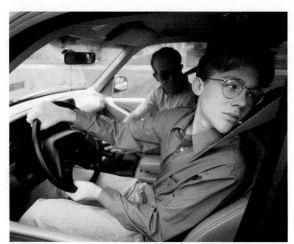

When people are first learning a complex skill, such as driving a car, they must give it their full attention. Eventually, they can drive without thinking much about it and can easily carry on a conversation with passengers at the same time.

neural circuits that produce a particular response. Clearly, the circuits that are responsible for instrumental conditioning begin in various regions of the sensory association cortex, where perception takes place, and end in the motor association cortex of the frontal lobe, which controls movements. But what pathways are responsible for these connections, and where do the synaptic changes responsible for the learning take place?

There are two major pathways between the sensory association cortex and the motor association cortex: direct transcortical connections (connections from one area of the cerebral cortex to another) and connections via the basal ganglia and thalamus. Both of these pathways appear to be involved in instrumental conditioning, but they play different roles.

In conjunction with the hippocampal formation the transcortical connections are involved in the acquisition of episodic memories—complex perceptual memories of sequences of events that we witness or are described to us. (The acquisition of these types of memories is discussed in the last section of this chapter.) The transcortical connections are also involved in the acquisition of complex behaviors that involve deliberation or instruction. For example, a person learning to drive a car with a manual transmission might say, "Let's see, push in the clutch, move the shift lever to the left and then away from me—there, it's in gear—now let the clutch come up—oh! It died—I should have given it more gas. Let's see, clutch down, turn the key. . . ." A memorized set of rules (or an instructor sitting next to us) provides a script for us to follow. Of course, this process does not have to be audible or even involve actual movements of the speech muscles; a person can think in words with neural activity that does not result in overt behavior.

At first, performing a behavior through observation or by following a set of rules is slow and awkward—and because so much of the brain's resources are involved with recalling the rules and applying them to our behavior, we cannot respond to other stimuli in the environment; we must ignore events that might distract us. But then, with practice, the behavior becomes much more fluid. Eventually, we perform it without thinking and can easily do other things at the same time, such as carrying on a conversation with passengers as we drive our car.

Evidence suggests that as learned behaviors become automatic and routine, they are "transferred" to the basal ganglia. The process seems to work like this. As we deliberately perform a complex behavior, the basal ganglia receive information about the stimuli that are present and the responses we are making. At first the basal ganglia are passive "observers" of the situation, but as the behaviors are repeated again and again, the basal ganglia begin to learn what to do. Eventually, they take over most of the details of the process, leaving the transcortical circuits free to do something else. We need no longer think about what we are doing.

The neostriatum—the caudate nucleus and the putamen—receives sensory information from all regions of the cerebral cortex. It also receives information from the frontal lobes about movements that are planned or are actually in progress. (So as you can see, the basal ganglia have all the information they need to monitor the progress of someone learning to drive a car.) The outputs of the caudate nucleus and the putamen are sent to another part of the basal ganglia: the globus pallidus. The outputs of this structure are sent to the frontal cortex: to the premotor and supplementary motor cortex, where plans for movements are made, and to the primary motor cortex, where they are executed. (See *Figure 12.18*.)

Studies with laboratory animals have found that lesions of the basal ganglia disrupt instrumental conditioning but do not affect other forms of learning. For example, Fernandez-Ruiz et al. (2001) destroyed the portions of the caudate nucleus and putamen that receive visual information from the ventral stream. They found that although the lesions did not disrupt visual perceptual learning, they impaired the monkeys' ability to learn to make a visually guided operant response.

Williams and Eskandar (2006) trained monkeys to move a joystick in a particular direction (left, right, forward, or backward) when they saw a particular visual stimulus. Correct responses were reinforced with a sip of fruit juice. As the monkeys learned the task, the rate of firing of single neurons in the caudate nucleus increased. In fact, the activity of caudate neurons was correlated with the animals' rate of learning. When the investigators increased the activation of caudate neurons through low-intensity, high-frequency electrical stimulation during the reinforcement period, the monkeys learned a particular stimulus-response association more quickly. These results provide further evidence for the role of the basal ganglia in instrumental conditioning.

As we saw in the previous section, long-term potentiation appears to play a critical role in classical conditioning. This form of synaptic plasticity appears to be involved in instrumental conditioning, as well. Packard and Teather (1997) found that blocking NMDA receptors in the basal ganglia with an injection of AP5 disrupted learning guided by a simple visual cue.

FIGURE 12.18

The Basal Ganglia and Their Connections

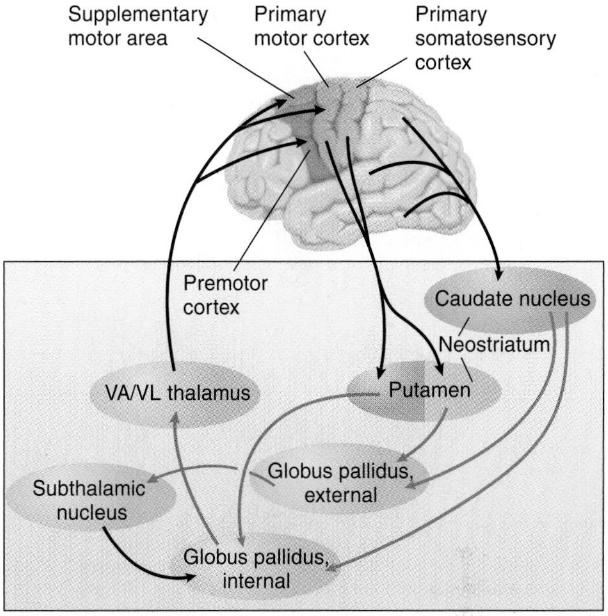

Reinforcement

Learning provides a means for us to profit from experience—to make responses that provide favorable outcomes. When good things happen (that is, when reinforcing stimuli occur), reinforcement mechanisms in the brain become active, and the establishment of synaptic changes is facilitated. The discovery of the existence of such reinforcement mechanisms occurred by accident.

Neural Circuits Involved in Reinforcement

In 1954, James Olds, a young assistant professor, and Peter Milner, a graduate student, attempted to determine whether electrical stimulation of the reticular formation would facilitate maze learning in rats. They planned to turn on the stimulator briefly each time an animal reached a choice point in the maze. First, however, they had to be certain that that the stimulation was not aversive, because an aversive stimulus would undoubtedly interfere with learning. As Olds reported,

> I applied a brief train of 60-cycle sine-wave electrical current whenever the animal entered one corner of the enclosure. The animal did not stay away from that corner, but rather came back quickly after a brief sortie which followed the first stimulation and came back even more quickly after a briefer sortie which followed the second stimulation. By the time the third electrical stimulus had been applied the animal seemed indubitably to be "coming back for more." (Olds, 1973, p. 81)

Realizing that they were on to something big, Olds and Milner decided to drop their original experiment and study the phenomenon they had discovered. Subsequent research discovered that although there are several different reinforcement mechanisms, the activity of dopaminergic neurons plays a particularly important role in reinforcement. As we saw in Chapter 4, the mesolimbic system of

FIGURE 12.19

The Ventral Tegmental Area and the Nucleus Accumbens.   Sections through a rat brain show the location of these regions.

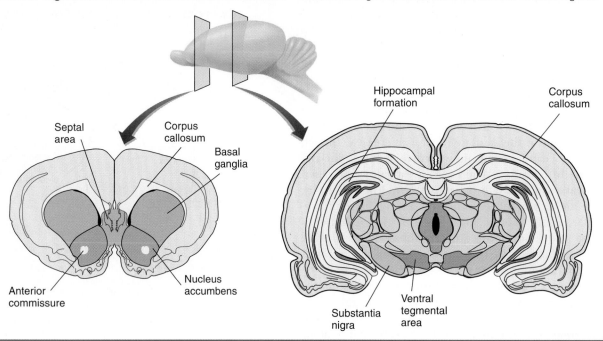

Adapted from Swanson, L. W. *Brain Maps: Structure of the Rat Brain*. New York: Elsevier, 1992.

FIGURE 12.20

Dopamine and Reinforcement.   Release of dopamine in the nucleus accumbens, measured by microdialysis, occurs when a rat pressed a lever that delivered electrical stimulation to the ventral tegmental area.

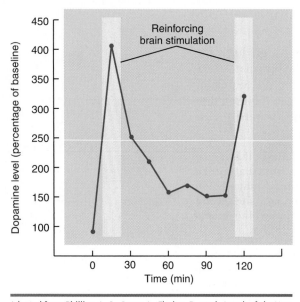

Adapted from Phillips, A. G., Coury, A., Fiorino, D., et al. *Annals of the New York Academy of Sciences*, 1992, *654*, 199–206.

dopaminergic neurons begins in the **ventral tegmental area (VTA)** of the midbrain and projects rostrally to several forebrain regions, including the amygdala, hippocampus, and **nucleus accumbens (NAC)**. This nucleus is located in the basal forebrain rostral to the preoptic area and immediately adjacent to the septum. (In fact, the full name of this region is the *nucleus accumbens septi*, or "nucleus leaning against the septum.") (See *Figure 12.19*.) Neurons in the NAC project to the ventral part of the basal ganglia, which, as we just saw, are involved in learning. The mesocortical system also plays a role in reinforcement. This system also begins in the ventral tegmental area but projects to the prefrontal cortex, the limbic cortex, and the hippocampus.

Chapter 5 described a research technique called *microdialysis*, which enables an investigator to analyze the contents of the interstitial fluid within a specific region of the brain. Researchers using this method have shown that reinforcing electrical stimulation of the ventral tegmental area or the administration of cocaine or amphetamine causes the release of dopamine in the nucleus accumbens (Moghaddam and Bunney, 1989; Nakahara et al., 1989; Phillips et al., 1992). (See *Figure 12.20*.) Microdialysis studies have also found that the presence of natural reinforcers, such as water, food, or a sex partner, stimulates the release of dopamine in the nucleus accumbens. Thus, the effects of reinforcing brain stimulation seem to be similar in many ways to those of natural reinforcers.

Although microdialysis probes are not placed in the brain of humans for experimental purposes, functional imaging studies have shown that reinforcing events activate the human nucleus accumbens. For example, Knutson et al. (2001) found that the nucleus accumbens became more active (and, presumably, dopamine was being released there) when people were presented with stimuli that indicated that they would be receiving money. Aharon et al. (2001) found that young heterosexual men would press a lever that presented pictures of beautiful women (but not handsome men) and that when they saw these pictures, the activity of the nucleus accumbens increased.

Functions of the Reinforcement System

A reinforcement system must perform two functions: detect the presence of a reinforcing stimulus (that is, recognize that something good has just happened) and strengthen the connections between the neurons that detect the discriminative stimulus (such as the sight of a lever) and the neurons that produce the instrumental response (a lever press). (Refer to *Figure 12.2*.)

Reinforcement occurs when neural circuits detect a reinforcing stimulus and cause the activation of dopaminergic neurons in the ventral tegmental area. Detection of a reinforcing stimulus is not a simple matter; a stimulus that serves as a reinforcer on one occasion may fail to do so on another. For example, the presence of food will reinforce the behavior of a hungry animal but not that of an animal that has just eaten. Thus, the reinforcement system is not automatically activated when particular stimuli are present; its activation also depends on the physiological state of the animal.

In general, if a stimulus causes the animal to engage in an appetitive behavior (that is, if it approaches the stimulus rather than runs away from it), that stimulus can reinforce the animal's behavior. When that stimulus occurs, it activates the brain's reinforcement mechanism, and the link between the discriminative stimulus and the instrumental response is strengthened. For example, a functional imaging study by Knutson and Adcock (2005) found that anticipation of a reinforcing stimulus (the opportunity to win some money) increased the activation of the ventral tegmentum and some of its projection regions (including the nucleus accumbens) in humans. The investigators also found that the subjects were more likely to remember pictures that they had seen while they were anticipating the chance to win some money.

The prefrontal cortex provides an important input to the ventral tegmental area. The terminal buttons of the axons connecting these two areas secrete glutamate, an excitatory neurotransmitter, and the activity of these synapses makes dopaminergic neurons in the ventral tegmental area fire in a bursting pattern, which greatly increases the amount of dopamine they secrete in the nucleus accumbens (Gariano and Groves, 1988). The prefrontal cortex is generally involved in devising strategies, making plans, evaluating progress made toward goals, and judging the appropriateness of one's own behavior. Perhaps the prefrontal cortex turns on the reinforcement mechanism when it determines that the ongoing behavior is bringing the organism nearer to its goals—that the present strategy is working.

How, exactly, does the release of dopamine facilitate the synaptic changes responsible for instrumental conditioning? In a review of the literature, Wise (2004) concluded that the release of dopamine in a variety of brain locations affects learning in a variety of tasks and that dopamine plays a critical role in long-lasting long-term potentiation and long-term depression in many brain regions, including the basal ganglia, amygdala, and frontal cortex. As we saw earlier, studies have shown that long-term potentiation is essential for instrumental conditioning and that dopamine is an essential ingredient in long-lasting long-term potentiation.

ventral tegmental area (VTA) A group of dopaminergic neurons in the ventral midbrain whose axons form the mesolimbic and mesocortical systems; plays a critical role in reinforcement.

nucleus accumbens (NAC) A nucleus of the basal forebrain near the septum; receives dopamine-secreting terminal buttons from neurons of the ventral tegmental area and is thought to be involved in reinforcement and attention.

InterimSummary

Instrumental Conditioning

Instrumental conditioning entails the strengthening of connections between neural circuits that detect stimuli and neural circuits that produce responses. One of the locations of these changes appears to be the basal ganglia, especially the changes responsible for learning of automated and routine behaviors. The basal ganglia receive sensory information and information about plans for movement from the neocortex. Instrumental conditioning activates the basal ganglia and damage to the basal ganglia or infusion of a drug that blocks NMDA receptors there disrupts instrumental conditioning.

Olds and Milner discovered that rats would perform a response that caused electrical current to be delivered through an electrode placed in their brain; thus, the stimulation was reinforcing. Although several neurotransmitters may play a role in reinforcement, one is particularly important: dopamine. The cell bodies of the most important system of dopaminergic neurons are located in the ventral tegmental area, and their axons project to the nucleus accumbens, prefrontal cortex, limbic cortex, and hippocampus.

Microdialysis studies have also shown that natural and artificial reinforcers stimulate the release of dopamine in the nucleus accumbens, and functional imaging studies have shown that reinforcing stimuli activate the nucleus accumbens in humans. The dopaminergic reinforcement system appears to be activated by reinforcers or stimuli that predict the occurrence of a reinforcer. Dopamine induces synaptic plasticity by facilitating associative long-term potentiation.

Thought Questions

Have you ever been working hard on a problem and suddenly thought of a possible solution? Did the thought make you feel excited and happy? What would we find if we had a microdialysis probe in your nucleus accumbens?

Relational Learning

So far, this chapter has discussed relatively simple forms of learning, which can be understood as changes in circuits of neurons that detect the presence of particular stimuli or as strengthened connections between neurons that analyze sensory information and those that produce responses. However, most forms of learning are more complex; most memories of real objects and events are related to other memories. Seeing a photograph of an old friend may remind you of the sound of the person's name and of the movements you have to make to pronounce it. You may also be reminded of things you have done with your friend: places you have visited, conversations you have had, experiences you have shared. Each of these memories can contain a series of events, complete with sights and sounds, that you will be able to recall in the proper sequence. Obviously, the neural circuits in the visual association cortex that recognize your friend's face are connected to circuits in many other parts of the brain, and these circuits are connected to many others. This section discusses research on relational learning, which includes the establishment and retrieval of memories of events, episodes, and places.

Human Anterograde Amnesia

One of the most dramatic and intriguing phenomena caused by brain damage is *anterograde amnesia*, which, at first glance, appears to be the inability to learn new information. However, when we examine the phenomenon more carefully, we find that the basic abilities of perceptual learning, stimulus–response learning, and motor learning are intact but that complex relational learning, of the type just described, is gone. This section discusses the nature of anterograde amnesia in humans and its anatomical basis. The section that follows discusses related research with laboratory animals.

The term **anterograde amnesia** refers to difficulty in learning new information. A person with pure anterograde amnesia can remember events that occurred in the past, from the time before the brain damage occurred, but cannot retain information about events encountered *after* the damage. In contrast, **retrograde amnesia**

anterograde amnesia Amnesia for events that occur after some disturbance to the brain, such as head injury or certain degenerative brain diseases.

retrograde amnesia Amnesia for events that preceded some disturbance to the brain, such as a head injury or electroconvulsive shock.

refs to the inability to remember events that happened *before* the brain damage occurred. (See *Figure 12.21*.) Pure antero- grade amnesia is rare; usually, there is also a retrograde amne- sia for events that occurred for a period of time before the brain damage occurred.

In 1889, Sergei Korsakoff, a Russian physician, first described a severe memory impairment caused by brain dam- age, and the disorder was given his name. The most profound symptom of **Korsakoff's syndrome** is a severe anterograde amnesia: The patients appear to be unable to form new memo- ries, although they can still remember old ones. They can con- verse normally and can remember events that happened long before their brain damage occurred, but they cannot remember events that happened afterward. The brain damage that causes Korsakoff's syndrome is usually (but not always) a result of chronic alcohol abuse.

Another symptom of Korsakoff's syndrome is **confabulation**. When people with this disorder are asked about events that occurred recently, they often describe a fic- titious event rather than simply saying, "I don't remember." (Notice that *confabulate* has the same root as *fable*.) Confabulations can contain mixtures of events that really occurred, or they can be completely imaginary. People who confabulate are not deliberately trying to deceive; they appear to believe that what they are saying really occurred. I will discuss confabulation in the epilogue to this chapter.

Anterograde amnesia can also be caused by damage to the temporal lobes. Scoville and Milner (1957) reported that bilateral removal of the medial temporal lobe produced a memory impairment in humans that was apparently identical to that seen in Korsakoff's syndrome. H. M., the man described in the prologue to this chapter, received the surgery in an attempt to treat his severe epilepsy, which could not be controlled even by high doses of anticonvulsant medication. The epilepsy appears to have been caused by a head injury he received when he was struck by a bicycle at age 9 (Corkin et al., 1997).

The surgery successfully treated H. M.'s seizure disorder, but it became appar- ent that the operation had produced a serious memory impairment. Further inves- tigation revealed that the critical site of damage was the hippocampus. Once it was known that bilateral medial temporal lobectomy causes anterograde amnesia, neu- rosurgeons stopped performing this operation and are now careful to operate on only one temporal lobe.

H. M.'s history and memory deficits were described in the chapter prologue (Milner, Corkin, and Teuber, 1968; Milner, 1970; Corkin et al., 1981). Because of his relatively pure amnesia, his memory deficit was extensively studied. Milner and her colleagues based the following conclusions on his pattern of deficits:

1. *The hippocampus is not the location of long-term memories, nor is it necessary for the retrieval of long-term memories.* If it were, H. M. would not have been able to remember events from early in his life, he would not know how to talk, he would not know how to dress himself, and so on.
2. *The hippocampus is not the location of immediate (short-term) memories.* If it were, H. M. would not be able to carry on a conversation, because he would not remember what the other person said long enough to think of a reply.
3. *The hippocampus is involved in converting immediate (short-term) memories into long- term memories.* This conclusion is based on a particular hypothesis of memory function: that our immediate memory of an event is retained by neural activity and that long-term memories consist of relatively permanent biochemical or structural changes in neurons. The conclusion seems a reasonable explanation for the fact that when presented with new information, H. M. seems to under- stand it and remember it as long as he thinks about it but that a permanent record of the information is just never made.

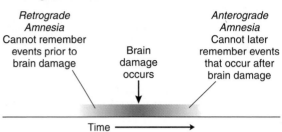

FIGURE 12.21

A Schematic Definition of Retrograde Amnesia and Anterograde Amnesia

Retrograde Amnesia
Cannot remember events prior to brain damage

Brain damage occurs

Anterograde Amnesia
Cannot later remember events that occur after brain damage

Time ———→

Korsakoff's syndrome Permanent anterograde amnesia caused by brain damage, usually resulting from chronic alcoholism.

confabulation The reporting of memories of events that did not take place without the intention to deceive; seen in people with Kor- sakoff's syndrome.

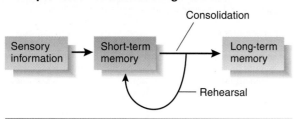

A Simple Model of the Learning Process

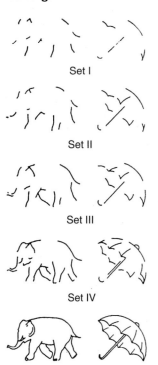

Examples of Broken Drawings

Set I

Set II

Set III

Set IV

Set V

Reprinted with permission of author and publisher from Gollin, E. S. Developmental studies of visual recognition of incomplete objects. *Perceptual and Motor Skills*, 1960, *11*, 289–298.

mypsychkit

Animation 12.4
Implicit Memory Tasks

consolidation The process by which short-term memories are converted into long-term memories.

As we will see, these three conclusions are too simple. Subsequent research on patients with anterograde amnesia indicates that the facts are more complicated—and more interesting—than they first appeared to be. But to appreciate the significance of the findings of more recent research, we must understand these three conclusions and remember the facts that led to them.

Most psychologists believe that learning consists of at least two stages: short-term memory and long-term memory. They conceive of short-term memory as a means of storing a limited amount of information temporarily and long-term memory as a means of storing an unlimited amount (or at least an enormously large amount) of information permanently. We can remember a new item of information (such as a telephone number) for as long as we want to by engaging in a particular behavior: rehearsal. However, once we stop rehearsing the information, we might or might not be able to remember it later; that is, the information might or might not get stored in long-term memory.

The simplest model of the memory process says that sensory information enters short-term memory, rehearsal keeps it there, and eventually, the information makes its way into long-term memory, where it is permanently stored. The conversion of short-term memories into long-term memories has been called **consolidation**, because the memories are "made solid," so to speak. (See *Figure 12.22*.)

Now you can understand the original conclusions of Milner and her colleagues: If H. M.'s short-term memory were intact and if he could remember events from before his operation, then the problem must have been that consolidation had not taken place. Thus, the role of the hippocampal formation in memory is consolidation—converting short-term memories to long-term memories.

Spared Learning Abilities

H. M.'s memory deficit was striking and dramatic. However, when he and other patients with anterograde amnesia were studied more carefully, it became apparent that the amnesia did not represent a total failure in learning ability. When the patients are appropriately trained and tested, we find that they are capable of three of the four major types of learning described earlier in this chapter: perceptual learning, stimulus–response learning, and motor learning. A review by Spiers, Maguire, and Burgess (2001) summarized 147 cases of anterograde amnesia that are consistent with the descriptions that follow.

First, let us consider perceptual learning. Figure 12.23 shows two sample items from a test of the ability to recognize broken drawings; note how the drawings are successively more complete. (See *Figure 12.23*.) Subjects are first shown the least complete set (set I) of each of twenty different drawings. If they do not recognize a figure (and most people do not recognize set I), they are shown more complete sets until they identify it. One hour later, the subjects are tested again for retention, starting with set I. When H. M. was given this test and was retested an hour later, he showed considerable improvement (Milner, 1970). When he was retested 4 months later, he *still* showed this improvement. His performance was not as good as that of normal control subjects, but he showed unmistakable evidence of long-term retention. (You can try the broken drawing task and some other tasks that people with anterograde amnesia can successfully learn by running *MyPsychKit 12.4, Implicit Memory Tasks*.)

Johnson, Kim, and Risse (1985) found that patients with anterograde amnesia could learn to recognize faces and melodies. The researchers played unfamiliar melodies from Korean songs to amnesic patients and found that when they were tested later, the patients preferred these melodies to ones they had not heard before. The experimenters also presented photographs of two men along with stories of their lives: One man was said to be dishonest, mean, and vicious; the other was said to be nice enough to invite home to dinner. (Half of the patients heard that one of the men was the bad one, and the other half heard that the other man was.) Twenty days later, the amnesic patients said they liked the picture of the "nice" man better than that of the "nasty" one.

Investigators have also succeeded in demonstrating stimulus–response learning by H. M. and other amnesic subjects. For example, Woodruff-Pak (1993) found that H. M. and another patient with anterograde amnesia could acquire a classically conditioned eyeblink response. H. M. even showed retention of the task 2 years later: He acquired the response again in one-tenth the number of trials that were needed previously. Sidman, Stoddard, and Mohr (1968) successfully trained patient H. M. on an instrumental conditioning task—a visual discrimination task in which pennies were given for correct responses.

Finally, several studies have demonstrated motor learning in patients with anterograde amnesia. For example, Reber and Squire (1998) found that subjects with anterograde amnesia could learn a sequence of button presses in a *serial reaction time task*. They sat in front of a computer screen and watched an asterisk appear—apparently randomly—in one of four locations. Their task was to press the one of four buttons that corresponded to the location of the asterisk. As soon as they did so, the asterisk moved to a new location, and they pressed the corresponding button. (See *Figure 12.24*.)

Although experimenters did not say so, the sequence of button presses specified by the moving asterisk was not random. For example, it might be DBCACBDCBA, a ten-item sequence that is repeated continuously. With practice, subjects become faster and faster at this task. It is clear that their rate increases because they have learned the sequence, because if the sequence is changed, their performance decreases. The amnesic subjects learned this task just as well as normal subjects did.

A study by Cavaco et al. (2004) tested amnesic patients on a variety of tasks modeled on real-world activities, such as weaving, tracing figures, operating a stick that controlled a video display, and pouring water into small jars. Both amnesic patients and normal subjects did poorly on these tasks at first, but their performance improved through practice. Thus, as you can see, patients with anterograde amnesia are capable of a variety of tasks that require perceptual learning, stimulus–response learning, and motor learning.

Declarative and Nondeclarative Memories

If amnesic patients can learn tasks like these, you might ask, why do we call them *amnesic*? The answer is this: Although the patients can learn to perform these tasks, they do not remember anything about having learned them. They do not remember the experimenters, the room in which the training took place, the apparatus that was used, or any events that occurred during the training. Although H. M. learned to recognize the broken drawings, he denied that he had ever seen them before. Although the amnesic patients in the study by Johnson, Kim, and Risse learned to like some of the Korean melodies better, they did not recognize that they had heard them before, nor did they remember having seen the pictures of the two young men. Although H. M. successfully acquired a classically conditioned eyeblink response, he did not remember the experimenter, the apparatus, or the headband he wore that held the device that delivered a puff of air to his eye.

In the experiment by Sidman, Stoddard, and Mohr, although H. M. learned to make the correct response (press a panel with a picture of a circle on it), he was unable to recall having done so. In fact, once H. M. had learned the task, the experimenters interrupted him, had him count his pennies (to distract him for a little while), and then asked him to say what he was supposed to do. He seemed puzzled by the question; he had absolutely no idea. But when they turned on the stimuli again, he immediately made the correct response. Finally, although the amnesic subjects in Reber and Squire's study obviously learned the sequence of button

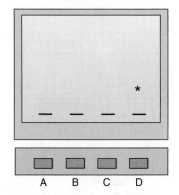

FIGURE 12.24

The Serial Reaction Time Task.   In the procedure of the study by Reber and Squire (1998), subjects pressed the button in a sequence indicated by movement of the asterisk on the computer screen.

DBCACBDCBA

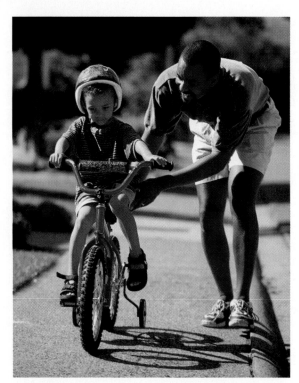

Learning to ride a bicycle is a combination of stimulus–response learning and motor learning, both of which are nondeclarative in nature. Remembering when we learned to ride a bicycle is an episodic memory, a form of relational learning.

presses, they were completely unaware that there was, in fact, a sequence; they thought that the movement of the asterisk was random.

The distinction between what people with anterograde amnesia can and cannot learn is obviously important because it reflects the basic organization of the learning process. Clearly, there are at least two major categories of memories. Psychologists have given them several different names. For example, some investigators (Eichenbaum, Otto, and Cohen, 1992; Squire, 1992) suggest that patients with anterograde amnesia are unable to form **declarative memories**, which have been defined as those that are "explicitly available to conscious recollection as facts, events, or specific stimuli" (Squire, Shimamura, and Amaral, 1989, p. 218). The term *declarative* obviously comes from *declare*, which means "to proclaim; to announce." The term reflects the fact that patients with anterograde amnesia cannot talk about experiences that they have had since the time of their brain damage. Thus, according to Squire and his colleagues, declarative memory is memory of events and facts that we can think and talk about.

Declarative memories are not simply verbal memories. For example, think about some event in your life, such as your last birthday. Think about where you were, when the event occurred, what other people were present, what events occurred, and so on. Although you could describe ("declare") this episode in words, the memory itself would not be verbal. In fact, it would probably be more like a video clip running in your head: one whose starting and stopping points—and fast forwards and rewinds—you could control.

The other category of memories, often called **nondeclarative memories**, includes instances of perceptual, stimulus–response, and motor learning that we are not necessarily conscious of. (Some psychologists refer to these two categories as *explicit* and *implicit* memories, respectively.) Nondeclarative memories appear to operate automatically. They do not require deliberate attempts on the part of the learner to memorize something. They do not seem to include facts or experiences; instead, they control behaviors. For example, think about when you learned to ride a bicycle. You did so quite consciously and developed declarative memories about your attempts: who helped you learn, where you rode, how you felt, how many times you fell, and so on—but you also formed nondeclarative stimulus–response and motor memories; *you learned to ride.* You learned to make automatic adjustments with your hands and body that keep your center of gravity above the wheels.

The acquisition of specific behaviors and skills is probably the most important form of implicit memory. Driving a car, turning the pages of a book, playing a musical instrument, dancing, throwing and catching a ball, sliding a chair backward as we get up from the dinner table—all of these skills involve coordination of movements with sensory information received from the environment and from our own moving body parts. We do not need to be able to describe these activities in order to perform them. We may not even be aware of all the movements we make while we are performing them.

declarative memory Memory that can be verbally expressed, such as memory for events in a person's past.

nondeclarative memory Memory whose formation does not depend on the hippocampal formation; a collective term for perceptual, stimulus–response, and motor memory.

Patient E. P. developed a profound anterograde amnesia when he was stricken with a case of viral encephalitis that destroyed much of his medial temporal lobe. Bayley, Frascino, and Squire (2005) taught patient E. P. to point to a particular member of each of a series of eight pairs of objects. He eventually learned to do so, but he had no explicit memory of which objects were correct. When asked why he chose a particular object, he said, "It just seems that's the one. It's here (pointing to head) somehow or another and the hand goes for it . . . I can't say memory. I just feel this is the one. . . . It's just jumping out at me. 'I'm the one. I'm the one.'" (Bayley, Frascino, and Squire, 2005, p. 551). Clearly, he learned a nondeclarative stimulus–response task without at the same time acquiring any declarative memories about what he had learned.

Table 12.1 lists the declarative and nondeclarative memory tasks described so far. (See *Table 12.1.*)

Anatomy of Anterograde Amnesia

The phenomenon of anterograde amnesia—and its implications for the nature of relational learning—has led investigators to study this phenomenon in laboratory animals. However, before I review this research (which has provided some very interesting results), we should examine the brain damage that produces anterograde amnesia. One fact is clear: Damage to the hippocampus or to regions of the brain that supply its inputs and receive its outputs causes anterograde amnesia.

As we saw earlier in this chapter, the hippocampal formation consists of the dentate gyrus, the CA fields of the hippocampus itself, and the subiculum (and its subregions). The most important input to the hippocampal formation is the entorhinal cortex; neurons there have axons that terminate in the dentate gyrus, CA3, and CA1. The entorhinal cortex receives its inputs from the amygdala, various regions of the limbic cortex, and all association regions of the neocortex, either directly or via two adjacent regions of limbic cortex: the **perirhinal cortex** and the **parahippocampal cortex**. The outputs of the hippocampal system come primarily from field CA1 and the subiculum. Most of these outputs are relayed back through the entorhinal, perirhinal, and parahippocampal cortex to the same regions of association cortex that provide inputs. (See *Figure 12.25.*)

Role of the Hippocampal Formation in Memory Consolidation

As we saw earlier in this chapter, the hippocampus is not the location of either short-term or long-term memories; after all, patients with damage to the hippocampal formation can remember events that happened before their brain

TABLE 12.1	Examples of Declarative and Nondeclarative Memory Tasks	
Declarative Memory Tasks		
Remembering past experiences		
Learning new words		
Finding way in new environment		
Nondeclarative Memory Tasks	**Type of Learning**	
Broken drawings	Perceptual	
Recognizing faces	Perceptual (and stimulus–response?)	
Recognizing melodies	Perceptual	
Classical conditioning (eyeblink)	Stimulus–response	
Instrumental conditioning (choose circle)	Stimulus–response	
Sequence of button presses	Motor	

perirhinal cortex A region of limbic cortex adjacent to the hippocampal formation that, along with the parahippocampal cortex, relays information between the entorhinal cortex and other regions of the brain.

parahippocampal cortex A region of limbic cortex adjacent to the hippocampal formation that, along with the perirhinal cortex, relays information between the entorhinal cortex and other regions of the brain.

FIGURE 12.25

Cortical Connections of the Hippocampal Formation.   The figure shows (a) a view of the base of a monkey's brain and (b) connections with the cerebral cortex.

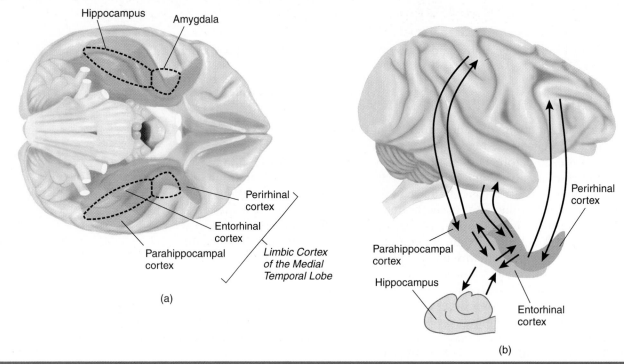

(a)

(b)

became damaged, and their short-term memory is relatively normal. The hippocampal formation, however, clearly plays a role in the process through which declarative memories are formed. Most researchers believe that the process works something like this: The hippocampus receives information about what is going on from the sensory and motor association cortices and from some subcortical regions, such as the basal ganglia and amygdala. It processes this information and then, through its *efferent* connections with these regions, modifies the memories that are being consolidated there, linking them together in ways that will permit us to remember the relationships among the elements of the memories; for example, the order in which events occurred, the context in which we perceived a particular item, and so on. Without the hippocampal formation we would be left with individual, isolated memories without the linkage that makes it possible to remember—and think about—episodes and contexts.

If the hippocampus does modify memories as they are being formed, then experiences that lead to declarative memories should activate the hippocampal formation. In fact, several studies have found this prediction to be true. In general, pictorial or spatial information activates the right hippocampal formation, and verbal information activates the left hippocampal formation. For example, Brewer et al. (1998) found that activation of the right hippocampal formation was related to people's ability to remember complex color photos, and Alkire et al. (1998) found that activation of the left hippocampal formation was related to people's ability to remember a list of words.

As we saw, anterograde amnesia is usually accompanied by retrograde amnesia—the inability to remember events that occurred for a period of time before the brain damage occurred. The duration of the retrograde amnesia appears to be related to the amount of damage to the medial temporal lobe (Squire and Bayley, 2007; Kirwan et al., 2008). The fact that retrograde amnesia extends back for a lim-

FIGURE 12.26

Changing Roles of Hippocampus and Prefrontal Cortex in Memory.   A functional imaging study found that (a) the role of the ventromedial prefrontal cortex increased over time, and (b) the role of the hippocampus decreased over time.

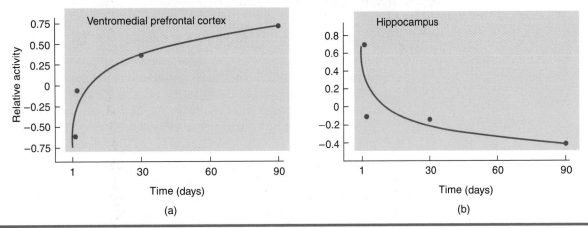

(a)   (b)

Adapted from Takashima, A., Petersson, K. M., Rutters, F., et al. *Proceedings of the National Academy of Sciences, USA*, 2006, *103*, 756–761.

ited period of time suggests that a gradual process controlled by the hippocampal formation transforms memories located elsewhere in the brain. Until this transformation is complete, the hippocampal formation is required for the retrieval of these memories. Later, retrieval of these memories can be accomplished even if the hippocampal formation has been damaged. A functional imaging study by Takashima et al. (2006) supports this hypothesis. The investigators had normal subjects look at—and try to memorize—320 different photographs of landscapes. Later that day, 1 day later, 1 month later, and 3 months later, the investigators presented photographs that included a mixture of new photographs and a sample of the photographs they had previously seen and asked the subjects to identify which ones were familiar to them. Takashima and her colleagues found that initially, hippocampal activation correlated with the subjects' memory of the photographs they had previously seen. However, as time went on, the hippocampal activation decreased, and the activation of the prefrontal cortex increased. (See *Figure 12.26.*) The investigators concluded that the hippocampus played a role in retrieval of early memories, but that this task was transferred to the prefrontal cortex as time went on. They suggested that it is unlikely that the memories for the photographs were actually stored in the prefrontal cortex but hypothesized that this region, with its rich connections with other regions of the cerebral cortex, is involved in organizing and linking information stored in other regions of the cerebral cortex.

Episodic and Semantic Memories

Declarative memories come in at least two forms: episodic and semantic. **Episodic memories** involve context; they include information about when and under what conditions a particular episode occurred and the order in which the events in the episode took place. Episodic memories are specific to a particular time and place, because a given episode—by definition—occurs only once. **Semantic memories** involve facts, but they do not include information about the context in which the facts were learned. In other words, semantic memories are less specific than episodic memories. For example, knowing that the sun is a star involves a less specific memory than being able to remember when, where, and from whom you learned this fact. Semantic memories can be acquired gradually, over time. Episodic memories must be learned all at once.

episodic memory Memory of a collection of perceptions of events organized in time and identified by a particular context.

semantic memory A memory of facts and general information.

Another patient, A. M., developed a progressive degenerative disorder of the lateral temporal cortex that disrupted his semantic memory but left his episodic memory intact (Murre, Graham, and Hodges, 2001). This syndrome is known as *semantic dementia.*

Examiner: Can you remember April last year?

A. M.: April last year, that was the first time, and eh, on the Monday, for example, they were checking all my whatsit, and that was the first time, when my brain was, eh, shown, you know, you know that bar of the brain (indicates left), not the, the other one was okay, but that was lousy, so they did that and then doing everything like that, like this and probably a bit better than I am just now (indicates scanning by moving his hands over his head). (Murre, Graham, and Hodges, 2001, p. 651)

Patient A. M.'s loss of semantic information had a profound effect on his everyday activities. He seemed not to understand functions of commonplace objects. For example, he held a closed umbrella horizontally over his head during a rainstorm and brought his wife a lawnmower when she had asked for a stepladder. He put sugar into a glass of wine and put yogurt on a raw defrosting salmon steak and ate it. He nevertheless showed some surprisingly complex behaviors. Because he could not be trusted to drive a car, his wife surreptitiously removed the car keys from his key ring. He noticed their absence, and rather than complaining to her (presumably, he realized that would be fruitless), he surreptitiously removed the car keys from *her* key ring, went to a locksmith, and had a duplicate set made.

Although his semantic memory was severely damaged, his episodic memory was surprisingly good. The investigators reported that even when his dementia had progressed to the point at which he was scoring at chance levels on a test of semantic information, he answered a phone call that was meant for his wife, who was out of the house. When she returned later, he remembered to tell her about the call.

The hippocampal formation and the limbic cortex of the medial temporal lobe appear to be involved in the consolidation and retrieval of declarative memories, both episodic and semantic, but the study of people with localized brain damage suggest that the semantic memories themselves appear to be stored in the neocortex; in particular, in the neocortex of the anterolateral temporal lobe. Pobric, Jefferies, and Lambon Ralph (2007) found that transcranial magnetic stimulation of the left anterior temporal lobe, which disrupted the normal neural activity of this region, produced the symptoms of semantic dementia. The subjects had difficulty naming pictures of objects and understanding the meanings of words, but they had no trouble performing other, nonsemantic, tasks such as naming six-digit numbers and matching large numbers according to their approximate size. Also, a functional imaging study by Rogers et al. (2006) recorded activation of the anterolateral temporal lobes when people performed a picture-naming task.

Specific evidence for a role of the hippocampus and medial temporal cortex in episodic memory comes from a functional imaging study by Lehn et al. (2009). Lehn and her colleagues had people watch a movie they had not seen before. Later, while their brains were being scanned, the subjects were shown sets of isolated screen shots taken from different scenes and were asked to indicate the order in which these scenes appeared in the movie. Functional imaging revealed extensive activation in the medial temporal lobe. In fact, activation in the right hippocampus was correlated with the accuracy of the subjects' recall of the correct sequence.

Spatial Memory

I mentioned earlier in this chapter that patient H. M. has not been able to find his way around his present environment. Although spatial information need not be declared (we can demonstrate our topographical memories by successfully getting from place to place), people with anterograde amnesia are unable to consolidate information about the location of rooms, corridors, buildings, roads, and other important items in their environment.

Bilateral medial temporal lobe lesions produce the most profound impairment in spatial memory, but significant deficits can be produced by damage that is limited to the right hemisphere. For example, Luzzi et al. (2000) reported the case of a man with a lesion of the right parahippocampal gyrus who lost his ability to find his way around a new environment. The only way he could find his room was by counting doorways from the end of the hall or by seeing a red napkin that was located on top of his bedside table.

Functional imaging studies have shown that the right hippocampal formation becomes active when a person is remembering or performing a navigational task. For example Maguire, Frackowiak, and Frith (1997) had London taxi drivers describe the routes they would take in driving from one location to another. Functional imaging performed during their description of the route showed activation of the right hippocampal formation. London taxi drivers undergo extensive training to learn how to navigate efficiently in that city; in fact, this training takes about 2 years, and the drivers receive their license only after passing a rigorous set of tests. We would expect that this topographical learning would produce some changes in various parts of their brains, including their hippocampal formation. In fact, Maguire et al. (2000) found that the volume of the posterior hippocampus of London taxi drivers was larger than that of control subjects. Furthermore, the longer an individual taxi driver had spent in this occupation, the larger was the volume of the right posterior hippocampus.

Iaria et al. (2003) trained subjects on a computerized virtual reality program that permitted them to learn a maze that could be learned two ways: through observation of distant spatial cues or by memorization of a series of turns. About half of the subjects spontaneously used spatial cues, and the other half spontaneously learned to make a sequence of turns. Functional imaging showed that the hippocampus was activated in subjects who followed the *spatial strategy* and the caudate nucleus was activated in subjects who followed the *response strategy*. In addition, a structural MRI study by Bohbot et al. (2007) found that people who tended to follow a spatial strategy in a virtual maze had a larger-than-average hippocampus, and people who tended to follow a response strategy had a larger-than-average caudate nucleus. (You will recall that the caudate nucleus, part of the basal ganglia, plays a role in stimulus-response learning.) Figure 12.27 shows the relationship between performance on test trials that could only be performed by using a response strategy. As you can see, the larger a person's caudate nucleus is (and the smaller a person's hippocampus is), the fewer errors that person made. (See *Figure 12.27*.)

Relational Learning in Laboratory Animals

The discovery that hippocampal lesions produced anterograde amnesia in humans stimulated interest in the exact role that this structure plays in the learning process. To pursue this interest, researchers have developed tasks that require relational learning, and on such tasks laboratory animals with hippocampal lesions show memory deficits, just as humans do.

Spatial Perception and Learning

As we saw, hippocampal lesions disrupt the ability to keep track of and remember spatial locations. For example, H. M. never learned to find his way home when his parents moved after his surgery. Laboratory animals show similar problems in navigation. Morris et al. (1982) developed a task that has been adopted by other

FIGURE 12.27

Spatial and Response Strategies. The figure shows the relation between the volume of gray matter of (a) the caudate nucleus and (b) the hippocampus and errors made on test trials in a virtual maze that could only be learned by using a response strategy. Increased density of the caudate nucleus (a) was associated with better performance, and increased density of the hippocampus (b) was associated with poorer performance.

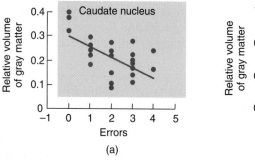
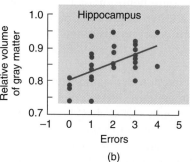

(a)   (b)

From Bohbot, V. D., Lerch, J., Thorndycraft, B., Iaria, G., and Zijdenbos, A. *Journal of Neuroscience,* 2007, *27,* 10078–10083. Reprinted with permission.

researchers as a standard test of rodents' spatial abilities. The task requires rats to find a particular location in space solely by means of visual cues external to the apparatus. The "maze" consists of a circular pool, 1.3 meters in diameter, filled with a mixture of water and something to increase the opacity of the water, such as powdered milk. The water hides the location of a small platform, situated just beneath the surface of the liquid. The experimenters put the rats into the water and let them swim until they encountered the hidden platform and climbed onto it. They released the rats from a new position on each trial. After a few trials normal rats learned to swim directly to the hidden platform from wherever they were released.

The Morris water maze requires relational learning; to navigate around the maze, the animals get their bearings from the relative locations of stimuli located outside the maze—furniture, windows, doors, and so on, but the maze can be used for nonrelational, stimulus–response learning too. If the animals are always released at the same place, they learn to head in a particular direction—say, toward a particular landmark they can see above the wall of the maze (Eichenbaum, Stewart, and Morris, 1990).

If rats with hippocampal lesions are always released from the same place, they learn this nonrelational, stimulus–response task about as well as normal rats do. However, if they are released from a new position on each trial, they swim in what appears to be an aimless fashion until they finally encounter the platform. (See *Figure 12.28.*)

Place Cells in the Hippocampal Formation

One of the most intriguing discoveries about the hippocampal formation was made by O'Keefe and Dostrovsky (1971), who recorded the activity of individual pyramidal cells in the hippocampus as an animal moved around the environment. The experimenters found that some neurons fired at a high rate only when the rat was in a particular location. Different neurons had different *spatial receptive fields;* that is, they responded when the animals were in different locations. A particular neuron might fire twenty times per second when the animal was in a particular location but only a few times per hour when the animal was located elsewhere. For obvious reasons these neurons were named **place cells**.

When a rat is placed in a symmetrical chamber, where there are few cues to distinguish one part of the apparatus from another, the animal must keep track of its

place cell A neuron that becomes active when the animal is in a particular location in the environment; most typically found in the hippocampal formation.

FIGURE 12.28

The Morris Water Maze.   (a) Environmental cues present in the room provide information that permits the animals to orient themselves in space. (b) Variable and fixed start positions. Normally, rats are released from a different position on each trial. If they are released from the same position every time, the rats can learn to find the hidden platform through stimulus–response learning. (c) The graphs show the performance of normal rats and rats with hippocampal lesions using variable or fixed start positions. Hippocampal lesions impair acquisition of the relational task. (d) This part shows representative samples of the paths followed by normal rats and rats with hippocampal lesions on the relational task (variable start positions).

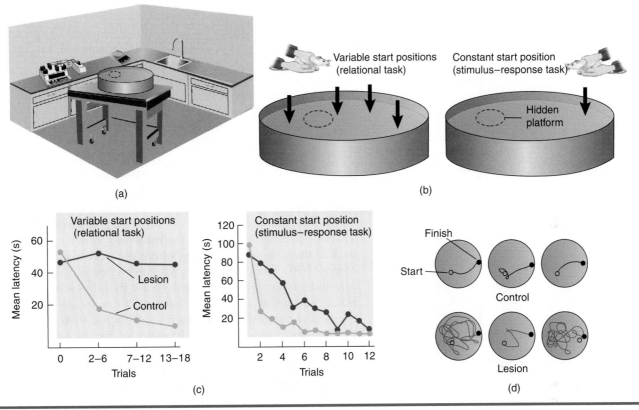

Adapted from Eichenbaum, H. *Nature Reviews: Neuroscience*, 2000, *1*, 41–50. Data from Eichenbaum et al., 1990.

location from objects it sees (or hears) in the environment outside the maze. Changes in these items affect the firing of the rats' place cells as well as their navigational ability. When experimenters move the stimuli as a group, maintaining their relative positions, the animals simply reorient their responses accordingly. However, when the experimenters interchange the stimuli so that they are arranged in a new order, the animals' performance (and the firing of their place cells) is disrupted. (Imagine how disoriented you might be if you entered a familiar room and found that the windows, doors, and furniture were in new positions.)

The fact that neurons in the hippocampal formation have spatial receptive fields does not mean that each neuron encodes a particular location. Instead, this information is undoubtedly represented by particular *patterns* of activity in circuits of large numbers of neurons within the hippocampal formation. In rodents most hippocampal place cells are found in the dorsal hippocampus, which corresponds to the posterior hippocampus in humans (Best, White, and Minai, 2001).

Evidence indicates that firing of hippocampal place cells appears to reflect the location where an animal "thinks" it is. Skaggs and McNaughton (1998) constructed an apparatus that contained two nearly identical chambers connected by a corridor. Each day, rats were placed in one of the chambers, and a cluster of electrodes in the animals' brains recorded the activity of hippocampal place cells. Each rat was always

FIGURE 12.29

Spatial Memory. The apparatus shown here was used in the study by Skaggs and McNaughton (1998). Because the rat was normally placed in the north chamber, its hippocampal place cells responded as if it were there when it was placed in the south chamber one day. However, once it stuck its head into the corridor, it saw that the other chamber was located to its right, so it "realized" that it had just been in the south chamber. From then on, the pattern of firing of the hippocampal place cells accurately reflected the chamber in which the animal was located.

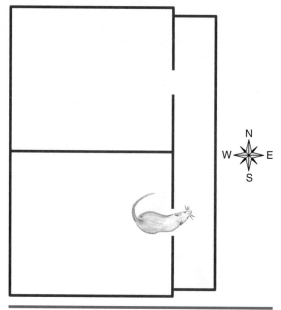

placed in the same chamber each day. Some of the place cells showed similar patterns of activity in each of the chambers, and some showed different patterns, which suggests that the hippocampus "realized" that there were two different compartments but also "recognized" the similarities between them. Then, on the last day of the experiment, the investigators placed the rats in the other chamber of the apparatus. For example, if a rat was usually placed in the north chamber, it was placed in the south chamber. The firing pattern of the place cells in at least half of the rats indicated that the hippocampus "thought" it was in the usual chamber—the one to the north. However, once the rat left the chamber and entered the corridor, it saw that it had to turn to the left to get to the other chamber and not to the right. The animal apparently realized its mistake, because for the rest of that session the neurons fired appropriately. They displayed the "north" pattern in the north chamber and the "south" pattern in the south chamber. (See *Figure 12.29.*)

The activity of circuits of hippocampal place cells provide information about more than space. Wood et al. (2000) trained rats on a spatial alternation task in a T-maze. The task required the rats to enter the left and the right arms on alternate trials; when they did so, they received a piece of food in goal boxes located at the ends of the arms of the T. Corridors led from the goal boxes back to the stem of the T-maze, where the next trial began. (See *Figure 12.30.*) Wood and her colleagues recorded from field CA1 pyramidal cells and, as expected, found that different cells fired when the rat was in different parts of the maze. However, two-thirds of the neurons fired differentially in the stem of the T on left-turn and right-turn trials. In other words, the cells not only encoded the rat's location in the maze, but also signaled whether the rat was going to turn right or turn left after it got to the choice point. Thus, pyramidal cells in CA1 encode both the current location and the intended destination.

Role of the Hippocampal Formation in Memory Consolidation

Several experiments indicate that the hippocampal formation plays a role in consolidation of relational memories. For example, Maviel et al. (2004) trained mice in a Morris water maze and tested later for their memory of the location of the platform. Just before testing the animal's performance, the investigators temporarily inactivated specific regions of the animals' brains with intracerebral infusions of lidocaine, a local anesthetic. If the hippocampus was inactivated 1 day after training, the mice showed no memory of the task. However, if the hippocampus was inactivated 30 days after training, their performance was normal. In contrast, inactivation of several regions of the cerebral cortex impaired memory retrieval 30 days after training, but not 1 day after training. These findings indicate that the hippocampus is required for recalling newly learned spatial information but not information learned 30 days previously. The findings also suggest that sometime during these 30 days the cerebral cortex takes on a role in retention of this information. (*See Figure 12.31.*)

As we saw in Chapter 8, slow-wave sleep facilitates the consolidation of declarative memories in human subjects, while REM sleep facilitates the consolidation of nondeclarative memories. One advantage of recording place cells in the hippocampus while animals perform a spatial task is that the investigators can detect different patterns of activity in these cells that change as the animals move through different environments. Lee and Wilson (2002) implanted an array of microelectrodes in field CA1 of rats, and were able to record from twenty-four to fifty-seven different

FIGURE 12.30

More than Spatial Information   Rats were trained to turn right and turn left at the end of the stem of the T-maze on alternate trials. The firing patterns of hippocampal place cells with spatial receptive fields in the stem of the maze were different on trials during which the animals subsequently turned left or right.

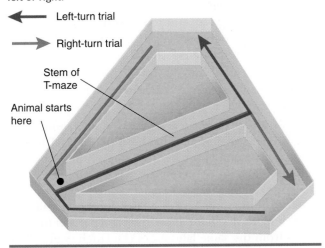

Adapted from Wood, E. R., Dudchenko, P. A., Robitsek, R. J., and Eichenbaum, H. *Neuron*, 2000, *27*, 623–633.

FIGURE 12.31

A Schematic Description of the Experiment by Maviel et al. (2004)   Learning was disrupted by temporary inactivation of the hippocampus 1 day after training or temporary inactivation of the cortex 30 days after training.

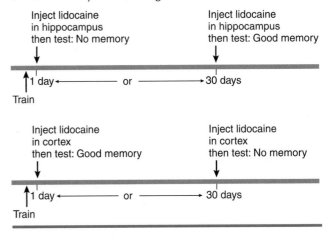

neurons simultaneously in each animal. The rats ran through straight or U-shaped tracks, at the ends of which they found a piece of chocolate. The investigators recorded the sequences of place cell activity in field CA1 as the animals ran. They also recorded the activity of these cells while the animals slept. They found that particular cells had particular spatial receptive fields, so that as the animals ran through the tracks, particular sequences of cell firing were seen. Recordings made after training showed the same patterns of activity while the animals engaged in slow-wave sleep. Presumably, these patterns indicate a replay of the animals' behavior as they moved through their environment and obtained the food, and facilitate consolidation of the memories of these episodes.

Reconsolidation of Memories

What happens to memories of events as time goes on? Clearly, if we learn something new about a particular subject, our memories pertaining to that subject must somehow be modified. For example, as mentioned earlier in this chapter, if a friend gets a new hairstyle or replaces glasses with contact lenses, our visual memory of that person will change accordingly. If you learn more about something—for example, the layout of a previously unfamiliar neighborhood—you will acquire a larger and larger number of interconnected memories. These examples indicate that memories can be altered or connected to newer memories. In recent years, researchers have been investigating a phenomenon known as *reconsolidation*, which appears to involve modification of long-term memories.

In fact, studies have found that long-term, well-consolidated relational memories are also susceptible to disruption. Presumably, a process of **reconsolidation**, which involves neural processes similar to those responsible for the original consolidation, makes it possible for established memories to be altered or attached to new information (Nader, 2003). Events that interfere with consolidation also interfere with reconsolidation and can even erase memories or at least make them inaccessible. For example, Debiec, LeDoux, and Nader (2002) trained rats on a relational

reconsolidation A process of consolidation of a memory that occurs subsequent to the original consolidation that can be triggered by a reminder of the original stimulus; thought to provide the means for modifying existing memories.

FIGURE 12.32

A Schematic Description of the Experiment by Deviec et al. (2002)

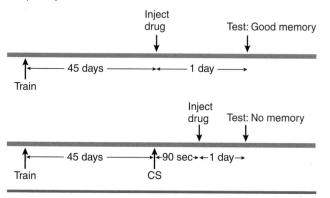

fear-conditioning task that required participation of the hippocampus. If a drug that interfered with protein synthesis was infused into the hippocampus immediately after training, consolidation did not occur. If the drug was infused 45 days later, no effect was seen. Apparently, the memory had already been consolidated. However, if the memory was reactivated 45 days later by presenting the CS that had been part of the original learning session and then the drug was injected into the hippocampus, the animals showed amnesia for the training when they were tested later. (See *Figure 12.32*.)

Role of Long-Term Potentiation in Memory

Earlier in this chapter we saw how synaptic connections could be quickly modified in the hippocampal formation, leading to long-term potentiation or long-term depression. Are these changes in synaptic strength related to the role the hippocampus plays in learning?

The answer is clearly "yes." For example, researchers have developed targeted mutations of the gene responsible for the production of NMDA receptors which, as we saw earlier, are responsible for long-term potentiation in several parts of the hippocampal formation. Two studies from the same laboratory (McHugh et al., 1996; Tsien, Huerta, and Tonegawa, 1996) produced a targeted mutation against the NMDA receptor gene that affected only the CA1 pyramidal cells. NMDA receptors in these neurons failed to develop; in all other parts of the brain these receptors were normal. Figure 12.33 shows photomicrographs of slices through the hippocampus of a normal mouse and a knockout mouse that were stained for the presence of the messenger RNA for the NMDA receptor. As you can see, the NMDA receptor is missing in the CA1 field of the mouse with the targeted mutation. (See *Figure 12.33*.)

As you might expect, the experimenters found that the lack of NMDA receptors prevented the establishment of long-term potentiation in field CA1 in the mice with the targeted mutation. Although the pyramidal cells of CA1 did show spatial receptive fields, these fields were larger and less focused than those shown by cells in normal animals. In addition, the knockout mice learned a Morris water maze much more slowly than did mice whose CA1 neurons contained NMDA receptors.

In summary, experimental evidence indicates that the participation of the hippocampal formation in learning involves long-term potentiation.

FIGURE 12.33

Absence of NMDA Receptors in Field CA1.
Photomicrographs of sections through the hippocampus show the location of messenger RNA responsible for the production of NMDA receptors in (a) a normal mouse and (b) a mouse with the targeted mutation (CA1 knockout). The effects of the targeted mutation (knockout) of the NMDA receptor gene is expressed only in the field CA1 of the hippocampus. Ctx = neocortex, CA1 = hippocampus field CA1, DG = dentate gyrus.

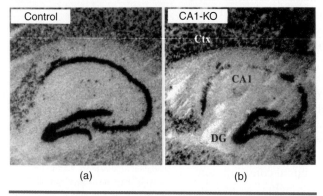

(a)   (b)

Reprinted from *Cell, 87*, Tsien, J. Z., Huerta, P. T., and Tonegawa, S., The Essential Role of Hippocampal CA1 NMDA Receptor–Dependent Synaptic Plasticity in Spatial Memory, 1327–1338, Copyright 1996, with permission from Elsevier.

Role of Hippocampal Neurogenesis in Learning

As we saw in Chapter 3, new neurons can be produced in the hippocampus of the adult brain. Stem cells located in the subgranular zone of the hippocampus divide and give rise to granule cells, which migrate into the dentate gyrus and extend axons that form connections with other neurons in the dentate gyrus and with neurons in field CA3 (Kempermann, Wiskott, and Gage, 2004).

Gould et al. (1999) trained rats on two versions of the Morris water maze: one requiring relational learning and one requiring only stimulus–response learning.

Training on the relational task, involving the hippocampus, doubled the number of newborn neurons in the dentate gyrus. Training on the stimulus–response task, not involving the hippocampus, had no effect on neurogenesis. Evidence suggests that new neurons in the dentate gyrus participate in learning. Jessberger and Kempermann (2003) trained mice on a relational learning task in a Morris water maze and found an increase in fos protein in newly formed dentate gyrus neurons, which indicates that the neurons had been activated by the experience.

Schmidt-Hieber, Jonas, and Bischofberger (2004) found that it was easier to establish associative long-term potentiation in newly formed neurons than in older neurons. They suggest that neurogenesis could be a mechanism that facilitates synaptic plasticity by providing a continuously available pool of neurons to participate in the formation of new memories.

Kempermann, Wiskott, and Gage (2004) noted that although learning experiences increase the number of new neurons in the hippocampus, maturation of these neurons and the establishment of their connections with other neurons take a considerable amount of time; thus, enhanced neurogenesis is of benefit to the animal only on a long-term basis. We do not yet understand the exact role of neurogenesis in learning and adaptation, nor can we explain why neurogenesis takes place in only two regions, the olfactory bulb and the hippocampus. If neurogenesis is useful in these places, why does it not also occur elsewhere in the brain?

InterimSummary

Relational Learning

Brain damage can produce anterograde amnesia, which consists of the inability to remember events that happen after the damage occurs, even though short-term memory (such as that needed to carry on a conversation) is largely intact. The patients also have a retrograde amnesia of several years' duration but can remember events from the distant past. Anterograde amnesia can be caused by chronic alcoholism (Korsakoff's syndrome) or bilateral damage to the medial temporal lobes.

The first explanation for anterograde amnesia was that the ability of the brain to consolidate short-term memories into long-term memories was damaged. However, ordinary perceptual, stimulus–response, and motor learning do not appear to be impaired; people can learn to recognize new stimuli, they are capable of instrumental and classical conditioning, and they can acquire motor memories. However, they are not capable of *declarative learning*—of describing events that happen to them. The amnesia has also been called a deficit in explicit memory. An even more descriptive term—one that applies to laboratory animals as well as to humans—is *relational learning*.

Although other structures may be involved, researchers are now confident that the primary cause of anterograde amnesia is damage to the hippocampal formation or to its inputs and outputs. The hippocampal formation receives information from other regions of the brain, processes this information, and then, through its *efferent* connections with these regions, modifies the memories that are being consolidated there, linking them together in ways that will permit us to remember the relationships among the elements of the memories.

Declarative memories come in at least two forms. Episodic memories are specific to a particular time and place, whereas semantic memories involve facts but not information about the context in which they were learned. Hippocampal lesions impair episodic memories. Lesions of the lateral temporal cortex can disrupt semantic memories.

Damage to the hippocampal formation disrupts spatial memory. The most profound deficits are caused by bilateral damage, but damage to the right hemisphere also impairs performance. Functional imaging studies have shown that performance of spatial tasks increases activity in the right hippocampal formation. The brains of London taxi drivers contain a larger-than-average right posterior hippocampus.

Studies with laboratory animals indicate that damage to the hippocampal formation disrupts the ability to learn spatial relations. For example, rats with hippocampal damage cannot learn the Morris water maze unless they are always released from the same place in the maze, which turns the task into one of stimulus–response learning. The hippocampal formation contains place cells—neurons that respond when the animal is in a particular location, which implies that the hippocampus contains neural networks that keep track of the relationships among stimuli in the environment that define the animal's location. Neurons in the hippocampal formation reflect where an animal "thinks" it is. Place cells encode more than space; they can include information about the response that the animal will perform next.

Research has shown that the hippocampal formation plays a role in memory consolidation. Inactivation of the dorsal hippocampus prevents consolidation if it occurs 1 day after learning a Morris water maze task but has no effect if it occurs 30 days later. In contrast, inactivation of regions of the cerebral cortex disrupts performance if it occurs 30 days after training but has no effect if it occurs 1 day after training. Slow-wave sleep facilitates the consolidation of declarative memories, and REM sleep facilitates the consolidation of nondeclarative memories. During slow-wave sleep, place cells in field CA1 of rats replay the sequence of activity that they showed while navigating in an environment in the laboratory.

Memories can be altered or connected to newer memories—a process known as reconsolidation. When a long-term memory is reactivated by stimuli that provide a "reminder" of the original experience, the memories become susceptible to events that interfere with consolidation, such as the administration of a drug that inhibits protein synthesis.

Learning involves long-term potentiation. When rats are trained in a maze, synaptic connections in the hippocampus are strengthened. A targeted mutation against the NMDA receptor gene that affects only field CA1 disrupts long-term potentiation and the ability to learn the Morris water maze.

The dentate gyrus is one of the two places in the brain where adult stem cells can divide and give rise to new neurons. These neurons establish connections with neurons in field CA3 and appear to participate in learning. Their ability to undergo long-term potentiation more easily than older neurons suggests that they facilitate the formation of new memories.

Thought Question

Although we can live only in the present, our memories are an important aspect of our identities. What do you think it would be like to have a memory deficit like H. M.'s? Imagine having no recollection of over 30 years of experiences. Imagine being surprised every time you see yourself in the mirror and discover someone who is more than 30 years older than you believe yourself to be.

⦂ EPILOGUE   What Causes Confabulation?

Recollecting a memory is a creative process. We do not simply retrieve stored information the way we might check a fact in a book; instead, we take fragmentary information and *interpret* what that information means. Suppose that you are waiting for a bus on a cold, rainy day. As you stand there, musing, you realize that you forgot to pay your rent, which was due several days ago. You resolve to do so as soon as you get home. In fact, you imagine yourself sitting down and writing a check, putting it in an envelope, and carrying it to the mailbox on the corner. However, you meet a friend on the bus, and the interesting conversation you have wipes the thought of paying the rent from your mind. That night, just as you are falling asleep, you suddenly think about the rent. You have a vague memory of writing a check and posting it, but as you think about it more, you realize that you must not have done so, because you remember thinking how glad you were not to have to go out again as you put your wet raincoat away. On further reflection you realize that the memory of writing the check and posting it is simply a memory of your having *thought about* doing so.

You will recall that one of the symptoms of Korsakoff's syndrome is confabulation—the reporting of memories of events that did not really occur. Some of these events are plausible, but some of them are contradicted by other information and cannot possibly be true. However, the stories always contain elements of true events—and people sometimes act on their false beliefs (Schnider, 2003). For example, a 58-year-old woman believed that she was at home, and not in a hospital, and insisted that she had to feed her baby—even though her "baby" was really 30 years old. An accountant actually left the hospital because he believed that a taxi was waiting to take him to a meeting. As Schnider notes, patients who confabulate do not try to answer questions unrelated to information contained in their memory. For example, they will not try to answer questions about fictitious people, places, or objects (Where is Premola? Who is Princess Lolita? What is a waterknube?). Schnider suggests that patients who confabulate have difficulty suppressing irrelevant memories of past events that are evoked by stimuli in the present. He notes that it is often impossible to convince patients that their confabulations are not real. For example, it was easier to convince the woman who wanted to feed her baby that the baby had already been fed than to convince her that the baby is grown up. Similarly, it was easier to convince the accountant that the meeting had been postponed than that no meeting had been scheduled.

A study by Benson et al. (1996) suggests that confabulation may be caused by brain damage that disrupts the normal functions of the prefrontal cortex. The investigators reported the case of a man who developed Korsakoff's syndrome, complete with confabulation. Neuropsychological testing found symptoms that indicate frontal lobe dysfunction, and a PET scan revealed hypoactivity of the medial and orbital prefrontal cortex. Four months later, the confabulation was gone, the neuropsychological tests did not show frontal lobe symptoms, and another PET scan revealed that the activity of the prefrontal cortex was back to normal. O'Connor et al. (1996) reported a case with complementary findings: A patient who had been amnesic for years had a close-head injury and suddenly began confabulating. Neuropsychological testing found evidence for frontal lobe dysfunction.

Johnson and Raye (1998) suggested that one of the functions of the frontal lobes is to help evaluate the plausibility of a proposi-tion or an ambiguous perception. When information is uncertain, the frontal lobes become involved in retrieving memories that might help us to evaluate whether a given interpretation makes sense.

Key Concepts

THE NATURE OF LEARNING

1. Learning takes many forms. The most important categories appear to be perceptual learning, stimu-lus–response learning, motor learning, and rela-tional learning.
2. The Hebb rule describes the synaptic change that appears to be responsible for stimulus–response learning: If an initially weak synapse repeatedly fires at the same time that the postsynaptic neuron fires, the synapse will become strengthened.

SYNAPTIC PLASTICITY: LONG-TERM POTENTIATION AND LONG-TERM DEPRESSION

3. Long-term potentiation occurs when axons in the hippocampal formation are repeatedly stimulated.
4. Associative long-term potentiation appears to follow the Hebb rule and understanding it may help us understand the physiological basis of learning.
5. The special properties of NMDA receptors as both voltage- and neurotransmitter-dependent account for associative long-term potentiation.
6. The entry of calcium into dendritic spines activates enzymes that cause the insertion of AMPA receptors into the postsynaptic membrane and initiate bio-chemical and structural changes in the synapse.

PERCEPTUAL LEARNING

7. Learning to recognize complex stimuli involves changes in the association cortex of the appropriate sensory modality.

CLASSICAL CONDITIONING

8. Study of the role of the amygdala and associated structures in learning conditioned emotional responses has furthered our understanding of the physiological basis of classical conditioning.

INSTRUMENTAL CONDITIONING

9. The basal ganglia appear to be involved in the reten-tion of learned behaviors that have become auto-matic and routine.
10. Electrical stimulation of several parts of the brain can reinforce an animal's behavior.
11. Reinforcing brain stimulation and natural rein-forcers are effective because they cause the activa-tion of neurons in the mesolimbic and mesocortical systems, which release dopamine in the nucleus accumbens, prefrontal cortex, limbic cortex, and hippocampus.
12. Drugs that block dopaminergic transmission in the nucleus accumbens block the reinforcing effects of electrical stimulation of the brain.

RELATIONAL LEARNING

13. Damage to the hippocampal formation causes a syndrome of anterograde amnesia, in which people can still learn to perform perceptual, stimulus–response, or motor learning tasks but can no longer learn to find their way in new environments or describe episodes from their lives that occur after the time of the brain damage.
14. Studies with laboratory animals suggest that the hip-pocampal formation facilitates relational learning by recognizing contexts and coordinating learning that takes place in other parts of the brain.
15. The hippocampus is involved in reconsolidation (modification of existing memories). Neurogenesis may play a role in hippocampal memory functions.

Suggested Readings

Best, P. J., White, A. M., and Minai, A. Spatial processing in the brain: The activity of hippocampal place cells. *Annual Review of Neuroscience*, 2001, *24*, 459–486.

Gazzaniga, M. S. *The Mind's Past.* Berkeley: University of Cali-fornia Press, 1998.

Lisman, J., Schulman, H., and Cline, H. The molecular basis of CaMKII function in synaptic and behavioural memory. *Nature Reviews: Neuroscience*, 2002, *3*, 175–190.

Redish, A. D. *Beyond the Cognitive Map: From Place Cells to Episodic Memory.* Cambridge, MA: MIT Press, 1999.

Schacter, D. L. *Searching for Memory: The Brain, the Mind, and the Past.* New York: Basic Books, 1996.

Squire, L. R., and Kandel, E. R. *Memory: From Mind to Molecules.* New York: Scientific American Library, 1999.

Squire, L. R., Stark, C. E., and Clark, R. E. The medial temporal lobe. *Annual Review of Neuroscience,* 2004, *27,* 279–306.

Additional Resources

Visit www.mypsychkit.com for additional review and practice of the material covered in this chapter. Within MyPsychKit, you can take practice tests and receive a customized study plan to help you review. Dozens of animations, tutorials, and Web links are also available. You can even review using the interactive electronic version of this textbook. You will need to register for MyPsychKit. See www.mypsychkit.com for complete details.

chapter
13 : Human Communication

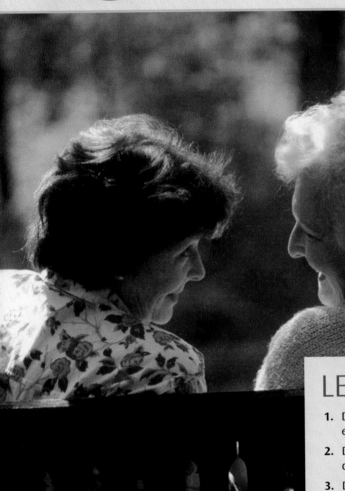

LEARNING OBJECTIVES

1. Describe the use of subjects with brain damage in the study of language and explain the concept of lateralization.

2. Describe Broca's aphasia and the three major speech deficits that result from damage to Broca's area: agrammatism, anomia, and articulation difficulties.

3. Describe the symptoms of Wernicke's aphasia, pure word deafness, and transcortical sensory aphasia and explain how they are related.

4. Discuss the brain mechanisms that underlie our ability to understand the meanings of words and to express our own thoughts and perceptions in words.

5. Describe the symptoms of conduction aphasia and anomic aphasia and the brain damage that produces them.

6. Discuss research on aphasia in deaf people.

7. Discuss research on the brain mechanisms of prosody—the use of rhythm and emphasis in speech—and stuttering.

8. Describe pure alexia and explain why this disorder is caused by damage to two specific parts of the brain.

9. Describe whole-word and phonetic reading and discuss three acquired dyslexias: surface dyslexia, phonological dyslexia, and direct dyslexia.

10. Explain the relationship between speaking and writing and describe the symptoms of phonological dysgraphia, orthographic dysgraphia, and semantic (direct) dysgraphia.

11. Describe research on the neurological basis of developmental dyslexias.

Dr. D. presented the case. "Mr. S. had two strokes about 10 years ago, which damaged both temporal lobes. His hearing, tested by an audiologist, is in the normal range. But as you will see, his speech comprehension is deficient."

Actually, as we soon saw, it was nonexistent. Mr. S. was ushered into the conference room and shown an empty chair at the head of the table, where we could all see and hear him. He looked calm and unworried; in fact, he seemed to be enjoying himself, and it occurred to me that this was probably not the first time he had been the center of attention. I had read about the syndrome I was about to see, and I knew that it was very rare.

"Mr. S., will you tell us how you are feeling?" asked Dr. D.

The patient turned his head at the sound of his voice and said, "Sorry, I can't understand you."

"*How are you feeling?*" he asked in a loud voice.

"Oh, I can hear you all right, I just can't understand you. Here," he said, handing Dr. D. a pencil and a small pad of paper.

Dr. D. took the pencil and paper and wrote something. He handed them back to Mr. S., who looked at it and said, "Fine. I'm just fine."

"Will you tell us about what you have been doing lately?" asked Dr. D. Mr. S. smiled, shook his head, and handed him the paper and pencil again.

"Oh sure," he said after reading the new question, and he proceeded to tell us about his garden and his other hobbies. "I don't get much from television unless there are a lot of close-ups, where I can read their lips. I like to listen to music on the radio, but, of course, the lyrics don't mean too much to me!" He laughed at his own joke, which had probably already seen some mileage.

"You mean that you can read lips?" someone asked.

Mr. S. immediately turned toward the sound of the voice and said, "What did you say? Say it slow, so I can try to read your lips." We all laughed, and Mr. S. joined us when the question was repeated slowly enough for him to decode. Another person tried to ask him a question, but apparently his Spanish accent made it impossible for Mr. S. to read his lips.

Suddenly, the phone rang. We all, including Mr. S., looked up at the wall where it was hanging. "Someone else had better get that," he said. "I'm not much good on the phone."

After Mr. S. had left the room, someone observed that although Mr. S.'s speech was easy to understand, it seemed a bit strange. "Yes," said a speech therapist, "he almost sounds like a deaf person who has learned to talk but doesn't get the pronunciation of the words just right."

Dr. D. nodded and played a tape for us. "This recording was made a few months after his strokes, 10 years ago." We heard the same voice, but this time it sounded absolutely normal.

"Oh," said the speech therapist. "He has lost the ability to monitor his own speech, and over the years he has forgotten some of the details of how various words are pronounced."

"Exactly," said Dr. D. "The change has been a gradual one."

Verbal behaviors constitute one of the most important classes of human social behavior. Our cultural evolution has been possible because we can talk and listen, write and read. Language enables our discoveries to be cumulative; knowledge gained by one generation can be passed on to the next.

The basic function of verbal communication is seen in its effects on other people. When we talk to someone, we almost always expect our speech to induce the person to engage in some sort of behavior. Sometimes, the behavior is of obvious advantage to us, as when we ask for an object or for help in performing a task. At other times we are simply asking for a social exchange: some attention and perhaps some conversation. Even "idle" conversation is not idle, because it causes another person to look at us and say something in return.

This chapter discusses the neural basis of verbal behavior: talking, understanding speech, reading, and writing.

Speech Production and Comprehension: Brain Mechanisms

Our knowledge of the physiology of language has been obtained primarily by observing the effects of brain lesions on people's verbal behavior. The most important category of speech disorders is **aphasia**, a primary disturbance in the comprehension or production of speech, caused by brain damage. Not all speech disturbances are aphasias; a patient must have difficulty comprehending, repeating, or producing meaningful speech, and this difficulty must not be caused by simple sensory or motor deficits or by lack of motivation. For example, an inability to speak caused by deafness or paralysis of the speech muscles is not considered to be aphasia. In addition, the deficit must be relatively isolated; that is, the patient must appear to be aware of what is happening in his or her environment and to comprehend that others are attempting to communicate.

Another source of information about the physiology of language comes from studies using functional imaging devices. In recent years, researchers have used PET and functional MRI to gather information about language processes from normal subjects. In general, these studies have confirmed or complemented what we have learned by studying patients with brain damage.

> **aphasia** Difficulty in producing or comprehending speech not caused by deafness or a simple motor deficit; caused by brain damage.

Lateralization

Verbal behavior is a *lateralized* function; most language disturbances occur after damage to the left side of the brain, whether people are left-handed or right-handed. Using an ultrasonic procedure to measure changes in cerebral blood flow while people performed a verbal task, Knecht et al. (2000) assessed the relationship between handedness and lateralization of speech mechanisms in people without any known brain damage. They found that right-hemisphere speech dominance was seen in only 4 percent of right-handed people, in 15 percent of ambidextrous people, and in 27 percent of left-handed people. If the left hemisphere is malformed or damaged early in life, then language dominance is very likely to pass to the right hemisphere (Vikingstad et al., 2000). Because the left hemisphere of approximately 90 percent of the total population is dominant for speech, you can assume that the brain damage described in this chapter is located in the left (speech-dominant) hemisphere unless I say otherwise.

Although the circuits that are *primarily* involved in speech comprehension and production are located in one hemisphere (almost always, the left hemisphere), it would be a mistake to conclude that the other hemisphere plays no role in speech. When we hear and understand words, and when we talk about or think about our own perceptions or memories, we are using neural circuits besides those directly involved in speech. Thus, these circuits, too, play a role in verbal behavior. For example, damage to the right hemisphere makes it difficult for a person to read maps, perceive spatial relations, and recognize complex geometrical forms. People with such damage also have trouble talking about things like maps and complex geometrical forms or understanding what other people have to say about them. The right hemisphere also appears to be involved in organizing a narrative—selecting and assembling the elements of what we want to say (Gardner et al., 1983). As we saw in Chapter 10, the right hemisphere is involved in the expression and recognition of emotion in the tone of voice. As we shall see in this chapter, it is also involved in control of *prosody*—the normal rhythm and stress found in speech. Therefore, both hemispheres of the brain have a contribution to make to our language abilities.

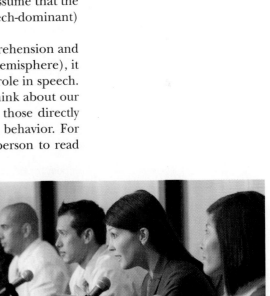

The first requirement of the ability to meaningful speech is having something to say.

FIGURE 13.1

Assessment of Aphasia. The drawing of the kitchen story is part of the Boston Diagnostic Aphasia Test.

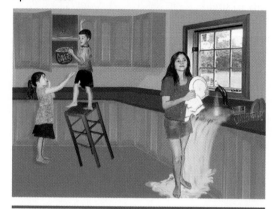

Speech Production

Being able to talk—that is, to produce meaningful speech—requires several abilities. First, the person must have something to talk about. Let us consider what this means. We can talk about something that is currently happening or something that happened in the past. In the first case we are talking about our perceptions: things we are seeing, hearing, feeling, smelling, and so on. In the second case we are talking about our memories of what happened in the past. Both perceptions of current events and memories of events that occurred in the past involve brain mechanisms in the posterior part of the cerebral hemispheres (the occipital, temporal, and parietal lobes). Thus, this region is largely responsible for our having something to say.

Given that a person has something to say, actually doing so requires some additional brain functions. As we shall see in this section, the conversion of perceptions, memories, and thoughts into speech makes use of neural mechanisms located in the frontal lobes.

Damage to a region of the inferior left frontal lobe (Broca's area) disrupts the ability to speak: It causes **Broca's aphasia**. This disorder is characterized by slow, laborious, and nonfluent speech. When trying to talk with patients who have Broca's aphasia, most people find it hard to resist supplying the words the patients are obviously groping for. But although they often mispronounce words, the ones they manage to come out with are usually meaningful. The posterior part of the cerebral hemispheres has something to say, but the damage to the frontal lobe makes it difficult for the patients to express these thoughts.

People with Broca's aphasia find it easier to say some types of words than others. They have great difficulty saying the little words with grammatical meaning, such as *a, the, some, in,* or *about.* These words are called **function words**, because they have important grammatical functions. The words that they do manage to say are almost entirely **content words**—words that convey meaning, including nouns, verbs, adjectives, and adverbs, such as *apple, house, throw,* or *heavy.*

Here is a sample of speech from a man with Broca's aphasia, who is trying to describe the scene shown in *Figure 13.1.* As you will see, his words are meaningful, but what he says is certainly not grammatical. The dots indicate long pauses.

kid. . . . kk . . . can . . . candy . . . cookie . . . candy . . . well I don't know but it's writ . . . easy does it . . . slam . . . early . . . fall . . . men . . . many no . . . girl. Dishes . . . soap . . . soap . . . water . . . water . . . falling pah that's all . . . dish . . . that's all.
Cookies . . . can . . . candy . . . cookies cookies . . . he . . . down . . . That's all. Girl . . . slipping water . . . water . . . and it hurts . . . much to do . . . Her . . . clean up . . . Dishes . . . up there . . . I think that's doing it. (Obler and Gjerlow, 1999, p. 41)

Broca's aphasia A form of aphasia characterized by agrammatism, anomia, and extreme difficulty in speech articulation.

function word A preposition, article, or other word that conveys little of the meaning of a sentence but is important in specifying its grammatical structure.

content word A noun, verb, adjective, or adverb that conveys meaning.

Broca's area A region of frontal cortex, located just rostral to the base of the left primary motor cortex, that is necessary for normal speech production.

People with Broca's aphasia can comprehend speech much better than they can produce it. In fact, some observers have said that their comprehension is unimpaired, but as we will see, this is not quite true. Broca (1861) suggested that this form of aphasia is produced by a lesion of the frontal association cortex, just anterior to the face region of the primary motor cortex. Subsequent research proved him to be essentially correct, and we now call the region **Broca's area.** (See *Figure 13.2.*)

Lesions that produce Broca's aphasia are certainly centered in the vicinity of Broca's area. However, damage that is restricted to the cortex of Broca's area does not appear to produce Broca's aphasia; the damage must extend to surrounding regions of the frontal lobe and to the underlying subcortical white matter (H. Damasio, 1989; Naeser et al., 1989). In addition, there is evidence that lesions of the basal ganglia—especially the head of the caudate nucleus—can also produce a Broca-like aphasia (Damasio, Eslinger, and Adams, 1984).

Watkins and her colleagues (Watkins, Dronkers, and Vargha-Khadem, 2002; Watkins et al., 2002) studied three generations of the KE family, half of whose members are affected by a severe speech and language disorder caused by the mutation of a single gene found on chromosome 7. The primary deficit appears to involve the ability to perform the sequential movements necessary for speech, but the affected people also have difficulty repeating sounds they hear and forming the past tense of verbs. The mutation causes abnormal development of the caudate nucleus and the left inferior frontal cortex, including Broca's area.

What do the neural circuits in and around Broca's area do? Wernicke (1874) suggested that Broca's area contains motor memories—in particular, *memories of the sequences of muscular movements that are needed to articulate words.* Talking involves rapid movements of the tongue, lips, and jaw, and these movements must be coordinated with each other and with those of the vocal cords; thus, talking requires some very sophisticated motor control mechanisms. Obviously, circuits of neurons somewhere in our brain will, when properly activated, cause these sequences of movements to be executed. Because damage to the inferior caudal left frontal lobe (including Broca's area) disrupts the ability to articulate words, this region is a likely candidate for the location of these "programs." The fact that this region is directly connected to the part of the primary motor cortex that controls the muscles used for speech certainly supports this conclusion.

However, the speech functions of the left frontal lobe include more than programming the movements used to speak. Broca's aphasia is much more than a deficit in pronouncing words. In general, three major speech deficits are produced by lesions in and around Broca's area: *agrammatism, anomia,* and *articulation difficulties.* Although most patients with Broca's aphasia will have all of these deficits to some degree, their severity can vary considerably from person to person—presumably, because their brain lesions differ. You can also hear the voice of an agrammatic patient and one with articulation difficulties in *MyPsychKit 13.1, Voices of Aphasia: Broca's Aphasia* .

Agrammatism refers to a patient's difficulty in using grammatical constructions. This disorder can appear all by itself, without any difficulty in pronouncing words (Nadeau, 1988). As we saw, people with Broca's aphasia rarely use function words. In addition, they rarely use grammatical markers such as *-ed* or auxiliaries such as *have* (as in *I have gone*). For some reason, they *do* often use *-ing*, perhaps because this ending converts a verb into a noun.

FIGURE 13.2

Speech Areas.   This figure shows the location of the primary speech areas of the brain. (Wernicke's area will be described later.)

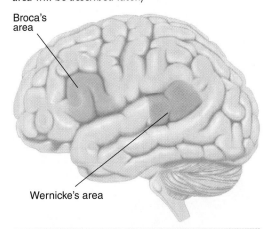

Broca's area

Wernicke's area

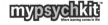

Animation 13.1
Voices of Aphasia: Broca's Aphasia

A study by Saffran, Schwartz, and Marin (1980) illustrates this difficulty. The following quotations are from agrammatic patients attempting to describe pictures:

Picture of a boy being hit in the head by a baseball

The boy is catch . . . the boy is hitch . . . the boy is hit the ball. (Saffran, Schwartz, and Marin, 1980, p. 229)

Picture of a girl giving flowers to her teacher

Girl . . . wants to . . . flowers . . . flowers and wants to. . . . The woman . . . wants to. . . . The girl wants to . . . the flowers and the woman. (Saffran, Schwartz, and Marin, 1980, p. 234)

So far, I have described Broca's aphasia as a disorder in speech *production.* In an ordinary conversation Broca's aphasics seem to understand everything that is said to

agrammatism One of the usual symptoms of Broca's aphasia; a difficulty in comprehending or properly employing grammatical devices, such as verb endings and word order.

FIGURE 13.3

Assessment of Grammatical Ability. This is an example of the stimuli used in the experiment by Schwartz, Saffran, and Marin (1980).

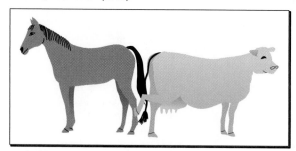

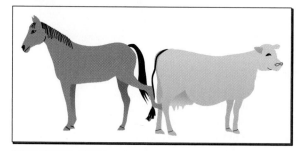

them. They appear to be irritated and annoyed by their inability to express their thoughts well, and they often make gestures to supplement their scanty speech. The striking disparity between their speech and their comprehension often leads people to assume that their comprehension is normal, but it is not. Schwartz, Saffran, and Marin (1980) showed Broca's aphasics pairs of pictures in which agents and objects of the action were reversed: for example, a horse kicking a cow and a cow kicking a horse, a truck pulling a car and a car pulling a truck, and a dancer applauding a clown and a clown applauding a dancer. As they showed each pair of pictures, they read the subject a sentence, for example, *The horse kicks the cow.* The subjects' task was to point to the appropriate picture, indicating whether they understood the grammatical construction of the sentence. (See *Figure 13.3.*) They performed very poorly.

The correct picture in the study by Schwartz and her colleagues was specified by a particular aspect of grammar: word order. The agrammatism that accompanies Broca's aphasia appears to disrupt patients' ability to use grammatical information, including word order, to decode the meaning of a sentence. Thus, their deficit in comprehension parallels their deficit in production.

Functional-imaging studies by Opitz and Friederici (2003, 2007) found that Broca's area was activated when people were taught an artificial grammar, which supports the conclusion that this region is involved in learning grammatical rules—especially complex ones.

The second major speech deficit seen in Broca's aphasia is **anomia** ("without name"). Anomia refers to a word-finding difficulty, and because all aphasics omit words or use inappropriate ones, anomia is actually a primary symptom of *all* forms of aphasia. However, because the speech of Broca's aphasics lacks fluency, their anomia is especially apparent; their facial expression and frequent use of sounds like "uh" make it obvious that they are groping for the correct words.

The third major characteristic of Broca's aphasia is *difficulty with articulation.* Patients mispronounce words, often altering the sequence of sounds. For example, *lipstick* might be pronounced "likstip." People with Broca's aphasia recognize that their pronunciation is erroneous, and they usually try to correct it.

Speech Comprehension

Comprehension of speech obviously begins in the auditory system, which detects and analyzes sounds, but *recognizing* words is one thing; *comprehending* them—understanding their meaning—is another. Recognizing a spoken word is a complex perceptual task that relies on memories of sequences of sounds. This task appears to be accomplished by neural circuits in the middle and posterior portion of the superior temporal gyrus of the left hemisphere, a region that has come to be known as **Wernicke's area.** (Refer to *Figure 13.2.*)

Wernicke's Aphasia: Description

The primary characteristics of **Wernicke's aphasia** are poor speech comprehension and production of meaningless speech. Unlike Broca's aphasia, Wernicke's aphasia is fluent and unlabored; the person does not strain to articulate words and does not appear to be searching for them. The patient maintains a melodic line, with the voice rising and falling normally. When you listen to the speech of a person with Wernicke's aphasia, it appears to be grammatical. That is, the person uses function

anomia Difficulty in finding (remembering) the appropriate word to describe an object, action, or attribute; one of the symptoms of aphasia.

Wernicke's area A region of the auditory association cortex on the left temporal lobe of humans, which is important in the comprehension of words and the production of meaningful speech.

Wernicke's aphasia A form of aphasia characterized by poor speech comprehension and fluent but meaningless speech.

words such as *the* and *but* and employs complex verb tenses and subordinate clauses. However, the person uses few content words, and the words that he or she strings together just do not make sense.

In the extreme, the speech of a person with Wernicke's aphasia deteriorates into a meaningless jumble, illustrated by the following quotation:

> *Examiner:* What kind of work did you do before you came into the hospital?
>
> *Patient:* Never, now mista oyge I wanna tell you this happened when happened when he rent. His—his kell come down here and is—he got ren something. It happened. In thesse ropiers were with him for hi—is friend—like was. And it just happened so I don't know, he did not bring around anything. And he did not pay it. And he roden all o these arranjen from the pedis on from iss pescid. In these floors now and so. He hadn't had em round here. (Kertesz, 1981, p. 73)

Because of the speech deficit of people with Wernicke's aphasia, when we try to assess their ability to comprehend speech, we must ask them to use nonverbal responses. That is, we cannot assume that they do not understand what other people say to them just because they do not give the proper answer. A commonly used test of comprehension assesses their ability to understand questions by pointing to objects on a table in front of them. For example, they are asked to "Point to the one with ink." If they point to an object other than the pen, they have not understood the request. When tested this way, people with severe Wernicke's aphasia do indeed show poor comprehension. You can hear the speech of people with Wernicke's aphasia in *MyPsychKit 13.2, Voices of Aphasia: Wernicke's Aphasia*.

mypsychkit

Animation 13.2
Voices of Aphasia: Wernicke's Aphasia

Wernicke's Aphasia: Analysis

Because the superior temporal gyrus is a region of the auditory association cortex and because a comprehension deficit is so prominent in Wernicke's aphasia, this disorder has been characterized as a *receptive* aphasia. Wernicke suggested that the region that now bears his name is the location of *memories of the sequences of sounds that constitute words.* This hypothesis is reasonable; it suggests that the auditory association cortex of the superior temporal gyrus recognizes the sounds of words, just as the visual association cortex of the inferior temporal gyrus recognizes the sight of objects.

But why should damage to an area that is responsible for the ability to recognize spoken words disrupt people's ability to speak? In fact, it does not; Wernicke's aphasia, like Broca's aphasia, actually appears to consist of several deficits. The abilities that are disrupted include *recognition of spoken words, comprehension of the meaning of words*, and the *ability to convert thoughts into words.* Let us consider each of these abilities in turn.

Recognition: Pure Word Deafness   As I said in the introduction to this section, *recognizing* a word is not the same as *comprehending* it. If you hear a foreign word several times, you will learn to recognize it, but unless someone tells you what it means, you will not comprehend it. Recognition is a perceptual task; comprehension involves retrieval of additional information from memory.

Damage to the left temporal lobe can produce a disorder of auditory word recognition, uncontaminated by other problems. This syndrome is called **pure word deafness**. (Mr. S., the patient described in the chapter prologue, had this disorder. See *Figure 13.4.*) Although people with pure word deafness are not deaf, they cannot understand speech. As one patient put it, "I can hear you talking, I just can't understand what you're saying." Another said, "It's as if there were a bypass somewhere, and my ears were not connected to my voice" (Saffran, Marin, and

pure word deafness The ability to hear, to speak, and (usually) to read and write without being able to comprehend the meaning of speech; caused by damage to Wernicke's area or disruption of auditory input to this region.

Yeni-Komshian, 1976, p. 211). These patients can recognize nonspeech sounds such as the barking of a dog, the sound of a doorbell, and the honking of a horn. Often, they can recognize the emotion expressed by the intonation of speech even though they cannot understand what is being said. More significantly, their own speech is unimpaired. They can often understand what other people are saying by reading their lips. They can also read and write, and they sometimes ask people to communicate with them in writing. Clearly, pure word deafness is not an inability to comprehend the meaning of words; if it were, people with this disorder would not be able to read people's lips or read words written on paper. Functional imaging studies confirm that perception of speech sounds activates neurons in the auditory association cortex of the superior temporal gyrus (Scott et al., 2000).

Sharp, Scott, and Wise (2004) found that deficits in speech comprehension were produced by lesions of the superior temporal lobe that damaged the region that is activated when people hear intelligible speech. Figure 13.5 shows a computer-generated depiction of the overlap of lesions of patients with brain damage that interfered with speech perception. Compare the regions of greatest overlap, shown in yellow and green, in *Figure 13.5* with the region shown in *Figure 13.4*.

Apparently, two types of brain injury can cause pure word deafness: disruption of auditory input to Wernicke's area or damage to Wernicke's area itself. Disruption of auditory input can be produced by bilateral damage to the primary auditory cortex, or it can be caused by damage to the white matter in the left temporal lobes that cuts axons bringing auditory information from the primary auditory cortex to Wernicke's area (Poeppel, 2001; Stefanatos, Gershkoff, and Madigan, 2005). Either type of damage—disruption of auditory input or damage to Wernicke's area—disturbs the analysis of the sounds of words and hence pre-

FIGURE 13.5

Speech Comprehension. The scan shows the overlap in the lesions of nine patients with deficits of speech comprehension. Note the similarity of the region of greatest overlap (yellow and green) with the damaged region shown in Figure 13.4.

FIGURE 13.4

Pure Word Deafness. An MRI scan shows the damage to the superior temporal lobe of a patient with pure word deafness (arrow).

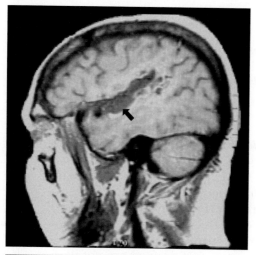

Gerry A. Stefanatos, Arthur Gershkoff, and Sean Madigan (2005). On pure word deafness, temporal processing, and the left hemisphere. *Journal of the International Neuropsychological Society, 11,* pp. 456–470, doi:10.1017/S1355617705050538. Reprinted with the permission of Cambridge University Press.

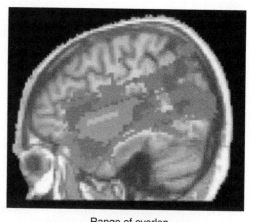

Range of overlap

From Sharp, D. J., Scott, S. K., and Wise, R. J. *Annals of Neurology*, 2004, *56*, 836–846. Reprinted with permission of John Wiley & Sons, Inc.

vents people from recognizing other people's speech. (See *Figure 13.6*.)

Our brains contain circuits of *mirror neurons*—neurons activated either when we perform an action or see another person performing particular grasping, holding, or manipulating movements or when we perform these movements ourselves (Gallese et al., 1996; Rizzolatti, Fogassi, and Gallese, 2001). Feedback from these neurons may help us to understand the intent of the actions of others. Although speech recognition is clearly an auditory event, research indicates that hearing words automatically engages brain mechanisms that control speech. In other words, these mechanisms appear also to contain mirror neurons that are activated by the sounds of words. Several investigators have suggested that feedback from subvocal articulation (very slight movements of the muscles involved in speech that do not actually cause obvious movement) facilitate speech recognition. Fadiga et al. (2002) had Italian-speaking subjects listen to real words and pronounceable nonwords that did or did not involve strong movement of the tongue. For example, the word *birra* ("beer") and the nonword *berro* require tongue movements, but the word *buffo* ("funny") and the nonword *biffo* do not. The investigators found that the excitability of the subjects' tongue muscles was increased only when they heard words that involved tongue movements. (See *Figure 13.7*.)

A functional imaging study by Schulz et al. (2005) found that the auditory cortex is strongly activated when people speak out loud but not when they whisper. The investigators suggest that this region—which is not activated during vocalization in the brains of other animals—is involved in self-monitoring of speech. Presumably, auditory feedback from our own voices helps to regulate our speech. As we saw in the chapter prologue, over a period of years, Mr. S.'s speech had lost its normal rhythm and stress, which underlines the importance of the monitoring of one's own speech.

Comprehension: Transcortical Sensory Aphasia   The other symptoms of Wernicke's aphasia—failure to comprehend the meaning of words and inability to express thoughts in meaningful speech—appear to be produced by damage that extends beyond Wernicke's area into the region that surrounds the posterior part of the lateral fissure, near the junction of the temporal, occipital, and parietal lobes. For want of a better term, I will refer to this region as the *posterior language area*. (See *Figure 13.8*.) The posterior language area appears to serve as a place for interchanging information between the auditory representation of words and the meanings of these words, stored as memories in the rest of the sensory association cortex.

Damage to the posterior language area alone, which isolates Wernicke's area from the rest of the posterior language area, produces a disorder known as **transcortical sensory aphasia**. (See *Figure 13.8*.) The difference between transcortical sensory aphasia and Wernicke's aphasia is that patients with transcortical sensory aphasia *can repeat what other people say to them;* therefore, they can recognize words. However, *they cannot comprehend the meaning of what they hear and repeat, nor can they produce meaningful speech of their own.* How can these people repeat what they hear? Because the posterior language area is damaged, repetition does not involve this part of the brain. Obviously, there must be a direct connection between Wernicke's area and Broca's area that bypasses the posterior language area. (See *Figure 13.8*.)

FIGURE 13.6

Brain Damage that Causes Pure Word Deafness

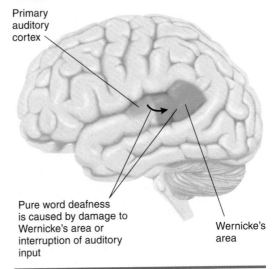

Primary auditory cortex

Pure word deafness is caused by damage to Wernicke's area or interruption of auditory input

Wernicke's area

transcortical sensory aphasia A speech disorder in which a person has difficulty comprehending speech and producing meaningful spontaneous speech but can repeat speech; caused by damage to the region of the brain posterior to Wernicke's area.

FIGURE 13.7

Mirror Neurons and Speech.   The graph shows excitability of tongue muscles when listening to syllables containing a sound produced by the tongue ("rr") or not produced by the tongue ("ff").

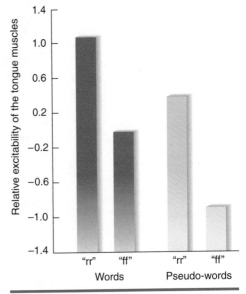

Adapted from Fadiga, L., Craighero, L., Buccino, G., and Rizzolatti, G. *European Journal of Neuroscience*, 2002, *15*, 399–402.

FIGURE 13.8

Transcortical Sensory Aphasia and Wernicke's Aphasia.   This schematic diagram shows the location and interconnections of the posterior language area and an explanation of its role in transcortical sensory aphasia and Wernicke's aphasia.

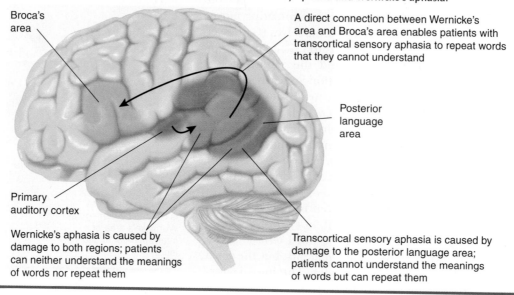

Broca's area

A direct connection between Wernicke's area and Broca's area enables patients with transcortical sensory aphasia to repeat words that they cannot understand

Posterior language area

Primary auditory cortex

Wernicke's aphasia is caused by damage to both regions; patients can neither understand the meanings of words nor repeat them

Transcortical sensory aphasia is caused by damage to the posterior language area; patients cannot understand the meanings of words but can repeat them

Geschwind, Quadfasel, and Segarra (1968) described a particularly interesting case of transcortical sensory aphasia. A woman sustained extensive brain damage from carbon monoxide produced by a faulty water heater. She spent several years in the hospital before she died, without ever saying anything meaningful on her own. She did not follow verbal commands or otherwise give signs of understanding them. However, she often repeated what was said to her. For example, if an examiner said "Please raise your right hand," she would reply "Please raise your right hand." The repetition was not parrotlike; she did not imitate accents different from her own, and if someone made a grammatical error while saying something to her, she sometimes repeated the sentence correctly, without the error. She could also recite poems if someone started them. For example, when an examiner said, "Roses are red, violets are blue," she continued with "Sugar is sweet and so are you." She could sing and would do so when someone started singing a song she knew. She even learned new songs from the radio while in the hospital. Remember, though, that she gave *no signs of understanding anything she heard or said*. This disorder, along with pure word deafness, clearly confirms the conclusion that *recognizing* spoken words and *comprehending* them are different processes and involve different brain mechanisms.

In conclusion, transcortical sensory aphasia can be seen as Wernicke's aphasia without a repetition deficit. To put it another way, the symptoms of Wernicke's aphasia consist of those of pure word deafness plus those of transcortical sensory aphasia. As I tell my students, WA = TSA + PWD. By simple algebra, TSA = WA − PWD, and so on. (Refer to *Figure 13.8*.)

What Is Meaning?   As we have seen, Wernicke's area is involved in the analysis of speech sounds and thus in the recognition of words. Damage to the posterior language area does not disrupt people's ability to recognize words, but it does disrupt their ability to *understand* words or to produce meaningful speech of their own. But what, exactly, do we mean by the word *meaning*? And what types of brain mechanisms are involved?

Words refer to objects, actions, or relationships in the world. Thus, the meaning of a word is defined by particular memories associated with it. For example, knowing the meaning of the word *tree* means being able to imagine the physical characteristics of trees: what they look like, what the wind sounds like blowing through their leaves, what the bark feels like, and so on. It also means knowing facts about trees: about their roots, buds, flowers, nuts, and wood and the chlorophyll in their leaves. These memories are stored not in the primary speech areas but in other parts of the brain, especially regions of the association cortex. Different categories of memories may be stored in particular regions of the brain, but they are somehow tied together, so hearing the word *tree* activates all of them. (As we saw in Chapter 12, the hippocampal formation is involved in this process of tying related memories together.)

In thinking about the brain's verbal mechanisms involved in recognizing words and comprehending their meaning, I find that the concept of a dictionary serves as a useful analogy. Dictionaries contain entries (the words) and definitions (the meanings of the words). In the brain we have at least two types of entries: auditory and visual. That is, we can look up a word according to how it sounds or how it looks (in writing). Let us just consider just one type of entry: the sound of a word. (I will discuss reading and writing later in this chapter.) We hear a familiar word and understand its meaning. How do we do so?

First, we must recognize the sequence of sounds that constitute the word; we find the auditory entry for the word in our "dictionary." As we saw, this entry appears in Wernicke's area. Next, the memories that constitute the meaning of the word must be activated. Presumably, Wernicke's area is connected—through the posterior language area—with the neural circuits that contain these memories. (See *Figure 13.9*.)

What evidence do we have that meanings of words are represented by neural circuits located in various regions of the association cortex? The best evidence comes from the fact that damage to particular regions of the sensory association cortex can damage particular kinds of information and thus abolish particular kinds of meanings.

FIGURE 13.9

The "Dictionary" in the Brain.   Wernicke's area contains the auditory entries of words; the meanings are contained as memories in the sensory association areas. Black arrows represent comprehension of words—the activation of memories that correspond to a word's meaning. Red arrows represent translation of thoughts or perceptions into words.

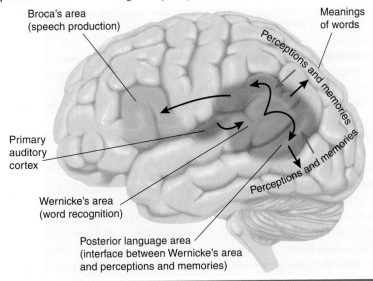

I met a patient who had recently had a stroke that damaged a part of her right parietal lobe that played a role in spatial perception. She was alert and intelligent and showed no signs of aphasia. However, she was confused about directions and other spatial relationships. When asked to, she could point to the ceiling and the floor, but she could not say which was *over* the other. Her perception of other people appeared to be entirely normal, but she could not say whether a person's head was at the *top* or *bottom* of the body.

I wrote a set of multiple-choice questions to test her ability to use words denoting spatial relations. The results of the test indicated that she did not know the meaning of words such as *up*, *down*, and *under* when they referred to spatial relationships, but she could use these words normally when they referred to nonspatial relations. For example, here are some of her incorrect responses when the words referred to spatial relations:

A tree's branches are *under* its roots.

The sky is *down*.

The ceiling is *under* the floor.

She made only ten correct responses on the sixteen-item test. In contrast, she got all eight items correct when the words referred to nonspatial relationships such as the following:

After exchanging pleasantries, they got *down* to business.

He got sick and threw *up*.

Damage to part of the association cortex of the *left* parietal lobe can produce an inability to name the body parts. The disorder is called **autotopagnosia**, or "poor knowledge of one's own topography." (I think a better name would have been *autotopanomia*, "poor naming of one's own topography" but, then, no one asked me to choose the term.) People who can otherwise converse normally cannot reliably point to their elbow, knee, or cheek when asked to do so and cannot name body parts when the examiner points to them. However, they have no difficulty understanding the meaning of other words.

As we saw in Chapter 12, lesions of the anterolateral temporal lobe result in *semantic dementia*—loss of semantic memories, including the names and even the functions of everyday objects. However, speech also conveys abstract concepts, some of them quite subtle. Studies of brain-damaged patients (Brownell et al., 1983, 1990) suggest that comprehension of the more subtle, figurative aspects of speech involves the right hemisphere in particular—for example, understanding the meaning behind proverbs such as "People who live in glass houses shouldn't throw stones" or the moral of stories such as the one about the race between the tortoise and the hare.

Functional imaging studies confirm these observations. Nichelli et al. (1995) found that judging the moral of Aesop's fables (as opposed to judging more superficial aspects of the stories) activated regions of the right hemisphere. Sotillo et al. (2005) found that a task that required comprehension of metaphors such as "green lung of the city" (that is, a park) activated the right superior temporal cortex. (See *Figure 13.10*.)

Repetition: Conduction Aphasia   As we saw earlier in this section, the fact that people with transcortical sensory aphasia can repeat what they hear suggests that there is a direct connection between Wernicke's area and Broca's area—and there is: the **arcuate fasciculus** ("arch-shaped bundle"). This bundle of axons appears to convey information about the *sounds* of words but not their *meanings*. The best evidence for this conclusion comes from a syndrome known as conduction aphasia, which is produced by damage to the inferior parietal lobe that extends into the subcortical white matter and damages the arcuate fasciculus (Damasio and Damasio, 1980). (See *Figure 13.11*.)

autotopagnosia   Inability to name body parts or to identify body parts that another person names.

arcuate fasciculus   A bundle of axons that connects Wernicke's area with Broca's area; damage causes conduction aphasia.

FIGURE 13.10

Evaluating Metaphors.   These images of neural activity in the right hemisphere were produced when the subjects evaluated the meaning of metaphors.

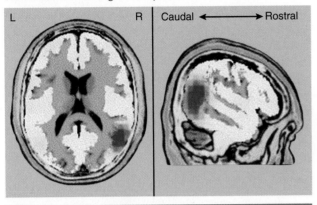

Reprinted from *Neuroscience Letters, 373*, Sotillo, M., Carretie, L., Hinojosa, J. A., et al., Neural Activity Associated with Metaphor Comprehension: Spatial Analysis, 5–9, Copyright 2004, with permission from Elsevier.

FIGURE 13.11

Conduction Aphasia.   MRI scans show the subcortical damage responsible for a case of conduction aphasia. This lesion damaged the arcuate fasciculus, a fiber bundle connecting Wernicke's area and Broca's area.

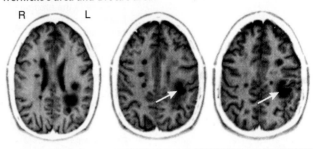

From Arnett, P. A., Rao, S. M., Hussain, M., et al. *Neurology*, 1996, *47*, 576–578. Reprinted with permission.

Conduction aphasia is characterized by meaningful, fluent speech; relatively good comprehension; but very poor repetition. For example, the spontaneous speech of patient L. B. (observed by Margolin and Walker, 1981) was excellent; he made very few errors and had no difficulty naming objects. He could repeat individual words but was unable to repeat nonwords such as *blaynge*. In addition, he could repeat a meaningful three-word phrase but not three unrelated words. People with conduction aphasia can repeat speech sounds that they hear *only if these sounds have meaning*. (You can hear this person's voice in *MyPsychKit 13.3, Voices of Aphasia: Conduction Aphasia.*)

Sometimes, when a person with conduction aphasia is asked to repeat a word, he or she says a word with the same meaning—or at least one that is related. For example, if the examiner says *house*, the patient may say *home*. If the examiner says *chair*, the patient may say *sit*. One patient made the following response when asked to repeat an entire sentence:

Examiner: The auto's leaking gas tank soiled the roadway.

Patient: The car's tank leaked and made a mess on the street.

The symptoms that are seen in transcortical sensory aphasia and conduction aphasia lead to the conclusion that there are pathways connecting the speech mechanisms of the temporal lobe with those of the frontal lobe. The direct pathway through the arcuate fasciculus simply conveys speech sounds from Wernicke's area to Broca's area. We use this pathway to repeat unfamiliar words—for example, when we are learning a foreign language or a new word in our own language or when we are trying to repeat a nonword such as *blaynge*. The second pathway, between the posterior language area and Broca's area, is indirect and is based on the *meaning* of words, not on the sounds they make. When patients with conduction aphasia hear a word or a sentence, the meaning of what they hear evokes some sort of image related to that meaning. (The patient in the previous example presumably imagined the sight of an automobile leaking fuel onto the pavement.) They are then able to describe that image, just as they would put their own thoughts into words. Of course, the words they choose might not be the same as the ones used by the person who spoke to them. (See *Figure 13.12*.)

A study by Catani, Jones, and ffytche (2005) provides the first anatomical evidence for the existence of the two pathways between Wernicke's area and Broca's area presented in Figure 13.13. The investigators used diffusion tensor MRI to

mypsychkit

Animation 13.3
Voices of Aphasia: Conduction Aphasia

conduction aphasia An aphasia characterized by an inability to repeat words that are heard but the ability to speak normally and comprehend the speech of others.

FIGURE 13.12

A Hypothetical Explanation of Conduction Aphasia. A lesion that damages the arcuate fasciculus disrupts transmission of auditory information, but not information related to meaning, to the frontal lobe.

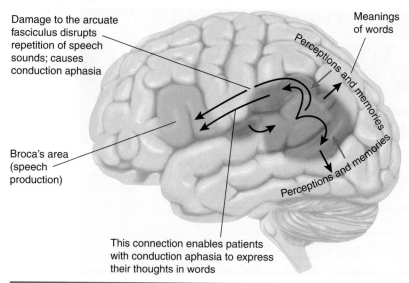

Damage to the arcuate fasciculus disrupts repetition of speech sounds; causes conduction aphasia

Meanings of words

Perceptions and memories

Broca's area (speech production)

Perceptions and memories

This connection enables patients with conduction aphasia to express their thoughts in words

trace large fiber bundles in the language regions of the brain. They found one deep pathway that directly connects these two regions and a shallower pathway that consists of two segments. The anterior segment connects Broca's area with the inferior parietal cortex, and the posterior segment connects Wernicke's area with the inferior parietal cortex. Damage to the direct pathway would be expected to produce conduction aphasia, whereas damage to the indirect pathway would be expected to spare the ability to repeat speech but would impair comprehension. (See *Figure 13.13*.)

The symptoms of conduction aphasia indicate that the connection between Wernicke's area and Broca's area appears to play an important role in short-term memory of words and speech sounds that have just been heard. Presumably, rehearsal of such information can be accomplished by "talking to ourselves" inside our head without actually having to say anything aloud. Imagining ourselves saying the word activates the region of Broca's area, whereas imagining that we are hearing it activates the auditory association area of the temporal lobe. These two regions, connected by means of the arcuate fasciculus (which contains axons traveling in *both* directions) circulate information back and forth, keeping the short-term memory alive. Baddeley (1993) refers to this circuit as the *phonological loop*.

Aziz-Zadeh et al. (2005) obtained evidence that we do use Broca's area when we talk to ourselves. The investigators applied transcranial magnetic stimulation (TMS) to Broca's area while people were silently counting the number of syllables in words presented on a screen. The parameters of stimulation that the investigators used disrupt overt (actual) speech. They found that it disrupted covert speech as well; the subjects took longer to count the syllables when the TMS was on.

FIGURE 13.13

Components of the Arcuate Fasciculus. A computer-generated reconstruction of the components of the arcuate fasciculus was obtained through diffusion tensor MRI.

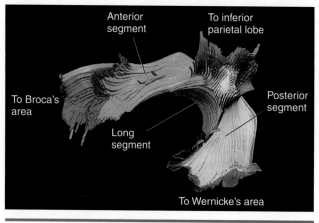

Anterior segment

To inferior parietal lobe

To Broca's area

Posterior segment

Long segment

To Wernicke's area

From Catani, M., Jones, D. K., and ffytche, D. H. *Annals of Neurology*, 2005, *57*, 8–16. Reprinted with permission.

Memory of Words: Anomic Aphasia

As I have already noted, anomia, in one form or other, is a hallmark of aphasia. However, one category of aphasia consists of almost pure anomia, the other symptoms being inconsequential. Speech of patients with anomic aphasia is fluent and grammatical, and their comprehension is excellent, but they have difficulty finding the appropriate words. They often employ **circumlocutions** (literally, "speaking in a roundabout way") to get around missing words. Anomic aphasia is different from Wernicke's aphasia. People with anomic aphasia can understand what other people say, and what those with anomic aphasia say makes perfect sense, even if they often choose roundabout ways to say it.

The following quotation is from a patient that some colleagues and I studied (Margolin, Marcel, and Carlson, 1985). We asked her to describe the kitchen picture shown earlier, in *Figure 13.1*. Her pauses, which are marked with three dots, indicate word-finding difficulties. In some cases, when she could not find a word, she supplied a definition instead (a form of circumlocution) or went off on a new track. I have added the words in brackets that I think she intended to use. (You can hear this person's voice on *MyPsychKit 13.4: Voices of Aphasia: Anomic Aphasia* .)

Examiner: Tell us about that picture.

Patient: It's a woman who has two children, a son and a daughter, and her son is to get into the . . . cupboard in the kitchen to get out [*take*] some . . . cookies out of the [*cookie jar*] . . . that she possibly had made, and consequently he's slipping [*falling*] . . . the wrong direction [*backward*] . . . on the . . . what he's standing on [*stool*], heading to the . . . the cupboard [*floor*] and if he falls backwards he could have some problems [*get hurt*], because that [*the stool*] is off balance.

Anomia has been described as a partial amnesia for words. It can be produced by lesions in either the anterior or posterior regions of the brain, but only posterior lesions produce a *fluent* anomia. The most likely location of lesions that produce anomia without the other symptoms of aphasia, such as comprehension deficits, agrammatism, or difficulties in articulation, is the left temporal or parietal lobe, usually sparing Wernicke's area. In the case of the woman just described, the damage included the left middle and inferior temporal gyri, which includes an important region of the visual association cortex. Wernicke's area was not damaged.

When my colleagues and I were studying the anomic patient, I was struck by the fact that she seemed to have more difficulty finding nouns than other types of words. I informally tested her ability to name actions by asking her what people shown in a series of pictures were doing. She made almost no errors in finding verbs. For example, although she could not say what a boy was holding in his hand, she had no trouble saying that he was *throwing* it. Similarly, she knew that a girl was *climbing* something but could not tell me the name of what she was climbing (a fence). Several studies have found that anomia for verbs (more correctly called *averbia*) is caused by damage to the frontal cortex, in and around Broca's area (Damasio and Tranel, 1993; Daniele et al., 1994; Bak et al., 2001). If you think about it, that makes sense. The frontal lobes are devoted to planning, organizing, and executing actions, so it should not surprise us that they are involved in the task of remembering the names of actions.

Several functional imaging studies have confirmed the importance of Broca's area and the region surrounding it in the production of verbs. For example, Hauk, Johnsrude, and Pulvermüller (2004) had subjects read verbs that related to movements of different parts of the body. For example, *bite*, *slap*, and *kick* involve movements of the face, arm, and leg, respectively. The investigators found that when the subjects read a verb, they saw activation in the regions of the motor cortex that

mypsychkit

Animation 13.4
Voices of Aphasia: Anomic Aphasia

circumlocution A strategy by which people with anomia find alternative ways to say something when they are unable to think of the most appropriate word.

FIGURE 13.14

Verbs and Movements.   The figure shows the relative activation of regions of the motor cortex that control movements of the face, arm, and leg when people read verbs that described movements of these regions, such as *bite*, *slap*, and *kick*.

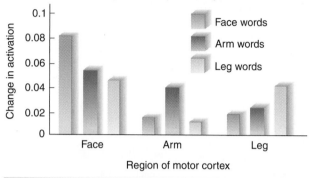

Reprinted from *Neuron, 41*, Hauk, 0., Johnsrude, I., and Pulvermuller, F., Somatotopic Representation of Action Words in Human Motor and Premotor Cortex, 301–307, Copyright 2004, with permission from Elsevier.

FIGURE 13.15

Mirror Neurons in Broca's Area.   PET scans show a region of the inferior left frontal lobe that was activated when a person saw a finger movement or imitated it. *Top:* Horizontal section. *Bottom:* Lateral view of left hemisphere.

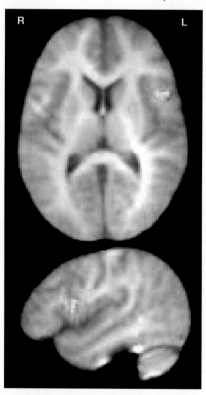

From Iacoboni, M., Woods, R. P., Brass, M., et al. *Science*, 1999, *286*, 2526–2528. Copyright © 1999. Reprinted with permission from AAAS.

controlled the relevant part of the body. (See *Figure 13.14*.) A similar study by Buccino et al. (2005) found that hearing sentences that involved hand movements (for example, *He turned the key*) activated the hand region of the motor cortex, and that hearing sentences that involved foot movements (for example, *He stepped on the grass*) activated the foot region. Presumably, thinking about particular actions activated regions that control these actions.

The picture I have drawn so far suggests that comprehension of speech includes a flow of information from Wernicke's area to the posterior language area to various regions of sensory and motor association cortex, which contain memories that provide meanings to words. Production of spontaneous speech involves the flow of information concerning perceptions and memories from the sensory and motor association cortex to the posterior language area to Broca's area. This model is certainly an oversimplification, but it is a useful starting point in conceptualizing basic mental processes. For example, thinking in words probably involves two-way communication between the speech areas and surrounding association cortex (and regions such as the hippocampus and medial temporal lobe, of course).

Aphasia in Deaf People

So far, I have restricted my discussion to brain mechanisms of spoken and written language, but communication among members of the Deaf community involves another medium: sign language. Sign language is expressed manually, by movements of the hands. Sign language is *not* English, nor is it French, Spanish, or Chinese. The most common sign language in North America is ASL—American Sign Language. ASL is a full-fledged language, having signs for nouns, verbs, adjectives, adverbs, and all the other parts of speech contained in oral languages. People can converse rapidly and efficiently by means of sign language, can tell jokes, and can even make puns based on the similarity between signs. They can also use their language ability to think in words.

Some researchers believe that in the history of our species, sign language preceded spoken language—that our ancestors began using gestures to communicate before they switched to speech. As mentioned earlier in this chapter, mirror neurons become active when we see or perform particular grasping, holding, or manipulating movements. Some of these neurons are found in Broca's area. Presumably, these neurons play an important role in learning to mimic another people's hand movements. Indeed, they might have been involved in the development of hand gestures used for communication in our ancestors, and they undoubtedly are used by deaf people when they communicate by sign language. A functional imaging study by Iacoboni et al. (1999) found that Broca's area was activated when people observed and imitated finger movements. (See *Figure 13.15*.)

Several studies have found a linkage between speech and hand movements, which supports the suggestion that the spoken language of present-day humans evolved from hand gestures. For example, Gentilucci (2003) had subjects speak the syllables *ba* or *ga* while they were watching him grasp objects of different sizes. When the experimenter grasped a large object, the subjects opened their mouths more and said the syllable more loudly than when he grasped a small one. These results suggest that the region of the

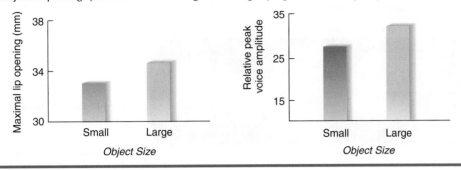

FIGURE 13.16

Links Between Hand and Mouth.   The graphs show lip opening and voice amplitude of subjects repeating syllables while watching someone grasping small and large objects.

Adapted from Gentilucci, M. *European Journal of Neuroscience*, 2003, *17*, 179–184.

brain that controls grasping is also involved in controlling speech movements. (See *Figure 13.16*.)

The grammar of ASL is based on its visual, spatial nature. For example, if a person makes the sign for *John* in one place and later makes the sign for *Mary* in another place, she can place her hand in the *John* location and move it toward the *Mary* location while making the sign for *love*. As you undoubtedly figured out for yourself, she is saying, "John loves Mary." The fact that the grammar of ASL is spatial suggests that aphasic disorders in deaf people who use sign language might be caused by lesions of the right hemisphere, which is primarily involved in spatial perception and memory. However, all the cases of deaf people with aphasia for signs reported in the literature so far have involved lesions of the left hemisphere (Hickok, Bellugi, and Klima, 1996). Functional imaging studies confirm these findings. For example, Pettito et al. (2000) found that when deaf signers produced meaningful signs, increased activity was seen in the left inferior frontal cortex—the region of Broca's area. When these subjects viewed signs made by others, they showed increased activity in the left superior temporal cortex. Therefore, sign language, like auditory and written language, appears to rely primarily on the left hemisphere for comprehension and expression. A study by Emmorey, Mehta, and Grabowski (2007) had both deaf and hearing subjects sign or say the names of objects they were shown. Activation was seen in the primary visual cortex and visual association cortex (inferior temporal cortex) and in Broca's area in both deaf and hearing subjects. In addition, two regions of the parietal cortex were specifically activated in deaf signers, presumably because of the spatially-oriented movements these subjects made.

Prosody: Rhythm, Tone, and Emphasis in Speech

When we speak, we do not merely utter words. Our speech has a regular rhythm and cadence; we give some words stress (that is, we pronounce them louder), and we vary the pitch of our voice to indicate phrasing and to distinguish between assertions and questions. In addition, we can impart information about our emotional state through the rhythm, emphasis, and tone of our speech. These rhythmic, emphatic, and melodic aspects of speech are referred to as **prosody**. The importance of these aspects of speech is illustrated by our use of punctuation symbols to indicate some elements of prosody when we write. For example, a comma indicates a short pause; a period indicates a longer one with an accompanying fall in the pitch of the voice; a question mark indicates a pause and a rise in the pitch of the voice; an exclamation mark indicates that the words are articulated with special emphasis; and so on.

prosody The use of changes in intonation and emphasis to convey meaning in speech besides that specified by the particular words; an important means of communication of emotion.

FIGURE 13.17

Listening to Normal Speech or its Prosodic Components. Functional MRI scans were made while subjects listened to normal speech (blue and green regions) or the prosodic elements of speech (orange and yellow regions).

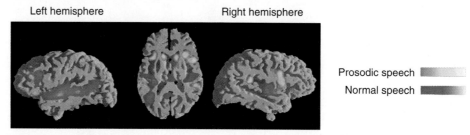

Left hemisphere   Right hemisphere

Prosodic speech
Normal speech

From Meyer, M., Alter, K., Friederici, A. D., et al. *Human Brain Mapping*, 2002, *17*, 73–88. Reprinted with permission.

The prosody of people with fluent aphasias, caused by posterior lesions, sounds normal. Their speech is rhythmical, with pauses after phrases and sentences, and has a melodic line. Even when the speech of a person with severe Wernicke's aphasia makes no sense, the prosody sounds normal. As Goodglass and Kaplan (1972) note, a person with Wernicke's aphasia may "sound like a normal speaker at a distance, because of his fluency and normal melodic contour of his speech." (Up close, of course, we hear the speech clearly enough to realize that it is meaningless.) In contrast, just as the lesions that produce Broca's aphasia destroy grammar, they also severely disrupt prosody. In patients with Broca's aphasia, articulation is so labored and words are uttered so slowly that there is little opportunity for the patient to demonstrate any rhythmic elements; and because of the relative lack of function words, there is little variation in stress or pitch of voice.

Evidence from studies of normal people and patients with brain lesions suggests that prosody is a special function of the right hemisphere. This function is undoubtedly related to the more general role of this hemisphere in musical skills and the expression and recognition of emotions: Production of prosody is rather like singing, and prosody often serves as a vehicle for conveying emotion.

In a functional imaging study by Meyer et al. (2002), subjects heard normal sentences or sentences that contained only the prosodic elements of speech with the meaningful sounds filtered out. As you can see in Figure 13.17, the meaningful components of speech primarily activated the left hemisphere (blue and green regions), whereas the prosodic components primarily activated the right hemisphere (orange and yellow regions). See *Figure 13.17.*)

Stuttering

Stuttering is a speech disorder characterized by frequent pauses, prolongations of sounds, or repetitions of sounds, syllables, or words that disrupt the normal flow of speech. Stuttering, which appears to be influenced by genetic factors, affects approximately 1 percent of the population and is three times more prevalent in men than in women (Brown et al., 2005). Stuttering seldom occurs when a person says a single word or is asked to read a list of words; it most often occurs at the beginning of a sentence, especially if the planned sentence is long or grammatically complex. This fact suggests that stuttering is a disorder of "selection, initiation, and execution of motor sequences necessary for fluent speech production" (Watkins et al., 2008, p. 50). Perhaps a person who stutters needs more time to plan the movements necessary for an utterance.

Stuttering is not a result of abnormalities in the neural circuits that contain the motor programs for speech. For example, stuttering is reduced or eliminated when a person reads aloud with another speaker, sings, or reads in cadence with a rhythmic stimulus. Brown et al. (2005) suggest that the source of the problem may be faulty auditory feedback from sounds of the stutterer's own speech. They note that a magnetoencephalographic (MEG) study by Salmelin et al. (2000) found disruptions in the normal timing of activation of brain regions involved in speech production.

Evidence in support of this suggestion includes the fact that delayed auditory feedback interferes with the speech of most fluent speakers but actually facilitates the speech of many people who stutter (Foundas et al., 2004a). *Delayed auditory feedback* is a procedure in which a person wearing headphones tries to speak normally while hearing his or her own voice, which has been electronically delayed, usually by 50–200 msec. (In fact, portable devices are commercially available that include a microphone, headphones, and an electronic device that provides the delay.) Certainly, if there were a problem with the control of articulation in people who stutter, delayed auditory feedback would not be expected to have any effect on their fluency.

A functional-imaging study by Watkins et al. (2008) increased activation in the insula, cerebellum, and midbrain, and decreased activation in the ventral premotor cortex, face region of the primary motor cortex and somatosensory cortex, and the superior temporal cortex. Watkins and her colleagues also used diffusion tensor imaging and found decreases in the white matter beneath the ventral premotor cortex of people who stuttered. They suggested that the axons in this white matter connect the ventral premotor cortex (involved in speaking) with regions of the superior temporal cortex and inferior parietal cortex that are involved in integrating the planning of speech with auditory feedback from one's own voice.

Neumann et al. (2005) provide further evidence that the apparently abnormal auditory feedback in stutterers is reflected in decreased activation of their temporal cortex. The authors used fMRI to measure the regional brain activation of stutterers reading sentences aloud during two sessions, one before and one after a successful 12-week course of fluency shaping therapy. Figure 13.18 shows that after the therapy, the activation of the temporal lobe—a region that both Brown et al. (2005) and Watkins et al. (2008) found to show decreased activation—was increased. (See *Figure 13.18*.)

FIGURE 13.18

Effects of Therapy for Stuttering.   A functional MRI scan shows regions of the superior temporal lobe that showed increased activity 1 year after a successful course of therapy for stuttering.

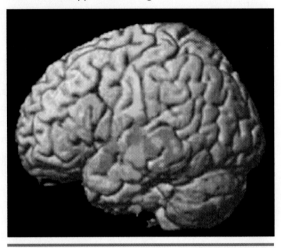

From Neumann, K., Preibisch, C., Euler, H. A., et al. *Journal of Fluency Disorders*, 2005, *30*, 23–39.

InterimSummary

Speech Production and Comprehension: Brain Mechanisms

Two regions of the brain are especially important in understanding and producing speech. Broca's area, in the left frontal lobe just rostral to the region of the primary motor cortex that controls the muscles of speech, is involved with speech production. This region contains memories of the sequences of muscular movements that produce words, each of which is connected with its auditory counterpart in the posterior part of the brain. Broca's aphasia—which is caused by damage to Broca's area, adjacent regions of the frontal cortex, and underlying white matter—consists of varying degrees of agrammatism, anomia, and articulation difficulties.

Wernicke's area, in the posterior superior temporal lobe, is involved with speech perception. The region just adjacent to Wer-

nicke's area, which I have called the posterior language area, is necessary for speech comprehension and the translation of thoughts into words. Presumably, Wernicke's area contains memories of the sounds of words, each of which is connected through the posterior language area with circuits that contain memories about the properties of the things the words denote and with circuits that are responsible for pronouncing the words. Damage restricted to Wernicke's area causes pure word deafness—loss of the ability to understand speech without loss of the ability to talk, read, and write. Wernicke's aphasia, caused by damage to Wernicke's area and the posterior language area, consists of poor speech comprehension, poor repetition, and production of fluent, meaningless speech. Transcortical sensory aphasia, caused by damage to the posterior speech area, consists of poor speech comprehension and production, but the patients can repeat what they hear. Thus, the symptoms of Wernicke's aphasia consist of those of transcortical sensory aphasia plus those of pure word deafness (WA = TSA + PWD). Feedback from mirror neurons that are activated when people hear the speech of other people may facilitate speech recognition. The right hemisphere plays a role in the more subtle, figurative aspects of speech.

The fact that people with transcortical sensory aphasia can repeat words that they cannot understand suggests that there is a direct connection between Wernicke's area and Broca's area. Indeed, there is: the arcuate fasciculus. Damage to this bundle of axons produces conduction aphasia: disruption of the ability to repeat exactly what was heard without disruption of the ability to comprehend or produce meaningful speech. A parallel pathway, consisting of an anterior and a posterior bundle that connect in the inferior parietal cortex, may be responsible for the ability of people with pure conduction aphasia to understand and paraphrase what they hear.

The meanings of words are our memories of objects, actions, and other concepts associated with them. These meanings are memories and are stored in the association cortex, not in the speech areas themselves. Anomic aphasia, caused by damage to the temporal or parietal lobes, consists of difficulty in word finding, particularly in naming objects. Brain damage can also disrupt the "definitions" as well as the "entries" in the mental dictionary; damage to specific regions of the association cortex effectively erases some categories of the meanings of words. Damage to Broca's area and surrounding regions disrupts the ability to name actions—to think of appropriate verbs. The right hemisphere plays a role in the more subtle, figurative aspects of speech.

The left hemisphere plays the more important role in the language abilities of deaf people who use sign language, just as it does in people who communicate acoustically. Gestural language may have been the precursor to vocal speech; mirror neurons in Broca's area are activated by hand movements.

Prosody includes changes in intonation, rhythm, and stress that add meaning, especially emotional meaning, to the sentences that we speak. The neural mechanisms that control the prosodic elements of speech appear to be in the right hemisphere.

Stuttering appears to be cause by abnormalities in neural circuits that are involved in feedback and planning and initiating speech, not in the circuits that contain the motor programs for articulation. Functional imaging indicates deficient auditory feedback produced by the stutterer's own voice. Delayed auditory feedback, which impairs the speech of most fluent speakers, often facilitates the speech of stutterers.

Because so many terms and symptoms were described in this section, I have provided a table that summarizes them. (See *Table 13.1*.)

Thought Questions

1. Suppose that you were asked to determine the abilities and deficits of people with aphasia. What tasks would you include in your examination to test for the presence of particular deficits?

2. What are the thoughts of a person with severe Wernicke's aphasia like? These people produce speech having very little meaning. Can you think of any ways in which you could test these people to find out whether their thoughts were any more coherent than their words?

TABLE 13.1   Aphasic Syndromes Produced by Brain Damage

Disorder	Areas of Lesion	Spontaneous Speech	Comprehension	Repetition	Naming
Wernicke's aphasia	Posterior portion of superior temporal gyrus (Wernicke's area) and posterior language area	Fluent	Poor	Poor	Poor
Pure word deafness	Wernicke's area or its connection with primary auditory cortex	Fluent	Poor	Poor	Good
Broca's aphasia	Frontal cortex rostral to base of primary motor cortex (Broca's area)	Nonfluent	Good	Poor[a]	Poor
Conduction aphasia	White matter beneath parietal lobe superior to lateral fissure (arcuate fasciculus)	Fluent	Good	Poor	Good
Anomic aphasia	Various parts of parietal and temporal lobes	Fluent	Good	Good	Poor
Transcortical sensory aphasia	Posterior language area	Fluent	Poor	Good	Poor

[a]May be better than spontaneous speech.

Disorders of Reading and Writing

Reading and writing are closely related to listening and talking; thus, oral and written language abilities have many brain mechanisms in common. This section discusses the neural basis of reading and writing disorders. As you will see, the study of these disorders has provided us with some useful and interesting information.

Pure Alexia

Dejerine (1892) described a remarkable syndrome, which we now call **pure alexia**, or sometimes *pure word blindness* or *alexia without agraphia*. His patient had a lesion in the visual cortex of the left occipital lobe and the posterior end of the corpus callosum. The patient could still write, although he had lost the ability to read. In fact, if he was shown some of his own writing, he could not read it.

Several years ago, some colleagues and I studied a man with pure alexia who discovered his ability to write in an interesting way. A few months after he sustained a head injury that caused his brain damage, he and his wife were watching a service person repair their washing machine. The patient wanted to say something privately to his wife, so he picked up a pad of paper and jotted a note. As he was handing it to her, they suddenly realized with amazement that although he could not read, he was able to write! His wife brought the note to their neurologist, who asked the patient to read it. Although he remembered the gist of the message, he could not read the words. Unfortunately, I do not have that note, but Figure 13.19 shows the writing of another person with pure alexia. (See *Figure 13.19*.)

FIGURE 13.19

Pure Alexia. This letter was written to Dr. Elizabeth Warrington by a patient with pure alexia. The letter reads as follows: "Dear Dr. Warrington, Thank you for your letter of September the 16th. I shall be pleased to be at your office between 10–10:30 am on Friday 17th october. I still find it very odd to be able to write this letter but not to be able to read it back a few minutes later. I much appreciate the opportunity to see you. Yours sincerely, Harry X."

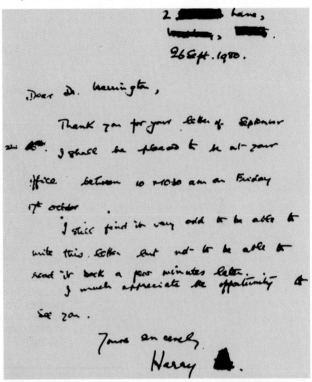

From McCarthy, R. A., and Warrington, E. K. *Cognitive Neuropsychology: A Clinical Introduction*. San Diego: Academic Press, 1990. Reprinted with permission from Elsevier Ltd.

Although patients with pure alexia cannot read, they can recognize words that are spelled aloud to them; therefore, they have not lost their memories of the spellings of words. Pure alexia is obviously a perceptual disorder; it is similar to pure word deafness, except that the patient has difficulty with visual input, not auditory input. The disorder is caused by lesions that prevent visual information from reaching the extrastriate cortex of the left hemisphere (Damasio and Damasio, 1983, 1986). Figure 13.20 explains why Dejerine's original patient could not read. (*MyPsychKit 13.5, Pure Alexia*, also illustrates the brain damage responsible for this disorder.) The first diagram shows the pathway that visual information would take if a person had damage *only to the left primary visual cortex*. In this case the person's right visual field would be blind; he or she would see nothing to the right of the fixation point. However, people with this disorder can read. Their only problem is that they must look to the right of each word so that they can see all of it, which means that they read somewhat more slowly than someone with full vision.

Let us trace the flow of visual information for a person with this brain damage. Information from the left side of the visual field is transmitted to the right striate cortex (primary visual cortex) and then to regions of the right visual association cortex. From there, the information crosses the posterior corpus callosum and is

Animation 13.5
Pure Alexia

pure alexia Loss of the ability to read without loss of the ability to write; produced by brain damage.

FIGURE 13.20

Pure Alexia. In this schematic diagram, red arrows indicate the flow of information that has been interrupted by brain damage. (a) The route followed by information as a person with damage to the left primary visual cortex reads aloud. (b) Additional damage to the posterior corpus callosum interrupts the flow of information and produces pure alexia.

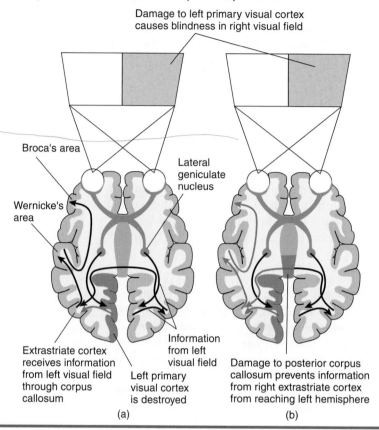

Damage to left primary visual cortex causes blindness in right visual field

Broca's area

Lateral geniculate nucleus

Wernicke's area

Extrastriate cortex receives information from left visual field through corpus callosum

Left primary visual cortex is destroyed

Information from left visual field

Damage to posterior corpus callosum prevents information from right extrastriate cortex from reaching left hemisphere

(a)   (b)

transmitted to the left visual association cortex, where it is analyzed further. (I will describe these regions later.) The information is then transmitted to speech mechanisms located in the left frontal lobe. Thus, the person can read the words aloud. (See *Figure 13.20a*.)

The second diagram shows Dejerine's patient. Notice how the additional lesion of the corpus callosum prevents visual information concerning written text from reaching the posterior left hemisphere. Without this information, the patient cannot read. (See *Figure 13.20b*.)

Mao-Draayer and Panitch (2004) reported the case of a man with multiple sclerosis who displayed the symptoms of pure alexia after sustaining a lesion that damaged both the subcortical white matter of the left occipital lobe and the posterior corpus callosum. As you can see in Figure 13.21, the lesions are in precisely the locations that Dejerine predicted would cause this syndrome. (See *Figure 13.21*.)

I must note that the diagrams shown in Figure 13.20 are as simple and schematic as possible. They illustrate only the pathway involved in seeing a word and pronouncing it, and they ignore neural structures that would be involved in understanding its meaning. As we will see later in this chapter, evidence from patients with brain lesions indicates that seeing and pronouncing words can take place independently of understanding them. Thus, although the diagrams are simplified, they are not unreasonable, given what we know about the neural components of the reading process.

Toward an Understanding of Reading

Reading involves at least two different processes: direct recognition of the word as a whole and sounding it out letter by letter. When we see a familiar word, we normally recognize it and pronounce it—a process known as **whole-word reading**. (With very long words we might instead perceive segments of several letters each.) The second method, which we use for unfamiliar words, requires recognition of individual letters and knowledge of the sounds they make. This process is known as **phonetic reading**.

Evidence for our ability to sound out words is easy to obtain. In fact, you can prove to yourself that phonetic reading exists by trying to read the following words:

glab   trisk   chint

Well, as you could see, they are not really words, but I doubt that you had trouble pronouncing them. Obviously, you did not *recognize* them, because you probably never saw them before. Therefore, you had to use what you know about the sounds that are represented by particular letters (or groups of letters, such as *ch*) to figure out how to pronounce the words.

The best evidence that proves that people can read words without sounding them out, using the whole-word method, comes from studies of patients with acquired dyslexias. *Dyslexia* means "faulty reading." *Acquired* dyslexias are those caused by damage to the brains of people who already know how to read. In contrast, *developmental* dyslexias refer to reading difficulties that become apparent when children are learning to read. Developmental dyslexias, which may involve anomalies in brain circuitry, are discussed in a later section.

Figure 13.22 illustrates some elements of the reading processes. The diagram is an oversimplification of a very complex process, but it helps to organize some of the facts that investigators have obtained. It considers only reading and pronouncing single words, not understanding the meaning of text. When we see a familiar word, we normally recognize it as a whole and pronounce it. If we see an unfamiliar word or a pronounceable nonword, we must try to read it phonetically. (See *Figure 13.22*.)

Investigators have reported several types of acquired dyslexias, and I will describe three of them in this section: surface dyslexia, phonological dyslexia, and direct dyslexia. **Surface dyslexia** is a deficit in whole-word reading. The term *surface* reflects the fact that people with this disorder make errors related to the visual appearance of the words and to pronunciation rules, not to the meaning of the words, which is metaphorically "deeper" than the appearance.

Because patients with surface dyslexia have difficulty recognizing words as a whole, they are obliged to sound them out. Thus, they can easily read words with regular spelling, such as *hand*, *table*, or *chin*. However, they have difficulty reading words with irregular spelling, such as *sew*, *pint*, and *yacht*. In fact, they may read these words as *sue*, *pinnt*, and *yatchet*. They have no difficulty reading pronounceable nonwords,

FIGURE 13.21

Pure Alexia in a Patient with Multiple Sclerosis.   The damage corresponds to that shown in Figure 13.20(b).

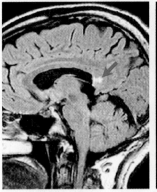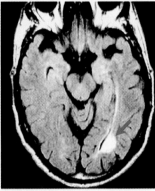

From Mao-Draayer, Y, and Panitch, H. *Multiple Sclerosis 10*(6), pp. 705–707, copyright © 2004. Reprinted by permission of SAGE.

whole-word reading Reading by recognizing a word as a whole; "sight reading."

phonetic reading Reading by decoding the phonetic significance of letter strings; "sound reading."

surface dyslexia A reading disorder in which a person can read words phonetically but has difficulty reading irregularly spelled words by the whole-word method.

FIGURE 13.22

Model of the Reading Process.   In this simplified model, whole-word reading is used for most familiar words and phonetic reading is used for unfamiliar words and for nonwords such as *glab*, *trisk*, or *chint*.

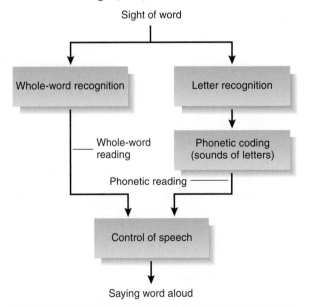

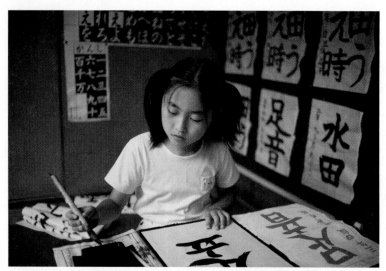

Japanese writing uses two forms of characters, which encode information phonetically or nonphonetically.

such as *glab, trisk,* and *chint.* Because people with surface dyslexia cannot recognize whole words by their appearance, they must, in effect, listen to their own pronunciation to understand what they are reading. If they read the word *pint* and pronounce it *pinnt,* they will say that it is not an English word (which it is not, pronounced that way). If the word is one member of a homophone, it will be impossible to understand it unless it is read in the context of a sentence. For example, if you hear the single word "pair" without additional information, you cannot know whether the speaker is referring to *pair, pear,* or *pare.* Thus, a patient with surface dyslexia who reads the word *pair* might say, ". . . it could be two of a kind, apples and . . . or what you do with your fingernails" (Gurd and Marshall, 1993, p. 594). (See *Figure 13.23.*)

The symptoms of **phonological dyslexia** are opposite those of surface dyslexia: People with this disorder can read by the whole-word method but cannot sound words out. Thus, they can read words that they are already familiar with but have great difficulty figuring out how to read unfamiliar words or pronounceable non-words (Beauvois and Dérouesné, 1979; Dérouesné and Beauvois, 1979). (In this context, *phonology*—loosely translated as "laws of sound"—refers to the relation between letters and the sounds they represent.) People with phonological dyslexia may be excellent readers if they had already acquired a good reading vocabulary before their brain damage occurred.

Phonological dyslexia provides further evidence that whole-word reading and phonological reading involve different brain mechanisms. Phonological reading, which is the only way we can read nonwords or words we have not yet learned, entails some sort of letter-to-sound decoding. Obviously, phonological reading of English requires more than decoding of the sounds produced by single letters, because, for example, some sounds are transcribed as two-letter sequences (such as *th* or *sh*) and the addition of the letter *e* to the end of a word lengthens an internal vowel (*can* becomes *cane*). (See *Figure 13.24.*)

The Japanese language provides a particularly interesting distinction between phonetic and whole-word reading. The Japanese language makes use of two kinds of written symbols. *Kanji* symbols are pictographs, adopted from the Chinese language (although they are pronounced as Japanese words). Thus, they represent concepts by means of visual symbols but do not provide a guide to their pronunciation. Reading words expressed in kanji symbols is analogous, then, to whole-word reading. *Kana* symbols are phonetic representations of syllables; thus, they encode acoustical information. These symbols are used primarily to represent foreign words or Japanese words that the average reader would be unlikely to recognize if they were represented by their kanji symbols. Reading words expressed in kana symbols is obviously phonetic.

Studies of Japanese people with localized brain damage have shown that the reading of kana and kanji symbols involves different brain mechanisms (Iwata, 1984; Sakurai et al., 1994; Sakurai, Ichikawa, and Mannen, 2001). Difficulty reading kanji symbols is a form of surface dyslexia, whereas difficulty reading kana symbols is a form of phonological dyslexia. What regions are involved in these two kinds of reading?

Evidence from lesion and functional imaging studies with readers of English, Chinese, and Japanese suggest that the process of whole-word reading follows the ventral stream of the visual system to the fusiform gyrus, located on the base of the

phonological dyslexia A reading disorder in which a person can read familiar words but has difficulty reading unfamiliar words or pronounceable nonwords.

visual word-form area (VWFA) A region of the fusiform gyrus on the base of the temporal lobe that plays a critical role in whole-word recognition.

FIGURE 13.23

Surface Dyslexia.   In this hypothetic example, whole-word reading is damaged; only phonetic reading remains.

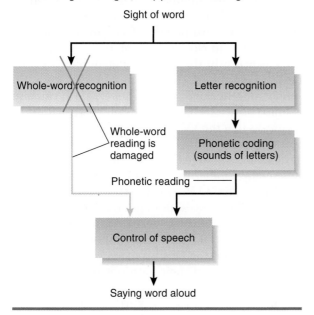

FIGURE 13.24

Phonological Dyslexia.   In this hypothetical example, phonetic reading is damaged; only whole-word reading remains.

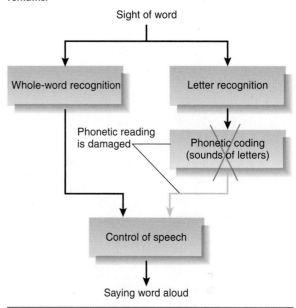

temporal lobe. For example, functional imaging studies by Thuy et al. (2004) and Liu et al. (2008) found that the reading of kanji words or Chinese characters (whole-word reading) activated the left fusiform gyrus. This region has come to be known as the **visual word-form area (VWFA)**. As we saw in Chapter 6, this region is also involved in the perception of faces and other shapes that require expertise to distinguish—and certainly, recognizing whole words or kanji symbols requires expertise. Phonological reading appears to follow the dorsal stream to the region around the junction of the inferior parietal lobe and the superior temporal lobe (the temporoparietal cortex) and then follows a fiber bundle from this region to the inferior frontal cortex—which includes Broca's area (Sakurai et al., 2000; Jobard, Crivello, and Tzourio-Mazoyer, 2003; Thuy et al., 2004; Tan et al., 2005). The fact that phonological reading involves Broca's area suggests that it may actually involve articulation—that we sound out words not so much by "hearing" them in our heads as by feeling ourselves pronounce them silently to ourselves. Once words are identified—by either means—their meaning must be accessed, which means that the two pathways converge on regions of the brain involved in recognition of word meaning, grammatical structure, and semantics. (See *Figure 13.25*.)

Let's consider the role of the VWFA. Obviously, some parts of the visual association cortex must be involved in perceiving written words. You will recall from Chapter 6 that visual agnosia is a perceptual deficit in which people with bilateral damage to the visual association cortex cannot recognize objects by sight. However, people with visual agnosia can still read, which means that the perceptual analysis of objects and words involves at least some different brain mechanisms. This fact is both interesting and puzzling. Certainly, the ability to read cannot have shaped the evolution of the human brain, because the invention of writing is only a few thousand years old, and until very recently, the vast majority of the world's population was illiterate. Thus, reading and object recognition use brain mechanisms that undoubtedly existed long before the invention of writing. However, just as experience seeing faces affects the development of the fusiform face area in the right hemisphere, experience learning to read words undoubtedly affects the development of the visual word-form area—which, probably not coincidentally, is found in

FIGURE 13.25

Phonological and Whole-Word Reading. A schematic diagram showing the brain regions primarily involved in (a) phonological reading and (b) whole-word reading.

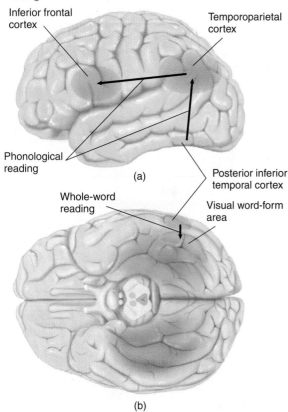

Inferior frontal cortex

Temporoparietal cortex

Phonological reading

(a)

Posterior inferior temporal cortex

Whole-word reading

Visual word-form area

(b)

direct dyslexia A language disorder caused by brain damage in which the person can read words aloud without understanding them.

the fusiform cortex of the left hemisphere (McCandliss, Cohen, and Dehaene, 2003).

The fusiform face area of the right hemisphere has the ability to quickly recognize unique configurations of people's eyes, noses, lips, and other features of their faces even when the differences between two people's faces are very similar. For example, parents and close friends of identical twins can see at a glance which twin they are looking at. Similarly, the VWFA of the left hemisphere can recognize a word even if it closely resembles another one. (See *Figure 13.26.*) It can also quickly recognize words written in different *typestyles*, fonts or CASES. This means that the VWFA can recognize whole words with different shapes; certainly, chair and CHAIR do not look the same. It takes an experienced reader the same amount of time to read equally familiar three-letter words and six-letter words (Nazir, Jacobs, and O'Regan, 1998), which means that the whole word reading process does not have to identify the letters one at a time, just as the face-recognition process in the right fusiform cortex does not have to identify each feature of a face individually before the face is recognized. Instead, we recognize several letters and their locations relative to each other.

A functional-imaging study by Vinckier et al. (2007) investigated the means by which the brain recognizes whole words. First, I need to provide some definitions. A *bigram* is a sequence of two letters. *Frequent* bigrams are two-letter sequences that are often encountered in a particular language. For example, the bigram *SH* often occurs in English. In contrast, *LQ* is an *infrequent* bigram. *Quadrigrams* are strings of four letters and can be classified as frequent or infrequent. Now to the study. Vinckier and his colleagues had adult readers look at the following stimuli: (1) strings of false fonts (nonsensical letter-like symbols); (2) strings of infrequent letters; (3) strings that contained infrequent bigrams; (4) strings that contained frequent bigrams; (5) strings that contained frequent quadrigrams; and (6) real words. (See *Figure 13.27* for examples of these stimuli.)

Functional imaging showed that some brain regions were activated by all of the visual stimuli, including letter-like symbols, some were activated by letters but not symbols, . . . and so on, up to regions that were activated by real words. The most selective region included the left anterior fusiform cortex, which was activated only

FIGURE 13.26

Subtle Differences in Written Words. Unless you can read Arabic, Hindi, or Mandarin, you will probably have to examine these words carefully to find the small differences. However, as a reader of English, you will immediately recognize the words "car" and "ear."

English	Arabic	Hindi	Mandarin
cars ears	زمان رمان pomegranate time/era	आज आजा today come	夫 天 man sky

Adapted from Devlin, J. T., Jamison, H. L., Gonnerman, L. M., and Matthews, P. M. *Journal of Cognitive Neuroscience*, 2006, *18*, 911–922.

FIGURE 13.27

Stimuli Used in a Test of Word Recognition. These examples of stimuli were used in the experiment by Vinckier et al. (2007). *Mouton* is the French word for "sheep." (The experiment took place in France.)

Types of stimuli

False font	Infrequent letters	Frequent letters	Frequent bigrams	Frequent quadrigrams	Words
⅂Ꙩ∩+∏Ꝓ	JZWYWK	QOADTQ	QUMBSS	AVONIL	MOUTON

Examples

by actual words. In fact, as Figure 13.28 shows, the scans revealed a posterior-to-anterior gradient of selectivity, from symbol to whole word, along the base of the left occipital and temporal lobes. A second, smaller, gradient was seen in Broca's area. Presumably, this gradient represented phonetic reading—decoding of the sounds represented by the stimuli that the subjects viewed. Note that very little activity was produced by letter-like symbols (shown in red) in Broca's area. This makes sense, because there is no way to pronounce these symbols. (See *Figure 13.28*.)

Many studies have found that damage to the VWFA produces surface dyslexia; that is, impairment of whole-word reading. A study by Gaillard et al. (2006) combined fMRI and lesion evidence from a single subject that provides evidence that the left fusiform cortex does, indeed, contain this region. A patient with a severe seizure disorder became a candidate for surgery aimed at removal of a seizure focus. Before the surgery was performed, the patient viewed printed words and pictures of faces, houses, and tools while his brain was being scanned. He was warned that the seizure focus was located in a region that played a critical role in reading, but his symptoms were so severe that he elected to undergo the surgery. As expected, the surgery produced a deficit in whole-word reading. A combination of structural and functional imaging revealed that the lesion—a very small one—was located in the fusiform gyrus, the location of the VWFA. (See *Figure 13.29*.)

What about phonological reading? I mentioned earlier that Thuy et al. (2004) found that phonological reading activated the left temporoparietal cortex and Broca's area. A meta-analysis of 35 neuroimaging studies by Jobard, Crivello, and Tzourio-Mazoyer (2003) found that phonological reading activates the left temporoparietal region and Broca's area.

As we saw earlier in this chapter, recognizing a spoken word is different from understanding it. For example, patients with transcortical sensory aphasia can repeat what is said to them even though they show no signs of understanding what they hear or say. The same is true for reading. **Direct dyslexia** resembles transcortical sensory aphasia, except that the words in question are written, not spoken (Schwartz, Marin, and Saffran, 1979; Lytton and Brust, 1989; Gerhand, 2001). Patients with direct dyslexia are able to read aloud *even though they cannot understand the words they are saying*. After sustaining a stroke that damaged his left frontal and temporal lobes, Lytton and Brust's patient lost the ability to communicate verbally; his speech was meaningless, and he was unable to comprehend what other people said to him. However, he could read words with which he was already familiar. He could *not* read pronounceable nonwords; therefore, he had lost the ability to read phonetically. His comprehension deficit seemed complete; when the investigators presented him with a word and several pictures, one of which corresponded to the word, he read the word correctly but had no idea what picture went with it. Gerhand's patient showed a similar pattern of

FIGURE 13.28

Word Recognition in the VWFA.   The scan shows regions of the brain that selectively responded to letter-like symbols, infrequent letters, frequent letters, bigrams, quadrigrams, and words. This range is indicated by colors that range from red to violet. Response gradients were seen in the VWFA (visual word-form area) and in Broca's area.

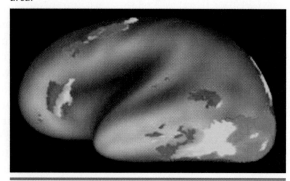

Reprinted from *Neuron, 55*, Vinckier, F., Dehaene, S., Jobert, A., et al., Hierarchical Coding of Letter Strings in the Ventral Stream: Dissecting the Inner Organization of the Visual Word-Form System, 143–156, Copyright 2007, with permission from Elsevier.

FIGURE 13.29

Effects of VWFA Lesion.   The scans show responses of brain regions to words, faces, houses, and tools before and after surgical removal of a small region of the VWFA. Note that the response to words (dark blue) is lost, but responses to faces, houses, and tools remains. The lesion is indicated by the green arrowheads.

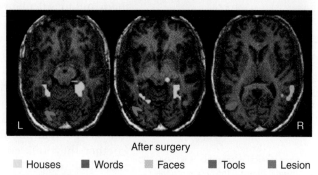

Before surgery

After surgery

■ Houses   ■ Words   ■ Faces   ■ Tools   ■ Lesion

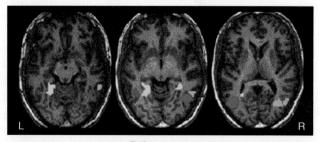

Reprinted from *Neuron, 50*, Gaillard, R., Naccache, L., Pinel, P., et al., Direct Intracranial, fMRI, and Lesion Evidence for the Causal Role of Left Inferotemporal Cortex in Reading, 191–204, Copyright 2006, with permission from Elsevier.

deficits, except that she was able to read phonetically: She could sound out pronounceable nonwords. These findings indicate that the brain regions responsible for phonetic reading and whole-word reading are each independently connected with brain regions responsible for speech.

Toward an Understanding of Writing

Writing depends on a knowledge of the words that are to be used, along with the proper grammatical structure of the sentences they are to form. Therefore, if a patient is unable to express him- or herself by speech, we should not be surprised to see a writing disturbance (*dysgraphia*) as well. In addition, most cases of dyslexia are accompanied by dysgraphia.

One type of writing disorder involves difficulties in motor control—in directing the movements of a pen or pencil to form letters and words. Investigators have reported surprisingly specific types of writing disorders that fall into this category. For example, some patients can write numbers but not letters, some can write uppercase letters but not lowercase letters, some can write consonants but not vowels, some can write cursively but not print uppercase letters, and others can write letters normally but have difficulty placing them in an orderly fashion on the page (Cubelli, 1991; Alexander, Fischer, and Friedman, 1992; Margolin and Goodman-Schulman, 1992; Silveri, 1996).

Many regions of the brain are involved in writing. For example, damage that produces various forms of aphasia will produce impairments in writing that are similar to those seen in speech. Organization of the motor aspects of writing involves the dorsal parietal lobe and the premotor cortex. These regions (and the primary motor cortex, of course) become activated when people engage in writing, and damage to these regions impairs writing (Otsuki et al., 1999; Katanoda, Yoshikawa, and Sugishita, 2001; Menon and Desmond, 2001). A functional imaging study by Rijntjes et al. (1999) had people sign their names with either their index finger or their big toe. In both cases, doing so activated the premotor cortex that controlled movements of the hand. This finding suggests that when we learn to make a complex series of movements, the relevant information is stored in regions of the motor association cortex that control the part of the body that is being used but that this information can be used to control similar movements in other parts of the body.

A more basic type of writing disorder involves problems in the ability to spell words, as opposed to problems with making accurate movements of the fingers. I will devote the rest of this section to this type of disorder. Like reading, writing (or, more specifically, spelling) involves more than one method. The first is related to audition. When children acquire language skills, they first learn the sounds of words, then learn to say them, then learn to read, and then learn to write. Undoubtedly, reading and writing depend heavily on the skills that are learned earlier. For example, to write most words, we must be able to "sound them out in our heads"; that is, to hear them and to articulate them subvocally. If you want to demonstrate this to yourself, try to write a long word such as *antidisestablishmentarianism* from memory and see whether you can do it without saying the word to yourself. If you recite a poem or sing a song to yourself under your breath at the same time, you will see that the writing comes to a halt.

A second way of writing involves transcribing an image of what a particular word looks like—copying a visual mental image. Have you ever looked off into the distance to picture a word so that you can remember how to spell it? Some people are not very good at phonological spelling and have to write some words down to see whether they look correct. This method obviously involves *visual* memories, not acoustical ones.

Neurological evidence supports these speculations. Brain damage can impair the first of these methods: phonetic writing. This deficit is called **phonological dys-**

phonological dysgraphia A writing disorder in which the person cannot sound out words and write them phonetically.

graphia (Shallice, 1981). (*Dysgraphia* refers to a writing deficit, just as *dyslexia* refers to a reading deficit.) People with this disorder are unable to sound out words and write them phonetically. Thus, they cannot write unfamiliar words or pronounceable nonwords, such as the ones presented in the section on reading. They can, however, visually imagine familiar words and then write them. Phonological dysgraphia appears to be caused by damage to regions of the brain involved in phonological processing and articulation. Damage to Broca's area, the ventral precentral gyrus, and the insula cause this disorder, and phonological spelling tasks activate these regions (Omura et al., 2004; Henry et al., 2007).

Orthographic dysgraphia is just the opposite of phonological dysgraphia: It is a disorder of visually based writing. People with orthographic dysgraphia can *only* sound words out; thus, they can spell regular words such as *care* or *tree*, and they can write pronounceable nonsense words. However, they have difficulty spelling irregular words such as *half* or *busy* (Beauvois and Dérouesné, 1981); they may write *haff* or *bizzy*. Orthographic dysgraphia (impaired phonological writing), like surface dyslexia, is caused by damage to the VWFA on the base of the temporal lobe (Henry et al., 2007).

Figure 13.30 shows the brain damage that causes phonological and orthographic dysgraphia. (See **Figure 13.30**.)

As we saw in the section on reading, some patients (those with direct dyslexia) can read aloud without being able to understand what they are reading. Similarly, some patients can write words that are dictated to them even though they cannot understand these words (Roeltgen, Rothi, and Heilman, 1986; Lesser, 1989). Of course, they cannot communicate by means of writing, because they cannot translate their thoughts into words. (In fact, because most of these patients have sustained extensive brain damage, their thought processes themselves are severely disturbed.) Some of these patients can even spell pronounceable nonwords, which indicates that their ability to spell phonetically is intact. Roeltgen et al. (1986) referred to this disorder as *semantic agraphia*, but perhaps the term *direct dysgraphia* would be more appropriate, because of the parallel with direct dyslexia.

Developmental Dyslexias

Some children have great difficulty learning to read and never become fluent readers, even though they are otherwise intelligent. Specific language learning disorders, called **developmental dyslexias**, tend to occur in families, a finding that suggests a genetic (and hence biological) component. The concordance rate of monozygotic twins ranges from 84 percent to 100 percent, and that of dizygotic twins ranges from 20 percent to 35 percent (Démonet, Taylor, and Chaix, 2004). Linkage studies suggest that the chromosomes 1, 2, 3, 6, 15, and 18 may contain genes responsible for different components of this disorder (Deffenbacher et al., 2004).

As we saw earlier, the fact that written language is a recent invention means that natural selection could not have given us brain mechanisms whose only role is to interpret written language. Therefore, we should not expect that developmental dyslexia involves only deficits in reading. Indeed, researchers have found a variety of

FIGURE 13.30

Phonological Dysgraphia and Orthographic Dysgraphia.   The scans show the overlap in the lesions of (a) thirteen patients with phonological dysgraphia and (b) eight patients with orthographic dysgraphia. The highest degree of overlap is indicated in red and the lowest degree is indicated in purple. Phonological dysgraphia was caused by damage centered on Broca's area, and orthographic dysgraphia was caused by damage centered on the VWFA in the left fusiform gyrus.

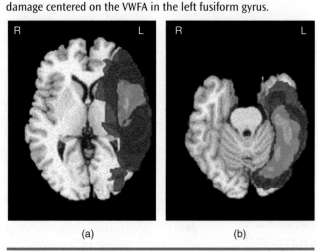

(a)   (b)

Reprinted from *Brain and Language, 100*, Henry, M. L., Beeson, P. M., Stark, A. J., and Rapcsak, S. Z. , The Role of Left Perisylvian Cortical Regions in Spelling, 44–52, Copyright 2007, with permission from Elsevier.

orthographic dysgraphia A writing disorder in which the person can spell regularly spelled words but not irregularly spelled ones.

developmental dyslexia A reading difficulty in a person of normal intelligence and perceptual ability; of genetic origin or caused by prenatal or perinatal factors.

language deficits that do not directly involve reading. One common deficit is deficient phonological awareness. That is, people with developmental dyslexia have difficulty blending or rearranging the sounds of words that they hear (Eden and Zeffiro, 1998). For example, they have difficulty recognizing that if we remove the first sound from "cat," we are left with the word "at." They also have difficulty distinguishing the order of sequences of sounds (Helenius, Uutela, and Hari, 1999). Problems such as these might be expected to impair the ability to read phonetically. Dyslexic children also tend to have great difficulty in writing: They make spelling errors, they show poor spatial arrangements of letters, they omit letters, and their writing tends to have weak grammatical development (Habib, 2000).

Developmental dyslexia is a heterogeneous and complex trait; thus, it undoubtedly has more than one cause. However, most studies that have closely examined the nature of the impairments seen in people with developmental dyslexia have found phonological impairments to be most common. For example, a study of sixteen dyslexics by Ramus et al. (2003) found that all had phonological deficits. Ten of the people also had auditory deficits, four also had a motor deficit, and two also had a visual deficit. These deficits—especially auditory deficits—aggravated the people's difficulty in reading but did not appear to be primarily responsible for the difficulty. Five of the people had only phonological deficits, and these deficits were sufficient to interfere with their ability to read.

Some evidence has been obtained from functional imaging that suggests that the brains of dyslexics process written information differently than do proficient readers (Shaywitz et al., 2002; Hoeft et al., 2007). The scans showed decreased activation of the VWFA and the left temporoparietal and occipitotemporal cortex. The scans also showed *hyperactivation* of the left inferior frontal cortex, including Broca's area. Presumably, the activation of Broca's area reflected an effort to decode the phonology of the incomplete information being received from the poorly functioning regions of the more posterior brain regions involved in reading.

Most languages—including English—contain many irregular words. For example, consider *cough, rough, bough,* and *through.* Because there is no phonetic rule that describes how these words are to be pronounced, readers of English are obliged to memorize them. In fact, the forty sounds that distinguish English words can be spelled in up to 1120 different ways. In contrast, Italian is much more regular; this language contains twenty-five different sounds that can be spelled in only thirty-three combinations of letters (Helmuth, 2001). Paulesu et al. (2001) found that developmental dyslexia is rare among people who speak Italian and is much more common among speakers of English and French (another language with many irregular words). Paulesu and his colleagues identified college students with a history of dyslexia from Italy, France, and Great Britain. The Italian dyslexics were much harder to find, and their disorders were much less severe than those of their English-speaking and French-speaking counterparts. However, functional imaging revealed that when all three groups were asked to read, their scans all showed the same pattern of activation: a decrease in the activity of the left occipitotemporal cortex—the same general region that Shaywitz et al. (2002) identified.

Paulesu and his colleagues (2001) concluded that the brain anomalies that cause dyslexia are similar in the three countries they studied but that the regularity of Italian spelling made it much easier for potential dyslexics in Italy to learn to read. By the way, other "dyslexia-friendly" languages include Spanish, Finnish, Czech, and Japanese. One of the authors of this study, Chris D. Frith, cites the case of an Australian boy who lived in Japan. He learned to read Japanese normally but was dyslexic in English (Recer, 2001). If the spelling of words in the English language were regularized (for example, *frend* instead of *friend, frate* instead of *freight, coff* instead of *cough*), many children who develop dyslexia under the present system would develop into much better readers. Somehow, I don't foresee that happening in the near future.

InterimSummary

Disorders of Reading and Writing

Brain damage can produce reading and writing disorders. Pure alexia is caused by lesions that produce blindness in the right visual field and that destroy fibers of the posterior corpus callosum.

Research in the past few decades has discovered that acquired reading disorders (dyslexias) can fall into one of several categories, and the study of these disorders has provided neuropsychologists and cognitive psychologists with thought-provoking information that has helped them to understand the brain mechanisms involved in reading. Analysis of written words appears to begin in the left posterior inferior temporal cortex. Phonological information is then analyzed by the temporoparietal cortex and Broca's area, whereas word-form information is analyzed by the visual word form area, located in the fusiform cortex. Surface dyslexia is a loss of whole-word reading ability. Phonological dyslexia is loss of the ability to read phonetically. Reading of kana (phonetic) and kanji (pictographic) symbols by Japanese people is equivalent to phonetic and whole-word reading, and damage to different parts of the brain interfere with these two forms of reading. Direct dyslexia is analogous to transcortical sensory aphasia; the patients can read words aloud but cannot understand what they are reading. Some can read both real words and pronounceable nonwords, so both phonetic and whole-word reading can be preserved.

Brain damage can disrupt writing ability by impairing people's ability to form letters—or even specific types of letters, such as uppercase or lowercase letters or vowels. The dorsal parietal cortex appears to be the most critical region for knowledge of the movements that produce letters. Other deficits involve the ability to spell words. We normally use two different strategies to spell words: phonetic (sounding the word out) and visual (remembering how it looks on paper). Two types of dysgraphia—phonological and orthographic—represent difficulties in implementing phonetic and visual strategies, respectively. The existence of these two disorders indicates that several different brain mechanisms are involved in the process of writing. In addition, some patients have a deficit parallel to direct dyslexia: They can write words they can no longer understand.

Developmental dyslexia is a hereditary condition that may involve abnormal development of parts of the brain that play a role in language. Most developmental dyslexics have difficulty with phonological processing—of spoken words as well as written ones. Functional imaging studies report that decreased activation of the VWFA and the left occipitotemporal and temporoparietal cortex, and hyperactivation of Broca's area may be involved in developmental dyslexia. Children who learn to read languages that have writing with regular correspondence between spelling and pronunciation (such as Italian) are much less likely to become dyslexic than those who learn to read languages with irregular spelling (such as English or French). A better understanding of the components of reading and writing may help us to develop effective teaching methods that will permit people with dyslexia to take advantage of the abilities that they do have.

Table 13.2 summarizes the disorders that were described in this section.

Thought Questions

Suppose someone close to you suffered a head injury that caused phonological dyslexia. What would you do to try to help this person read better? (It would probably be best to build on the person's remaining abilities.) Suppose this person needed to learn to read some words that he or she had never seen before. How would you help the person to do so?

TABLE 13.2   Reading and Writing Disorder Produced by Brain Damage

Reading Disorder	Whole-Word Reading	Phonetic Reading	Remarks
Pure alexia	Poor	Poor	Can write
Surface dyslexia	Poor	Good	
Phonological dyslexia	Good	Poor	
Direct dyslexia	Good	Good	Cannot comprehend words
Writing Disorder	Whole-Word Writing	Phonetic Writing	
Phonological dysgraphia	Good	Poor	
Orthographic dysgraphia	Poor	Good	
Semantic agraphia (direct dysgraphia)	Good	Good	Cannot comprehend words

EPILOGUE

Speech Sounds and the Left Hemisphere

Mr. S., the man described in the chapter prologue, had pure word deafness. As you learned in this chapter, pure word deafness is a perceptual deficit that does not affect people's general language abilities, nor does it affect their ability to recognize nonspeech sounds.

What is involved in the analysis of speech sounds? Just what tasks does the auditory system have to accomplish? What are the differences in the functions of the auditory association cortex of the left and right hemispheres? Most researchers believe that the left hemisphere is primarily involved in judging the timing of the components of rapidly changing complex sounds, whereas the right hemisphere is primarily involved in judging more slowly changing components, including melody. Evidence suggests that the most crucial aspect of speech sounds is timing, not pitch. We can recognize words whether they are conveyed by the low pitch of a man or the high pitch of a woman or child. If you listen to *MyPsychKit 13.6, Speech Perception*, you will hear that we can understand speech from which the almost all tonal information has been removed, leaving only some noise modulated by the rapid stops and starts that characterize human speech sounds. On the other hand, emphasis or the emotional state of the speaker is conveyed by the pitch and melody of speech and by much slower changes in rhythm. In other words, the sounds that convey the identity of words are very brief, whereas those that convey prosody (either for emphasis or for the expression of emotion) are of longer duration. (As we saw, the right hemisphere is specialized for recognition of prosody.) Studies of patients with pure word deafness have shown that the patients can distinguish between different vowels but not between different consonants, especially between different stop consonants, such as /t/, /d/, /k/, or /p/. (Linguists represent speech sounds by putting letters or special phonetic symbols between pairs of slashes.) Patients with pure word deafness *can* generally recognize consonants with a long duration, such as /s/, /z/, or /f/. (Say these consonants to yourself, and you will hear how different they sound from the first four examples.) Therefore, the auditory system of the left hemisphere appears to be particularly specialized for the recognition of acoustical events of short duration (Phillips and Farmer, 1990; Stefanatos, Gershkoff, and Madigan, 2005).

Several studies have found deficits in auditory perception of nonspeech sounds that support this conclusion (Phillips and Farmer, 1990). For example, normal subjects can perceive a series of clicks as being separate events when they are separated by only 1 to 3 msec; in contrast, patients with pure word deafness require a separation of 15 to 30 msec. In addition, although normal subjects can count clicks that are presented at a rate of up to nine to eleven per second, patients with pure word deafness cannot count clicks presented faster than two per second. One study reported that a patient with pure word deafness could no longer understand messages in Morse code, although he could still *send* messages that way. Thus, his deficit was perceptual, not motor.

mypsychkit

Animation 13.6
Speech Perception

Key Concepts

SPEECH PRODUCTION AND COMPREHENSION: BRAIN MECHANISMS

1. Broca's area, located in the left frontal lobe, is important in articulating words and producing and understanding grammatical constructions.
2. Wernicke's area, located in the auditory association cortex of the left hemisphere, is important in recognizing the sounds of words.
3. Comprehension of speech involves connections between Wernicke's area and memories that define words. These memories are located in the sensory association cortex, and the connections are made via the posterior language area.
4. Conduction aphasia occurs when Wernicke's area and Broca's area can no longer communicate directly.
5. Prosody—the use of rhythm and emphasis in speech—involves the right hemisphere. Stuttering may be caused by deficient auditory monitoring of one's own speech.

DISORDERS OF READING AND WRITING

6. Brain damage can produce a variety of reading and writing disorders. Study of these disorders is helping investigators discover the brain functions necessary for these behaviors.
7. Reading takes two forms: whole-word and phonetic. Writing can be based on memories of the sounds the words make or their visual shape.
8. Developmental dyslexia may be a genetic disorder that results in abnormal development of the brain regions involved in language abilities.

Suggested Readings

Davis, G. A. *Aphasiology: Disorders and Clinical Practice*. Boston: Allyn and Bacon, 2000.

Démonet, J.-F., Taylor, M. J., and Chaix, Y. Developmental dyslexia. *Lancet*, 2004, *363*, 1451–1460.

Démonet, J.-F., Thierry, G., and Cardebat, D. Renewal of the neurophysiology of language: Functional neuroimaging. *Physiological Review*, 2005, *85*, 49–95.

Obler, L. K., and Gjerlow, K. *Language and the Brain*. Cambridge, England: Cambridge University Press, 1999.

Sarno, M. T. *Acquired Aphasia*, 3rd ed. New York: Academic Press, 1998.

Shaywitz, S. E., and Shaywitz, B. A. Dyslexia (specific reading disability). *Biological Psychiatry*, 2005, *57*, 1301–1309.

Additional Resources

Visit www.mypsychkit.com for additional review and practice of the material covered in this chapter. Within MyPsychKit, you can take practice tests and receive a customized study plan to help you review. Dozens of animations, tutorials, and Web links are also available. You can even review using the interactive electronic version of this textbook. You will need to register for MyPsychKit. See www.mypsychkit.com for complete details.

chapter 14

Neurological Disorders

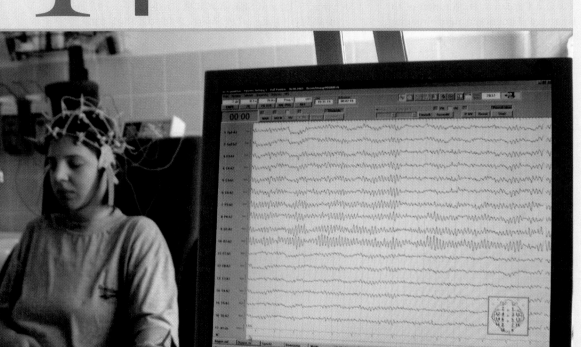

LEARNING OBJECTIVES

1. Discuss the causes, symptoms, and treatment of brain tumors, seizure disorders, and cerebrovascular accidents.

2. Discuss developmental disorders resulting from toxic chemicals, inherited metabolic disorders, and Down syndrome.

3. Discuss research on the role of misfolded prion proteins in the transmissible spongiform encephalopathies.

4. Discuss the causes, symptoms, and available treatments for the degeneration of the basal ganglia that occurs in Parkinson's disease and Huntington's disease.

5. Discuss the causes, symptoms, and potential treatments for the brain degeneration caused by Alzheimer's disease, amyotrophic lateral sclerosis, and multiple sclerosis.

6. Discuss the causes, symptoms, and available treatments for encephalitis, dementia caused by the AIDS virus, and meningitis.

Mrs. R., a divorced, 50-year-old elementary school teacher, was sitting in her car, waiting for a traffic light to change. Suddenly, her right foot began to shake. Afraid that she would inadvertently press the accelerator and lurch forward into the intersection, she quickly grabbed the shift lever and switched the transmission into neutral. Now her lower leg was shaking, then her upper leg as well. With horrified fascination she felt her body, then her arm, begin to shake in rhythm with her leg. The shaking slowed and finally stopped. By this time the light had changed to green, and the cars behind her began honking at her. She missed that green light, but by the time the light changed again, she had recovered enough to put the car in gear and drive home.

Mrs. R. was frightened by her experience and tried in vain to think what she might have done to cause it. The next evening, some close friends visited her apartment for dinner. She found it hard to concentrate on their conversation and thought of telling them about her spell, but she finally decided not to bring up the matter. After dinner, while she was clearing the dishes off the table, her right foot began shaking again. This time she was standing up, and the contractions—much more violent than before—caused her to fall. Her friends, seated in the living room, heard the noise and came running to see what had happened. They saw Mrs. R. lying on the floor, her legs and arms held out stiffly before her, vibrating uncontrollably. Her head was thrown back and she seemed not to hear their anxious questions. The convulsion soon ceased; less than a minute later, Mrs. R. regained consciousness but seemed dazed and confused.

Mrs. R. was brought by ambulance to a hospital. After learning about her first spell and hearing her friends describe the convulsion, the emergency room physician immediately called a neurologist, who ordered a CT scan. The scan showed a small, circular white spot right where the neurologist expected it, between the frontal lobes, above the corpus callosum. Two days later, a neurosurgeon removed a small benign tumor, and Mrs. R. made an uneventful recovery.

When my colleagues and I met Mrs. R., we saw a pleasant, intelligent woman, much relieved to know that her type of brain tumor rarely produces brain damage if it is removed in time. Indeed, although we tested her carefully, we found no signs of intellectual impairment.

Although the brain is the most protected organ, many pathological processes can damage it or disrupt its functioning. Because much of what we have learned about the functions of the human brain has been gained by studying people with brain damage, you have already encountered many neurological disorders in this book: movement disorders, such as Parkinson's disease; perceptual disorders, such as visual agnosia and blindness caused by damage to the visual system; language disorders such as aphasia, alexia, and agraphia; and memory disorders, such as Korsakoff's syndrome. This chapter describes the major categories of the neuropathological conditions that the brain can sustain—tumors, seizure disorders, cerebrovascular accidents, disorders of development, degenerative disorders, and disorders caused by infectious diseases—and discusses the behavioral effects of these conditions and their treatments.

Tumors

A **tumor** is a mass of cells whose growth is uncontrolled and that serves no useful function. Some tumors are **malignant**, or cancerous, and others are **benign** ("harmless"). The major distinction between malignancy and benignancy is whether the tumor is *encapsulated*: whether there is a distinct border between the mass of tumor cells and the surrounding tissue. If there is such a border, the tumor is benign; the surgeon can cut it out, and it will not regrow. However, if the tumor grows by *infiltrating* the surrounding tissue, there will be no clear-cut border between the tumor and normal tissue. If the surgeon removes the tumor, some cells may be missed, and these cells will produce a new tumor. In addition, malignant tumors often give rise to **metastases**. A metastasizing tumor will shed cells, which then travel

tumor A mass of cells whose growth is uncontrolled and that serves no useful function.

malignant tumor A cancerous (literally, "harm-producing") tumor; lacks a distinct border and may metastasize.

benign tumor (*bee nine*) A noncancerous (literally, "harmless") tumor; has a distinct border and cannot metastasize.

metastasis (*meh tass ta sis*) The process by which cells break off of a tumor, travel through the vascular system, and grow elsewhere in the body.

FIGURE 14.1

Meningioma. This photograph of a slice of a human brain, shows how a large nonmalignant tumor (a meningioma) has displaced the right side of the brain toward the left. (The dashed line indicates the location of the midline.) The right lateral ventricle is almost completely occluded.

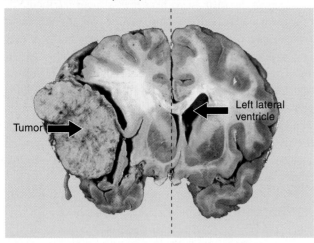

Courtesy of A. D'Agostino, Good Samaritan Hospital, Portland, Oregon.

FIGURE 14.2

Glioma. This photograph of a slice of a human brain, shows a large glioma located in the basal ganglia, which has invaded both the left and right lateral ventricles.

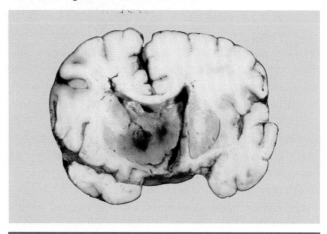

Courtesy of A. D'Agostino, Good Samaritan Hospital, Portland, Oregon.

through the bloodstream, lodge in capillaries, and serve as seeds for the growth of new tumors in different locations in the body.

Tumors damage brain tissue by two means: compression and infiltration. Obviously, *any* tumor growing in the brain, malignant or benign, can produce neurological symptoms and threaten the patient's life. Even a benign tumor occupies space and thus pushes against the brain. The compression can directly destroy brain tissue, or it can do so indirectly by blocking the flow of cerebrospinal fluid and causing hydrocephalus. Even worse are malignant tumors, which cause both compression and infiltration. As a malignant tumor grows, it invades the surrounding region and destroys cells in its path. Figure 14.1 illustrates the compressive effect of a large nonmalignant tumor. As you can see, the tumor has displaced the lateral and third ventricles. (See *Figure 14.1*.)

TABLE 14.1 Types of Brain Tumors

Gliomas

    Glioblastoma multiformae (poorly differentiated glial cells)

    Astrocytoma (astrocytes)

    Ependymoma (ependymal cells that line ventricles)

    Medulloblastoma (cells in roof of fourth ventricle)

    Oligodendrocytoma (oligodendrocytes)

Meningioma (cells of the meninges)

Pituitary adenoma (hormone-secreting cells of the pituitary gland)

Neurinoma (Schwann cells or cells of connective tissue covering cranial nerves)

Metastatic carcinoma (depends on nature of primary tumor)

Angioma (cells of blood vessels)

Pinealoma (cells of pineal gland)

Tumors do not arise from neurons, because mature neurons are not capable of dividing. Instead, they arise from other cells found in the brain or from metastases originating elsewhere in the body. The most common types are listed in Table 14.1. (See *Table 14.1*.) The most serious types of tumors are metastases and the **gliomas** (derived from various types of glial cells), which are usually very malignant and fast growing. Figures 14.2 shows a glioma located in the basal ganglia. (See *Figure 14.2*.) Some tumors are sensitive to radiation and can be destroyed by a beam of radiation focused on them. Usually, a neurosurgeon first removes as much of the tumor as possible, and then the remaining cells are targeted by the radiation.

The chapter prologue described a woman whose sudden onset of seizures suggested the presence of a tumor near the top of the primary motor cortex. Indeed, she had a **meningioma**, an encapsulated, benign tumor consisting of cells that constitute the dura mater or arachnoid membrane. Such tumors tend to originate in the part of the dura mater that is found between the two cerebral hemispheres or along the tentorium, the sheet of dura mater that lies between the occipital lobes and the cerebellum. (See *Figure 14.3*.)

Seizure Disorders

Because of negative connotations that were acquired in the past, some physicians prefer not to use the term *epilepsy*. Instead, they use the phrase **seizure disorder** to refer to a condition that has many causes. Seizure disorders constitute the second most important category of neurological disorders, following stroke. At present, approximately 2.5 million people in the United States have a seizure disorder. A *seizure* is a period of sudden, excessive activity of cerebral neurons. Sometimes, if neurons that make up the motor system are involved, a seizure can cause a **convulsion**, which is wild, uncontrollable activity of the muscles. However, not all seizures cause convulsions; in fact, most do not. In ancient religious traditions, seizures were considered to be God's punishment or the work of demons. However, as early as the 5th century B.C., Hippocrates noted that head injuries to soldiers and gladiators sometimes led to seizures like the ones he saw in his patients, which suggested that seizures had a physical cause (Hoppe, 2006).

Table 14.2 presents a summary of the most important categories of seizure disorders. Two distinctions are important: *partial* versus *generalized* seizures and *simple* versus *complex* ones. **Partial seizures** have a definite *focus*, or source of irritation: typically, a scarred region caused by an old injury, or a developmental abnormality such as a malformed blood vessel. The neurons that become involved in the seizure are restricted to a small part of the brain. **Generalized seizures** are widespread, involving most of the brain. In many cases they grow from a focus, but in some cases their origin is not discovered. Simple and complex seizures are two categories of partial seizures. **Simple partial seizures** often cause *changes* in consciousness but do not cause *loss* of consciousness. In contrast, because of their particular location and severity, **complex partial seizures** lead to loss of consciousness. (See *Table 14.2*.)

The most severe form of seizure is a **tonic-clonic** seizure (sometimes called a *grand mal* seizure). This seizure is generalized, and because it includes the motor systems of the brain, it is accompanied by convulsions. Often, before having a tonic-clonic seizure, a person has warning symptoms, such as changes in mood or perhaps a few sudden jerks of muscular activity upon awakening. (Almost everyone sometimes experiences these jolts while falling asleep.) A few seconds before the seizure occurs, the person often experiences an **aura**, which is presumably caused by excitation of neurons surrounding a seizure focus. This excitation has effects similar to those that would be produced by electrical stimulation of the region. Obviously, the nature of an aura varies according to the location of the focus. For example, because structures in the temporal lobe are involved in the control of emotional

FIGURE 14.3

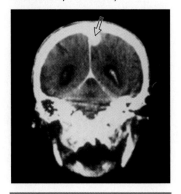

Meningioma. The CT scan of a brain shows the presence of a meningioma (round white spot indicated by the arrow).

Courtesy of J. McA. Jones, Good Samaritan Hospital, Portland, Oregon.

glioma (*glee oh mah*) A cancerous brain tumor composed of one of several types of glial cells.

meningioma (*men in jee oh ma*) A benign brain tumor composed of the cells that constitute the meninges.

seizure disorder The preferred term for epilepsy.

convulsion A violent sequence of uncontrollable muscular movements caused by a seizure.

partial seizure A seizure that begins at a focus and remains localized, not generalizing to the rest of the brain.

generalized seizure A seizure that involves most of the brain, as contrasted with a partial seizure, which remains localized.

simple partial seizure A partial seizure, starting from a focus and remaining localized, that does not produce loss of consciousness.

complex partial seizure A partial seizure, starting from a focus and remaining localized, that produces loss of consciousness.

tonic-clonic seizure A generalized, tonic-clonic seizure, which results in a convulsion.

aura A sensation that precedes a seizure; its exact nature depends on the location of the seizure focus.

TABLE 14.2 The Classification of Seizure Disorders

I. Generalized seizures (with no apparent local onset)
  A. Tonic-clonic (grand mal)
  B. Absence (petit mal)
  C. Atonic (loss of muscle tone, temporary paralysis)

II. Partial seizures (starting from a focus)
  A. Simple (no major change in consciousness)
    1. Localized motor seizure
    2. Motor seizure, with progression of movements as seizure spreads along the primary motor cortex
    3. Sensory (somatosensory, visual, auditory, olfactory, vestibular)
    4. Psychic (forced thinking, fear, anger, etc.)
    5. Autonomic (sweating, salivating, etc.)
  B. Complex (with altered consciousness)
    Includes 1–5, as above

III. Partial seizures (simple or complex) evolving to generalized cortical seizure: Starts as IIA or IIB, then becomes a grand mal seizure

behaviors, seizures that originate from a focus located there often begin with feelings of fear and dread or, occasionally, euphoria.

The beginning of a tonic-clonic seizure is called the **tonic phase**. All the patient's muscles contract forcefully. The arms are rigidly outstretched, and the person may make an involuntary cry as the tense muscles force air out of the lungs. (At this point the patient is completely unconscious.) The patient holds a rigid posture for about 15 seconds, and then the **clonic phase** begins. (*Clonic* means "agitated.") The muscles begin trembling, then start jerking convulsively—quickly at first, then more and more slowly. Meanwhile, the eyes roll, the patient's face is contorted with violent grimaces, and the tongue may be bitten. Intense activity of the autonomic nervous system manifests itself in sweating and salivation. After about 30 seconds, the patient's muscles relax; only then does breathing begin again. The patient falls into a stuporous, unresponsive sleep, which lasts for about 15 minutes. After that the patient may awaken briefly but usually falls back into an exhausted sleep that may last for a few hours.

Other types of seizures are far less dramatic. Partial seizures involve relatively small portions of the brain. The symptoms can include sensory changes, motor activity, or both. For example, a simple partial seizure that begins in or near the motor cortex can involve jerking movements that begin in one place and spread throughout the body as the excitation spreads along the precentral gyrus. In the chapter prologue I described such a progression, caused by a seizure triggered by a meningioma. The tumor was pressing against the "foot" region of the left primary motor cortex. When the seizure began, it involved the foot; as it spread, it began involving the other parts of the body. (See *Figure 14.4*.) Mrs. R.'s first spell was a simple partial seizure, but her second one—much more severe—would be classed as a complex partial seizure, because she lost consciousness. A seizure beginning in the occipital lobe may produce visual symptoms such as spots of color, flashes of light, or temporary blindness; one originating in the parietal lobe can evoke somatosensations, such as feelings of pins and needles or heat and cold. Seizures in the temporal lobes may cause hallucinations that include old memories; presumably, neural

tonic phase The first phase of a tonic-clonic seizure, in which all of the patient's skeletal muscles are contracted.

clonic phase The phase of a tonic-clonic seizure in which the patient shows rhythmic jerking movements.

circuits involved in these memories are activated by the spreading excitation. Depending on the location and extent of the seizure, the patient may or may not lose consciousness.

Children are especially susceptible to seizure disorders. Many of them do not have tonic-clonic episodes but instead have very brief seizures that are referred to as spells of **absence**. During an absence seizure, which is a *generalized* seizure disorder, they stop what they are doing and stare off into the distance for a few seconds, often blinking their eyes repeatedly. (These spells are also sometimes referred to as *petit mal* seizures.) During this time they are unresponsive, and they usually do not notice their attacks. Because absence seizures can occur up to several hundred times each day, they can disrupt a child's performance in school. Unfortunately, many of these children are considered to be inattentive and unmotivated unless the disorder is diagnosed.

Seizures can have serious consequences: They can cause brain damage. Approximately 50 percent of patients with seizure disorders show evidence of damage to the hippocampus. The amount of damage is correlated with the number and severity of seizures the patient has had. Significant hippocampal damage can be caused by a single episode of **status epilepticus**, a condition in which the patient undergoes a series of seizures without regaining consciousness. The damage appears to be caused by an excessive release of glutamate during the seizure (Thompson et al., 1996).

Seizures have many causes. The most common cause is scarring, which may be produced by an injury, a stroke, a developmental abnormality in the brain, or the irritating effect of a growing tumor. For injuries the development of seizures can take a considerable amount of time. Often, a person who receives a head injury from an automobile accident will not start having seizures until several months later.

Various drugs and infections that cause a high fever can also produce seizures. High fevers are most common in children, and approximately 3 percent of children under the age of 5 years sustain seizures associated with fevers (Berkovic et al., 2006). In addition, seizures are commonly seen in alcohol or barbiturate addicts who suddenly stop taking the drug; the sudden release from the inhibiting effects of the alcohol or barbiturate leaves the brain in a hyperexcitable condition. In fact, this condition is a medical emergency because it can be fatal.

Genetic factors contribute to the incidence of seizure disorders (Berkovic et al., 2006). Nearly all of the genes that have been identified as playing a role in seizure disorders control the production of ion channels, which is not surprising, considering the fact that ion channels control the excitability of the neural membrane, and are responsible for the propagation of action potentials. However, most seizure disorders are caused by nongenetic factors. In the past, many cases were considered to be *idiopathic* (of unknown causes, or literally "one's own suffering"). However, the development of MRIs with more and more resolution and sensitivity has meant that small brain abnormalities responsible for triggering seizures are more likely to be seen.

Seizure disorders are treated with anticonvulsant drugs, many of which work by increasing the effectiveness of inhibitory synapses. Most disorders respond well enough that the patient can lead a normal life. In a few instances drugs provide little or no help. Sometimes, seizure foci remain so irritable that despite drug treatment, brain surgery is required. The surgeon removes the region of the brain

Primary Motor Cortex and Seizures.   Mrs. R.'s seizure began in the foot region of the primary motor cortex, and as the seizure spread, more and more parts of her body became involved.

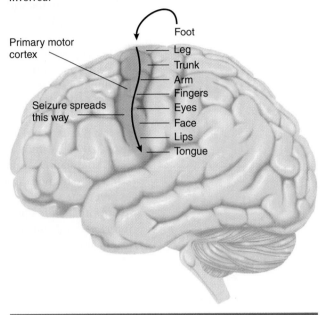

absence   A type of seizure disorder often seen in children; characterized by periods of inattention, which are not subsequently remembered; also called *petit mal* seizure.

status epilepticus   A condition in which a patient undergoes a series of seizures without regaining consciousness.

surrounding the focus (usually located in the medial temporal lobe). Most patients recover well, with their seizures eliminated or greatly reduced in frequency. Mrs. R.'s treatment, described in the chapter prologue was a different matter; in her case the removal of a meningioma eliminated the source of the irritation and ended her seizures. No healthy brain tissue was removed.

Many patients with seizure disorders obtain relief from seizures by following a *ketogenic diet* (Sinha and Kossoff, 2005). Most of the calories on such a diet come from fats, with a moderate amount from proteins and a very low amount from carbohydrates. A person on such a regime must adhere strictly to the diet, because a single meal rich in carbohydrates increases the risk of having a seizure. This diet leads to the production of *ketones*—compounds that are produced by the liver through the breakdown of fats when the blood level of glucose is low. In such a condition, the brain is nourished primarily by ketones. The benefits of a ketogenic diet have been known for at least 80 years, but only recently have researchers begun to investigate how it works (Rho, 2008). A study with rats by Garriga-Canut et al. (2006) administered daily electrical stimulation of the perforant path, the major fiber bundle that brings information to the hippocampus. This treatment eventually establishes seizures, presumably in much the same way as head injuries often establish seizure disorders several weeks or months later. The investigators found that administration of 2-DG, a drug that interferes with glucose metabolism, reduced the occurrence of seizures. They also found that the 2-DG caused changes in the levels of several neurochemicals, which may provide clues to aid in the search for more effective anti-seizure drugs.

Cerebrovascular Accidents

You have already learned about the *effects* of cerebrovascular accidents, or *strokes*, in earlier chapters. For example, we saw that strokes can produce impairments in perception, emotional recognition and expression, memory, and language. This section will describe only their causes and treatments.

The incidence of strokes in the United States is approximately 600,000 per year. The likelihood of having a stroke is related to age; the probability doubles each decade after 45 years of age and reaches 1–2 percent per year by age 75 (Wolfe, Cobb and D'Agostino, 1992). The two major types of strokes are *hemorrhagic* and *obstructive*. **Hemorrhagic strokes** are caused by bleeding within the brain, usually from a malformed blood vessel or from one weakened by high blood pressure. The blood that seeps out of the defective blood vessel accumulates within the brain, putting pressure on the surrounding brain tissue and damaging it. **Obstructive strokes**—those that plug up a blood vessel and prevent the flow of blood—can be caused by thrombi or emboli. (Loss of blood flow to a region is called **ischemia**, from the Greek *ischein*, "to hold back," and *haima*, "blood.") A **thrombus** is a blood clot that forms in blood vessels, especially in places where their walls are already damaged. Sometimes, thrombi become so large that blood cannot flow through the vessel, causing a stroke. People who are susceptible to the formation of thrombi are often advised to take a drug such as aspirin, which helps to prevent clot formation. An **embolus** is a piece of material that forms in one part of the vascular system, breaks off, and is carried through the bloodstream until it reaches an artery too small to pass through. It lodges there, damming the flow of blood through the rest of the vascular tree (the "branches" and "twigs" arising from the artery). Emboli can consist of a variety of materials, including bacterial debris from an infection in the lining of the heart or pieces broken off from a blood clot. As we will see in a later section, emboli can introduce a bacterial infection into the brain. (See *Figure 14.5*.)

Strokes produce permanent brain damage, but depending on the size of the affected blood vessel, the amount of damage can vary from negligible to massive. If

hemorrhagic stroke A cerebrovascular accident caused by the rupture of a cerebral blood vessel.

obstructive stroke A cerebrovascular accident caused by occlusion of a blood vessel.

ischemia (*is kee mee uh*) The interruption of the blood supply to a region of the body.

thrombus A blood clot that forms within a blood vessel, which may occlude it.

embolus (*emm bo lus*) A piece of matter (such as a blood clot, fat, or bacterial debris) that dislodges from its site of origin and occludes an artery; in the brain an embolus can lead to a stroke.

FIGURE 14.5

Strokes.   This figure shows: (a) formation of thrombi and emboli; (b) an intracerebral hemorrhage.

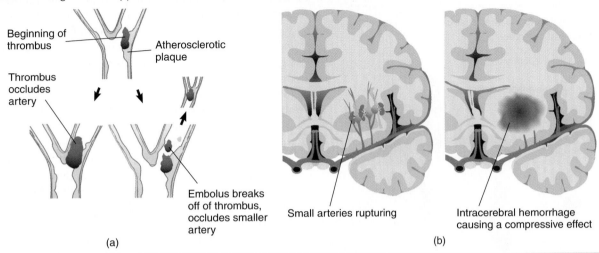

Beginning of thrombus

Atherosclerotic plaque

Thrombus occludes artery

Embolus breaks off of thrombus, occludes smaller artery

Small arteries rupturing

Intracerebral hemorrhage causing a compressive effect

(a)

(b)

a hemorrhagic stroke is caused by high blood pressure, medication is given to reduce blood pressure. If a stroke is caused by weak and malformed blood vessels, brain surgery may be used to seal off the faulty vessels to prevent another hemorrhage. If a thrombus was responsible for the stroke, anticoagulant drugs will be given to make the blood less likely to clot, reducing the likelihood of another stroke. If an embolus broke away from a bacterial infection, antibiotics will be given to suppress the infection.

What, exactly, causes the death of neurons when the blood supply to a region of the brain is interrupted? We might expect that the neurons will simply starve to death because they lose their supply of glucose and of oxygen to metabolize it. However, research indicates that the immediate cause of neuron death is the presence of excessive amounts of glutamate. In other words, the damage produced by loss of blood flow to a region of the brain is actually an excitotoxic lesion, just like one produced in a laboratory animal by the injection of a chemical such as kainic acid. (See Koroshetz and Moskowitz, 1996, for a review.)

Researchers have sought ways to minimize the amount of brain damage caused by strokes. One approach has been to administer drugs that dissolve blood clots in an attempt to reestablish circulation to an ischemic brain region. This approach has met with some success. Administration of a clot-dissolving drug called *tPA* (tissue plasminogen activator) after the onset of a stroke has clear benefits if it is given within 3 hours (NINDS, 1995). However, more recent research indicates that although tPA helps to dissolve blood clots and restore cerebral circulation, it also has toxic effects in the central nervous system. tPA is neurotoxic if it is able to cross the blood–brain barrier and reach the interstitial fluid. Evidence suggests that in cases of severe stroke, in which the blood–brain barrier is damaged, tPA increases excitotoxicity, further damages the blood–brain barrier, and may even cause cerebral hemorrhage (Benchenane et al., 2004; Klaur et al., 2004).

As you undoubtedly know, vampire bats live on the blood of other warm-blooded animals. They make a small incision in a sleeping animal's skin with their sharp teeth and lap up the blood with their tongues. One compound in their saliva acts as a local

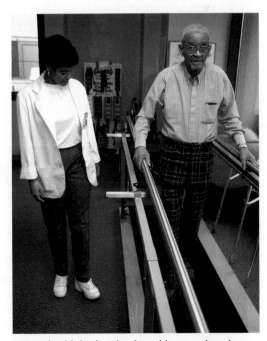

Research with both animals and humans has shown that exercise and sensory stimulation facilitate recovery of functions lost as a result of brain damage.

FIGURE 14.6

Desmoteplase in Treatment of Strokes. The graph shows the effects of desmoteplase and a placebo on restoration of cerebral blood flow to the affected area (*reperfusion*) and favorable clinical outcome.

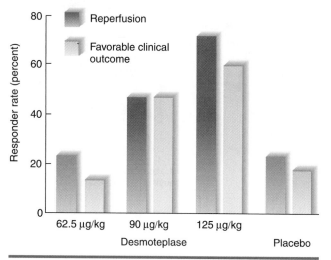

Adapted from Hacke, W., Albers, G., Al-Rawi, Y., et al. *Stroke*, 2005, *36*, 66–73.

FIGURE 14.7

Atherosclerotic Plaque. An angiogram shows an obstruction in the internal carotid artery caused by an atherosclerotic plaque.

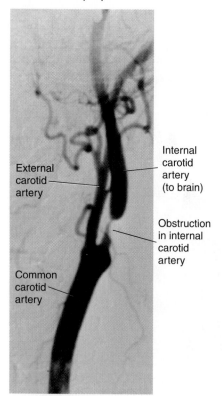

From Stapf, C., and Mohr, J. P. *Annual Review of Medicine*, 2002, *53*, 453–475. Reprinted with permission.

anesthetic and keeps the animal from awakening. Another compound (and this is the one we are interested in) acts as an anticoagulant, preventing the blood from clotting. The name of this enzyme is *Desmodus rotundus plasminogen activator* (DSPA), otherwise known as *desmoteplase.* (*Desmodus rotundus* is the Latin name for the vampire bat.) Research with laboratory animals indicate that unlike tPA, desmoteplase causes no excitotoxic injury when injected directly into the brain (Reddrop et al., 2005). A phase II placebo-controlled, double-blind clinical trial of desmoteplase (Hacke et al., 2005) found that desmoteplase restored blood flow and reduced clinical symptoms in a majority of patients if given up to 9 hours after the occurrence of a stroke. (See *Figure 14.6.*)

How can strokes be prevented? Risk factors that can be reduced by medication or changes in lifestyle include high blood pressure, cigarette smoking, diabetes, and high blood levels of cholesterol. The actions we can take to reduce these risk factors are well known, so I need not describe them here. *Atherosclerosis*, a process in which the linings of arteries develop a layer of plaque, deposits of cholesterol, fats, calcium, and cellular waste products, is a precursor to heart attacks (myocardial infarction) and obstructive stroke, caused by clots that form around atherosclerotic plaques in cerebral and cardiac blood vessels. Atherosclerotic plaques often form in the internal carotid artery—the artery that supplies most of the blood flow to the cerebral hemispheres. These plaques can cause severe narrowing of the interior of the artery, greatly increasing the risk of a massive stroke. This narrowing can be visualized in an angiogram, produced by injecting a radiopaque dye into the blood and examining the artery with a computerized X-ray machine. (See *Figure 14.7.*) If the narrowing is severe, a *carotid endarterectomy* can be performed. The surgeon makes an incision in the neck that exposes the carotid artery, inserts a shunt in the artery, cuts the artery open, removes the plaque, and sews the artery back again (and the neck too, of course). Endarterectomy has been shown to reduce the risk of stroke by 50 percent in people under 75 years of age.

An even more effective—and possibly safer—surgical treatment involves the placement of a *stent* in a seriously narrowed carotid artery (Yadav et al., 2004). An arterial stent is an implantable device made of a metal mesh that is used to expand and hold open a partially occluded artery. The stent consists of a mesh tube made of springy metal collapsed inside a *catheter*—a flexible plastic tube. The surgeon cuts open a large artery in the groin and passes the catheter through large arteries up to the neck until the stent reaches the occlusion in the carotid artery. The end of the catheter holds a filter shaped like a collapsed parachute. When the catheter is retracted, the stent expands, opening the narrowed artery. The filter also springs open, catching any debris that is dislodged from the plaque, which would otherwise travel through the bloodstream and get trapped in a small artery, causing an infarct. The filter is then withdrawn, and the cannula is removed, leaving the expanded stent in place to keep the artery open. (See *Figure 14.8.*)

Depending on the location of the brain damage, people who have strokes will receive physical therapy, and perhaps speech therapy, to help them recover from their disability. Several studies have shown that exercise and sensory stimulation can facilitate recovery from the effects of brain damage (Cotman, Berchtold, and Christie, 2007). For example, Taub et al. (2006) studied patients with strokes that impaired their ability to use one arm

FIGURE 14.8

An Arterial Stent. The figure shows the placement of a stent in an obstructed internal carotid artery.

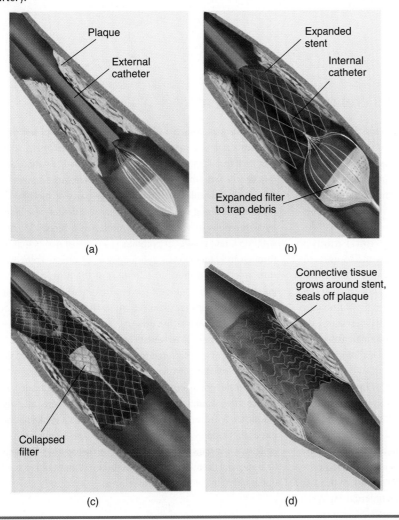

(a)

Plaque

External catheter

(b)

Expanded stent

Internal catheter

Expanded filter to trap debris

(c)

Collapsed filter

(d)

Connective tissue grows around stent, seals off plaque

and hand. They put the *unaffected* arm in a sling for 14 days and gave the patients training sessions during which the patients were forced to use the impaired arm. A placebo group received cognitive, relaxation, and physical fitness exercises for the same amount of time. This procedure (which is called *constraint-induced movement therapy*) produced long-term improvement in the patients' ability to use the affected arm, apparently by changing connections of the primary motor cortex (Liepert et al., 2000). (See *Figure 14.9.*)

In some cases of brain damage or spinal cord damage, patients are unable to perform useful limb movements, even after intensive therapy. In such cases, investigators have attempted to devise brain-computer interfaces that permit the patient to control electronic and mechanical devices to perform useful actions. Developers of such interfaces have implanted arrays of microelectrodes directly into the patient's motor cortex and have applied surface electrodes to measure changes in EEG activity transmitted through the skull and scalp.

FIGURE 14.9

Constraint-Induced Movement Therapy The graph shows the effects of CI therapy and placebo therapy on the use of a limb whose movement was impaired by a stroke.

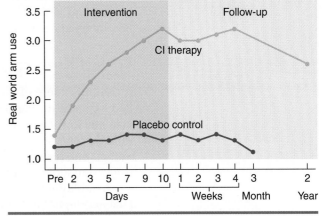

Adapted from Taub, E., Uswatte, F., King, D. K., et al. *Stroke*, 2006, *37*, 1045–1049.

These devices, while still experimental, permit patients to move prosthetic hands, perform actions with multi-jointed robotic arms, and move the cursor of a computer display and operate the computer (Wolpaw and McFarland, 2004; Hochberg et al., 2006).

InterimSummary

Tumors, Seizure Disorders, and Cerebrovascular Accidents

Neurological disorders have many causes. Brain tumors are caused by the uncontrolled growth of various types of cells *other than neurons*. They can be benign or malignant. Benign tumors are encapsulated and thus have a distinct border; when one is surgically removed, the surgeon has a good chance of getting all of it. Tumors produce brain damage by compression and, in the case of malignant tumors, infiltration.

Seizures are periodic episodes of abnormal electrical activity of the brain. Partial seizures are localized, beginning with a focus—usually, some scar tissue caused by previous damage or a tumor. When they begin, they often produce an aura, consisting of particular sensations or changes in mood. Simple partial seizures do not produce profound changes in consciousness; complex partial seizures do. Generalized seizures may or may not originate at a single focus, but they involve most of the brain. Some seizures involve motor activity; the most serious are the convulsions that accompany tonic-clonic generalized seizures. The convulsions are caused by involvement of the brain's motor systems; the patient first shows a tonic phase, consisting of a few seconds of rigidity, and then a clonic phase, consisting of rhythmic jerking. Absence seizures, also called petit mal seizures, are common in children. These generalized seizures are characterized by periods of inattention and temporary loss of awareness. Seizures are treated with anticonvulsant drugs and, in the case of intractable seizure disorders caused by an abnormal focus, by

seizure surgery, which usually involves the medial temporal lobe. (Seizure surgery is described in the chapter epilogue.) A ketogenic diet high in fat, moderate in protein, and low in carbohydrate, also relieves the symptoms of seizure disorders in some patients.

Cerebrovascular accidents damage parts of the brain through rupture of a blood vessel or occlusion (obstruction) of a blood vessel by a thrombus or embolus. A thrombus is a blood clot that forms within a blood vessel. An embolus is a piece of debris that is carried through the bloodstream and lodges in an artery. Emboli can arise from infections within the chambers of the heart or can consist of pieces of thrombi. The best current treatment for stroke is administration of a drug that dissolves clots. Tissue plasminogen activator (tPA) must be given within 3 hours of the onset of the stroke and in some cases appears to cause brain damage on its own. Desmoteplase, an enzyme secreted in the saliva of vampire bats, is effective up to 9 hours after a stroke and does not appear to cause brain damage. Carotid endarterectomy or insertion of a carotid stent can reduce the likelihood of a stroke in people with atherosclerotic plaque that obstruct the carotid arteries. After a stroke has occurred, physical therapy can facilitate recovery and minimize a patient's deficits. Constraint-induced movement therapy has been shown to be especially useful in restoring useful movement of limbs following unilateral damage to the motor cortex.

Disorders of Development

As you will see in this section, brain development can be affected adversely by the presence of toxic chemicals during pregnancy and by genetic abnormalities, both hereditary and nonhereditary. In some instances the result is mental retardation.

Toxic Chemicals

A common cause of mental retardation is the presence of toxins that impair fetal development during pregnancy. For example, if a woman contracts rubella (German measles) early in pregnancy, the toxic chemicals released by the virus interfere with the chemical signals that control normal development of the brain. Most women who receive good health care will be immunized for rubella to prevent them from contracting it during pregnancy.

In addition to the toxins produced by viruses, various drugs can adversely affect fetal development. For example, mental retardation can be caused by the ingestion of alcohol during pregnancy—especially during the third to fourth week (Sulik,

FIGURE 14.10

Facial Malformations in Fetal Alcohol Syndrome.   The photographs show a child with fetal alcohol syndrome, along with magnified views of mouse fetuses: (a) fetus whose mother received alcohol during pregnancy and (b) normal mouse fetus.

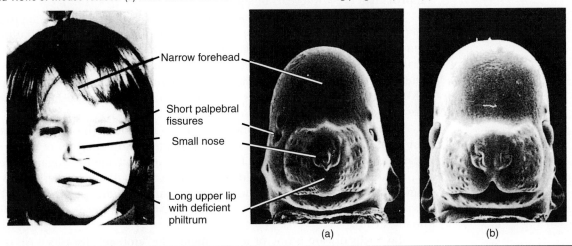

Narrow forehead

Short palpebral fissures

Small nose

Long upper lip with deficient philtrum

(a)   (b)

Photographs courtesy of Katherine K. Sulik.

2005). Babies born to alcoholic women are typically smaller than average and develop more slowly. Many of them exhibit **fetal alcohol syndrome**, which is characterized by abnormal facial development and deficient brain development. Figure 14.10 shows photographs of the faces of a child with fetal alcohol syndrome, of a mouse fetus whose mother was fed alcohol during pregnancy, and of a normal mouse fetus. As you can see, alcohol produces similar abnormalities in the offspring of both species. The facial abnormalities are relatively unimportant, of course. Much more serious are the abnormalities in the development of the brain. (See *Figure 14.10.*)

A woman need not be an alcoholic to impair the development of her offspring; some investigators believe that fetal alcohol syndrome can be caused by a single alcoholic binge during a critical period of fetal development. Now that we recognize the dangers of this syndrome, pregnant women are advised to abstain from alcohol (and from other drugs not specifically prescribed by their physicians) while their bodies are engaged in the task of sustaining the development of another human being.

Inherited Metabolic Disorders

Several inherited "errors of metabolism" can cause brain damage or impair brain development. Normal functioning of cells requires intricate interactions among countless biochemical systems. As you know, these systems depend on enzymes, which are responsible for constructing or breaking down particular chemical compounds. Enzymes are proteins and therefore are produced by mechanisms involving the chromosomes, which contain the recipes for their synthesis. "Errors of metabolism" are genetic abnormalities in which the recipe for a particular enzyme is in error, so the enzyme cannot be synthesized. If the enzyme is a critical one, the results can be very serious.

There are at least a hundred different inherited metabolic disorders that can affect the development of the brain. The most common and best-known is called **phenylketonuria (PKU)**. This disease is caused by an inherited lack of an enzyme that converts phenylalanine (an amino acid) into tyrosine (another amino acid). Excessive amounts of phenylalanine in the blood interfere with the myelinization of neurons in the central nervous system. Much of the myelinization of the cerebral

fetal alcohol syndrome A birth defect caused by ingestion of alcohol by a pregnant woman; includes characteristic facial anomalies and faulty brain development.

phenylketonuria (PKU) (*fee nul kee ta new ree uh*) A hereditary disorder caused by the absence of an enzyme that converts the amino acid phenylalanine to tyrosine; the accumulation of phenylalanine causes brain damage unless a special diet is implemented soon after birth.

hemispheres takes place after birth. Thus, when an infant born with PKU receives foods containing phenylalanine, the amino acid accumulates, and the brain fails to develop normally. The result is severe mental retardation, with an average IQ of approximately 20 by 6 years of age.

Fortunately, PKU can be treated by putting the infant on a low-phenylalanine diet. The diet keeps the blood level of phenylalanine low, and myelinization of the central nervous system takes place normally. Diagnosing PKU immediately after birth is imperative so that the infant's brain is never exposed to high levels of phenylalanine. Consequently, many governments have passed laws that mandate a PKU test for all newborn babies. The test is inexpensive and accurate, and it has prevented many cases of mental retardation.

Some other inherited metabolic disorders cannot yet be treated successfully. For example, **Tay-Sachs disease**, which occurs mainly in children of Eastern European Jewish descent, causes the brain to swell and damage itself against the inside of the skull and against the folds of the dura mater than encase it. The neurological symptoms begin by 4 months of age and include an exaggerated startle response to sounds, listlessness, irritability, spasticity, seizures, dementia, and finally, death.

Tay-Sachs disease is one of several metabolic "storage" disorders. All cells contain sacs of material encased in membrane, called lysosomes ("dissolving bodies"). These sacs constitute the cell's rubbish-removal system; they contain enzymes that break down waste substances that cells produce in the course of their normal activities. The broken-down waste products are then recycled (used by the cells again) or excreted. Metabolic storage disorders are genetic errors of metabolism in which one or more vital enzymes are missing. Because of this, particular kinds of waste products cannot be destroyed by the lysosomes, so they accumulate. The lysosomes get larger and larger, the cells get larger and larger, and eventually the brain begins to swell and become damaged.

Researchers investigating hereditary errors of metabolism hope to prevent or treat these disorders in several ways. Some, like PKU, will be treated by avoiding a constituent of the diet that cannot be tolerated. Others will be treated by administering a substance that the body requires. Still others may be cured some day by the techniques of genetic engineering. Viruses infect cells by inserting their own genetic material into them and thus taking over the cells' genetic machinery, using it to reproduce themselves. Researchers hope to develop genetically modified viruses that will "infect" an infant's cells with genetic information that is needed to produce the enzymes that the cells lack, leaving the rest of the cells' functions intact.

Down Syndrome

Down syndrome is a congenital disorder that results in abnormal development of the brain, producing mental retardation in varying degrees. *Congenital* does not necessarily mean *hereditary*; it simply refers to a disorder that one is born with. Down syndrome is caused not by the inheritance of a faulty gene but by the possession of an extra twenty-first chromosome. The syndrome is closely associated with the mother's age; in most cases something goes wrong with some of her ova, resulting in the presence of two (rather than one) twenty-first chromosomes. When fertilization occurs, the addition of the father's twenty-first chromosome makes three, rather than two. The extra chromosome presumably causes biochemical changes that impair normal brain development. The development of *amniocentesis*, a procedure whereby some fluid is withdrawn from a pregnant woman's uterus through a hypodermic syringe, has allowed physicians to identify fetal cells with chromosomal abnormalities and thus to determine whether the fetus carries Down syndrome.

Tay-Sachs disease A heritable, fatal, metabolic storage disorder; lack of enzymes in lysosomes causes accumulation of waste produces and swelling of cells of the brain.

Down syndrome A disorder caused by the presence of an extra twenty-first chromosome, characterized by moderate to severe mental retardation and often by physical abnormalities.

Down syndrome, described in 1866 by John Langdon Down, occurs in approximately 1 out of 700 births. An experienced observer can recognize people with this disorder; they have round heads; thick, protruding tongues that tend to keep the mouth open much of the time; stubby hands; short stature; low-set ears; and somewhat slanting eyelids. They are slow to learn to talk, but most do talk by 5 years of age. The brain of a person with Down syndrome is approximately 10 percent lighter than that of a normal person, the convolutions (gyri and sulci) are simpler and smaller, the frontal lobes are small, and the superior temporal gyrus (the location of Wernicke's area) is thin. After age 30, the brain develops abnormal microscopic structures and begins to degenerate. Because this degeneration resembles that of Alzheimer's disease, it will be discussed in the next section.

A study by Fernandez et al. (2007) found that repeated low-dose injections of picrotoxin or pentylenetetrazole, drugs that serve as GABA antagonists, increased both long-term potentiation and performance on declarative learning tasks of a strain of mice that serve as a genetic model for Down syndrome. The drugs appeared to improve the animals' cognitive performance by suppressing excessive inhibition that is seen in their brains.

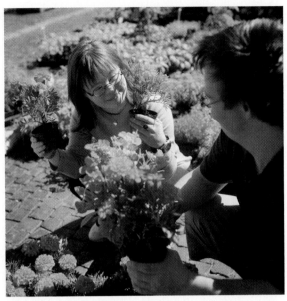

People with Down syndrome, caused by the presence of an extra twenty-first chromosome, are often only mildly retarded, and many of them can function well with only minimal supervision.

InterimSummary

Disorders of Development

Developmental disorders can result in brain damage serious enough to cause mental retardation. During pregnancy the fetus is especially sensitive to toxins, such as alcohol or chemicals produced by some viruses. Several inherited metabolic disorders can also impair brain development. For example, phenylketonuria is caused by the lack of an enzyme that converts phenylalanine into tyrosine. Brain damage can be averted by feeding the infant a diet low in phenylalanine, so early diagnosis is essential. Storage disorders, such as Tay-Sachs disease, are caused by the inability of cells to destroy waste products within the lysosomes, which causes the cells to swell and eventually die. So far, these disorders cannot be treated. Down syndrome is produced by the presence of an extra twenty-first chromosome. The brain development of people with Down syndrome is abnormal, and after age 30, their brains develop features similar to those of people with Alzheimer's disease. A study with an animal model of Down syndrome suggests that administration of GABA antagonists might be useful.

Degenerative Disorders

Many disease processes cause degeneration of the cells of the brain. Some of these conditions injure particular kinds of cells, a fact that provides the hope that research will uncover the causes of the damage and find a way to halt it and prevent it from occurring in other people.

Transmissible Spongiform Encephalopathies

The outbreak of bovine spongiform encephalopathy (BSE, or "mad cow disease") in Great Britain in the late 1980s and early 1990s brought a peculiar form of brain disease to public attention. BSE is a **transmissible spongiform encephalopathy (TSE)**— a fatal contagious brain disease ("encephalopathy") whose degenerative process

transmissible spongiform encephalopathy (TSE) A contagious brain disease whose degenerative process gives the brain a sponge-like appearance; caused by accumulation of misfolded prion protein.

FIGURE 14.11

Bovine Spongiform Encephalopathy and Creutzfeldt-Jakob Disease. The graph shows the number of cases of BSE in cattle and variant Creutzfeldt-Jakob disease in humans in Great Britain between 1988 and March 31, 2008.

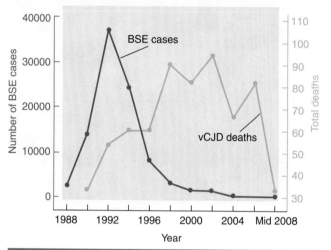

Data from OIE-World Organisation for Animal Health and the CJD Surveillance Unit.

gives the brain a sponge-like (or Swiss cheese-like) appearance. Besides BSE, these diseases include Creutzfeldt-Jakob disease, fatal familial insomnia, and kuru, which affect humans, and scrapie, which primarily affects sheep. Scrapie cannot be transmitted to humans, but BSE can, and it produces a variant of Creutzfeldt-Jakob disease. (See *Figure 14.11*.)

Unlike other transmissible diseases, TSEs are caused not by microorganisms, but by simple proteins, which have been called **prions**, or "protein infectious agents" (Prusiner, 1982). Prion proteins are found primarily in the membrane of neurons, where they are believed to play a role in synaptic function. They are resistant to levels of heat that denature normal proteins, which explains why cooking meat from cattle with BSE does not destroy the infectious agent. The sequence of amino acids of normal prion protein (PrPc) and infectious prion (PrPSc) are identical. How, then, can two proteins with the same amino acid sequences have such different effects? The answer is that the functions of proteins are determined largely by their three-dimensional shapes. The only difference between PrPc and PrPSc is the way the protein is folded. Once misfolded PrPSc is introduced into a cell, it causes normal PrPc to become misfolded too, and the process of this transformation ultimately kills them. (See Hetz et al., 2003, for a review.)

A familial form of Creutzfeldt-Jakob disease is transmitted as a dominant trait, caused by a mutation of the *PRNP* gene located on the short arm of chromosome 20, which codes for the human prion protein gene. However, most cases of Creutzfeldt-Jakob disease are **sporadic**. That is, they occur in people without a family history of prion protein disease. Prion protein diseases are unique not only because they can be transmitted by means of a simple protein, but also because they can also be genetic or sporadic—and the genetic and sporadic forms can be transmitted to others. The most common form of transmission of Creutzfeldt-Jakob disease in humans is through transplantation of tissues such as dura mater or corneas, harvested from cadavers of people who were infected with a prion disease. One form of human prion protein disease, kuru, was transmitted through cannibalism: Out of respect to their recently departed relatives, members of a South Pacific tribe ate their brains and sometimes thus contracted the disease. This practice has since been abandoned.

A study by Steele et al. (2006) suggests that normal prion protein plays a role in neural development and differentiation in fetuses and neurogenesis in adults. Steele and his colleagues produced a genetically engineered strain of mice that produced increased amounts of PrPc and found increased numbers of proliferating cells in the subventricular zone, and more neurons in the dentate gyrus, compared with normal mice. Mice with a targeted mutation of the prion protein gene had fewer proliferating cells. Málaga-Trillo et al. (2009) found that a targeted mutation against the prion protein gene in zebra fish produced serious developmental anomalies.

Mallucci et al. (2003) created a genetically modified mouse strain whose neurons produced an enzyme at 12 weeks of age that destroyed normal prion protein. When the animals were a few weeks of age, the experimenters infected them with misfolded mouse scrapie prions. Soon thereafter, the animals began to develop spongy holes in their brains, indicating that they were infected with mouse scrapie. Then, at 12 weeks, the enzyme became active and started destroying normal PrPc. Although analysis showed that glial cells in the brain still contained misfolded PrPSc, the disease process stopped. Neurons stopped making normal PrPc, which

prion (*pree* on) A protein that can exist in two forms that differ only in their three-dimensional shape; accumulation of misfolded prion protein is responsible for transmissible spongiform encephalopathies.

sporadic disease A disease that occurs rarely and is not obviously caused by heredity or an infectious agent.

FIGURE 14.12

Experimental Treatment of a Prion Protein Infection.   Neural death was prevented and early spongiosis was reversed in scrapie-infected mice after a genetically engineered enzyme began to destroy PrPc at 12 weeks of age. Arrows point to degenerating neurons in mice without the prion-destroying enzyme. Spongiosis is seen as holes in the brain tissue (*arrowheads*).

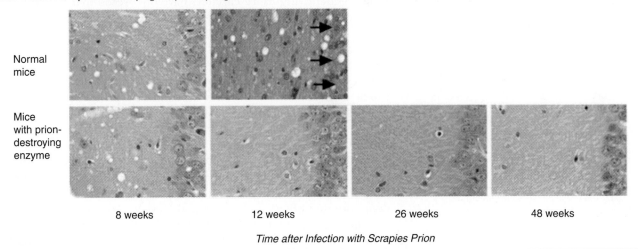

Normal mice

Mice with prion-destroying enzyme

8 weeks   12 weeks   26 weeks   48 weeks

Time after Infection with Scrapies Prion

From Mallucci, G., Dickinson, A., Linehan, J., Klöhn, P. C., et al. *Science*, 2003, *302*, 871–874. Copyright © 2003. Reprinted with permission from AAAS.

could no longer be converted into PrPSc, so the mice went on to live normal lives. The disease process continued to progress in mice without the special enzyme, and these animals soon died. The authors concluded that the process of conversion of PrPc to PrPSc is what kills cells. The mere presence of PrPSc in the brain (found in nonneuronal cells) does not cause the disease. Figure 14.12 shows the development of spongiform degeneration and its disappearance after the PrPc-destroying enzyme became active at 12 weeks of age. (See *Figure 14.12.*)

How might misfolded prion protein kill neurons? As we will see later in this chapter, the brains of people with several other degenerative diseases, including Parkinson's disease, Alzheimer's disease, amyotrophic lateral sclerosis, and Huntington's disease contain aggregations of misfolded proteins (Soto, 2003). As we saw in Chapter 3, cells contain the means by which they can commit suicide—a process known as *apoptosis*. Apoptosis can be triggered either externally, by a chemical signal telling the cell it is no longer needed (for example, during development), or internally, by evidence that biochemical processes in the cell have become disrupted so that the cell is no longer functioning properly. Perhaps the accumulation of misfolded, abnormal proteins provides such a signal. Apoptosis involves production of "killer enzymes" called **caspases**. Mallucci et al. (2003) suggest that inactivation of caspase-12, the enzyme that appears to be responsible for the death of neurons infected with PrPSc, may provide a treatment that could arrest the progress of transmissible spongiform encephalopathies. Let's hope they are right.

Parkinson's Disease

One of the most common degenerative neurological disorders, Parkinson's disease, is caused by degeneration of the nigrostriatal system—the dopamine-secreting neurons of the substantia nigra that send axons to the basal ganglia. Parkinson's disease is seen in approximately 1 percent of people over 65 years of age. The primary symptoms of Parkinson's disease are muscular rigidity, slowness of movement, a resting tremor, and postural instability.

Examination of the brains of patients who had Parkinson's disease shows, of course, the near-disappearance of nigrostriatal dopaminergic neurons. Many

caspase A "killer enzyme" that plays a role in apoptosis, or programmed cell death.

Lewy Bodies. A photomicrograph of the substantia nigra of a patient with Parkinson's disease shows a Lewy body, indicated by the arrow.

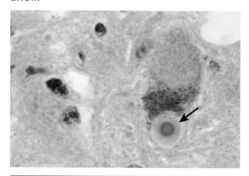

Photograph courtesy of Dr. Don Born, University of Washington.

Lewy body Abnormal circular structures with a dense core consisting of α-synuclein protein; found in the cytoplasm of nigrostriatal neurons in people with Parkinson's disease.

α-synuclein A protein normally found in the presynaptic membrane, where it is apparently involved in synaptic plasticity. Abnormal accumulations are apparently the cause of neural degeneration in Parkinson's disease.

toxic gain of function Said of a genetic disorder caused by a dominant mutation that involves a faulty gene that produces a protein with toxic effects.

parkin A protein that plays a role in ferrying defective or misfolded proteins to the proteasomes; mutated parkin is a cause of familial Parkinson's disease.

loss of function Said of a genetic disorder caused by a recessive gene that fails to produce a protein that is necessary for good health.

proteasome An organelle responsible for destroying defective or degraded proteins within the cell.

ubiquitin A protein that attaches itself to faulty or misfolded proteins and thus targets them for destruction by proteasomes.

surviving dopaminergic neurons show **Lewy bodies**, abnormal circular structures found with the cytoplasm. Lewy bodies have a dense protein core, surrounded by a halo of radiating fibers (Forno, 1996). (See *Figure 14.13*.) Although most cases of Parkinson's disease do not appear to have genetic origins, researchers have discovered that the mutation of a particular gene located on chromosome 4 will produce this disorder (Polymeropoulos et al., 1996). This gene produces a protein known as α-**synuclein**, which is normally found in the presynaptic terminals and is thought to be involved in synaptic transmission in dopaminergic neurons (Moore et al., 2005). The mutation produces what is known as a **toxic gain of function** because it produces a protein that results in effects that are toxic to the cell. Mutations that cause toxic gain of function are normally dominant because the toxic substance is produced whether one or both members of the pair of chromosomes contains the mutated gene. Abnormal α-synuclein becomes misfolded and forms aggregations, especially in dopaminergic neurons (Goedert, 2001). The dense core of Lewy bodies consists primarily of these aggregations, along with neurofilaments and synaptic vesicle proteins.

Another hereditary form of Parkinson's disease is caused by mutation of a gene on chromosome 6 that produces a gene that has been named **parkin** (Kitada et al., 1998). This mutation causes a **loss of function**, which makes it a recessive disorder. If a person carries a mutated parkin gene on only one chromosome, the normal allele on the other chromosome can produce a sufficient amount of normal parkin for normal cellular functioning. Normal parkin plays a role in ferrying defective or misfolded proteins to the **proteasomes**—organelles responsible for destroying these proteins (Moore et al., 2005). This mutation permits high levels of defective protein to accumulate in dopaminergic neurons and ultimately damage them. Figure 14.14 illustrates the role of parkin in the action of proteasomes. Parkin assists in the tagging of abnormal or misfolded proteins with numerous molecules of **ubiquitin**, a small, compact globular protein. Ubiquitination (as this process is called) targets the abnormal proteins for destruction by the proteasomes, which break them down into their constituent amino acids. Defective parkin fails to ubiquinate abnormal proteins, and they accumulate in the cell, eventually killing it. For some reason, dopaminergic neurons are especially sensitive to this accumulation. (See *Figure 14.14*.)

The overwhelming majority of the cases of this Parkinson's disease (approximately 95 percent) are sporadic. That is, they occur in people without a family history of Parkinson's disease. What, then, triggers the accumulation of α-synuclein and the destruction of dopaminergic neurons? Research suggests that Parkinson's disease may be caused by toxins present in the environment, by faulty metabolism, or by unrecognized infectious disorders. For example, the insecticides rotenone and paraquat can also cause Parkinson's disease—and, presumably, so can other unidentified toxins. All of these chemicals inhibit mitochondrial functions, which leads to the aggregation of misfolded α-synuclein, especially in dopaminergic neurons. These accumulated proteins eventually kill the cells (Dawson and Dawson, 2003).

As we saw in Chapter 4, the standard treatment for Parkinson's disease is L-DOPA, the precursor of dopamine. An increased level of L-DOPA in the brain causes a patient's remaining dopaminergic neurons to produce and secrete more dopamine and, for a time, alleviates the symptoms of the disease. However, this compensation does not work indefinitely; eventually, the number of nigrostriatal dopaminergic neurons declines to such a low level that the symptoms become worse. In addition, high levels of L-DOPA produce side effects by acting on dopaminergic systems other than the nigrostriatal system. Some patients—especially those whose symptoms began when they were relatively young—become bedridden, scarcely able to move.

Another drug, deprenyl, is often given to patients with Parkinson's disease, usually in conjunction with L-DOPA. As we saw in the prologue and epilogue of Chapter 4, several people acquired the symptoms of Parkinson's disease after taking an illicit drug contaminated with MPTP. Subsequent studies with laboratory animals revealed that the toxic effects of this drug could be prevented by administration of deprenyl, a drug that inhibits the activity of the enzyme MAO-B. The original rationale for administering deprenyl to patients with Parkinson's disease was that it might prevent unknown toxins from producing further damage to dopaminergic neurons. In addition, Kumar and Andersen (2004) note that there is an age-related increase in MAO-B activity that might increase the level of oxidative stress in dopaminergic neurons. The intracellular breakdown of dopamine by MAO-B causes the formation of hydrogen peroxide, which can damage cells. Thus, a beneficial effect of MAO-B inhibitors might be to decrease normal, age-related oxidative stress. In addition, Czerniczyniec, Bostamante, and Arnaiz-Lores (2007) found that deprenyl increased mitochondrial functions in the brains of mice. Ironically, cigarette smokers have a lower incidence of Parkinson's disease, perhaps because compounds in tobacco inhibit MAO-B activity (Fowler et al., 2003). Of course, the increased incidence of lung cancer, emphysema, and other smoking-related diseases far outweighs any potential beneficial effects on the incidence of Parkinson's disease.

Neurosurgeons have developed three stereotaxic procedures designed to alleviate the symptoms of Parkinson's disease that no longer respond to treatment with L-DOPA. The first one, transplantation of fetal tissue, attempts to reestablish the secretion of dopamine in the neostriatum. The tissue is obtained from the substantia nigra of aborted human fetuses and implanted into the caudate nucleus and putamen by means of stereotaxically guided needles. As we saw in Chapter 5, PET scans have shown that dopaminergic fetal cells are able to grow in their new host and secrete dopamine, reducing the patient's symptoms—at lease, initially. In a study of thirty-two patients with fetal tissue transplants, Freed (2002) found that those whose symptoms had previously responded to L-DOPA were most likely to benefit from the surgery. Presumably, these patients had a sufficient number of basal ganglia neurons with receptors that could be stimulated by the dopamine secreted by either the medication or the transplanted tissue. Unfortunately, many transplant patient later developed severe, persistent *dyskinesias*—troublesome and often painful involuntary movements. As a result, transplants of dopaminergic fetal cells are no longer recommended (Olanow et al., 2003).

One potential source of dopaminergic neurons could come from cultures of neural stem cells—undifferentiated cells that have the ability, if appropriately stimulated, to develop into a variety of types of cells, not just dopaminergic neurons (Snyder and Olanow, 2005). A significant advantage of human neural stem cells is that large numbers of cells could be transplanted, thus increasing the numbers of surviving cells in the patients' brains. Redmond et al. (2007) produced parkinsonian symptoms in monkeys through injections of MPTP that destroyed most of the animals' nigrostriatal dopaminergic neurons. The investigators then implanted

FIGURE 14.14

The Role of Parkin in Parkinson's Disease. Parkin is involved in the destruction of abnormal or misfolded proteins by the ubiquitin-proteasome system. If parkin is defective because of a mutation, abnormal or misfolded proteins cannot be destroyed, so they accumulate in the cell. If α-synuclein is defective because of a mutation, parkin is unable to tag it with ubiquitin, and it accumulates in the cell.

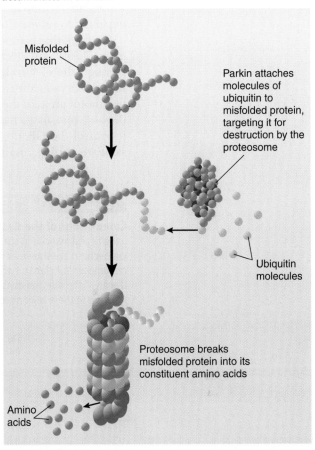

Misfolded protein

Parkin attaches molecules of ubiquitin to misfolded protein, targeting it for destruction by the proteosome

Ubiquitin molecules

Proteosome breaks misfolded protein into its constituent amino acids

Amino acids

neural stem cells into the caudate nucleus and found that the stem cells differentiated not just into DA-secreting neurons, but also into astrocytes and other cells that protect and repair neurons. The implants also had a functional impact: The monkeys' motor behavior improved.

The second stereotaxic procedure involves destruction of the **internal division of the globus pallidus (GP$_i$)**. The output of the GP$_i$ which is directed through the thalamus to the motor cortex, is inhibitory. The decreased release of dopamine in the caudate nucleus and putamen that is seen in patients with Parkinson's disease causes an *increase* in the activity of the GP$_i$. Thus, damage to the GP$_i$ might be expected to relieve the symptoms of Parkinson's disease. (See *Figure 14.15.*)

In fact, that is exactly what happens (Graybiel, 1996; Lai et al., 2000). Neurosurgeons insert an electrode into the GP$_i$ and then pass radiofrequency current through the electrode that heats and destroys the brain tissue. PET studies have found that after the surgery, the metabolic activity in the premotor and supplementary motor areas of the frontal lobes, normally depressed in patients with Parkinson's disease, returns to normal levels (Grafton et al., 1995). This result indicates that lesions of the GP$_i$ do indeed release the motor cortex from inhibition. Using the same reasoning, neurosurgeons have also successfully treated the symptoms of

---

FIGURE 14.15

Connections of the Basal Ganglia   This schematic shows the major connections of the basal ganglia and associated structures. Excitatory connections are shown as black lines; inhibitory connections are shown as red lines. Many connections, such as the inputs to the substantia nigra, are omitted for clarity. Two regions that have been targets of stereotaxic surgery for Parkinson's disease—the internal division of the globus pallidus and the subthalamus—are outlined in gray. Damage to these regions reduces inhibitory input to the thalamus and facilitates movement.

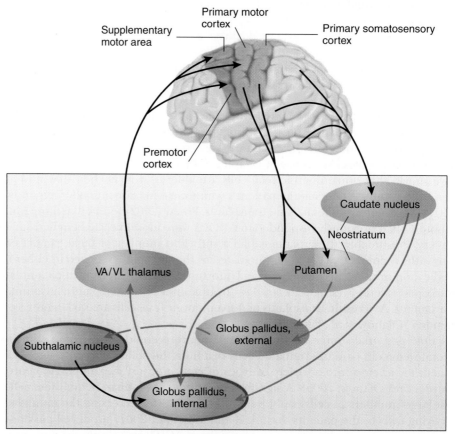

internal division of the globus pallidus (**GPi**) A division of the globus pallidus that provides inhibitory input to the motor cortex via the thalamus; sometimes stereotaxically lesioned to treat the symptoms of Parkinson's disease.

FIGURE 14.16

Gene Therapy of Parkinson's Disease.   The gene for GAD, the enzyme responsible for biosynthesis of GABA, was delivered to cells in the subthalamic nucleus of patients with Parkinson's disease by means of a genetically modified virus. Functional MRI scans show (a) decreased activation of the subthalamic nucleus and (b) increased activation of the supplementary motor area. The graph (c) shows the relation between changes in the activation of the supplementary motor area and symptoms of Parkinson's disease.

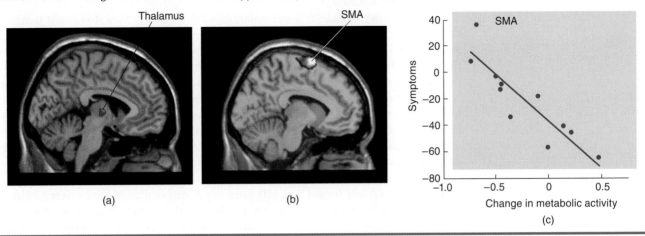

(a)   (b)   (c)

Reprinted from *The Lancet, 369*, Kaplitt, M. G., Feigin, A., Tang, C., et al., Safety and Tolerability of Gene Therapy with an Adeno-Associated Virus (AAV) Borne GAD Gene for Parkinson's Disease: An Open Label, Phase I Trial, 2097–2105, Copyright 2007, with permission from Elsevier.

Parkinson's disease by targeting the subthalamus, which provides an excitatory input to the GP_i.

The third stereotaxic procedure aimed at relieving the symptoms of Parkinson's disease involves implanting electrodes in the subthalamic nucleus and attaching a device that permits the patient to electrically stimulate the brain through the electrodes. According to some studies, deep brain stimulation is as effective as brain lesions in suppressing tremors and has fewer adverse side effects (Simuni et al., 2002; Speelman et al., 2002). The fact that either lesions or stimulation alleviates tremors suggests that the stimulation has an inhibitory effect on neurons in the subthalamic nucleus.

Kaplitt et al. (2007) developed a remarkable procedure that might provide an alternate (or supplement) to deep brain stimulation. In a clinical trial designed to assess the safety of the new procedure, Kaplitt and his colleagues injected a genetically modified virus into the subthalamic nucleus of patients with Parkinson's disease that delivered a gene for GAD, the enzyme responsible for the biosynthesis of the major inhibitory neurotransmitter, GABA. The production of GAD turned some of the excitatory, glutamate-producing neurons in the subthalamic nucleus into inhibitory, GABA-producing neurons. As a result, the activity of the GP_i decreased, the activity of the supplementary motor area increased, and the symptoms of the patients improved. (See *Figure 14.16*.)

Huntington's Disease

Another basal ganglia disease, **Huntington's disease**, is caused by degeneration of the caudate nucleus and putamen. Whereas Parkinson's disease causes a poverty of movements, Huntington's disease causes uncontrollable ones, especially jerky limb movements. The movements of Huntington's disease look like fragments of purposeful movements but occur involuntarily. This disease is progressive, includes cognitive and emotional changes, and eventually causes death, usually within 10–15 years after the symptoms begin.

The symptoms of Huntington's disease usually begin in the person's thirties and forties but can sometimes begin in the early twenties. The first signs of neural

Huntington's disease An inherited disorder that causes degeneration of the basal ganglia; characterized by progressively more severe uncontrollable jerking movements, writhing movements, dementia, and finally death.

degeneration occur in the putamen, in a specific group of inhibitory neurons—GABAergic medium spiny neurons. Damage to these neurons removes some inhibitory control exerted on the premotor and supplementary motor areas of the frontal cortex. Loss of this control leads to involuntary movements. As the disease progresses, neural degeneration is seen in many other regions of the brain, including the cerebral cortex.

Huntington's disease is a hereditary disorder, caused by a dominant gene on chromosome 4. In fact, the gene has been located, and its defect has been identified as a repeated sequence of bases that code for the amino acid glutamine (Collaborative Research Group, 1993). This repeated sequence causes the gene product—a protein called **huntingtin (htt)**—to contain an elongated stretch of glutamine. Abnormal htt becomes misfolded and forms aggregations that accumulate in the nucleus. Longer stretches of glutamine are associated with patients whose symptoms began at a younger age, a finding that indicates that this abnormal portion of the huntingtin molecule is responsible for the disease. These facts suggest that the mutation causes the disease through a toxic gain of function; that abnormal htt causes harm. In fact, the cause of death of neurons in Huntington' disease is apoptosis. Li et al. (2000) found that HD mice lived longer if they were given a caspase inhibitor, which suppresses apoptosis. Abnormal htt may trigger apoptosis by impairing the function of the ubiquitin-protease system, which activates caspase (Hague, Klaffke, and Bandmann, 2005).

At present there is no treatment for the disorder. However, a study by DiFiglia et al. (2007) suggests a possible approach. The investigators used a genetically modified virus to deliver a mutant human htt gene into the striatum and overlying cortex of mice, which caused the development of neuropathology and motor deficits. DiFiglia and her colleagues then injected a small interfering RNA (siRNA) into the striatum that blocked the transcription of the htt genes—and hence the production of mutant htt—in this region. The treatment decreased the size of inclusion bodies in striatal neurons, prolonged the life of the striatal neurons, and reduced the animals' motor symptoms.

Alzheimer's Disease

Several neurological disorders result in **dementia**, a deterioration of intellectual abilities resulting from an organic brain disorder. A common form of dementia is called **Alzheimer's disease**, which occurs in approximately 10 percent of the population above the age of 65 and almost 50 percent of people older than 85 years. It is characterized by progressive loss of memory and other mental functions. At first, people may have difficulty remembering appointments and sometimes fail to think of words or other people's names. As time passes, they show increasing confusion and increasing difficulty with tasks such as balancing a checkbook. The memory deficit most critically involves recent events, and thus it resembles the anterograde amnesia of Korsakoff's syndrome. If people with Alzheimer's disease venture outside alone, they are likely to get lost. They eventually become bedridden, then become completely helpless, and finally succumb (Terry and Davies, 1980).

Alzheimer's disease produces severe degeneration of the hippocampus, entorhinal cortex, neocortex (especially the association cortex of the frontal and temporal lobes), nucleus basalis, locus coeruleus, and raphe nuclei. Figure 14.17 shows photographs of the brain of a patient with Alzheimer's disease and of a normal brain. You can see how much wider the sulci are in the patient's brain, especially in the frontal and temporal lobes, indicating substantial loss of cortical tissue. (See *Figure 14.17.*)

Earlier, I mentioned that the brains of patients with Down syndrome usually develop abnormal structures that are also seen in patients with Alzheimer's disease: *amyloid plaques* and *neurofibrillary tangles*. **Amyloid plaques** are extracellular deposits that consist of a dense core of a protein known as **β-amyloid** (usually referred to as

huntingtin (htt) A protein that may serve to facilitate the production and transport of brain-derived neurotrophic factor. Abnormal huntingtin is the cause of Huntington's disease.

dementia (*da men* sha) A loss of cognitive abilities such as memory, perception, verbal ability, and judgment; common causes are multiple strokes and Alzheimer's disease.

Alzheimer's disease A degenerative brain disorder of unknown origin; causes progressive memory loss, motor deficits, and eventual death.

amyloid plaque An extracellular deposit containing a dense core of β-amyloid protein surrounded by degenerating axons and dendrites and activated microglia and reactive astrocytes.

β-amyloid (Aβ) (*amm i loyd*) A protein found in excessive amounts in the brains of patients with Alzheimer's disease.

FIGURE 14.17

Alzheimer's Disease.   The figure shows (a) a lateral view of the right side of the brain of a person with Alzheimer's disease. (Rostral is to the right; dorsal is up.) Note that the sulci of the temporal lobe and parietal lobe are especially wide, indicating degeneration of the neocortex (*arrowheads*). The figure also shows (b) a lateral view of the right side of a normal brain.

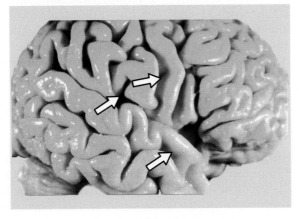
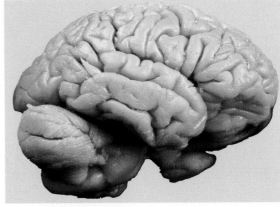

(a)   (b)

Photo of diseased brain courtesy of A. D'Agostino, Good Samaritan Hospital, Portland, Oregon; photo of normal brain © Dan McCoy/Rainbow.

Aβ), surrounded by degenerating axons and dendrites, along with activated microglia and reactive astrocytes, cells that are involved in destruction of damaged cells. Eventually, the phagocytic glial cells destroy the degenerating axons and dendrites, leaving only a core of β-amyloid.

Neurofibrillary tangles consist of dying neurons that contain intracellular accumulations of twisted filaments of hyperphosphorylated **tau protein**. Normal tau protein serves as a component of microtubules, which provide the cells' transport mechanism. During the progression of Alzheimer's disease, excessive amounts of phosphate ions become attached to strands of tau protein, thus changing its molecular structure. Abnormal filaments are seen in the soma and proximal dendrites of pyramidal cells in the cerebral cortex, which disrupt transport of substances within the cell, and the cell dies, leaving behind a tangle of protein filaments. (See *Figure 14.18*.)

Formation of amyloid plaques is caused by the production of a defective form of Aβ. The production of Aβ takes several steps. First, a gene encodes the production of the **β-amyloid precursor protein (APP)**, a chain of approximately 700 amino acids. APP is then cut apart in two places by enzymes known as **secretases** to produce Aβ. The first, β-secretase, cuts the "tail" off of an APP molecule. The second, γ-secretase (gamma-secretase), cuts the "head" off. The result is a molecule of Aβ that contains either forty or forty-two amino acids. (See *Figure 14.19*.)

The location of the second cut of the APP molecule by γ-secretase determines which form is produced. In normal brains, 90 to 95 percent of the Aβ molecules are of the short form; the other 5 to 10 percent are of the long form. In patients with Alzheimer's disease, the proportion of long Aβ rises to as much as 40 percent of the total. High concentrations of the long form have a tendency to fold themselves improperly and form aggregations, which have toxic effects on the cell. (As we saw earlier in this chapter, abnormally folded prions and α-synuclein proteins form aggregations that cause brain degeneration.) Small amounts of long Aβ can easily

FIGURE 14.18

Microscopic Features of Alzheimer's Disease.   The photomicrographs from deceased patients with Alzheimer's disease show (a) an amyloid plaque, filled with β-amyloid protein and (b) neurofibrillary tangles.

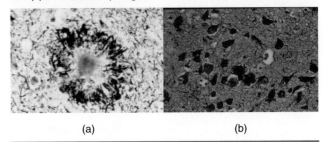

(a)   (b)

Photos courtesy of D. J. Selkoe, Brigham and Women's Hospital, Boston, Massachusetts.

neurofibrillary tangle (*new row fib ri lair y*) A dying neuron containing intracellular accumulations of twisted filaments of tau protein that formerly served as the cell's internal skeleton.

tau protein A protein that normally serves as a component of microtubules, which provide the cell's transport mechanism.

β-amyloid precursor protein (APP) A protein produced and secreted by cells that serves as the precursor for β-amyloid protein.

secretase (*see cre tayss*) A class of enzymes that cut the β-amyloid precursor protein into smaller fragments, including β-amyloid.

FIGURE 14.19

β-Amyloid Protein.   The schematic shows the production of β-amyloid protein (Aβ) from the amyloid precursor protein.

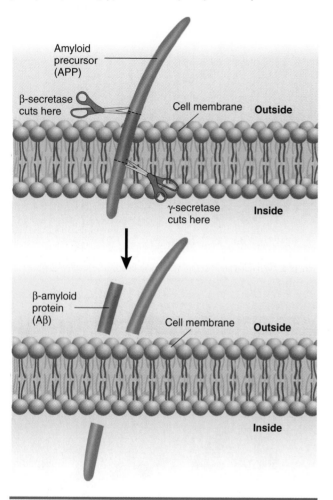

presenilin (*pree sen **ill** in*) A protein produced by a faulty gene that causes β-amyloid precursor protein to be converted to the abnormal short form; may be a cause of Alzheimer's disease.

apolipoprotein E (ApoE) (*ay po lye po **proh** teen*) A glycoprotein that transports cholesterol in the blood and plays a role in cellular repair; presence of the E4 allele of the apoE gene increases the risk of late-onset Alzheimer's disease.

be cleared from the cell. The molecules are given a ubiquitin tag that marks them for destruction, and they are transported to the proteasomes, where they are rendered harmless. However, this system cannot keep up with abnormally high levels of production of long Aβ.

Acetylcholinergic neurons in the basal forebrain are among the first cells to be affected in Alzheimer's disease. Aβ serves as a ligand for the *p75 neurotrophin receptor*, a receptor that normally responds to stress signals and stimulates apoptosis (Sotthibundhu et al., 2008). Basal forebrain ACh neurons contain high levels of this receptors; thus, once the level of long-form Aβ reach a sufficiently high lever, these neurons begin to die.

Figure 14.20 shows the abnormal accumulation of Aβ in the brain of a person with Alzheimer's disease. Klunk and his colleagues (Klunk et al., 2003; Mathis et al., 2005) developed a chemical that binds with Aβ and readily crosses the blood–brain barrier. They gave the patient and a healthy control subject an injection of a radioactive form of this chemical and examined their brains with a PET scanner. You can see the accumulation of the protein in the patient's cerebral cortex. (See *Figure 14.20*.) The ability to measure the levels of Aβ in the brains of Alzheimer's patients will enable researchers to evaluate the effectiveness of potential treatments for the disease. If such a treatment is devised, the ability to identify the accumulation of Aβ early in the development of the disease will make it possible to begin a patient's treatment before significant degeneration—and the accompanying decline in cognitive abilities—has occurred.

Research has shown that at least some forms of Alzheimer's disease appear to run in families and thus appear to be hereditary. Because the brains of people with Down syndrome (caused by an extra twenty-first chromosome) also contain deposits of Aβ, some investigators hypothesized that the twenty-first chromosome may be involved in the production of this protein. In fact, St. George-Hyslop et al. (1987) found that chromosome 21 *does* contains the gene that produces APP.

Since the discovery of the APP gene, several studies found specific mutations of this gene that produce familial Alzheimer's disease (Martinez et al., 1993; Farlow et al., 1994). In addition, other studies have found numerous mutations of two **presenilin** genes, found on chromosomes 1 and 14, that also produce Alzheimer's disease. Abnormal APP and presenilin genes all cause the defective long form of Aβ to be produced (Hardy, 1997). The two presenilin proteins, PS1 and PS2, appear to be subunits of γ-secretase, which is not a simple enzyme but consists of a large multiprotein complex (De Strooper, 2003).

Yet another genetic cause of Alzheimer's disease is a mutation in the gene for **apolipoprotein E (ApoE)**, a glycoprotein that transports cholesterol in the blood and also plays a role in cellular repair. One allele of the ApoE gene, known as E4, increases the risk of late-onset Alzheimer's disease, apparently by interfering with the removal of the long form of Aβ from the extracellular space in the brain (Roses, 1997; Price and Sisodia, 1998; Mahley and Rall, 2000). Another allele, ApoE2, may actually protect people from developing Alzheimer's disease (Wilhelmus et al., 2005). Traumatic brain injury is also a serious risk factor for Alzheimer's disease. For example, examination of the brains of people who have sustained closed head injuries (including those that occur during prize fights) often reveals a widespread distribution of amyloid plaques. Risk of Alzheimer's disease following traumatic brain injury is especially high in people who possess the ApoE4 allele (Lesné et al., 2005; Luukinen et al., 2005). Obesity, hypertension, high cholesterol levels, and diabetes are also risk factors, and these factors, too, are exacerbated by the presence of the ApoE4 allele (Martins et al., 2006).

Although the studies I have cited indicate that genetically triggered production of abnormal Aβ plays an important role in the development of Alzheimer's disease, the fact is that most forms of Alzheimer's disease are sporadic, not hereditary. So far, the strongest known nongenetic risk factor for Alzheimer's disease (other than age) is traumatic brain injury. Another factor, level of education, has also been shown to play an important role. The Religious Orders Study, supported by the U.S. National Institute on Aging, measures the cognitive performance of older Catholic clergy (priests, nuns, and monks) and examines their brains when they die. A report by Bennett et al. (2003) found a positive relationship between increased number of years of formal education and cognitive performance, even in people whose brains contained significant numbers of amyloid plaques. For example, people who had received some postgraduate education had significantly higher cognitive test scores than people with the same number of amyloid plaques but less formal education. Of course, it is possible that variables such as individual differences in cognitive ability affect the likelihood that a person will pursue advanced studies, and these differences, by themselves, could play an important role. In any case, engaging in vigorous intellectual activity (and adopting a lifestyle that promotes good general health) is probably the most important thing a person can do to stave off the development of dementia.

Billings et al. (2007) performed an experiment with *AD mice*—a strain of genetically modified mice that contain a mutant human gene for APP that leads to the development of Alzheimer's disease. The investigators began training the mice early in life on the water maze task, described in Chapter 12. The mice were trained at 3-month intervals between the ages of 2 to 18 months. The training delayed the accumulation of Aβ and led to a slower decline of the animals' performance. This study lends support to the conclusion that intellectual activity (if I can use that term for mice) delays the appearance of Alzheimer's disease.

Currently, the only approved pharmacological treatments for Alzheimer's disease are acetylcholinesterase inhibitors (donepezil, rivastigmine, and galantamine) and an NMDA receptor antagonist (memantine). Because acetylcholinergic neurons are among the first to be damaged in Alzheimer's disease and because these neurons play a role in cortical activation and memory, drugs that inhibit the destruction of ACh and hence enhance its activity have been found to provide a modest increase in cognitive activity of patients with this disease. However, these drugs have no effect on the process of neural degeneration and do not prolong patients' survival. Meantime, a noncompetitive NMDA receptor blocker, appears to produce a slight improvement in symptoms of dementia by retarding excitotoxic destruction of acetylcholinergic neurons caused by the entry of excessive amounts of calcium (Rogawski and Wenk, 2003).

Perhaps the most promising approaches to the prevention of Alzheimer's disease come from immunological research with AD mice. Schenk et al. (1999) and Bard et al. (2000) attempted to sensitize the immune system against Aβ. They injected AD mice with a vaccine that, they hoped, would stimulate the immune

FIGURE 14.20

Detection of β-Amyloid Protein.   The PET scans show the accumulation of β-amyloid protein (Aβ) in the brain of a patient with Alzheimer's disease. AD = Alzheimer's disease, MR = structural magnetic resonance image, [C-11]PIB PET = PET scan of the brain after an injection of a radioactive ligand for Aβ.

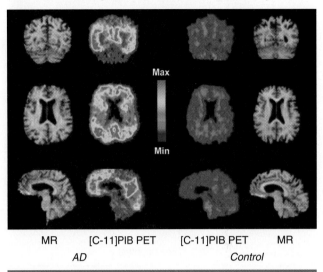

MR   [C-11]PIB PET   [C-11]PIB PET   MR
AD   *Control*

Courtesy of William Klunk, Western Psychiatric Institute and Clinic, Pittsburgh, Pennsylvania.

FIGURE 14.21

Immunization Against Aβ. The graph shows the effect of immunization against Aβ on the cognitive decline of patients who generated Aβ antibodies (successfully immunized patients) and those who did not (controls).

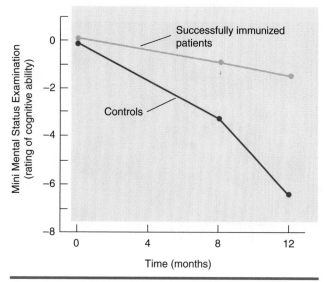

Adapted from Hock, C., Konietzko, U., Streffer, J. R., et al. *Neuron*, 2003, *38*, 547–554.

system to destroy Aβ. The treatment worked: The vaccine suppressed the development of amyloid plaques in the brains of mice that received the vaccine from an early age and halted or even reversed the development of plaques in mice that received the vaccine later in life.

A clinical trial with Alzheimer's patients attempted to destroy Aβ by sensitizing the patient's immune systems to the protein (Monsonego and Weiner, 2003). In a double-blind study, thirty patients with mild-to-moderate Alzheimer's disease were given injections of a portion of the Aβ protein. Twenty of these patients generated antibodies against Aβ, which slowed the course of the disease, presumably because their immune systems began destroying Aβ in their brain and reducing the neural destruction caused by the accumulation of this protein. Hock et al. (2003) compared the cognitive abilities of the patients who generated Aβ antibodies to those who did not. As Figure 14.21 shows, antibody production significantly reduced cognitive decline. (See *Figure 14.21*.)

One of the patients whose immune system generated antibodies against Aβ died of a pulmonary embolism (a blood clot in a blood vessel serving the lungs). Nicoll et al. (2003) examined this patient's brain and found evidence that the immune system had removed Aβ from many regions of the cerebral cortex. Unfortunately, the injections of the Aβ antigen caused an inflammatory reaction in the brains of 5 percent of the patients, so the clinical trial was terminated.

A study by Nikolic et al. (2007) used a different method to try to induce the immune system to attack Aβ. They vaccinated normal and AD mice with Aβ by injecting the protein in their skin. The vaccinations stimulated the mice's immune system to produce Aβ antibodies. No neuropathology was seen in any of the animals, and the numbers of Aβ plaques in the brain decreased.

Amyotrophic Lateral Sclerosis

Amyotrophic lateral sclerosis (ALS) is a degenerative disorder that attacks spinal cord and cranial nerve motor neurons (Bruijn, Miller, and Cleveland, 2004). The incidence of this disease is approximately 5 in 100,000. The symptoms include spasticity (increased tension of muscles, causing stiff and awkward movements), exaggerated stretch reflexes, progressive weakness and muscular atrophy, and, finally, paralysis. Death usually occurs 5 to 10 years after the onset of the disease as a result of failure of respiratory muscles. The muscles that control eye movements are spared. Cognitive abilities are rarely affected.

Ten percent of the cases of ALS are hereditary; the other 90 percent are sporadic. Of the hereditary cases, 10 to 20 percent are caused by a mutation in the gene that produces the enzyme *superoxide dismutase 1 (SOD1)*, found on chromosome 21. This mutation causes a toxic gain of function that leads to protein misfolding and aggregation, impaired axonal transport, and mitochondrial dysfunction. It also impairs glutamate reuptake into glial cells, which increases extracellular levels of glutamate and causes excitotoxicity in motor neurons (Bossy-Wetzel, Schwarzenbacher, and Lipton, 2004).

The only current pharmacological treatment for ALS is riluzole, a drug that reduces glutamate-induced excitotoxicity, probably by decreasing the release of glutamate. Clinical trials found that patients treated with riluzole lived an average of 1 to 3 months longer than those who received a placebo (Bensimon, Lacomblez, and Meininger, 1994). However, a study by Kaspar et al. (2003) using mice with a genet-

amyotrophic lateral sclerosis (ALS) A degenerative disorder that attacks the spinal cord and cranial nerve motor neurons.

ically engineered SOD1 mutation provides some hope of a more effective treatment, at least for familial ALS. The authors injected a harmless virus that contained a gene that causes the production of *insulin-like growth factor-1 (IGF-1)* into leg muscles of mice. The virus was taken up by terminal buttons of motor neurons and carried by means of retrograde axoplasmic flow to the cell bodies of these neurons, located in the ventral horn of the spinal cord. The inserted gene triggered the production of IGF-1, a protein that has been shown to prolong the lives of injured motor neurons, at least partly by blocking caspase activation. The animals lived 30 percent longer than mice treated with a placebo if the treatment started before the onset of physical symptoms and 18 percent longer if treatment was started after symptom onset. (See *Figure 14.22*.) The advantages of this treatment are that the virus used to insert the gene into the motor neurons is harmless to humans as well as mice and that the gene expression lasts for a long time. So far, the results of clinical trials with humans have been inconclusive (Mitchell, Wokke, and Borasio, 2007).

Multiple Sclerosis

Multiple sclerosis (MS) is an autoimmune demyelinating disease. At scattered locations within the central nervous system, myelin sheaths are attacked by the person's immune system, leaving behind hard patches of debris called *sclerotic plaques*. (See *Figure 14.23*.) The normal transmission of neural messages through the demyelinated axons is interrupted. Because the damage occurs in white matter located throughout the brain and spinal cord, a wide variety of neurological disorders are seen.

Multiple sclerosis afflicts women somewhat more frequently than men, and the disorder usually occurs in people in their late twenties or thirties. People who spend their childhood in places far from the equator are more likely to come down with the disease than are those who live close to the equator. Hence, it is likely that some disease contracted during a childhood spent in a region in which the virus is prevalent causes the person's immune system to attack his or her own myelin. Perhaps a

---

FIGURE 14.22

Gene Therapy for ALS. This graph shows the effect of delivery of a gene for insulin-like growth factor (IGF-1) into spinal motor neurons of mice with experimentally produced ALS. The therapy increased the average number of motor neurons seen in each section of tissue.

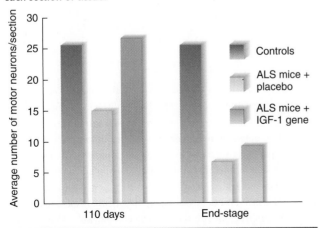

From Kaspar, B. K., Lladó, J., Sherkat, N., et al. *Science*, 2003, *301*, 839–842.
Copyright © 2003. Reprinted with permission from AAAS.

FIGURE 14.23

Multiple Sclerosis. In this slice of the brain of a person who had multiple sclerosis, the arrowheads point to sclerotic plaques in the white matter.

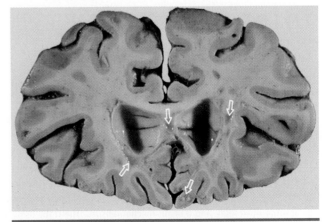

Courtesy of A. D'Agostino, Good Samaritan Hospital, Portland, Oregon.

virus weakens the blood–brain barrier, allowing myelin protein into the general circulation and sensitizing the immune system to it, or perhaps the virus attaches itself to myelin. In addition, people born during the late winter and early spring are at higher risk, which suggests that infections contracted by a pregnant woman (for example, a viral disease contracted during the winter) may also increase susceptibility to this disease. In any event, the process is a long-lived one, lasting for many decades.

Only two treatments for multiple sclerosis have shown any promise. The first is *interferon* β, a protein that modulates the responsiveness of the immune system. Administration of interferon β has been shown to reduce the frequency and severity of attacks and slow the progression of neurological disabilities in some patients with multiple sclerosis (Arnason 1999). However, the treatment is only partially effective.

Another partially effective treatment is *glatiramer acetate* (also known as copaxone or copolymer-1). Glatiramer acetate is a mixture of synthetic peptides composed from random sequences of the amino acids tyrosine, glutamate, alanine, and lysine. This compound was first produced in an attempt to induce the symptoms of multiple sclerosis in laboratory animals. An experimentally induced demyelinating disease known as *experimental allergic encephalitis (EAE)* can be produced in laboratory animals by injecting them with protein found in myelin. The immune system then becomes sensitized to myelin protein and attacks the animal's own myelin sheaths. Glatiramer acetate turned out to do just the opposite; rather than *causing* EAE, it *prevented* its occurrence, apparently by stimulating certain cells of the immune system to secrete anti-inflammatory chemicals such as *interleukin 4*, which suppress the activity of immune cells that would otherwise attack the patient's myelin (Farina et al., 2005). As you might expect, researchers tested glatiramer acetate in people with MS and found that the drug reduced the symptoms of patients who showed the relapsing-remitting form of the disease: periodic occurrences of neurological symptoms followed by partial remissions. The drug is now approved for treatment of this disorder. A structural MRI study by Sormani et al. (2005) found a reduction of 20 to 54 percent in white-matter lesions in 95 percent of patients treated with glatiramer acetate.

Although interferon β and glatiramer acetate provide some relief, neither treatment halts the progression of MS. We still need better forms of therapy. Because the symptoms of MS are often episodic—new or worsening symptoms followed by partial recovery—patients and their families often attribute the changes in the symptoms to whatever has happened recently. For example, if the patient has taken a new medication or gone on a new diet and the symptoms get worse, the patient will blame the symptoms on the medication or diet. Conversely, if the patient gets better, he or she will credit the medication or diet.

InterimSummary

Degenerative Disorders

Transmissible spongiform encephalopathies such as Creutzfeldt-Jakob disease, scrapie, and bovine spongiform encephalopathy ("mad cow disease") are unique among contagious diseases: They are produced by a simple protein molecule, not by a virus or microbe. The sequence of amino acids of normal prion protein (PrPc) and infectious prion protein (PrPSc) are identical, but their three-dimensional shapes differ in the way that they are folded. Somehow, the presence of a misfolded prion protein in a neuron causes normal prion proteins to become misfolded, and a chain reaction ensues. The transforma-

tion of PrPc into PrPSc kills the cell, apparently by triggering apoptosis. Creutzfeldt-Jakob disease is heritable as well as transmissible, but the most common form is sporadic—of unknown origin. Normal prion protein may play a role in neural development and neurogenesis, which may in turn affect the establishment and maintenance of long-term memories.

Parkinson's disease is caused by degeneration of dopamine-secreting neurons of the substantia nigra that send axons to the basal ganglia. Study of rare hereditary forms of Parkinson's disease reveals that the death of these neurons is caused by the aggregation of misfolded protein, α-synuclein. One mutation produces defective α-synuclein, and another produces defective parkin, a protein that assists in the tagging of abnormal proteins for destruction by the proteasomes. The accumulation of α-synuclein can also be triggered by some toxins, which suggests that nonhereditary forms of the disease may be caused by toxic substances present in the environment. Treatment of Parkinson's disease includes administration of L-DOPA, implantation of fetal dopaminergic neurons in the basal ganglia, stereotaxic destruction of a portion of the globus pallidus or subthalamus, and implantation of electrodes that enable the patient to electrically stimulate the subthalamus. Fetal transplants of dopaminergic neurons have turned out to be less successful than they had initially appeared to be, but transplants of neural stem cells shows more promise. A trial of gene therapy designed to reduce excitation in the subthalamic nucleus obtained promising results.

Huntington's disease, an autosomal-dominant hereditary disorder, produces degeneration of the caudate nucleus and putamen. Mutated huntingtin misfolds and forms aggregations that accumulate in the nucleus of GABAergic neurons in the putamen. The primary effect of mutated huntingtin appears to be a toxic gain of function that triggers apoptosis. An animal study that transferred small interfering RNA targeted against the htt gene suggested that this approach might be fruitful.

Alzheimer's disease, another degenerative disorder, involves much more of the brain; the disease process eventually destroys most of the hippocampus and cortical gray matter. The brains of affected individuals contain many amyloid plaques, which contain a core of misfolded long-form Aβ protein surrounded by degenerating axons and dendrites, and neurofibrillary tangles, composed of dying neurons that contain intracellular accumulations of twisted filaments of tau protein. Hereditary forms of Alzheimer's disease involve defective genes for the amyloid precursor protein (APP), for the secretases that cut APP into smaller pieces, or for apolipoprotein E (ApoE), a glycoprotein involved in transport of cholesterol and the repair of cell membranes. A promising treatment is vaccination against Aβ, and transcutaneous administration of the antigen may provide a way to avoid triggering an inflammatory reaction. Temporary reduction of symptoms is seen in some patients who are treated with anticholinergic drugs or drugs that serve as NMDA antagonists. Exercise and intellectual stimulation appear to delay the onset of Alzheimer's disease; obesity, high cholesterol levels, and diabetes are significant risk factors.

Amyotrophic lateral sclerosis is a degenerative disorder that attacks motor neurons. Ten percent of the cases are hereditary, caused by a mutation of the gene for SOD1; the other 90 percent are sporadic. The only pharmacological treatment is riluzole, a drug that reduces glutamate-induced excitotoxicity. A virally introduced gene for IGF-1 has shown promise in an animal model of ALS.

Multiple sclerosis, a demyelinating disease, is characterized by periodic attacks of neurological symptoms, usually with partial remission between attacks. The damage appears to be caused by the body's immune system, which attacks the protein contained in myelin. Most investigators believe that a viral infection early in life somehow sensitizes the immune system to myelin protein. The only effective treatments for MS are interferon β and glatiramer acetate, a mixture of synthetic peptides that appears to stimulate certain immune cells to secrete anti-inflammatory chemicals.

Disorders Caused by Infectious Diseases

Several neurological disorders can be caused by infectious diseases, transmitted by bacteria, fungi or other parasites, or viruses. The most common are encephalitis and meningitis. **Encephalitis** is an infection that invades the entire brain. The most common cause of encephalitis is a virus that is transmitted by mosquitoes, which pick up the infectious agent from horses, birds, or rodents. The symptoms of acute encephalitis include fever, irritability, and nausea, often followed by convulsions, delirium, and signs of brain damage, such as aphasia or paralysis. Unfortunately, there is no specific treatment besides supportive care, and between 5 and 20 percent of the cases are fatal; 20 percent of the survivors show some residual neurological symptoms.

Encephalitis can also be caused by the **herpes simplex virus**, which is the cause of cold sores (or "fever blisters") that most people develop in and around their mouth from time to time. Normally, the viruses live quietly in the *trigeminal nerve ganglia* nodules on the fifth cranial nerve that contain the cell bodies of somatosensory neurons that serve the face. The viruses proliferate periodically, traveling down to the ends of nerve fibers, where they cause sores to develop in mucous membrane. Unfortunately, they occasionally (but rarely) go the other way into the brain. Herpes encephalitis is a serious disease; the virus attacks the frontal and temporal lobes in particular and can severely damage them.

Two other forms of viral encephalitis are probably already familiar to you: polio and rabies. **Acute anterior poliomyelitis** ("polio") has fortunately been very rare in

encephalitis (*en seff a lye tis*) An inflammation of the brain; caused by bacteria, viruses, or toxic chemicals.

herpes simplex virus (*her peez*) A virus that normally causes cold sores near the lips but that can also cause brain damage.

acute anterior poliomyelitis (*poh lee oh my a lye tis*) A viral disease that destroys motor neurons of the brain and spinal cord.

developed countries since the development of vaccines that immunize people against the disease. The virus causes specific damage to motor neurons of the brain and spinal cord: neurons in the primary motor cortex; in the motor nuclei of the thalamus, hypothalamus, and brain stem; in the cerebellum; and in the ventral horns of the gray matter of the spinal cord. Undoubtedly, these motor neurons contain some chemical substance that either attracts the virus or in some way makes the virus become lethal to them.

Rabies is caused by a virus that is passed from the saliva of an infected mammal directly into a person's flesh by means of a bite wound. The virus travels through peripheral nerves to the central nervous system and there causes severe damage. It also travels to peripheral organs, such as the salivary glands, which makes it possible for the virus to find its way to another host. The symptoms include a short period of fever and headache, followed by anxiety, excessive movement and talking, difficulty in swallowing, movement disorders, difficulty in speaking, seizures, confusion, and, finally, death within 2 to 7 days of the onset of the symptoms. The virus has a special affinity for cells in the cerebellum and hippocampus, and damage to the hippocampus probably accounts for the emotional changes that are seen in the early symptoms.

Fortunately, the incubation period for rabies lasts up to several months while the virus climbs through the peripheral nerves. (If the bite is received in the face or neck, the incubation time will be much shorter because the virus has a smaller distance to travel before it reaches the brain.) During the incubation period a person can receive a vaccine that will confer an immunity to the disease; the person's own immune system will destroy the virus before it reaches the brain.

Several infectious diseases cause brain damage even though they are not primarily diseases of the central nervous system. One such disease is acquired immune deficiency syndrome (AIDS). Records of autopsies have revealed that at least 75 percent of people who died of AIDS show evidence of brain damage (Levy and Bredesen, 1989). The brain damage often results in a syndrome called *AIDS dementia complex*, which is characterized by damage to synapses and death of neurons in the hippocampus, cerebral cortex, and basal ganglia (Mattson, Haughey, and Nath, 2005). The brain damage leads to a loss of cognitive and motor functions and is the leading cause of cognitive decline in people under 40 years of age. At first the patients may become forgetful, they may think and reason more slowly, and they may have word-finding difficulties (anomia). Eventually, they may become almost mute. Motor deficits may begin with tremor and difficulty in making complex movement but then may progress so much that the patient becomes bedridden (Maj, 1990).

For several years, researchers have been puzzled by the fact that although AIDS certainly causes neural damage, neurons are not themselves infected by the HIV virus (the organism responsible for the disease). Instead, ADC is caused by the glycoprotein *gp120* envelope that coats the RNA that is responsible for the AIDS infection. The gp120 binds with other proteins that trigger apoptosis—cell suicide (Mattson, Haughey, and Nath, 2005; Alirezaei et al., 2007).

Another category of infectious diseases of the brain actually involves inflammation of the meninges, the layers of connective tissue that surround the central nervous system. **Meningitis** can be caused by viruses or bacteria. The symptoms of all forms include headache, a stiff neck, and, depending on the severity of the disorder, convulsions, confusion or loss of consciousness, and sometimes death. The stiff neck is one of the most important symptoms. Neck movements cause the meninges to stretch; because they are inflamed, the stretch causes severe pain. Therefore, the patient resists having his or her neck moved.

The most common form of viral meningitis usually does not cause significant brain damage. However, various forms of bacterial meningitis do. The usual cause is spread of a middle-ear infection into the brain, introduction of an infection into the brain from a head injury, or the presence of emboli that have dislodged from a bac-

rabies A fatal viral disease that causes brain damage; usually transmitted through the bite of an infected animal.

meningitis (*men in jy tis*) An inflammation of the meninges; can be caused by viruses or bacteria.

terial infection present in the chambers of the heart. Such an infection is often caused by unclean hypodermic needles; therefore, drug addicts are at particular risk for meningitis (as well as many other diseases). The inflammation of the meninges can damage the brain by interfering with circulation of blood or by blocking the flow of cerebrospinal fluid through the subarachnoid space, causing hydrocephalus. In addition, the cranial nerves are susceptible to damage. Fortunately, bacterial meningitis can usually be treated effectively with antibiotics. Of course, early diagnosis and prompt treatment are essential, because neither antibiotics nor any other known treatment can repair a damaged brain.

InterimSummary

Disorders Caused by Infectious Diseases

Infectious diseases can damage the brain. Encephalitis, usually caused by a virus, affects the entire brain. One form is caused by the herpes simplex virus, which infects the trigeminal nerve ganglia of most of the population. This virus tends to attack the frontal and temporal lobes. The polio virus attacks motor neurons in the brain and spinal cord, resulting in motor deficits or even paralysis. The rabies virus, acquired by an animal bite, travels through peripheral nerves and attacks the brain, particularly the cerebellum and hippocampus. An AIDS infection can also produce brain damage when the gp120 protein envelope of the HIV virus binds with other proteins that trigger apoptosis. Meningitis is an infection of the meninges, caused by viruses or bacteria. The bacterial form, which is usually more serious, is generally caused by an ear infection, a head injury, or an embolus from a heart infection.

EPILOGUE Seizure Surgery

Mrs. R.'s surgery was performed to remove a noncancerous brain tumor that, incidentally, produced seizures. As mentioned in this chapter, neurosurgeons occasionally perform surgery specifically to remove brain tissue that contains a seizure focus. Such an operation, called *seizure surgery*, is performed only when drug therapy is unsuccessful.

Because seizure surgery often involves the removal of a substantial amount of brain tissue (usually from one of the temporal lobes), we might expect it to cause behavioral deficits—but in most cases the reverse is true: People's performance on tests of neuropsychological functioning usually *improves*. How can the removal of brain tissue improve a person's performance?

The answer is provided by looking at what happens in the brain not *during* seizures but *between* them. The seizure focus, usually a region of scar tissue, irritates the brain tissue surrounding it, causing increased neural activity that tends to spread to adjacent regions. Between seizures this increased excitatory activity is held in check by a compensatory increase in inhibitory activity. That is, inhibitory neurons in the region surrounding the seizure focus become more active. (This phenomenon is known as *interictal inhibition; ictus* means "stroke" in Latin.) A seizure occurs when the excitation overcomes the inhibition.

The problem is that the compensatory inhibition does more than hold the excitation in check; it also suppresses the normal functions of a rather large region of brain tissue surrounding the seizure focus. Thus, even though the focus may be small, its effects are felt over a much larger area even between seizures. Removing the seizure focus and some surrounding brain tissue eliminates the source of the irritation and makes the compensatory inhibition unnecessary. Freed from interictal inhibition, the brain tissue located near the site of the former seizure focus can now function normally, and the patient's neuropsychological abilities will show an improvement.

As mentioned, seizures often occur after a head injury, but only after a delay of several months. The cause of the delay is related to some properties of neurons that make learning possible. Goddard (1967) implanted electrodes in the brains of rats and administered a brief, weak electrical stimulus once a day. At first the stimulation produced no effects, but after several days the stimulation began to trigger small, short seizures. As days went by, the seizures became larger and longer until the animal was finally having full-blown clonic-tonic convulsions. Goddard called the phenomenon *kindling*, because it resembled the way a small fire can be kindled to start a larger one.

Kindling appears to be analogous to learning, and it presumably involves changes in synaptic strength like those seen in long-term potentiation. It can most easily be induced in the temporal lobe, which is the place where seizure foci are most likely to occur. The probable reason for the delayed occurrence of seizures after a head injury is that it takes time for kindling to occur. The irritation produced by the brain injury eventually causes increased synaptic strength in excitatory synapses located nearby.

Kindling has become an animal model of focal-seizure disorders, and it has proved useful in research on the causes and treatment of these disorders. For example, Silver, Shin, and McNamara (1991) produced seizure foci in rats through kindling and compared the effects of some commonly used medications on both seizures (the electrical events within the brain) and convulsions (the motor manifestations of the seizures). They found that one of the drugs they tested prevented the convulsions but left seizures intact, whereas another prevented both seizures and convulsions. Because each seizure is capable of producing some brain damage through overstimulation of neurons (especially those in the hippocampal formation, which become especially active during a seizure), the goal of medical treatment should be the elimination of seizures, not simply the convulsions that accompany them. Research with the animal model of kindling will undoubtedly contribute to the effective treatment of focal-seizure disorders.

Key Concepts

TUMORS

1. Brain tumors are uncontrolled growths of cells other than neurons within the skull that damage normal tissue by compression or infiltration.

SEIZURE DISORDERS

2. Seizures are periodic episodes of abnormal neural firing, which can produce a variety of symptoms. They usually originate from a focus, but some have no apparent source of localized irritation.

CEREBROVASCULAR ACCIDENTS

3. Cerebrovascular accidents, hemorrhagic or obstructive in nature, produce localized brain damage. The two most common sources of obstructive strokes are emboli and thrombi.

DISORDERS OF DEVELOPMENT

4. Developmental disorders can be caused by drugs or disease-produced toxins, or by chromosomal or genetic abnormalities.

DEGENERATIVE DISORDERS

5. Several degenerative disorders of the nervous system, including transmissible spongiform encephalopathies, Parkinson's disease, Huntington's disease, Alzheimer's disease, amyotrophic lateral sclerosis, and multiple sclerosis, have received much attention from scientists in recent years. All of these diseases except multiple sclerosis appear to involve accumulations of abnormal proteins.

DISORDERS CAUSED BY INFECTIOUS DISEASES

6. Infectious diseases, either viral or bacterial, can damage the brain. The two most important infections of the central nervous system are encephalitis and meningitis, but with the rise of the AIDS epidemic, AIDS dementia complex has become more common.

Suggested Readings

Bossy-Wetzel, E., Schwarzenbacher, R., and Lipton, S. A. Molecular pathways to neurodegeneration. *Nature Medicine*, 2004, *10*, S2–S9.

Hardy, J. Toward Alzheimer therapies based on genetic knowledge. *Annual Review of Medicine*, 2004, *55*, 15–25.

Moore, D. J., West, A. B., Dawson, V. L., and Dawson, T. M. Molecular pathophysiology of Parkinson's disease. *Annual Review of Neuroscience*, 2005, *28*, 57–87.

Ropper, A. H., and Brown, R. H. *Adams and Victor's Principles of Neurology*, 8th ed. New York: McGraw-Hill Professional, 2005.

Weissmann, C., and Aguzzi, A. Approaches to therapy of prion diseases. *Annual Review of Medicine*, 2005, *56*, 321–344.

Additional Resources

Visit www.mypsychkit.com for additional review and practice of the material covered in this chapter. Within MyPsychKit, you can take practice tests and receive a customized study plan to help you review. Dozens of animations, tutorials, and Web links are also available. You can even review using the interactive electronic version of this textbook. You will need to register for MyPsychKit. See www.mypsychkit.com for complete details.

chapter 15

Schizophrenia, Affective Disorders, and Anxiety Disorders

LEARNING OBJECTIVES

1. Describe the symptoms of schizophrenia and discuss evidence concerning its heritability.

2. Summarize the dopamine hypothesis of schizophrenia and discuss drugs that alleviate or produce the positive symptoms of schizophrenia.

3. Describe evidence that schizophrenia may result from abnormal brain development.

4. Describe evidence linking both the positive and negative symptoms to decreased activity of the prefrontal cortex.

5. Describe the two major affective disorders, their heritability, and their physiological treatments.

6. Summarize the monoamine hypothesis of depression and review evidence for brain abnormalities in people with affective disorders.

7. Explain the role of circadian rhythms in affective disorders: the effects of REM sleep deprivation and total sleep deprivation and the symptoms and treatment of seasonal affective disorder.

8. Describe the symptoms, possible causes, and treatments of panic disorder, generalized anxiety disorder, and social anxiety disorder.

9. Describe the symptoms, possible causes, and treatments of obsessive-compulsive disorder.

PROLOGUE Anxiety Surgery

In 1935 the report of an experiment with a chimpanzee triggered events whose repercussions are still felt today. Jacobsen, Wolfe, and Jackson (1935) tested some chimpanzees on a behavioral task that requires the animal to remain quiet and remember the location of food that the experimenter has placed behind a screen. One animal, Becky, displayed a violent emotional reaction whenever she made an error while performing this task. "[When] the experimenter lowered . . . the opaque door to exclude the animal's view of the cups, she immediately flew into a temper tantrum, rolled on the floor, defecated, and urinated. After a few such reactions during the training period, the animal would make no further responses." After the chimpanzee's frontal lobes were removed, it became a model of good comportment. It "offered its usual friendly greeting, and eagerly ran from its living quarters to the transfer cage, and in turn went properly to the experimental cage. . . . If the animal made a mistake, it showed no evidence of emotional disturbance but quietly awaited the loading of the cups for the next trial" (Jacobsen, Wolfe, and Jackson, 1935, pp. 9–10).

These findings were reported at a scientific meeting in 1935, which was attended by Egas Moniz, a Portuguese neuropsychiatrist. He heard the report by Jacobsen and his colleagues and also one by Brickner (1936), which indicated that radical removal of the frontal lobes in a human patient (performed because of a tumor) did not appear to produce intellectual impairment; therefore, people could presumably get along without their frontal lobes. These two reports suggested to Moniz that "if frontal-lobe removal . . . eliminates frustrational behavior, why would it not be feasible to relieve anxiety states in man by surgical means?" (Fulton, 1949, pp. 63–64). In fact, Moniz persuaded a neurosurgeon to do so, and approximately one hundred operations were eventually performed under his supervision. In 1949 Moniz received the Nobel Prize for the development of this procedure.

Most of the discussion in this book has concentrated on the physiology of normal, adaptive behavior. The last two chapters summarize research on the nature and physiology of syndromes characterized by maladaptive behavior: mental disorders, autism, attention-deficit/hyperactivity disorder, stress disorders, and drug abuse. The symptoms of mental disorders include deficient or inappropriate social behaviors; illogical, incoherent, or obsessional thoughts; inappropriate emotional responses, including depression, mania, or anxiety; and delusions and hallucinations. Research in recent years indicates that many of these symptoms are caused by abnormalities in the brain, both structural and biochemical.

Schizophrenia

Description

Schizophrenia is a serious mental disorder that afflicts approximately 1 percent of the world's population. Its monetary cost to society is enormous; in the United States this figure exceeds that of the cost of all cancers (Thaker and Carpenter, 2001). Descriptions of symptoms in ancient writings indicate that the disorder has been around for thousands of years (Jeste et al., 1985). The major symptoms of schizophrenia are universal, and clinicians have developed criteria for reliably diagnosing the disorder in people of a wide variety of cultures (Flaum and Andreasen, 1990). *Schizophrenia* is probably the most misused psychological term in existence. The word literally means "split mind," but it does *not* imply a split or multiple personality. People often say that they "feel schizophrenic" about an issue when they really mean that they have mixed feelings about it. A person who sometimes wants to build a cabin in the wilderness and live off the land and at other times wants to take over the family insurance agency might be undecided, but he or she is not schizophrenic. The man who invented the term, Eugen Bleuler (1911/1950), intended it to refer to a break with reality caused by disorganization of the various functions of the mind, such that thoughts and feelings no longer worked together normally.

Schizophrenia is characterized by three categories of symptoms: positive, negative, and cognitive (Mueser and McGurk, 2004). **Positive symptoms** make themselves known by their presence. They include thought disorders, hallucinations, and delusions. A **thought disorder**—disorganized, irrational thinking—is probably the most important symptom of schizophrenia. Schizophrenics have great difficulty arranging their thoughts logically and sorting out plausible conclusions from absurd ones. In conversation they jump from one topic to another as new associations come up. Sometimes, they utter meaningless words or choose words for rhyme rather than for meaning. **Delusions** are beliefs that are obviously contrary to fact. Delusions of *persecution* are false beliefs that others are plotting and conspiring against oneself. Delusions of *grandeur* are false beliefs in one's power and importance, such as a conviction that one has godlike powers or has special knowledge that no one else possesses. Delusions of *control* are related to delusions of persecution; the belief (for example) that one is being controlled by others through such means as radar or tiny radio receivers implanted in one's brain.

The third positive symptom of schizophrenia is **hallucinations**, perceptions of stimuli that are not actually present. The most common schizophrenic hallucinations are auditory, but they can also involve any of the other senses. The typical schizophrenic hallucination consists of voices talking to the person. Sometimes, the voices order the person to do something; sometimes, they scold the person for his or her unworthiness; sometimes, they just utter meaningless phrases. Olfactory hallucinations are also fairly common; often they contribute to the delusion that others are trying to kill the person with poison gas. (See *Table 15.1.*)

In contrast to the positive symptoms, the **negative symptoms** of schizophrenia are known by the absence or diminution of normal behaviors: flattened emotional response, poverty of speech, lack of initiative and persistence, *anhedonia* (inability to experience pleasure), and social withdrawal. The **cognitive symptoms** of schizophrenia are closely related to the negative symptoms and may be produced by abnormalities in the same brain regions. These symptoms include difficulty in sustaining attention, low *psychomotor speed* (the ability to rapidly and fluently perform movements of the fingers, hands, and legs), deficits in learning and memory, poor abstract thinking, and poor problem solving. Negative symptoms and cognitive symptoms are not specific to schizophrenia; they are seen in many neurological disorders that involve brain damage, especially to the frontal lobes. As we will see later in this chapter, positive symptoms appear to involve excessive activity in some neural circuits that include dopamine as a neurotransmitter, and negative symptoms and cognitive symptoms appear to be caused by developmental or degenerative processes that impair the normal functions of some regions of the brain. (See *Table 15.1.*)

schizophrenia A serious mental disorder characterized by disordered thoughts, delusions, hallucinations, and often bizarre behaviors.

positive symptom A symptom of schizophrenia evident by its presence: delusions, hallucinations, or thought disorders.

thought disorder Disorganized, irrational thinking.

delusion A belief that is clearly in contradiction to reality.

hallucination Perception of a nonexistent object or event.

negative symptom A symptom of schizophrenia characterized by the absence of behaviors that are normally present: social withdrawal, lack of affect, and reduced motivation.

cognitive symptom A symptom of schizophrenia characterized by cognitive difficulties, such as deficits in learning and memory, poor abstract thinking, and poor problem solving.

TABLE 15.1 Positive, Cognitive, and Negative Symptoms of Schizophrenia		
Positive	**Negative**	**Cognitive**
Hallucinations	Flattened emotional response	Difficulty in sustaining attention
Thought disorders	Poverty of speech	Low psychomotor speed
Delusions	Lack of initiative and persistence	Deficits in learning and memory
Persecution	Anhedonia	Poor abstract thinking
Grandeur	Social withdrawal	Poor problem solving
Control		

The symptoms of schizophrenia typically appear gradually and insidiously, over a period of 3 to 5 years. Negative symptoms are the first to emerge, followed by cognitive symptoms. The positive symptoms follow several years later. As we will see later, this progression of symptoms provides some hints about the nature of the brain abnormalities that are responsible for them.

Heritability

One of the strongest pieces of evidence that schizophrenia is a biological disorder is that it appears to be heritable. Both adoption studies (Kety et al., 1968, 1994) and twin studies (Gottesman and Shields, 1982; Tsuang, Gilbertson, and Faraone, 1991) indicate that schizophrenia is a heritable trait.

If schizophrenia were a simple trait produced by a single gene, we would expect to see this disorder in at least 75 percent of the children of two schizophrenic parents if the gene were dominant. If it were recessive, *all* children of two schizophrenic parents should become schizophrenic. However, the actual incidence is less than 50 percent, which means either that several genes are involved or that having a "schizophrenia gene" imparts a *susceptibility* to develop schizophrenia, the disease itself being triggered by other factors.

So far, researchers have not yet located a "schizophrenia gene," although many candidates have been found. A review by Crow (2007) notes that evidence for linkage to susceptibility for schizophrenia has been reported for 21 of the 23 pairs of chromosomes, but many of the findings have not been replicated. So far, no single gene has been shown to cause schizophrenia, the way that mutations in the genes for γ-secretase or amyloid precursor protein apparently produce Alzheimer's disease. Walsh et al. (2008) suggest that a large number of rare mutations play a role in the development of schizophrenia. For example, mutations of *DISC1 (disrupted in schizophrenia 1)*, a gene involved in regulation of neuronal migration during development, have been found in some families with a high incidence of schizophrenia (Chubb et al., 2008). Mutations that affect neural differentiation and growth, guidance of axons during brain development, assembly of components of neurotransmitter receptors, and factors that control the formation of synapses could be responsible for susceptibility to schizophrenia in different families, and population-wide genetic studies would miss these mutations.

Pharmacology of Schizophrenia: The Dopamine Hypothesis

Pharmacological evidence suggests that the positive symptoms of schizophrenia are caused by a biochemical disorder. The explanation that has received the most attention from researchers is the *dopamine hypothesis*, which suggests that the positive symptoms of schizophrenia are caused by overactivity of synapses between dopaminergic neurons of the ventral tegmental area and neurons in the nucleus accumbens and amygdala.

Around the middle of the twentieth century, a French surgeon named Henri Laborit discovered that a drug used to prevent surgical shock seemed also to reduce anxiety. A French drug company developed a related compound called chlorpromazine, which seemed to be even more effective (Snyder, 1974). The discovery of the antipsychotic effects of chlorpromazine profoundly altered the way in which physicians treated schizophrenic patients and made prolonged hospital stays unnecessary for many of them (the patients, that is).

Since the discovery of chlorpromazine, many other drugs have been developed that relieve the positive symptoms of schizophrenia. These drugs were found to have one property in common: They block dopamine receptors (Creese, Burt, and Snyder, 1976; Strange, 2008).

Another category of drugs has the opposite effect, namely, *production* of the positive symptoms of schizophrenia. The drugs that can produce these symptoms have one known pharmacological effect in common: They act as dopamine agonists. These drugs include amphetamine, cocaine, and methylphenidate (which block the reuptake of dopamine) and L-DOPA (which stimulates the synthesis of dopamine). The symptoms that these drugs produce can be alleviated with antipsychotic drugs, a result that further strengthens the argument that the antipsychotic drugs exert their therapeutic effects by blocking dopamine receptors.

How might we explain the apparent link between overactivity of dopaminergic synapses and the positive symptoms of schizophrenia? Most researchers believe that the mesolimbic pathway, which begins in the ventral tegmental area and ends in the nucleus accumbens and amygdala, is likely to be involved in the symptoms of schizophrenia. As we saw in Chapter 12, the activity of dopaminergic synapses in the nucleus accumbens appears to be a vital link in the process of reinforcement.

The positive symptoms of schizophrenia also include disordered thinking and unpleasant, often terrifying delusions. The disordered thinking may be caused by disorganized attentional processes; the indiscriminate activity of the dopaminergic synapses in the nucleus accumbens makes it difficult for the patients to follow an orderly, rational thought sequence. Fibiger (1991) suggests that paranoid delusions may be caused by increased activity of the dopaminergic input to the amygdala. As we saw in Chapter 10, the central nucleus of the amygdala is involved with conditioned emotional responses elicited by aversive stimuli. The central nucleus receives a strong projection from the mesolimbic dopaminergic system, so Fibiger's suggestion is certainly plausible.

Recent years have seen the development of the *atypical antipsychotic medications*, which reduce both the positive symptoms and negative symptoms of schizophrenia—even those of many patients who were not significantly helped by the older antipsychotic drugs. Clozapine, the first of the atypical antipsychotic medications, has been joined by several others, including risperidone, olanzapine, ziprasidone, and aripiprazole. To understand how these drugs work, we first need to know more about the results of research on the neuropathology of schizophrenia, which brings us to the next section.

Schizophrenia as a Neurological Disorder

So far, I have been discussing the physiology of the positive symptoms of schizophrenia—principally, hallucinations, delusions, and thought disorders. These symptoms could very well be related to one of the known functions of dopaminergic neurons: reinforcement. However, the negative and cognitive symptoms of schizophrenia are very different. Whereas the positive symptoms are unique to schizophrenia (and to amphetamine or cocaine psychosis), the negative and cognitive symptoms are similar to those produced by brain damage caused by several different means. (In fact, some investigators do not distinguish between negative symptoms and cognitive symptoms.) Many pieces of evidence suggest that these symptoms of schizophrenia are indeed a result of brain abnormalities. As we will see, these abnormalities give rise to increased secretion of dopamine in the nucleus accumbens and the accompanying positive symptoms.

Evidence for Brain Abnormalities in Schizophrenia

Although schizophrenia has traditionally been labeled a psychiatric disorder, most patients with schizophrenia exhibit neurological symptoms that suggest the presence of brain damage—in particular, poor control of eye movements and unusual facial expressions (Stevens, 1982). In addition, many studies have found evidence of loss of brain tissue in CT and MRI scans of schizophrenic patients. In one of the ear-

FIGURE 15.1

Relative Ventricular Size in Chronic Schizophrenics and Controls

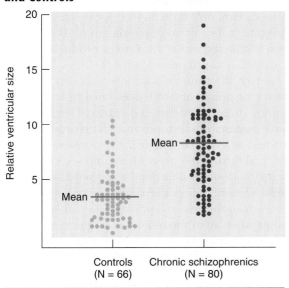

Adapted from Weinberger, D. R., and Wyatt, R. J., in *Schizophrenia as a Brain Disease*, edited by F. A. Henn and H. A. Nasrallah. New York: Oxford University Press, 1982.

FIGURE 15.2

Cerebral Gray Matter and Schizophrenia.   The graph shows changes in volume of cerebral gray matter with age in normal subjects and people with schizophrenia.

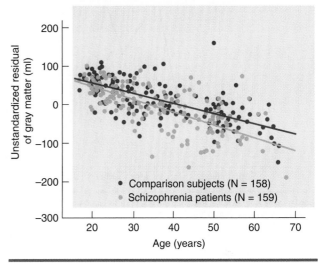

Adapted from Hulshoff-Pol, H. E., Schnack, H. G., Bertens, M. G. B. C., et al. *American Journal of Psychiatry*, 2002, *159*, 244–250.

liest studies, Weinberger and Wyatt (1982) obtained CT scans of eighty chronic schizophrenics and sixty-six normal controls of the same mean age (29 years). They found that the relative size of the lateral ventricles of the schizophrenic patients was more than twice as great as that of the normal control subjects. (See *Figure 15.1*.) The most likely cause of the enlarged ventricles is loss of brain tissue; thus, the CT scans provide evidence that chronic schizophrenia is associated with brain abnormalities. In fact, Hulshoff-Pol et al. (2002) found that although everyone loses some cerebral gray matter as they age, the rate of tissue loss is greater in schizophrenic patients. (See *Figure 15.2*.)

Possible Causes of the Brain Abnormalities

As we saw earlier, schizophrenia is a heritable disease, but its heritability is less than perfect. Why do fewer than half the children of parents with chronic schizophrenia become schizophrenic? Perhaps what is inherited is a defect that renders people susceptible to some environmental factors that adversely affect brain development or cause brain damage later in life. Let's look at the evidence concerning environmental factors that increase the risk of schizophrenia.

Epidemiological Studies   **Epidemiology** is the study of the distribution and causes of diseases in populations. Thus, epidemiological studies examine the relative frequency of diseases in groups of people in different environments and try to correlate the disease frequencies with factors that are present in these environments. Evidence from these studies indicates that the incidence of schizophrenia is related to several environmental factors:, season of birth, viral epidemics, and population density. Let's examine each of these factors in turn.

Many studies have shown that people born during the late winter and early spring are more likely to develop schizophrenia—a phenomenon known as the **seasonality effect**. For example, Kendell and Adams (1991) studied the month of birth of over 13,000 schizophrenic patients born in Scotland between 1914 and

epidemiology The study of the distribution and causes of diseases in populations.

seasonality effect The increased incidence of schizophrenia in people born during late winter and early spring.

FIGURE 15.3

The Seasonality Effect. The graph shows the number of schizophrenic births per 10,000 live births.

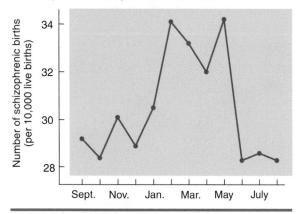

Based on data from Kendell, R. E., and Adams, W. *British Journal of Psychiatry*, 1991, *158*, 758–763.

1960. They found that disproportionately more patients were born in February, March, April, and May. (See *Figure 15.3*.)

What factors might be responsible for the seasonality effect? One possibility is that pregnant women may be more likely to contract a viral illness during a critical phase of their infants' development. The brain development of their fetuses may be adversely affected either by a toxin produced by the virus or by the mother's antibodies against the virus. As Pallast et al. (1994) noted, the winter flu season coincides with the second trimester of pregnancy of babies born in late winter and early spring. In fact, Kendell and Adams (1991) found that the relative number of schizophrenic births in late winter and early spring was especially high if the temperature was lower than normal during the previous autumn—a condition that keeps people indoors and favors the transmission of viral illnesses. Similarly, Eaton, Mortensen, and Frydenberg (2000) reported that schizophrenia is approximately three times higher in people who live in the middle of large cities than in those who live in rural areas, presumably because the transmission of infectious illnesses is facilitated by increased population density.

If the viral hypothesis is true, then an increased incidence of schizophrenia should be seen in babies born a few months after an influenza epidemic, whatever the season. Several studies have observed just that (Mednick, Machon, and Huttunen, 1990; Sham et al., 1992). A study by Brown et al. (2004) examined stored samples of blood serum that had been taken during pregnancy from mothers of children who later developed schizophrenia. They found elevated levels of interleukin-8, a protein secreted by cells of the immune system. The presence of this chemical indicates the presence of an infection or other inflammatory process, and supports the suggestion that maternal infections during the second trimester can increase the incidence of schizophrenia in the women's children. Presumably, some critical aspects of brain development occur during this time. Brown (2006) noted that research has found that maternal infection with at least two other infections diseases—rubella (German measles) and toxoplasmosis—are associated with in increased incidence of schizophrenia.

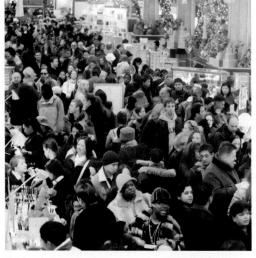

Epidemiological studies have provided important information about the possible causes of schizophrenia. For example, the fact that schizophrenia is more prevalent in crowded urban areas with cold winter climates suggests that viral infections may play a role.

Although cold weather and crowding may contribute to the seasonality effect by increasing the likelihood of infectious illness, another variable may also play a role: a vitamin D deficiency. Dealberto (2007) noted that Northern European researchers have observed a threefold increase in the incidence of schizophrenia in immigrants and the children of immigrants—especially in dark-skinned people. Vitamin D is a fat-soluble chemical that is produced in the skin by the action of ultraviolet rays on a chemical derived from cholesterol. People whose ancestors lived near the equator, where the sunlight is intense all year long, have dark skin, while those whose ancestors lived in more extreme latitudes (such as Northern Europeans) have light skin. The evolutionary change of the skin color of Northern Europeans from the original dark skin to light skin is an adaptation that permitted them to make more vitamin D in conditions of less-intense sunlight. When people with dark skin move to more northern regions, they and their offspring are likely to sustain a vitamin D deficiency because the pigment in their skin blocks much of the ultraviolet radiation. In addition, many people of African origin are lactose intolerant, and hence drink less milk, which is fortified with vitamin D. Because vitamin D plays an important role in brain development, this deficiency may be a risk factor for schizophrenia. These considerations suggest that at least some of the increased incidence of schizophrenia in city dwellers and those who live in cold climates may be attributable to a vitamin D deficiency. Some investigators have suggested that with the increased use of sunscreens, which can reduce the production of vitamin D by the skin by up to 98 percent, people should take daily vitamin D supplements to compensate for the decreased absorption of ultraviolet radiation by the skin (Tavera-Mendoza and White, 2007).

Evidence for Abnormal Brain Development   Both behavioral and anatomical evidence indicates that abnormal prenatal development is associated with schizophrenia. Let's first consider behavioral evidence. A study by Cannon et al. (1997) found that children who later became schizophrenic had poorer social adjustment and did more poorly in school. In 1972, 265 Danish children, aged 11 to 13 years, were videotaped briefly while eating lunch (Schiffman et al., 2004). Many of these children had a schizophrenic parent, which meant that many of them were at increased risk for developing schizophrenia. In 1991, the investigators examined the medical records of these children and determined which of them had developed schizophrenia. Raters, who did not know the identities of the children, found that those who later developed schizophrenia displayed less sociability and deficient psychomotor functioning. The results of these studies are consistent with the hypothesis that although the symptoms of schizophrenia are not normally seen in childhood, the early brain development of children who later become schizophrenic is not entirely normal.

Minor physical anomalies, such as a high-steepled palate, partial webbing of the two middle toes, or especially wide-set or narrow-set eyes, have also been shown to be associated with the incidence of schizophrenia (Schiffman et al., 2002). These differences were first reported in the late nineteenth century by Kraepelin, one of the pioneers in schizophrenia research. As Schiffman and his colleagues note, these anomalies provide evidence of factors that have adverse effects on development.

As we saw, the concordance rate of monozygotic twins for schizophrenia is less than 100 percent. In the past, most researchers assumed that discordance for schizophrenia in monozygotic twins must be caused by differential exposure to some environmental factors after birth. Not only are monozygotic twins genetically identical, but they also share the same intrauterine environment. Thus, because all prenatal factors should be identical, any differences must be a result of factors in the postnatal environment. However, some investigators have pointed out that the prenatal environment of monozygotic twins is *not* identical. In fact, there are two types of monozygotic twins: monochorionic and dichorionic. The formation of monozygotic twins occurs when the blastocyst (the developing organism) splits in two—when it clones itself. If twinning occurs before day 4, the two organisms develop independently, each forming its own placenta. (That is, the twins are *dichorionic*. The *chorion* is the outer layer of the blastocyst, which gives rise to the placenta.) If twinning occurs after day 4, the two organisms become *monochorionic*, sharing a single placenta. (See ***Figure 15.4***.)

The placenta transports nutrients to the developing organism from the mother's circulation and transports waste products to her, which she metabolizes in her liver or excretes in her urine. It also constitutes the barrier through which toxins or infectious agents must pass if they are to affect fetal development. The prenatal environments of monochorionic twins, who share a single placenta, are more similar than those of dichorionic twins. Thus, we might expect that the concordance rates for schizophrenia of *monochorionic* monozygotic twins should be higher than those of *dichorionic* monozygotic twins. In fact, they are. Davis, Phelps, and Bracha (1995) found that the concordance rate for schizophrenia was 10.7 percent in the dichorionic twins and 60 percent in the monochorionic twins. These results

FIGURE 15.4

Monozygotic Twins. This figure shows (a) monochorionic twins, sharing a single placenta, and (b) dichorionic twins, each with its own placenta.

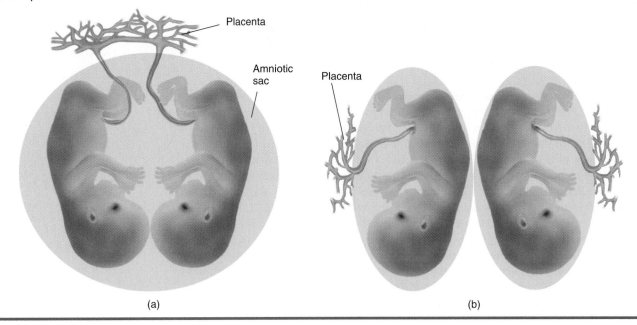

Placenta

Amniotic sac

Placenta

(a)

(b)

provide strong evidence for an interaction between heredity and environment during prenatal development.

Although studies have found that people who develop schizophrenia show some abnormalities even during childhood, the symptoms of schizophrenia itself rarely begin before late adolescence or early adulthood. If schizophrenia does begin during childhood, the symptoms are likely to be more severe. Figure 15.5 shows a graph of the ages of first signs of mental disorder in males and females diagnosed with schizophrenia. (See *Figure 15.5.*)

In a review of the literature, Woods (1998) notes that MRI studies suggest that schizophrenia is not caused by a degenerative process, as are Parkinson's disease, Huntington's disease, and Alzheimer's disease, in which neurons continue to die over a period of years. Instead, a sudden, rapid loss of brain volume typically occurs during young adulthood, with little evidence for continuing degeneration. This loss coincides with a much smaller decrease in volume of cortical gray matter that occurs even in normal young people. Perhaps the disease process of schizophrenia begins prenatally and then lies dormant until puberty, when the normal process of "synaptic pruning" that occurs at that time triggers degeneration of some population of neurons. A study by Cannon, Jones, and Murray (2002) comparing members of twins who were discordant for schizophrenia found that the loss of cortical gray matter was much greater in the twins with schizophrenia. They also found that changes in the volume of the dorsolateral prefrontal cor-

FIGURE 15.5

Age at First Sign of Psychotic Symptoms in Schizophrenic Patients

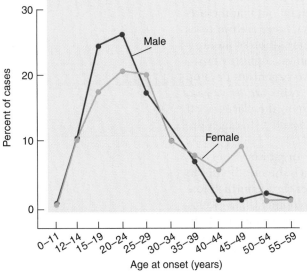

Adapted from Häfner H., Riecher-Rössler A., an der Heiden W., et al. *Psychological Medicine*, 1993, *23*, 925–940.

tex were most strongly influenced by hereditary factors. The next subsection of this chapter describes the significance of this finding.

Relationship Between Positive and Negative Symptoms: Role of the Prefrontal Cortex

As we saw, schizophrenia has positive, negative, and cognitive symptoms. The positive symptoms may be caused by hyperactivity of dopaminergic synapses, and the negative and cognitive symptoms may be caused by developmental or degenerative changes in the brain. Is there a relationship between these categories of schizophrenic symptoms? An accumulating amount of evidence suggests that the answer is yes.

Many studies have shown evidence from MRI scans and postmortem examination of brain tissue that schizophrenia is associated with abnormalities in many parts of the brain (Shenton et al., 2001). In recent years the prefrontal cortex has received a great deal of attention. Weinberger (1988) first suggested that the negative symptoms of schizophrenia are caused primarily by **hypofrontality**, decreased activity of the frontal lobes—in particular, of the dorsolateral prefrontal cortex. In fact, schizophrenic patients do poorly on neuropsychological tests that are sensitive to prefrontal damage. Figure 15.6 shows composite functional MRI scans from a study by MacDonald et al. (2005) of subjects with schizophrenia and normal comparison subjects taken while the people were performing a task that required concentration and focused attention. As you can see, the dorsolateral prefrontal cortex was activated in the normal subjects but not in the subjects with schizophrenia. (See *Figure 15.6.*)

What might produce the hypofrontality that so many studies have observed? Ironically, the cause might be a *decrease* in the release of dopamine in the prefrontal cortex. Dopamine plays an important role in the normal functioning of the prefrontal cortex; studies with monkeys indicate that destruction of the dopaminergic input to the prefrontal cortex lowers its metabolic rate and leads to cognitive dysfunctions (Brozowski et al., 1979). In fact, Sawaguchi and Goldman-Rakic (1994) found that injection of dopamine antagonists into the prefrontal cortex of monkeys caused behavioral deficits like those produced by prefrontal lesions.

As we saw in the discussion of the dopamine hypothesis of schizophrenia, dopamine agonists such as cocaine and amphetamine can cause positive symptoms of schizophrenia. Two other drugs, PCP (phencyclidine, also known as "angel dust") and ketamine ("Special K"), can cause all three types of symptoms of schizophrenia: positive, negative, and cognitive (Adler et al., 1999; Lahti et al., 2001; Avila et al., 2002). Because PCP and ketamine elicit the full range of the symptoms of schizophrenia, many researchers believe that studying the physiological and behavioral effects of these drugs will help to solve the puzzle of schizophrenia.

The negative and cognitive symptoms produced by ketamine and PCP are apparently caused by a decrease in the metabolic activity of the frontal lobes. Jentsch et al. (1997) administered PCP to monkeys twice a day for 2 weeks. Then, 1 week later, they tested the animals on a task that involved reaching around a barrier, which was performed poorly by monkeys with lesions of the prefrontal cortex. Normal monkeys performed well, but those that had been treated with PCP showed a severe deficit. (See *Figure 15.7.*)

As you might recall from Chapter 4, PCP is an indirect antagonist of NMDA-receptors. (So is ketamine.) By inhibiting the activity of NMDA receptors, PCP

FIGURE 15.6

Hypofrontality in Schizophrenia. The images show composite functional MRI scans of subjects with schizophrenia and normal comparison subjects taken while the people were performing a task that required concentration and focused attention. The schizophrenic subjects show deficient activation of the dorsolateral prefrontal cortex (hypofrontality).

Dorsal prefrontal cortex

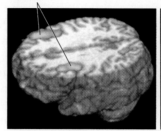 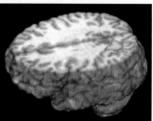

Normal subjects   Schizophrenic patients

From MacDonald, A. W., Carter, C. S., Kerns, J. G., et al. *American Journal of Psychiatry*, 2005, *162*, 475–484. Reprinted with permission from the American Journal of Psychiatry, (Copyright 2005). American Psychiatric Association.

hypofrontality Decreased activity of the prefrontal cortex; believed to be responsible for the negative symptoms of schizophrenia.

FIGURE 15.7

Chronic PCP Treatment and Perseveration.   The graphs show the effects of 2 weeks of PCP treatment on the performance of monkeys on a task that requires reaching around a barrier. An increased number of reaches toward the barrier is an indication of perseveration of an incorrect response.

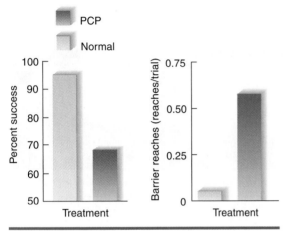

Adapted from Jentsch, J. D., Redmond, D. E., Elsworth, J. D., et al. *Science*, 1997, *277*, 953–955.

FIGURE 15.8

Prefrontal Inhibition of Dopamine Release.   The graph shows the effects of electrical stimulation of the prefrontal cortex on the release of dopamine in the nucleus accumbens (NAC), as measured by microdialysis.

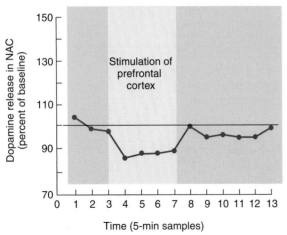

Adapted from Jackson, M. E., Frost, A. D., and Moghaddam, B. *Journal of Neurochemistry*, 2001, *78*, 920–923.

suppresses the activity of several regions of the brain—most notably, the dorsolateral prefrontal cortex. These drugs also decrease the level of dopamine utilization in this region (Elsworth et al., 2008), possibly as a result of the inhibitory effect on NMDA receptors. The hypoactivity of NMDA and dopamine receptors appear to play an important role in the production of negative and cognitive symptoms: Suppression of these receptors causes hypofrontality, which appears to be the primary cause of the symptoms. But why might hypoactivity of NMDA and dopamine receptors in the prefrontal cortex cause the positive symptoms of schizophrenia, which appear to be produced by *hyperactivity* of dopaminergic synapses in the nucleus accumbens?

Evidence indicates that these events are linked—that prefrontal hypoactivity causes hyperactivity of mesolimbic dopaminergic neurons. Excitatory glutamatergic neurons of the prefrontal cortex send axons to the ventral tegmental area, where they form synapses with dopaminergic neurons that project back to the prefrontal cortex. They also form synapses with GABA-secreting neurons in the ventral tegmental area that inhibit another set of dopaminergic neurons that project to the nucleus accumbens (Carr and Sesack, 2000). Jackson, Frost, and Moghaddam (2001) found that electrical stimulation of the prefrontal cortex inhibits the release of dopamine in the nucleus accumbens, as measured by microdialysis. (See *Figure 15.8*.) In contrast, Jentsch et al. (1998) found that infusion of PCP directly into the prefrontal cortex (which suppresses the activity of this region) increased the release of dopamine in the nucleus accumbens. Thus, decreased activation of the prefrontal cortex causes an increase in the release of dopamine in the nucleus accumbens.

We also saw that the atypical antipsychotic drug clozapine alleviates the positive, negative, and cognitive symptoms of schizophrenia. In a study with monkeys, Youngren et al. (1999) found that injections of clozapine, which cause an *increase* in the release of dopamine in the prefrontal cortex, also caused a *decrease* in the release of dopamine in the nucleus accumbens.

As we saw earlier in this chapter, schizophrenia has a gradual onset, beginning with negative symptoms followed shortly by cognitive symptoms and, several years later, the positive symptoms. The course of the disease and the evidence reviewed in this subsection suggest that a pathological process that typically occurs around late adolescence causes hypofrontality, which involves decreased activation of NMDA receptors. This hypofrontality causes negative and cognitive symptoms to emerge. As the hypofrontality becomes more severe, decreased output from the prefrontal cortex to the ventral tegmental area causes a decrease in dopaminergic transmission to the prefrontal cortex and an increase in dopaminergic transmission to the nucleus accumbens. The cognitive symptoms get worse, and the positive symptoms begin. (See *Figure 15.9*.)

What causes the hypofrontality that appears to be the first step in the development of schizophrenia? One possibility is the synaptic pruning that occurs during adolescence, which might decrease the activity of glutamatergic synapses below a critical value. If decreased activity of NMDA receptors in the prefrontal cortex causes the negative and cognitive symptoms of schizophrenia, then we might expect drugs that act as NMDA agonists to reduce these symptoms. Direct NMDA agonists (such as NMDA itself) cannot be used, because they increase the risk of seizures and might even cause brain damage through excitotoxicity. However, you might remember from Chapter 4 that NMDA receptors have several other sites to which ligands can bind, besides the glutamate site and the PCP site. Glycine and D-serine bind to one of these sites, where they act as indirect agonists. In fact, without the presence of glycine or D-serine, the ion channel of an NMDA receptor will not open, even if glutamate is present and the postsynaptic membrane is depolarized. Normally, adequate amounts of glycine or D-serine are present, but it is possible that administering glycine or D-serine—or glycine agonists such as *sarcosine*—might facilitate NMDA activity and reduce schizophrenic symptoms.

Several studies have found exactly that. (See Javitt, 2008 and Shim, Hammonds, and Kee, 2008, for reviews.) Figure 15.10 summarizes the results of ten studies that assessed the effects of glycine, D-serine, or sarcosine on the negative symptoms of schizophrenia. All but one study found an improvement in these symptoms. (See *Figure 15.10*.)

The research findings presented in this subsection explain why the "classic" antischizophrenic drugs fail to reduce negative and cognitive symptoms: One of the causes of these symptoms is decreased activity of dopamine receptors in the prefrontal cortex, and drugs that block dopamine receptors would, if anything, make these symptoms worse. What is different about the newer atypical antischizophrenic drugs that enables them to reduce all three categories of schizophrenic symptoms?

FIGURE 15.9

Hypofrontality and Schizophrenic Symptoms.   The diagram illustrates a hypothetical explanation for the role of hypofrontality in development of positive and negative symptoms of schizophrenia.

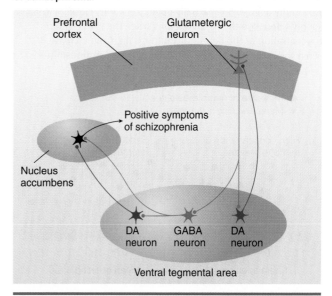

FIGURE 15.10

Treatment of Schizophrenia with NMDA Agonists.   The graph shows the results of ten studies that treated schizophrenic patients with an NMDA agonist (glycine, D-serine, or sarcosine). All but one study showed a reduction of symptoms with the treatment.

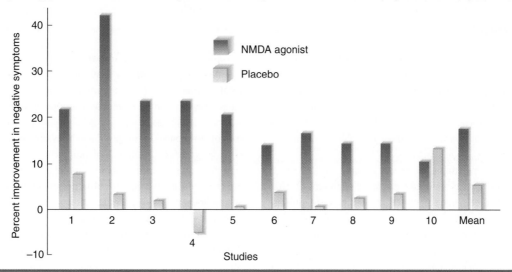

Adapted from Javitt, D. C. *Biological Psychiatry*, 2008, *63*, 6–8.

FIGURE 15.11

Effects of a Partial Agonist.   The diagram explains the differential effects of a partial agonist in regions of high and low concentrations of the normal ligand. Numbers beneath each receptor indicate the degree of opening of the ion channel: 1.0 = fully open, 0.5 = partially open, 0.0 = fully closed. Partial agonists decrease the mean opening when the extracellular concentration of the neurotransmitter is high and increase it when the extracellular concentration of the neurotransmitter is low.

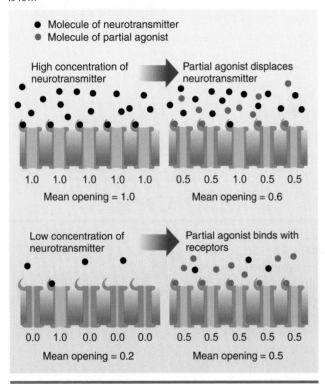

The atypical antischizophrenic drugs seem to do the impossible: They increase dopaminergic activity in the prefrontal cortex and reduce it in the nucleus accumbens. Let's examine the action of one of the newest atypical drugs, *aripiprazole* (Winans, 2003; Lieberman, 2004). Aripiprazole acts as a *partial agonist* at dopamine receptors. A **partial agonist** is a drug that has a very high affinity for a particular receptor but activates that receptor less than the normal ligand does. This means that in a patient with schizophrenia, aripiprazole serves as an antagonist in regions such as the nucleus accumbens, where too much dopamine is present, but serves as an agonist in regions such as the prefrontal cortex, where too little dopamine is present. Hence, this action appears to account for the ability of aripiprazole to reduce all three categories of schizophrenic symptoms. (See *Figure 15.11.*)

In the interest of clarity and brevity, I have been selective in my review of research on schizophrenia. This puzzling and serious disorder has stimulated many ingenious hypotheses and much research. Some hypotheses have been proved wrong; others have not yet been adequately tested. Possibly, future research will find that all of these hypotheses (including the ones discussed here) are incorrect or that one that I have not mentioned is correct. However, I am impressed with recent research, and I believe that we have real hope of finding the causes of schizophrenia in the near future. With the discovery of the causes we can hope for the discovery of methods of prevention and not just treatment.

InterimSummary

Schizophrenia

Researchers have made considerable progress in the past few years in their study of the physiology of mental disorders, but many puzzles still remain. Schizophrenia consists of positive, negative, and cognitive symptoms, the first involving the presence of unusual behavior and the latter two involving the absence or deficiency of normal behavior. Because schizophrenia is strongly heritable, its occurrence must be affected by biological factors.

The dopamine hypothesis, which was inspired by the findings that dopamine antagonists alleviate the positive symptoms of schizophrenia and that dopamine agonists increase or even produce them, states that the positive symptoms of schizophrenia are caused by hyperactivity of dopaminergic synapses. The involvement of dopamine in reinforcement could plausibly explain the positive effects of schizophrenia; inappropriately reinforced thoughts could persist and become delusions.

The fact that the negative and cognitive symptoms of schizophrenia are not alleviated by "classical" antipsychotic drugs poses an unsolved problem for the dopamine hypothesis. Atypical antipsychotic drugs, including clozapine, risperidone, olanzapine, ziprasidone, and aripiprazole, reduce positive symptoms as well as negative and cognitive ones, and they reduce the symptoms of some patients who are not helped by traditional antipsychotic medication. In addition, these drugs reduce positive symptoms as well as negative ones, and they reduce the symptoms of some patients who are not helped by traditional antipsychotic medication.

MRI scans and the presence of signs of neurological impairments indicate the presence of brain abnormalities in schizophrenic patients. Studies of the epidemiology of schizophrenia indicate that season of birth, a cold climate, viral epidemics during pregnancy, and population density all contribute to the occurrence of schizophrenia. The most sensitive period appears to occur during the second trimester of pregnancy. A vitamin D deficiency, caused by insufficient exposure to sunlight or insufficient intake of the vitamin itself, may at least partly account for the effects of season of birth, population density, a cold climate, and maternal nutrition. In addition, videos of young children who became schizophrenic reveal early abnormalities in movements and social behavior. More evidence is provided by the presence of an increased size of the lateral ventricles in schizophrenic patients. The increased concordance rate of monochorionic monozygotic twins indicates that hereditary and prenatal environmental factors may interact.

The symptoms of schizophrenia often emerge soon after puberty, when the brain is undergoing important maturational changes. Some investigators believe that the disease process of schizophrenia begins prenatally, lies dormant until puberty, and then causes a period of neural degeneration that causes the symptoms to appear.

The negative symptoms of schizophrenia appear to be a result of hypofrontality (decreased activity of the dorsolateral prefrontal cortex), which may be caused by a decreased release of dopamine in this region, perhaps in turn caused by decreased activation of glutamatergic NMDA receptors. Schizophrenic patients do poorly on tasks that require activity of the prefrontal cortex, and functional imaging studies indicate that the prefrontal cortex is hypoactive when the patients attempt to perform these tasks.

The drugs PCP and ketamine mimic both the positive and negative symptoms of schizophrenia. Long-term administration of PCP to monkeys disrupts their performance of a reaching task that requires the prefrontal cortex. Furthermore, the disruption is related to the decrease in prefrontal dopaminergic activity caused by the drug. Evidence suggests that hypofrontality causes an increase in the activity of dopaminergic neurons in the mesolimbic system, thus producing the positive symptoms of schizophrenia. Connections between the prefrontal cortex and the ventral tegmental area appear to be responsible for this phenomenon. Clozapine, an atypical antipsychotic drug, reduces hypofrontality, increases the performance of monkeys on the reaching task, and decreases the release of dopamine in the ventral tegmental area—and decreases both the positive and negative symptoms of schizophrenia. An even newer atypical antipsychotic drug, aripiprazole, serves as a partial agonist for dopamine receptors, increasing activation of DA receptors in regions that contain little dopamine (such as the prefrontal cortex) and decreasing activation of DA receptors in regions that contain excessive amounts of dopamine (such as the nucleus accumbens).

PCP and ketamine act as indirect antagonists for NMDA receptors. Glycine and D-serine, which serve as NMDA receptor agonists, reduce the negative symptoms of schizophrenia, providing further support for the PCP model of this disorder.

Thought Question

Suppose that a young schizophrenic woman insists on living in the streets and refuses to take antipsychotic medication. She is severely disturbed; she is undernourished and often takes intravenous drugs, which expose her to the risk of AIDS. Her parents have tried to get her to seek help, but she believes that they are plotting against her. Suppose further that we can predict with 90 percent accuracy that she will die within a few years. She is not violent, and she has never talked about committing suicide, so we cannot prove that her behavior constitutes an immediate threat to herself or to others. Should her parents be able to force her to receive treatment, or does she have an absolute right to be left alone, even if she is mentally ill?

Major Affective Disorders

Affect, as a noun, refers to feelings or emotions. Just as the primary symptom of schizophrenia is disordered thoughts, the **major affective disorders** (also called *mood disorders*) are characterized by disordered feelings.

Description

Feelings and emotions are essential parts of human existence; they represent our evaluation of the events in our lives. In a very real sense, feelings and emotions are what human life is all about. The emotional state of most of us reflects what is happening to us: Our feelings are tied to events in the real world, and they are usually the result of reasonable assessments of the importance these events have for our lives. However, for some people, affect becomes divorced from reality. These people have feelings of extreme elation (*mania*) or despair (*depression*) that are not justified by events in their lives. For example, depression that accompanies the loss of a loved one is normal, but depression that becomes a way of life—and will not respond to the sympathetic effort of friends and relatives or even to psychotherapy—is pathological. Depression has a prevalence of approximately 3 percent in men and 7 percent in women, which makes it the fourth leading cause of disability (Kessler et al., 2003).

partial agonist A drug that has a very high affinity for a particular receptor but activates that receptor less than the normal ligand does; serves as an agonist in regions of low concentration of the normal ligand and as an antagonist in regions of high concentrations.

major affective disorder A serious mood disorder; includes unipolar depression and bipolar disorder.

There are two principal types of major affective disorders. The first type is characterized by alternating periods of mania and depression—a condition called **bipolar disorder**. This disorder afflicts men and women in approximately equal numbers. Episodes of mania can last a few days or several months, but they usually take a few weeks to run their course. The episodes of depression that follow generally last three times as long as the mania. The second type is **major depressive disorder (MDD)**, characterized by depression without mania. This depression may be continuous and unremitting or, more typically, may come in episodes. Mania without periods of depression sometimes occurs, but it is rare.

Severely depressed people usually feel unworthy and have strong feelings of guilt. The affective disorders are dangerous; a person who suffers from a major affective disorder runs a considerable risk of death by suicide. According to Chen and Dilsaver (1996), 15.9 percent of people with MDD and 29.2 percent of people with bipolar disorder attempt to commit suicide. Schneider, Muller, and Philipp (2001) found that the rate of death by unnatural causes (not all suicides are diagnosed as such) for people with affective disorders was 28.8 times higher than expected for people of the same age in the general population. Depressed people have very little energy, and they move and talk slowly, sometimes becoming almost torpid. At other times, they may pace around restlessly and aimlessly. They may cry a lot. They are unable to experience pleasure and lose their appetite for food and sex. Their sleep is disturbed; they usually have difficulty falling asleep and awaken early and find it difficult to get to sleep again. Even their body functions become depressed; they often become constipated, and secretion of saliva decreases.

> [A psychiatrist] asked me if I was suicidal, and I reluctantly told him yes. I did not particularize—since there seemed no need to—did not tell him that in truth many of the artifacts of my house had become potential devices for my own destruction: the attic rafters (and an outside maple or two) a means to hang myself, the garage a place to inhale carbon monoxide, the bathtub a vessel to receive the flow from my opened arteries. The kitchen knives in their drawers had but one purpose for me. Death by heart attack seemed particularly inviting, absolving me as it would of active responsibility, and I had toyed with the idea of self-induced pneumonia—a long frigid, shirt-sleeved hike through the rainy woods. Nor had I overlooked an ostensible accident . . . by walking in front of a truck on the highway nearby. . . . Such hideous fantasies, which cause well people to shudder, are to the deeply depressed mind what lascivious daydreams are to persons of robust sexuality. (Styron, 1990, pp. 52–53)

Episodes of mania are characterized by a sense of euphoria that does not seem to be justified by circumstances. The diagnosis of mania is partly a matter of degree; one would not call exuberance and a zest for life pathological. People with mania usually exhibit nonstop speech and motor activity. They flit from topic to topic and often have delusions, but they lack the severe disorganization that is seen in schizophrenia. They are usually full of their own importance and often become angry or defensive if they are contradicted. Frequently, they go for long periods without sleep, working furiously on projects that are often unrealistic. (Sometimes, their work is fruitful; George Frideric Handel wrote *Messiah*, one of the masterpieces of choral music, during one of his periods of mania.)

Heritability

Evidence indicates that a tendency to develop an affective disorder is a heritable characteristic. (See Hamet and Tremblay, 2005, for a review.) For example, Rosenthal (1971) found that close relatives of people who suffer from affective psychoses are ten times more likely to develop these disorders than are people without afflicted relatives. Gershon et al. (1976) found that if one member of a set of monozygotic twins was afflicted with an affective disorder, the likelihood that the

bipolar disorder A serious mood disorder characterized by cyclical periods of mania and depression.

major depressive disorder (MDD) A serious mood disorder that consists of unremitting depression or periods of depression that do not alternate with periods of mania.

other twin was similarly afflicted was 69 percent. In contrast, the concordance rate for dizygotic twins was only 13 percent. The heritability of the affective disorders implies that they have a physiological basis.

Genetic studies have found evidence that genes on several chromosomes may be implicated in the development of the affective disorders, but the findings of most linkage studies have not been replicated (Hamet and Tremblay, 2005). As we will see later in this chapter, the strongest candidate is the gene for the serotonin transporter, which plays an important role in brain development. This gene is found on chromosome 17.

Biological Treatments

There are several established and experimental biological treatments for major depressive disorder: monoamine oxidase (MAO) inhibitors, drugs that inhibit the reuptake of norepinephrine or serotonin, electroconvulsive therapy (ECT), transcranial magnetic stimulation, deep brain stimulation, vagus nerve stimulation, bright-light therapy (phototherapy), and sleep deprivation. (Phototherapy and sleep deprivation are discussed in a later section of this chapter.) Bipolar disorder can be treated by lithium and some anticonvulsant drugs. The fact that these disorders often respond to biological treatment provides additional evidence that they have a physiological basis. Furthermore, the fact that lithium is effective in treating bipolar affective disorder but not major depressive disorder suggests that there is a fundamental difference between these two illnesses (Soares and Gershon, 1998).

Before the 1950s there was no effective drug treatment for depression. In the late 1940s clinicians noticed that some drugs used for treating tuberculosis seemed to elevate the patient's mood. Researchers subsequently found that a derivative of these drugs, iproniazid, reduced symptoms of psychotic depression (Crane, 1957). Iproniazid inhibits the activity of MAO, which destroys excess monoamine transmitter substances within terminal buttons. Thus, the drug increases the release of dopamine, norepinephrine, and serotonin. Other MAO inhibitors were soon discovered. Unfortunately, MAO inhibitors can have harmful side effects, so they must be used with caution.

Fortunately, another class of antidepressant drugs was soon discovered that did not have these side effects: the **tricyclic antidepressants**. These drugs were found to inhibit the reuptake of 5-HT and norepinephrine by terminal buttons. By retarding reuptake, the drugs keep the neurotransmitter in contact with the postsynaptic receptors, thus prolonging the postsynaptic potentials. Thus, both the MAO inhibitors and the tricyclic antidepressant drugs are monoaminergic agonists.

Since the discovery of the tricyclic antidepressants, other drugs have been discovered that have similar effects. The most important of these are the **specific serotonin reuptake inhibitors (SSRI)**, whose action is described by their name. These drugs (for example, fluoxetine [Prozac], citalopram [Celexa], and paroxetine [Paxil]) are widely prescribed for their antidepressant properties and for their ability to reduce the symptoms of obsessive-compulsive disorder and social phobia (described later in this chapter). Recently, another class of antidepressant drugs have been developed, the **serotonin and norepinephrine reuptake inhibitors (SNRI)**, which do what their name indicates. These drugs have fewer nonspecific actions, and therefore fewer side effects, than the tricyclic antidepressants, which also have effects on both norepinephrine and serotonin reuptake (Stahl et al., 2005). The category of SNRIs includes milnacipran, duloxetine, and venlafaxine, with relative effects on 5-HT and noradrenergic transporters of 1:1, 1:10, and 1:30, respectively.

Another biological treatment for depression has an interesting history. Early in the twentieth century, a physician named von Meduna noted that psychotic patients who were also subject to epileptic seizures showed improvement immediately after each attack. He reasoned that the violent storm of neural activity in the brain that

tricyclic antidepressant A class of drugs used to treat depression; inhibits the reuptake of norepinephrine and serotonin but also affects other neurotransmitters; named for the molecular structure.

specific serotonin reuptake inhibitor (SSRI) An antidepressant drug that specifically inhibits the reuptake of serotonin without affecting the reuptake of other neurotransmitters.

serotonin and norepinephrine reuptake inhibitor (SNRI) An antidepressant drug that specifically inhibits the reuptake of norepinephrine and serotonin without affecting the reuptake of other neurotransmitters.

FIGURE 15.12

A Patient Being Prepared for Electroconvulsive Therapy

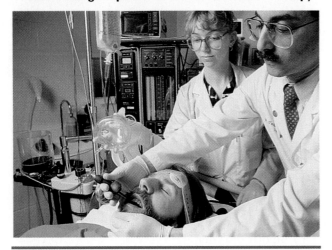

Will and Deni McIntyre/Photo Researchers, Inc.

constitutes an epileptic seizure somehow improved the patients' mental condition. He developed a way to produce seizures by administering a drug, but the procedure was dangerous to the patient. In 1937, Ugo Cerletti, an Italian psychiatrist, developed a less dangerous method for producing seizures (Cerletti and Bini, 1938). He had previously learned that the local slaughterhouse applied a jolt of electricity to animals' heads to stun them before killing them. The electricity appeared to produce a seizure that resembled an epileptic attack. He decided to attempt to use electricity to induce a seizure more safely.

Cerletti tried the procedure on dogs and found that an electrical shock to the skull did produce a seizure and that the animals recovered with no apparent ill effects. He then used the procedure on humans and found it to be safer than the chemical treatment that was previously used. As a result of Cerletti's experiments, **electroconvulsive therapy (ECT)** became a common treatment for mental illness. Before a person receives ECT, he or she is anesthetized and is given a drug similar to curare, which paralyzes the muscles, preventing injuries that might be produced by a convulsion. (Of course, the patient is attached to a respirator until the effects of this drug wear off.) Electrodes are placed on the patient's scalp (most often to the nonspeech-dominant hemisphere, to avoid damaging verbal memories), and a jolt of electricity triggers a seizure. Usually, a patient receives three treatments per week until maximum improvement is seen, which usually involves six to twelve treatments. The effectiveness of ECT has been established by placebo studies, in which some patients are anesthetized but not given shocks (Weiner and Krystal, 1994). Although ECT was originally used for a variety of disorders, including schizophrenia, we now know that its usefulness is limited to treatment of mania and depression. (See *Figure 15.12.*)

Even when depressed patients respond to treatment with antidepressant drugs, they do not do so immediately; improvement in symptoms is not usually seen before 2 to 3 weeks of drug treatment. In contrast, the effects of ECT are more rapid. A few seizures induced by ECT can often snap a person out of a deep depression within a few days. Although prolonged and excessive use of ECT causes brain damage, resulting in long-lasting impairments in memory (Squire, 1974), the judicious use of ECT during the interim period before antidepressant drugs become effective has undoubtedly saved the lives of some suicidal patients.

How does ECT exert its antidepressant effect? It has been known for a long time that seizures have an anticonvulsant effect: ECT decreases brain activity and raises the seizure threshold of the brain, making it less likely for another seizure to occur (Sackeim et al., 1983; Nobler et al., 2001). The increased seizure threshold appears to be caused by an increased release of GABA and neuropeptide Y (Bolwig, Woldbye, and Mikkelsen, 1999; Sanacora et al., 2003). These changes may also be responsible for reducing the symptoms of depression.

Researchers have investigated another procedure designed to provide some of the benefits of ECT without introducing the risk of cognitive impairments or memory loss. As we saw in Chapter 5, transcranial magnetic stimulation (TMS) is accomplished by applying a strong localized magnetic field into the brain by passing an electrical current through a coil of wire placed on the scalp. The magnetic field induces an electrical current in the brain. Several studies suggested that TMS applied to the prefrontal cortex reduces the symptoms of depression without producing any apparent cognitive deficits (Padberg and Moller, 2003; Fitzgerald, 2004). However, a review of the literature by Mitchell and Loo (2006) concluded that

electroconvulsive therapy (ECT) A brief electrical shock, applied to the head, that results in an electrical seizure; used therapeutically to alleviate severe depression.

although studies have obtained statistically significant results, the size of the effect is generally too small to be clinically significant.

Preliminary research suggests that direct electrical stimulation of the brain (deep brain stimulation) may also be a useful therapy for treatment-resistant depression (Mayberg et al., 2005; Lozano et al., 2008). The investigators implanted stimulating electrodes just below the **subgenual anterior cingulate cortex (subgenual ACC)**, a region of the medial prefrontal cortex. If you look at a sagittal view of the corpus callosum, you will see that the front of this structure looks like a bent knee—*genu*, in Latin. The subgenual ACC is located below the "knee" at the front of the corpus callosum. Response to the stimulation began soon, and it increased with time. One month after surgery, 35 percent of the patients showed an improvement in symptoms, and 10 percent showed a complete remission. Six months after surgery, 60 percent showed improvement, and 35 percent showed remission.

Another experimental treatment for depression, electrical stimulation of the vagus nerve, shows some promise of reducing the symptoms of depression (Groves and Brown, 2005). Vagus nerve stimulation provides an indirect form of brain stimulation. It is painless and does not elicit seizures; in fact, the procedure was originally developed as a treatment to prevent seizures in patients with seizure disorders. The stimulation is accomplished by means of an implanted device similar to the one used for deep brain stimulation, described in the section on Parkinson's disease in Chapter 14, except that the stimulating electrodes are attached to the vagus nerve. Approximately 80 percent of the axons in the vagus nerve are afferent, so electrical stimulation of the vagus nerve activates several regions of the brain stem. A review of the literature by Daban et al. (2008) concluded that the procedure showed promise in treatment of patients with treatment-resistant depression, but that further double-blind clinical trials are needed to confirm its efficacy.

Functional imaging studies have shown that the both vagus nerve stimulation and deep brain stimulation cause a progressive decrease in the activity of several brain regions, including the subgenual ACC (Lozano et al., 2008; Pardo et al., 2008). As we will see later in this chapter, other research implicates this region in the development of depression. (See *Figure 15.13*.)

The therapeutic effect of **lithium**, the drug used to treat bipolar affective disorders, is very rapid. This drug, which is administered in the form of lithium carbonate, is most effective in treating the manic phase of a bipolar affective disorder; once the mania is eliminated, depression usually does not follow (Gerbino, Oleshansky, and Gershon, 1978; Soares and Gershon, 1998). Some clinicians and investigators have referred to lithium as psychiatry's wonder drug: It does not suppress normal feelings of emotions, but it leaves patients able to feel and express joy and sadness in response to events in their lives. Similarly, it does not impair intellectual processes; many patients have received the drug continuously for years without any apparent ill effects (Fieve, 1979). Between 70 and 80 percent of patients with bipolar disorder show a positive response to lithium within a week or two (Price and Heninger, 1994).

FIGURE 15.13

Effects of Deep-Brain Stimulation and Vagus Nerve Stimulation.   The scans show the effects of 3 months (a) and 6 months (b) of deep brain stimulation and the effects of 6 months (c) and 1 year (d) of vagus nerve stimulation of patients with treatment-resistant depression. All scans show evidence of decreased activity after treatment. "Warm" colors indicate increased activity and "cool" colors indicate decreased activity in (a) and (b).

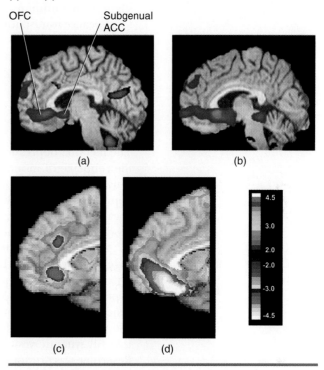

Reprinted from *Biological Psychiatry, 64*, Lozano, A. M., Mayberg, H. S., Giacobbe, P., et al., Subcallosal Cingulate Gyrus Deep Brain Stimulation for Treatment-Resistant Depression, 461–467, Copyright 2008; and from *NeuroImage, 42*, Pardo, J. V., Sheikh, S. A., Schwindt, G. C., et al., Chronic Vagus Nerve Stimulation for Treatment-Resistant Depression Decreases Resting Ventromedial Prefrontal Glucose Metabolism, 879–889, Copyright 2008, with permission from Elsevier.

subgenual anterior cingulate cortex (subgenual ACC) A region of the medial prefrontal cortex located below the "knee" at the front of the corpus callosum; plays a role in the symptoms of depression.

lithium A chemical element; lithium carbonate is used to treat bipolar disorder.

Researchers have found that lithium has many physiological effects, but they have not yet discovered the pharmacological effects of lithium that are responsible for its ability to eliminate mania (Phiel and Klein, 2001). Some suggest that the drug stabilizes the population of certain classes of neurotransmitter receptors in the brain (especially serotonin receptors), thus preventing wide shifts in neural sensitivity. Others have shown that lithium may increase the production of neuroprotective proteins that help to prevent cell death (Manji, Moore, and Chen, 2001). In fact, Moore et al. (2000) found that 4 weeks of lithium treatment for bipolar disorder increased the volume of cerebral gray matter in the patients' brains, a finding that suggests that lithium facilitates neural or glial growth.

Because some patients cannot tolerate the side effects of lithium and because of the potential danger of overdose, researchers have been searching for alternative medications for bipolar disorder. The most promising results have come from the use of anticonvulsants, such as lamotrigine, valproate, and carbamazepine (Grunze, 2005).

The Monoamine Hypothesis

The fact that depression can be treated with MAO inhibitors and drugs that inhibit the reuptake of monoamines suggested the **monoamine hypothesis**: Depression is caused by insufficient activity of monoaminergic neurons. Because the symptoms of depression are not relieved by potent dopamine agonists such as amphetamine or cocaine, most investigators have focused their research efforts on the other two monoamines: norepinephrine and serotonin.

As we saw earlier in this chapter, the dopamine hypothesis of schizophrenia was suggested by the fact that dopamine agonists can produce the symptoms of schizophrenia and dopamine antagonists can reduce them. Similarly, the monoamine hypothesis of depression was suggested by the fact that monoamine antagonists can produce the symptoms of depression and monoamine agonists can reduce them. As you will recall from Chapter 4, the drug *reserpine* blocks the activity of transporters that fill synaptic vesicles in monoaminergic terminals with the neurotransmitter. Reserpine was previously used to lower blood pressure by blocking the release of norepinephrine in muscles in the walls of blood vessels, which causes these muscles to relax. However, reserpine has a serious side effect: By interfering with the release of serotonin and norepinephrine in the brain, it can cause depression. In fact, in the early years of its use as a hypotensive agent, up to 15 percent of the people who received it became depressed (Sachar and Baron, 1979). As we can see, a monoamine antagonist produces the symptoms of depression, and monoamine agonists alleviate them.

Delgado et al. (1990) developed an ingenious approach to study the role of serotonin in depression—the **tryptophan depletion procedure**. They studied depressed patients who were receiving antidepressant medication and were currently feeling well. For 1 day they had the patients follow a low-tryptophan diet (for example, salad, corn, cream cheese, and a gelatin dessert). Then the next day, the patients drank an amino acid "cocktail" that contained no tryptophan. The uptake of amino acids through the blood–brain barrier is accomplished by amino acid transporters. Because the patients' blood level of tryptophan was very low and that of the other amino acids was high, very little tryptophan found its way into the brain, and the level of tryptophan in the brain fell drastically. As you will recall, tryptophan is the precursor of 5-HT, or serotonin. Thus, the treatment lowered the level of serotonin in the brain.

Delgado and his colleagues found that the tryptophan depletion caused most of the patients to relapse back into depression. Then when they began eating a normal diet again, they recovered. These results strongly suggest that the therapeutic effect of at least some antidepressant drugs depends on the availability of serotonin in the brain.

monoamine hypothesis A hypothesis that states that depression is caused by a low level of activity of one or more monoaminergic synapses.

tryptophan depletion procedure A procedure involving a low-tryptophan diet and a tryptophan-free amino acid "cocktail" that lowers brain tryptophan and consequently decreases the synthesis of 5-HT.

Most investigators believe that the simple monoamine hypothesis, that depression is caused by low levels of norepinephrine or serotonin, is just that: too simple. The effects of tryptophan depletion certainly suggest that serotonin plays a role in depression, but depletion causes depression only in people with a personal or family history of depression. An acute decrease in serotonergic activity in healthy people with no family history of depression has no effect on mood. Thus, there appear to be physiological differences in the brains of the vulnerable people. Also, although SSRIs and SNRIs change the increase in the level of 5-HT or norepinephrine in the brain very rapidly, the drugs do not relieve the symptoms of depression until they have been taken for several weeks. This fact suggests that something other than a simple increase in monoaminergic activity is responsible for the normalization of mood. Many investigators believe that the increased extracellular levels of monoamines produced by administration of antidepressant drugs begin a chain of events that eventually produce changes in the brain that are ultimately responsible for antidepressant effect.

Evidence for Brain Abnormalities

In a review of the relevant literature, Drevets (2001) suggests that the amygdala and several regions of the prefrontal cortex play special roles in the development of depression. As we saw in Chapter 10, the amygdala is critically involved in the expression of negative emotions. Functional imaging studies indicate a 50 to 75 percent increase in blood flow and metabolism in the amygdala of depressed patients (Drevets et al., 1992; Links et al., 1996). A study by Abercrombie et al. (1998) found that the activity of the amygdala of depressed patients was positively correlated with the severity of their depression. In addition, the metabolic activity of the amygdala increases in normal subjects when they look at pictures of faces with expressions of sadness, and it also increases when depressed subjects remember episodes in their lives that made them sad (Drevets, 2000b; Liotti et al., 2002).

Drevets et al. (1997) found that the subgenual ACC shows a lower level of activation in depressed patients. As the bar graph in Figure 15.14 shows, the activity of this region *increases* during a manic episode in patients with bipolar disorder (Drevets et al., 1997). Thus the activity of this region decreases during times of negative mood and increases during times of positive mood. (See *Figure 15.14.*)

I mentioned earlier that two experimental therapies for treatment-resistant depression, deep-brain stimulation of the subgenual ACC and vagus nerve stimulation, decreased the activity of the subgenual ACC. These results appear to contradict the finding that the activity level of this region is *lower* in depressed people. So far, I have found no suggestions in the research literature that can explain the discrepancy, but at least all of the experiments point to the importance of the subgenual ACC. One other study suggested that this region plays a role in depression. A functional-imaging study by Siegle, Carter, and Thase (2006) found that depressed patients who initially exhibited a low response to emotional stimuli in the subgenual ACC and a high response in the amygdala responded best to cognitive behavior therapy. (Research has found that cognitive behavior therapy is the most effective form of psychotherapy for depression.)

In recent years, evidence has been accumulating that implicates the serotonin transporter in depression. A portion of the gene—the *promoter region*—for the 5-HT transporter (5-HTT) comes in two forms: short and long. Possession of a short allele on one or both chromosomes results in production of significantly decreased amounts of the 5-HT transporter. As we saw in Chapter 10, people with one or two short alleles show greater activation of the amygdala when they look at photographs of faces expressing anger or fear, which indicates an increased emotional response to negative stimuli. A longitudinal study by Caspi et al. (2003) followed 847 people over a period of more than 20 years, starting at 3 years of age, and recorded the occurrence of stressful events in their lives, including abuse during childhood,

FIGURE 15.14

Metabolic Rate of the Subgenual ACC in Mania and Depression. (a) The composite fMRI image shows decreased metabolic activity of this region in depressed patients. (b) The graph shows mean relative metabolic rate of the subgenual prefrontal cortex in normal controls and depressed and manic patients.

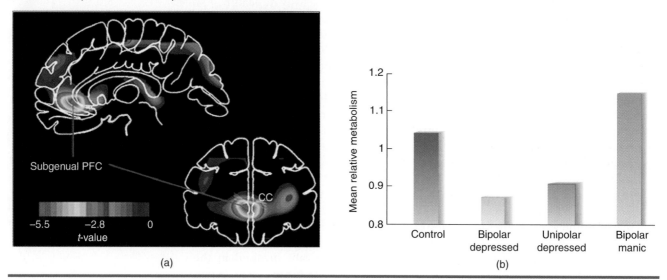

(a)　　　　　　　　　　　　　　　　(b)

Reprinted from *Current Opinion in Neurobiology, 11,* Drevets, W. C., Neuroimaging and Neuropathological Studies of Depression: Implications for the Cognitive-Emotional Features of Mood Disorders, 240–249, Copyright 2001, with permission from Elsevier.

romantic disasters, bereavements, illnesses, and job crises. The investigators found that the probability of major depression and suicidality increased with the number of stressful life events the people had experienced. Moreover, the increase was much greater for people with one or two copies of the short alleles for the 5-HTT promoter. This study shows clear evidence of an interaction between environment and genetics. (See *Figure 15.15.*)

FIGURE 15.15

Stressful Life Events, 5-HTT, and Depression. The graphs show the probability of (a) major depression and (b) suicide ideation or attempts as a function of number of previous stressful life events of people with two long alleles (L/L), one short allele (S/L), or two short alleles (S/S) of the promoter region of the 5-HT transporter gene.

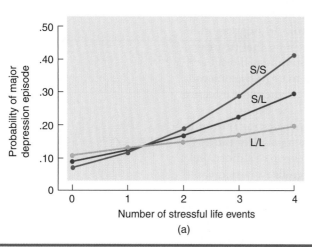
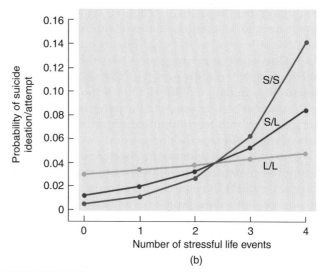

(a)　　　　　　　　　　　　　　　　(b)

Adapted from Caspi, A., Sugden, K., Moffitt, T. E., et al. *Science,* 2003, *301,* 386–389.

Other studies have confirmed the importance of the 5-HTT promoter to the development of depression. For example, Lee et al. (2004) found that depressed people with two long alleles who were treated with antidepressant drugs had a much better long-term outcome (up to 3 years) than did people with one or two short alleles.

What are the physiological effects of the long and short alleles of the 5-HTT promoter? It turns out that serotonin has important roles in prenatal development as well as in postnatal brain functions (Gaspar, Cases, and Maroteaux, 2003; Bonnin et al., 2007). In fact, some glutamatergic neurons in the hippocampus and anterior cingulate cortex take up serotonin during a brief period during development. Presumably, this uptake has effects on the development of these brain regions.

A structural and functional imaging study by Pezawas et al. (2005) suggests a mechanism that might explain the interaction between serotonin transporters and brain regions involved in mood. The investigators studied healthy people with no history of depression. They found that people with one or more short alleles had a 25 percent reduction in the gray matter of the region around the genu of the corpus callosum. The largest reduction was in the subgenual ACC. Figure 15.16 shows this finding. As we just saw, 5-HT is involved in prenatal development of the anterior cingulate cortex. Presumably, the possession of one or two short alleles of the 5-HTT promoter increases extracellular levels of 5-HT, affects prenatal development, and causes a reduction in the size of the subgenual ACC. (See *Figure 15.16*.)

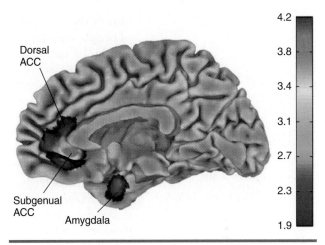

FIGURE 15.16

Gray Matter of the Amygdala and the Subgenual ACC. The scan shows reduction in the gray matter volume of the amygdala and subgenual anterior cingulate cortex (ACC) of normal subjects with one or two short alleles of the promoter region of the 5-HT transporter gene relative to subjects with two long alleles. "Hotter" colors indicate lower volume of brain tissue.

Reprinted by permission from Macmillan Publishers Ltd: *Nature Neuroscience*, Pezawas, L., Meyer-Linderberg, A., Drabant, E. M., et al., 5-HTTLPR polymorphism impacts human cingulate-amygdala interactions: A genetic susceptibility mechanism for depression, *8*, 828–834, copyright 2005.

Role of Neurogenesis

As we saw in Chapters 3 and 12, neurogenesis can take place in the dentate gyrus—a region of the hippocampal formation—in the adult brain. Several studies with laboratory animals have shown that stressful experiences that produce the symptoms of depression suppress hippocampal neurogenesis, and the administration of antidepressant treatments, including MAO inhibitors, tricyclic antidepressants, SSRIs, ECT, and lithium, increases neurogenesis. In addition, the delay in the action of antidepressant treatments is about the same length as the time it takes for newborn neurons to mature. Moreover, if neurogenesis is suppressed by a low-level dose of x-radiation, antidepressant drugs lose their effectiveness. (See Sahay and Hen, 2007, for a review.) It is tempting to conclude that decreased hippocampal neurogenesis is the cause (or one of the causes) of depression. However, Sapolsky (2004) points out that it is difficult to find a link between the known functions of the hippocampus and the possible causes of depression. For example, disorders of memory, not of affect, are seen in people with hippocampal damage. We do not yet have enough evidence to decide whether neurogenesis plays a role in depression or whether the relationship between the two is coincidental.

There is currently no way to measure the rate of neurogenesis in the human brain. So far, all the evidence about human neurogenesis has been by extrapolation from studies with laboratory animals. However, a study by Pereira et al. (2007) used an MRI procedure that permitted them to estimate the blood volume of particular regions of the hippocampal formation in both mice and humans. They found that exercise (running wheels for the mice, an aerobic exercise regimen for humans) increased the blood volume of the dentate gyrus—the region where neurogenesis takes place—in both species. (As we will see in the next section of this chapter, exercise is an effective treatment for depression.) Histological procedures verified that increased neurogenesis in the mouse brain correlated with the increased blood volume, which supports the suggestion that exercise induces neurogenesis in the human brain, as well. (See *Figure 15.17.*)

Role of Circadian Rhythms

One of the most prominent symptoms of depression is disordered sleep. The sleep of people with depression tends to be shallow; slow-wave delta sleep (stages 3 and 4) is reduced, and stage 1 is increased. Sleep is fragmented; people tend to awaken frequently, especially toward the morning. In addition, REM sleep occurs earlier, the first half of the night contains a higher proportion of REM periods, and REM sleep contains an increased number of rapid eye movements (Kupfer, 1976; Vogel et al., 1980). (See *Figure 15.18.*)

REM Sleep Deprivation

One of the most effective antidepressant treatments is sleep deprivation, either total or selective. Selective deprivation of REM sleep, accomplished by monitoring people's EEG and awakening them whenever they show signs of REM sleep, alleviates depression (Vogel et al., 1975, 1990). The therapeutic effect, like that of the antidepressant medications, occurs slowly, over the course of several weeks. Some patients show long-term improvement even after the deprivation is discontinued; thus, it is a practical as well as an effective treatment. In addition, regardless of their specific pharmacological effects, other treatments for depression suppress REM sleep, delaying its onset and decreasing its duration (Scherschlicht et al., 1982; Vogel et al., 1990; Grunhaus et al., 1997; Thase, 2000). These results suggest that an important effect of successful antidepressant treatment may be to suppress REM sleep, and the changes in mood may be a result of this suppression. However, at least one antidepressant drug has been shown in a double-blind, placebo-controlled study *not* to

FIGURE 15.17

Exercise and Neurogenesis. The scans show the effect of a program of aerobic exercise on the blood volume of regions of the human hippocampal formation. This measure serves as an indirect measure of neurogenesis: (a) subregions of the hippocampus (EC = entorhinal cortex, DG = dentate gyrus, SUB = subiculum). (b) This scan shows the regional blood volume; "hotter" colors indicate increased blood volume.

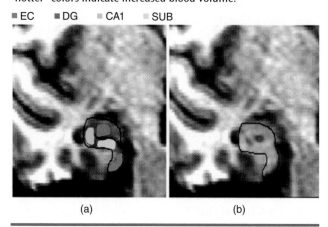

From Pereira, A. C., Huddleston, D. E., Brickman, A. M., et al. *Proceedings of the National Academy of Sciences, USA,* 2007, *104,* 5638–5643. Copyright 2007 National Academy of Sciences, U.S.A.

FIGURE 15.18

Sleep and Depression. The diagram illustrates patterns of the stages of sleep of a normal subject and of a patient with major depression. Note the reduced sleep latency, reduced REM latency, reduction in slow-wave sleep (stages 3 and 4), and general fragmentation of sleep (arrows) in the depressed patient.

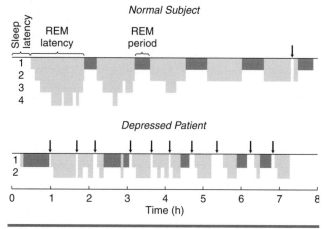

Reprinted from *Trends in Neurosciences, 8,* Gillin, J. C., and Borbely, A. A., Sleep: A Neurobiological Window on Affective Disorders, 537–542, Copyright 1985, with permission from Elsevier.

suppress REM sleep (Mayers and Baldwin, 2005). Thus, suppression of REM sleep cannot be the *only* way in which antidepressant drugs work.

Total Sleep Deprivation

Total sleep deprivation also has an antidepressant effect. Unlike specific deprivation of REM sleep, which takes several weeks to reduce depression, total sleep deprivation produces immediate effects (Wu and Bunney, 1990). Typically, the depression is lifted by the sleep deprivation but returns the next day, after a normal night's sleep. Wu and Bunney suggest that during sleep, the brain produces a chemical that has a *depressogenic* effect in susceptible people. During waking, this substance is gradually metabolized and hence inactivated. Some of the evidence for this hypothesis is presented in Figure 15.19. The data are taken from eight different studies (cited by Wu and Bunney, 1990) and show self-ratings of depression of people who did and did not respond to sleep deprivation. (Total sleep deprivation improves the mood of patients with major depression approximately two-thirds of the time.) (See *Figure 15.19.*)

Why do only some people profit from sleep deprivation? This question has not yet been answered, but several studies have shown that it is possible to predict who will profit and who will not (Riemann, Wiegand, and Berger, 1991; Haug, 1992; Wirz-Justice and Van den Hoofdakker, 1999). In general, depressed patients whose mood remains stable will probably not benefit from sleep deprivation, whereas those whose mood fluctuates probably will. The patients who are most likely to respond are those who feel depressed in the morning but then gradually feel better as the day progresses. In these people, sleep deprivation appears to prevent the depressogenic effects of sleep from taking place and simply permits the trend to continue. If you examine Figure 15.19, you can see that the responders were already feeling better by the end of the day. This improvement continued through the sleepless night and during the following day. The next night they were permitted to sleep normally, and their depression was back the following morning. As Wu and Bunney note, these data are consistent with the hypothesis that sleep produces a substance with a depressogenic effect. (See *Figure 15.19.*)

Although total sleep deprivation is not a practical method for treating depression (it is obviously impossible to keep people awake indefinitely), several studies suggest that *partial* sleep deprivation can hasten the beneficial effects of antidepressant drugs (Szuba, Baxter, and Fairbanks, 1991; Leibenluft and Wehr, 1992). Some investigators have found that *intermittent* total sleep deprivation (say, twice a week for 4 weeks) can have beneficial results (Papadimitriou et al., 1993).

Role of Zeitgebers

Yet another phenomenon relates depression to sleep and waking—or, more specifically, to the mechanisms that are responsible for circadian rhythms. Some people become depressed during the winter season, when days are short and nights are long (Rosenthal et al., 1984). The symptoms of this form of depression, called **seasonal affective disorder (SAD)**, are somewhat different from those of major depression; both forms

FIGURE 15.19

Antidepressant Effects of Sleep Deprivation.
The graph shows the mean mood rating of responding and nonresponding patients deprived of one night's sleep as a function of the time of day.

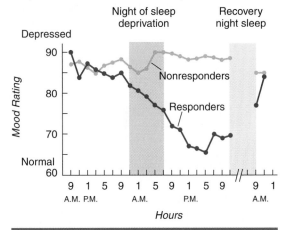

Adapted from Wu, J. C., and Bunney, W. E. *American Journal of Psychiatry*, Vol. 147, pp. 14–21, 1990.

seasonal affective disorder A mood disorder characterized by depression, lethargy, sleep disturbances, and craving for carbohydrates during the winter season when days are short.

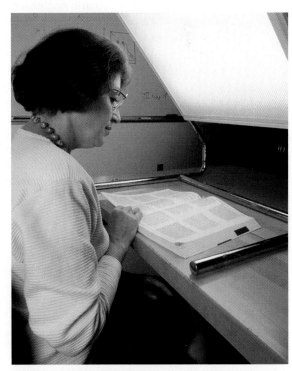

Seasonal affective disorder, which is provoked by the long nights and short days of winter, can be treated by daily exposure to bright lights.

FIGURE 15.20

Cycles of Sleep and Melatonin Secretion.   Normally, melatonin secretion begins in the evening, approximately 6 hours before the midpoint of sleep. Most people with seasonal affective disorder begin secreting melatonin earlier, showing a phase delay between cycles of melatonin and sleep. A few people with this disorder show a phase advance, with melatonin secretion beginning at a later time.

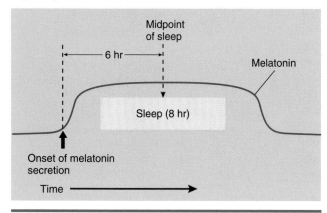

Adapted from Lewy, A. K., Lefler, B. J., Emens, J. S., and Bauer, V. K. *Proceedings of the National Academy of Sciences, USA*, 2006, *103*, 7414–7419.

phototherapy   Treatment of seasonal affective disorder by daily exposure to bright light.

include lethargy and sleep disturbances, but seasonal depression includes a craving for carbohydrates and an accompanying weight gain. (As you will recall, people with major depression tend to lose their appetite.)

Seasonal affective disorder, like MDD and bipolar disorder, appears to have a genetic basis. In a study of 6439 adult twins, Madden et al. (1996) found that seasonal affective disorder ran in families, and they estimated that at least 29 percent of the variance in seasonal mood disorders could be attributed to genetic factors.

Seasonal affective disorder can be treated by **phototherapy**: exposing people to bright light for several hours a day (Rosenthal et al., 1985; Stinson and Thompson, 1990). As you will recall, circadian rhythms of sleep and wakefulness are controlled by the activity of the suprachiasmatic nucleus of the hypothalamus. Light serves as a *zeitgeber*; that is, it synchronizes the activity of the biological clock to the day–night cycle.

According to Lewy et al. (2006), SAD is caused by a mismatch between cycles of sleep and cycles of melatonin secretion. Normally, secretion of melatonin begins in the evening, before people go to sleep. In fact, the time between the onset of melatonin secretion and the midpoint of sleep (halfway between falling asleep and waking up in the morning) is approximately 6 hours. People with SAD most often show a *phase delay* between cycles of melatonin and sleep; that is, the time interval between the onset of melatonin secretion and the midpoint of sleep is more than 6 hours. Exposure to bright light in the morning or administration of melatonin late in the afternoon (or, preferably, both treatments) advances the circadian cycle controlled by the biological clock in the suprachiasmatic nucleus. (These cycles were discussed in Chapter 8.) Those people with SAD who show a *phase advance* in their cycles can best be treated with exposure to bright light in the evening and administration of melatonin in the morning. (See *Figure 15.20.*) By the way, phototherapy has also been found to help patients with major depressive disorder, especially in conjunction with administration of antidepressant drugs (Terman, 2007).

Phototherapy is a safe and effective treatment for SAD. According to a study by Wirz-Justice et al. (1996), a special apparatus is not even needed. The authors found that a 1-hour walk outside each morning reduced the symptoms of seasonal affective disorder. They noted that even on an overcast winter day, the early morning sky provides considerably more illumination than normal indoor artificial lighting, so a walk outside increases a person's exposure to light. The exercise helps, too. Many studies (for example, Dunn et al., 2005) have shown that a program of exercise improves the symptoms of depression.

Interim Summary

Major Affective Disorders

The major affective disorders include bipolar disorder, with its cyclical episodes of mania and depression, and major depressive disorder. Heritability studies suggest that genetic anomalies are at least partly responsible for these disorders. MDD has been treated by several established or experimental biological treatments: MAO inhibitors, drugs that block the reuptake of norepinephrine and serotonin (tricyclic antidepressants, SSRIs, and SNRIs), ECT, TMS, deep brain stimulation, vagus nerve stimulation, and sleep deprivation.

Bipolar disorder can be successfully treated by lithium salts and anti-convulsant drugs.

The therapeutic effect of noradrenergic and serotonergic agonists and the depressant effect of reserpine, a monoaminergic antagonist, suggested the monoamine hypothesis of depression: that depression is caused by insufficient activity of monoaminergic neurons. Depletion of tryptophan (the precursor of 5-HT) in the brain causes a recurrence of depressive symptoms in depressed patients who were in remission, which lends further support to the conclusion that 5-HT plays a role in mood. However, although SSRIs have an immediate effect on serotonergic transmission in the brain, they do not relieve the symptoms of depression for several weeks, so the simple monoamine hypothesis appears not to be correct.

Functional imaging studies found an increased activity in the amygdala and a decreased activity in the subgenual ACC. Stressful life experiences increase the likelihood of depression in people with one or two short alleles of the 5-HT transporter promoter gene, and a better response to antidepressant treatment is seen in depressed people with two long alleles. Structural and functional imaging studies have found a decrease in the volume of the subgenual ACC, which presumably occurs because increased serotonergic activity associated with the presence of short alleles for the 5-HTT promoter affects prenatal brain development. Stressful experiences suppress hippocampal neurogenesis, and antidepressant treatments increase it. In addition, the effects of antidepressant treatments are abolished by suppression of neurogenesis.

Sleep disturbances are characteristic of affective disorders. In fact, total sleep deprivation rapidly (but temporarily) reduces depression in many people, and selective deprivation of REM sleep does so slowly (but more lastingly). In addition, almost all effective antidepressant treatments suppress REM sleep. A specific form of depression, seasonal affective disorder, can be treated by exposure to bright light. Clearly, the mood disorders are somehow linked to biological rhythms.

Thought Questions

A television commentator, talking in particular about the suicide of a young pop star and in general about unhappy youth, asked with exasperation, "What would all these young people be doing if they had real problems like a Depression, World War II, or Vietnam?" People with severe depression often try to hide their pain because they fear others will scoff at them and say that they have nothing to feel unhappy about. If depression is caused by abnormal brain functioning, are these remarks justified? How would you feel if you were severely depressed and people close to you berated you for feeling so sad and told you to snap out of it and quit feeling sorry for yourself? Do you think the expression of attitudes like this would decrease the likelihood of a depressed person committing suicide?

Anxiety Disorders

As we saw in the previous section of this chapter, the affective disorders are characterized by unrealistic extremes of emotion: depression or elation (mania). The **anxiety disorders** are characterized by unrealistic, unfounded fear and anxiety. This section describes three of the anxiety disorders that appear to have biological causes: panic disorder, generalized anxiety disorder, and social anxiety disorder. Although obsessive compulsive disorder has traditionally been classified as an anxiety disorder, it has different symptoms from the other three disorders and involves different brain regions, so it is discussed separately.

Panic Disorder, Generalized Anxiety Disorder, and Social Anxiety Disorder

Description

People with **panic disorder** suffer from episodic attacks of acute anxiety—periods of acute and unremitting terror that grip them for variable lengths of time, from a few seconds to a few hours. The prevalence of this disorder is just under 2 percent (Kessler et al., 2006). Women appear to be a little more than twice as likely as men to suffer from panic disorder (Eaton et al., 1994.) (See *Figure 15.21*.)

Panic attacks include many physical symptoms, such as shortness of breath, clammy sweat, irregularities in heartbeat, dizziness, faintness, and feelings of unreality. The victim of a panic attack often feels that he or she is going to die, and often seeks help in a hospital emergency room. Between panic attacks many people with panic disorder suffer from **anticipatory anxiety**—the fear that another panic attack will strike them. This anticipatory anxiety often leads to the development of a serious phobic disorder: **agoraphobia** (*agora* means "open space"). Agoraphobia can be

anxiety disorder A psychological disorder characterized by tension, overactivity of the autonomic nervous system, expectation of an impending disaster, and continuous vigilance for danger.

panic disorder A disorder characterized by episodic periods of symptoms such as shortness of breath, irregularities in heartbeat, and other autonomic symptoms, accompanied by intense fear.

anticipatory anxiety A fear of having a panic attack; may lead to the development of agoraphobia.

agoraphobia A fear of being away from home or other protected places.

Prevalence of Panic Disorder. The graph shows the percentage of men and women who receive a diagnosis of panic disorder earlier and later in life.

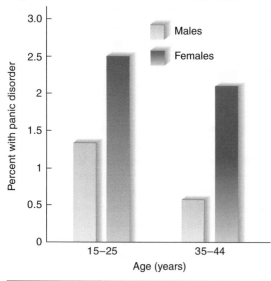

Based on data from Eaton, W. W., Kessler, R. C., Wittchen, H. U., and Magee, W. J. *American Journal of Psychiatry*, 1994, *151*, 413–420.

generalized anxiety disorder A disorder characterized by excessive anxiety and worry serious enough to cause disruption of people's lives.

social anxiety disorder A disorder characterized by excessive fear of being exposed to the scrutiny of other people that leads to avoidance of social situations in which the person is called on to perform.

severely disabling; some people with this disorder have stayed inside their homes for years, afraid to venture outside where they might have a panic attack in public.

The primary characteristics of **generalized anxiety disorder** are excessive anxiety and worry, difficulty in controlling these symptoms, and clinically significant signs of distress and disruption of their lives. The prevalence of generalized anxiety disorder is approximately 3 percent, and the incidence is approximately two times greater in women than in men.

Social anxiety disorder (also called *social phobia*) is a persistent, excessive fear of being exposed to the scrutiny of other people that leads to avoidance of social situations in which the person is called on to perform (such as speaking or performing in public). If such situations are unavoidable, the person experiences intense anxiety and distress. The prevalence of social anxiety disorder, which is equally likely in men and women, is approximately 5 percent.

Possible Causes

Family studies and twin studies indicate that panic disorder, generalized anxiety disorder, and social anxiety disorder all have a hereditary component (Hettema, Neale, and Kendler, 2001; Merikangas and Low, 2005). Panic attacks can be triggered in people with a history of panic disorder by a variety of treatments that activate the autonomic nervous system, such as injections of lactic acid (a by-product of muscular activity), yohimbine (an α_2 adrenoreceptor antagonist), doxapram (a drug used by anesthesiologists to increase breathing rate), or breathing air containing an elevated amount of carbon dioxide (Stein and Uhde, 1995). Lactic acid and carbon dioxide both increase heart rate and rate of respiration, just as exercise does; yohimbine has direct pharmacological effects on the nervous system.

As we also saw earlier in this chapter, the presence of one or two short alleles of the promoter region of the serotonin transporter (5-HTT) gene is associated with increased emotionality and susceptibility to depression, apparently because of differences in the structure and activity of the amygdala and the subgenual ACC. Evidence indicates that the presence of the short allele is also associated with higher levels of anxiety. Auerbach et al. (1999) found higher levels of negative emotionality in 2-month-old infants with two short alleles. Furmark et al. (2004) found that people with social anxiety disorder whose chromosomes contained one or two short alleles showed a greater increase levels of anxiety than people with two long alleles while they were anticipating speaking in front of an audience. In addition, functional imaging found that their amygdalas showed increased activations. (See *Figure 15.22*.) A study by Domschke et al. (2008) found that blushing (a symptom of social anxiety disorder) is more prevalent in people with social anxiety disorder whose chromosomes contain one or two short alleles of the 5-HTT promoter gene.

Functional imaging studies suggest that the amygdala and the cingulate, prefrontal, and insular cortices are involved in anxiety disorders. Monk et al. (2008) found that adolescents with generalized anxiety disorder showed increased activation of the amygdala and decreased activation of the ventrolateral prefrontal cortex while looking at angry faces. They also found evidence that activation of the ventromedial prefrontal cortex suppressed amygdala activation in healthy control subjects but not in those with anxiety disorder. Stein et al. (2007) found that college students with a high level of anxiety showed increased activation of the amygdala and the insular cortex, both of which correlated positively with students' anxiety measures.

FIGURE 15.22

Role of Short or Long Alleles of the 5-HTT Promotor Gene in Anxiety. The graph shows the percentage change in regional blood flow (a measure of local brain activation) of the right amygdala of patients with social phobia while they anticipated speaking in front of an audience. Open circles represent subjects with two short alleles.

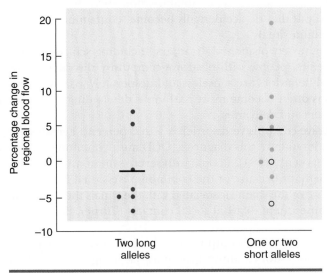

Adapted from Furmark, T., Tillfors, M., Garpenstrand, H., et al. *Neuroscience Letters*, 2004, *362*, 189–192.

FIGURE 15.23

Fluvoxamine and Panic Disorder. The graph shows the effects of fluvoxamine (an SSRI) on the severity of panic disorder.

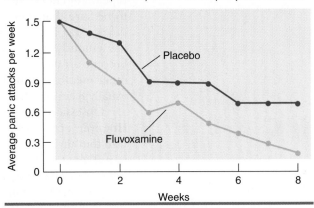

Adapted from Asnis, G. M., Hameedi, F. A., Goddard, A. W., et al. *Psychiatry Research*, 2001, *103*, 1–14.

Treatment

Anxiety disorders are sometimes treated with benzodiazepines. As we just saw, increased activity of the amygdala is a common feature of the anxiety disorders. The amygdala contains a high concentration of GABA$_A$ receptors, which are the target of the benzodiazepines. Paulus et al. (2005) found that administration of a benzodiazepine (lorazepam) decreased the activation of both the amygdala and the insula of subjects looking at emotional faces. Administration of flumazenil, a benzodiazepine antagonist (having an action *opposite* that of the benzodiazepine tranquilizers), produces panic in patients with panic disorder but not in control subjects (Nutt et al., 1990).

As we saw earlier, serotonin appears to play a role in depression. Much evidence suggests that serotonin plays a role in anxiety disorders too. Even though the symptoms of the anxiety disorders discussed in this subsection are very different from those of obsessive-compulsive disorder (described in the next subsection), specific serotonin reuptake inhibitors, which serve as potent serotonin agonists (such as fluoxetine), have become the first-line medications for treating all of these disorders—preferably in combination with cognitive behavior therapy (Asnis et al., 2001; Ressler and Mayberg, 2007). Figure 15.23 shows the effect of fluvoxamine, a serotonin reuptake inhibitor (SSRI), on the number of panic attacks in patients with panic disorder. (See *Figure 15.23*.)

Obsessive-Compulsive Disorder

Description

As the name implies, people with an **obsessive-compulsive disorder (OCD)** suffer from **obsessions**—thoughts that will not leave them—and **compulsions**—behaviors that they cannot keep from performing. Obsessions include concern or disgust with

obsessive-compulsive disorder (OCD) A mental disorder characterized by obsessions and compulsions.

obsession An unwanted thought or idea with which a person is preoccupied.

compulsion The feeling that one is obliged to perform a behavior, even if one prefers not to do so.

bodily secretions, dirt, germs, and such; fear that something terrible might happen; and a need for symmetry, order, or exactness. Most compulsions fall into one of four categories: *counting, checking, cleaning,* and *avoidance.* For example, people might repeatedly check burners on the stove to see that they are off and windows and locks to be sure that they are locked. Some people will wash their hands hundreds of times a day, even if their hands become covered with painful sores. Other people meticulously clean their house or endlessly wash, dry, and fold their clothes. Some become afraid to leave home because they fear contamination and refuse to touch other members of their family. If they do accidentally become "contaminated," they usually have lengthy purification rituals.

Obsessions are seen in a variety of mental disorders, including schizophrenia. However, unlike schizophrenics, people with obsessive-compulsive disorder recognize that their thoughts and behaviors are senseless and desperately wish that they would go away. Compulsions often become more and more demanding until they interfere with people's careers and daily lives.

The incidence of obsessive-compulsive disorder is 1 to 2 percent. Females are slightly more likely than males to have this diagnosis. OCD most commonly begins in young adulthood (Robbins et al., 1984). People with severe symptoms this disorder are unlikely to marry, perhaps because of the common obsessional fear of dirt and contamination or because of the shame associated with the rituals they are compelled to perform, which causes them to avoid social contacts (Turner, Beidel, and Nathan, 1985).

Some investigators believe that the compulsive behaviors seen in OCD are forms of species-typical behaviors—for example, grooming, cleaning, and attention to sources of potential danger—that are released from normal control mechanisms by a brain dysfunction (Wise and Rapoport, 1988). Fiske and Haslam (1997) suggest that the behaviors seen in OCD are simply pathological examples of a natural behavioral tendency to develop and practice social rituals. For example, people perform cultural rituals to mark transitions or changes in social status, to diagnose or treat illnesses, to restore relationships with deities, or to ensure the success of hunting or planting. Consider the following scenario (from Fiske and Haslam, 1997):

> Imagine that you are traveling in an unfamiliar country. Going out for a walk, you observe a man dressed in red, standing on a red mat in a red-painted gateway. . . . He utters the same prayer six times. He brings out six basins of water and meticulously arranges them in a symmetrical configuration in front of the gateway. Then he washes his hands six times in each of the six basins, using precisely the same motions each time. As he does this, he repeats the same phrase, occasionally tapping his right finger on his earlobe. Through your interpreter, you ask him what he is doing. He replies that there are dangerous polluting substances in the ground, . . . [and that] he must purify himself or something terrible will happen. He seems eager to tell you about his concerns. (p. 211)

Why is the man acting this way? Is he a priest following a sacred ritual or does he have OCD? Without knowing more about the spiritual rituals followed by the man's culture, we cannot say. Fiske and Haslam compared the features of OCD and other psychological disorders in descriptions of rituals, work, or other activities in fifty-two cultures. They found that the features of OCD were found in rituals in these cultures. The features of other psychological disorders were much less common. On the whole, the evidence suggests that the symptoms of OCD represent an exaggeration of natural human tendencies.

Zhong and Liljenquist (2006) found that even well-educated people in an industrialized country (students at Northwestern University, in the United States) apparently unknowingly considered cleansing rituals to "wash away their sins." The investigators had the subjects recall in detail either an ethical or an unethical deed they had committed in the past. Later, they were asked to complete some word fragments by filling in letters where blanks occurred. Some word fragments could be made into words that did or did not pertain to cleansing. For example, W _ _ H, SH _ _ ER, and S _ _ P could be *wash, shower,* and *soap,* or they could be *wish, shaker,* and *step.* The subjects who had told about a misdeed were much more likely to think of cleansing-related words. When offered a free gift—either a pencil or an antiseptic wipe—subjects who had told about a misdeed were more likely to chose the antiseptic wipe.

Possible Causes

Evidence suggests that OCD has a genetic origin. Several studies have found a greater concordance for obsessions and compulsions in monozygotic twins than in dizygotic twins (Hettema, Neale, and Kendler, 2001) At least two studies suggest that chromosome 9 contains a region associated with OCD (Hanna et al., 2002; Willour et al., 2004).

Not all cases of OCD have a genetic origin; the disorder sometimes occurs after brain damage caused by various means, such as birth trauma, encephalitis, and head trauma (Hollander et al., 1990; Berthier et al., 1996). In particular, the symptoms of OCD appear to be associated with damage to or dysfunction of the basal ganglia, cingulate gyrus, and prefrontal cortex (Giedd et al., 1995; Robinson et al., 1995).

Evidence suggests that infections illness can sometimes affect the basal ganglia and produce the symptoms of OCD. Bodner, Morshed, and Peterson (2001) reported the case of a 25-year-old man whose untreated sore throat (he lived in a religious group that prohibited antibiotics) developed into an autoimmune disease that produced obsessions and compulsions. The investigators found antibodies to a particular type of streptococcus bacterium in his blood, and MRI scans indicated abnormalities in the basal ganglia. An MRI study of thirty-four children with streptococcus-associated tics or OCD by Giedd et al. (2000) found an increase in the size of the basal ganglia that they attributed to an autoimmune inflammation of this region.

Several functional imaging studies have found evidence of increased activity in the frontal lobes and caudate nucleus in patients with OCD. A review by Whiteside, Port, and Abramowitz (2004) found that functional imaging studies consistently showed increased activity of the caudate nucleus and the prefrontal cortex. Guehl et al. (2008) inserted microelectrodes into the caudate nuclei of three patients with OCD who were being evaluated for neurosurgery. They found that two of the patients, who reported the presence of obsessive thoughts during the surgery, showed increased activity in neurons in the caudate nucleus. The third patient, who did not report obsessive thoughts, showed a lower rate of neural activity.

Treatment

A review by Saxena et al. (1998) described several studies that measured regional brain activity of OCD patients before and after successful treatment with drugs or cognitive behavior therapy. In general, the improvement in a patient's symptoms was correlated with a reduction in the activity of the caudate nucleus and prefrontal cortex. The fact that cognitive behavior therapy and drug therapy produced similar results is especially remarkable: It indicates that very different procedures may be bringing about physiological changes that alleviate a serious mental disorder.

As we saw in Chapter 10, the prefrontal cortex and the cingulate cortex are involved in emotional reactions, so it is not surprising to learn that they might be implicated in OCD. In fact, some patients with severe OCD have been successfully treated with **cingulotomy**—surgical destruction of specific fiber bundles in the subcortical frontal lobe, including the cingulum bundle (which connects the prefrontal and cingulate cortex with the limbic cortex of the temporal lobe) and a region that contains fibers that connect the basal ganglia with the prefrontal cortex

cingulotomy The surgical destruction of the cingulum bundle, which connects the prefrontal cortex with the limbic system; helps to reduce intense anxiety and the symptoms of obsessive-compulsive disorder.

(Ballantine et al., 1987; Mindus, Rasmussen, and Lindquist, 1994). These operations have a reasonably good success rate (Dougherty et al., 2002). Another reasonably successful surgical procedure, *capsulotomy*, destroys a region of a fiber bundle (the *internal capsule*) that connects the caudate nucleus with the medial prefrontal cortex (Rück et al., 2008). Of course, neurosurgery cannot be undone, so such procedures must be considered only as a last resort. As Rück and his colleagues reported, some patients suffer from adverse side effects after surgery, such as problems of planning, apathy, or difficulty inhibiting socially inappropriate behavior.

In one extraordinary case a patient performed his own psychosurgery. Solyom, Turnbull, and Wilensky (1987) reported the case of a young man with a serious OCD whose ritual hand washing and other behaviors made it impossible for him to continue his schooling or lead a normal life. Finding that his life was no longer worthwhile, he decided to end it. He placed the muzzle of a .22-caliber rifle in his mouth and pulled the trigger. The bullet entered the base of the brain and damaged the frontal lobes. He survived, and he was amazed to find that his compulsions were gone. Fortunately, the damage did not disrupt his ability to make or execute plans; he went back to school and completed his education, and he now has a job. His IQ was unchanged. Ordinary surgery would have been less hazardous and messy, but it could hardly have been more successful.

As we saw in Chapter 14, deep brain stimulation (DBS) has been found to be useful in treating the symptoms of Parkinson's disease. Because OCD, like Parkinson's disease, appears to involve abnormalities in the basal ganglia, several clinics have tried to use DBS of the basal ganglia or fiber tracts connected with them to treat this disorder. This form of therapy appears to reduce the symptoms of OCD in some patients (Abelson et al., 2005; Larson, 2008). Fontaine et al. (2004) reported the case of a man with both Parkinson's disease and severe OCD. Deep brain stimulation of the subthalamic nucleus relieved both his motor disability and his obsessive-compulsive symptoms. A significant benefit of this procedure is that unlike psychosurgical procedures that destroy brain tissue, it is reversible: If no benefit is obtained from the stimulation, the electrodes can be removed.

Three drugs are regularly used to treat the symptoms of OCD: clomipramine, fluoxetine, and fluvoxamine. These effective antiobsessional drugs are specific blockers of 5-HT reuptake; thus, they are serotonergic agonists. In general, serotonin has an inhibitory effect on species-typical behaviors, which has tempted several investigators to speculate that these drugs alleviate the symptoms of OCD by reducing the strength of innate tendencies for counting, checking, cleaning, and avoidance behaviors that may underlie this disorder. Brain regions that have been implicated in OCD, including the prefrontal cortex and the basal ganglia, receive input from serotonergic terminals (Lavoie and Parent, 1990; El Mansari and Blier, 1997).

The importance of serotonergic activity in inhibiting compulsive behaviors is underscored by three interesting compulsions: trichotillomania, onychophagia, and acral lick dermatitis. *Trichotillomania* is compulsive hair pulling. People with this disorder (almost always females) often spend hours each night pulling hairs out one by one, sometimes eating them (Rapoport, 1991). *Onychophagia* is compulsive nail biting, which in its extreme can cause severe damage to the ends of the fingers. (For those who are sufficiently agile, toenail biting is not uncommon.) Double-blind studies have shown that both of these disorders can be treated successfully by clomipramine, the drug of choice for OCD (Leonard et al., 1992).

Acral lick dermatitis is a disease of dogs, not humans. Some dogs will continuously lick at a part of their body, especially their wrist or ankle (called the *carpus* and the *hock*). The licking removes the hair and often erodes away the skin as well. The disorder seems to be genetic; it is seen almost exclusively in large breeds such as Great Danes, Labrador retrievers, and German shepherds, and it runs in families. A double-blind study found that clomipramine reduces this compulsive behavior (Rapoport, Ryland, and Kriete, 1992). (At first, when I read the term "double-blind" in the report by Rapoport and her colleagues, I was amused to think that the investigators were careful not to let the dogs learn whether they were receiving clomipramine or a placebo. Then I realized that, of course, it was the dogs' owners who had to be kept in the dark.)

We saw in the previous subsection that an NMDA receptor agonist, D-cycloserine, appears to be useful in treating the symptoms of anxiety disorders. This drug appears also to help in the treatment of the symptoms of OCD as well. A double-blind study by Kushner et al. (2007) found that compared with patients who received a placebo, patients who received D-cycloserine along with sessions of cognitive behavior therapy showed a more rapid decrease in their obsessive symptoms and were less likely to drop out of the treatment program. Presumably, the drug facilitated the extinction of the maladaptive thoughts and behaviors, just as it facilitates the extinction of conditioned emotional responses in patients with anxiety disorders.

InterimSummary

Anxiety Disorders

The anxiety disorders severely disrupt some people's lives. People with panic disorder periodically have panic attacks, during which they experience intense symptoms of autonomic activity and often feel as if they are going to die. Frequently, panic attacks lead to the development of agoraphobia, an avoidance of being away from a safe place, such as home. Family and twin studies have shown that panic disorder is at least partly heritable, which suggests that it has biological causes.

Panic attacks can be alleviated by the administration of a benzodiazepine, a finding that suggests that the disorder may involve decreased numbers of benzodiazepine receptors or an inadequate secretion of an endogenous benzodiazepine; a benzodiazepine *antagonist* can trigger a panic attack. Nowadays, the first choice of medical treatment for panic attacks is an SSRI. In addition, the presence of one or two short alleles are associated with increased activation of the amygdala and higher levels of anxiety. Functional imaging studies suggest that the amygdala and the cingulate, prefrontal, and insular cortices are involved in anxiety disorders.

Obsessive-compulsive disorder (OCD) is characterized by obsessions—unwanted thoughts—and compulsions—uncontrollable behaviors, especially those involving cleanliness and attention to danger. Some investigators believe that these behaviors represent overactivity of species-typical behavioral tendencies. OCD has a heritable basis. It can also be caused by birth trauma, encephalitis, and head injuries, especially when the basal ganglia are involved. A streptococcus infection can stimulate an autoimmune attack—presumably on the basal ganglia—that produces the symptoms of OCD.

Functional imaging studies indicate that people with OCD tend to show increased activity in the prefrontal cortex, cingulate cortex, and caudate nucleus. Drug treatment or behavior therapy that successfully reduces the symptoms of OCD generally reduces the activity of the prefrontal cortex and caudate nucleus. In severe cases of OCD that do not respond to other treatments, surgical procedures such as cingulotomy and capsulotomy may provide relief. Deep brain stimulation with implanted electrodes has been shown to be effective in some patients, and, unlike cingulotomy and capsulotomy, has the benefits of being reversible. The most effective drugs are SSRIs such as clomipramine. Some investigators believe that clomipramine and related drugs alleviate the symptoms of OCD by increasing the activity of serotonergic pathways that play an inhibitory role on species-typical behaviors. Three other compulsions—hair pulling, nail biting, and (in dogs) acral lick syndrome—are also suppressed by clomipramine.

Thought Questions

Most reasonable people would agree that a person with mental disorders cannot be blamed for his or her thoughts and behaviors. Most of us would sympathize with someone whose life is disrupted by panic attacks or obsessions and compulsions, and we would not see their plight as a failure of willpower. After all, whether these disorders are caused by traumatic experiences or brain abnormalities (or both), the afflicted person has not chosen to be the way he or she is. But what about less dramatic examples: Should we blame people for their shyness or hostility or other maladaptive personality traits? If, as many psychologists believe, people's personality characteristics are largely determined by their heredity (and thus by the structure and chemistry of their brains), what are the implications for our concepts of "blame" and "personal responsibility"?

EPILOGUE Prefrontal Lobotomy

In the chapter prologue I wrote that the repercussions of the 1935 meeting at which the results of the surgery on Becky the chimpanzee are still felt today. Since that time tens of thousands of people have received prefrontal lobotomies, primarily to reduce symptoms of emotional distress, and many of these people are still alive. At first the medical community welcomed the procedure because it provided their patients with relief from emotional anguish. Only after many years were careful studies performed on the side effects of the procedure. These studies showed that although patients did perform well on standard tests of intellectual ability, they showed serious changes in personality, becoming irresponsible and childish. They also lost the ability to carry out plans, and most were unemployable. Although pathological emotional reactions were eliminated, so were normal ones. Because of these findings, and because of the discovery of drugs and therapeutic methods that relieve the patients' symptoms without producing such drastic side effects, neurosurgeons eventually abandoned the prefrontal lobotomy procedure (Valenstein, 1986).

I should point out that the prefrontal lobotomies that were performed under Moniz's supervision and by the neurosurgeons who followed were not as drastic as the surgery performed by Jacobsen and his colleagues on Becky, the chimpanzee. In fact, no brain tissue was removed. Instead, the surgeons introduced various kinds of cutting devices into the frontal lobes and severed white matter (bundles of axons). One rather gruesome procedure did not even require an operating room; it could be performed in a physician's office. A *transorbital leucotome*, shaped like an ice pick, was introduced into the brain by passing it beneath the upper eyelid until the point reached the orbital bone above the eye. The instrument was hit with a mallet, driving it through the bone into the brain. The end was then swept back and forth so that it cut through the white matter. The patient often left the office within an hour.

Many physicians objected to the "ice pick" procedure because it was done blind (that is, the surgeon could not see just where the blade of the leucotome was located) and because it produced more damage than was necessary. Also, the fact that it was so easy and left no external signs other than a pair of black eyes may have tempted its practitioners to perform it too casually. In fact, at least twenty-five hundred patients underwent this form of surgery (Valenstein, 1986).

What we know today about the effects of prefrontal lobotomy—whether done transorbitally or by more conventional means—tells us that such radical surgery should never have been performed. For too long the harmful side effects were ignored. As we saw earlier in this chapter, neurosurgeons have developed a much restricted version of this surgery—cingulotomy—to treat intractable OCD. Fortunately, this procedure reduces the symptoms of OCD without producing such harmful side effects.

Key Concepts

SCHIZOPHRENIA

1. Schizophrenia is characterized by positive, negative, and cognitive symptoms.
2. Because a tendency to develop schizophrenia is heritable, biological factors appear to be important in the development of this disorder.
3. The effects of dopamine agonists and antagonists on the positive symptoms of schizophrenia gave rise to the dopamine hypothesis.
4. Evidence of brain abnormalities is found in people with schizophrenia. Many researchers believe that brain abnormalities seen early in life trigger pathological changes during adolescence and young adulthood.
5. Evidence suggests that the negative and cognitive symptoms of schizophrenia are primarily caused by decreased activity of the prefrontal cortex, which causes an increased release of dopamine in the nucleus accumbens and provokes the positive symptoms.

MAJOR AFFECTIVE DISORDERS

6. The major affective disorders include major depression and bipolar disorder. Evidence suggests that both types are heritable.
7. Biological treatments for unipolar depression include noradrenergic or serotonergic agonists, electroconvulsive therapy (ECT), transcranial magnetic stimulation (TMS), bright-light therapy (phototherapy), and sleep deprivation. Bipolar disorder can be effectively treated by lithium and some anticonvulsant drugs.
8. The monoamine hypothesis was suggested by the findings that monoaminergic agonists and antago-

nists affect the symptoms of the affective disorders and that depressive symptoms are provoked by dietary depletion of serotonin in people with a history of this disorder.

9. The presence of one or more short alleles of the 5-HTT promoter gene may be a predisposing factor for affective disorders. People with these alleles show more activation of the amygdala and less activation of the subgenual anterior cingulate cortex.

10. The affective disorders are related to sleep disturbances and can be relieved by REM sleep deprivation or total sleep deprivation. In addition, some people suffer from seasonal affective disorders. Thus, affective disorders may be caused by malfunctions of the neural systems that regulate circadian rhythms.

ANXIETY DISORDERS

11. The most common anxiety disorders are panic disorder, generalized anxiety disorder, and social anxiety disorder. Like depression, these disorders have a hereditary component and are more likely to occur in people who possess at least one short allele of the 5-HT transporter. Treatment includes administration of benzodiazepines and SSRIs.

12. Obsessive-compulsive disorder may be related to the species-typical behaviors of grooming, cleaning, and attention to danger. It has a hereditary component and appears to involve abnormalities or damage to the basal ganglia. It is treated with specific serotonin reuptake inhibitors such as clomipramine, which inhibit these behaviors in laboratory animals.

Suggested Readings

Aouizerate, B., Guehl, D., Cuny, E., Rougier, A., Biolac, B., Tignol, J., and Burbaud, P. Pathophysiology of obsessive-compulsive disorder: A necessary link between phenomenology, neuropsychology, imagery and physiology. *Progress in Neurobiology*, 2004, *72*, 195–221.

Barch, D. M. The cognitive neuroscience of schizophrenia. *Annual Review of Clinical Psychology*, 2005, *1*, 321–353.

Etkin, A., Pittenger, C., Polan, H. J., and Kandel, E. R. Toward a neurobiology of psychotherapy: Basic science and clinical applications. *Journal of Neuropsychiatry and Clinical Neurosciences*, 2005, *17*, 145–158.

Gordon, J. A., and Hen, R. Genetic approaches to the study of anxiety. *Annual Review of Neuroscience*, 2004, *27*, 193–222.

Gross, C., and Hen, R. The developmental origins of anxiety. *Nature Reviews Neuroscience*, 2004, *5*, 545–552.

Hasler, G., Drevets, W. C., Manji, H. K., and Charney, D. S. Discovering endophenotypes for major depression. *Neuropsychopharmacology*, 2004, *29*, 1765–1781.

Merikangas, K. R., and Low, N. C. Genetic epidemiology of anxiety disorders. *Handbook of Experimental Pharmacology*, 2005, *169*, 163–179.

Mueser, K. T., and McGurk, S. R. Schizophrenia. *The Lancet*, 2004, *363*, 2063–2072.

Southwick, S. M., Vythilingam, M., and Charney, D. S. The psychobiology of depression and resilience to stress: Implications for prevention and treatment. *Annual Review of Clinical Psychology*, 2005, *1*, 255–291.

Tsai, G., and Coyle, J. T. Glutamatergic mechanisms in schizophrenia. *Annual Review of Pharmacology and Toxicology*, 2002, *42*, 165–179.

Walker, E., Kestler, L., Bollini, A., and Hochman, K. M. Schizophrenia: Etiology and course. *Annual Review of Psychology*, 2004, *55*, 401–430.

Yudofsky, S. C., and Hales, R. E. *The American Psychiatric Publishing Textbook of Neuropsychiatry and Clinical Neurosciences*, 4th ed. Washington, DC: American Psychiatric Press, 2002.

Additional Resources

Visit www.mypsychkit.com for additional review and practice of the material covered in this chapter. Within MyPsychKit, you can take practice tests and receive a customized study plan to help you review. Dozens of animations, tutorials, and Web links are also available. You can even review using the interactive electronic version of this textbook. You will need to register for MyPsychKit. See www.mypsychkit.com for complete details.

chapter 16 : Autistic, Attention-Deficit/Hyperactivity, Stress, and Substance Abuse Disorders

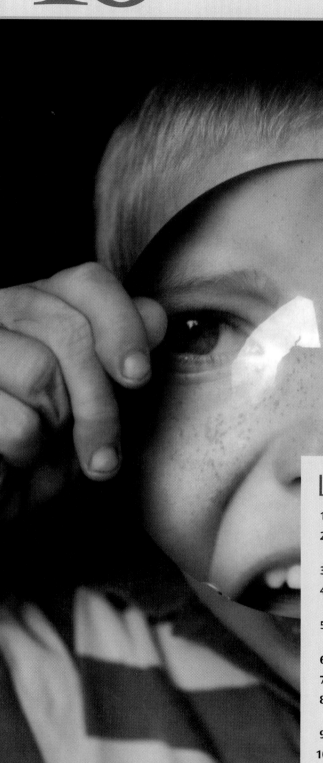

LEARNING OBJECTIVES

1. Describe the symptoms and possible causes of autism.

2. Describe the symptoms and possible causes of attention-deficit/hyperactivity disorder.

3. Describe the physiological responses to stress and their effects on health.

4. Discuss some of the long-term effects of stress, including posttraumatic stress disorder.

5. Discuss the interactions between stress, the immune system, and infectious diseases.

6. Review the general characteristics and consequences of addiction.

7. Discuss the neural mechanisms responsible for craving and relapse.

8. Describe the behavioral and pharmacological effects of opiates, cocaine, amphetamine, and nicotine.

9. Describe the behavioral and pharmacological effects of alcohol and cannabis.

10. Describe research on the role that heredity plays in addiction in humans.

11. Discuss methods of therapy for drug abuse.

John was beginning to feel that perhaps he would be able to get his life back together. It looked as though his drug habit was going to be licked. He had started taking drugs several years ago. At first, he had used them only on special occasions—mostly on weekends with his friends—but heroin proved to be his undoing. One of his acquaintances had introduced him to the needle, and John had found the rush so blissful that he couldn't wait a whole week for his next fix. Soon he was shooting up daily. Shortly after that, he lost his job and, to support his habit, began earning money through car theft and small-time drug dealing. As time went on, he needed more and more heroin at shorter and shorter intervals, which necessitated even more money. Eventually, he was arrested and convicted of selling heroin to an undercover agent.

The judge gave John the choice of prison or a drug rehabilitation program, and he chose the latter. Soon after starting the program, he realized that he was relieved to have been caught. Now that he was clean and could reflect on his life, he realized what would have become of him had he continued to take drugs. Withdrawal from heroin was not an experience he would want to live through again, but it turned out not to be as bad as he had feared. The counselors in his program told him to avoid his old neighborhood and to break contact with his old acquaintances, and he followed their advice. He had been clean for 8 weeks, he had a job, and he had met a woman who really seemed sympathetic. He knew that he hadn't completely kicked his habit, because every now and then, despite his best intentions, he found himself thinking about the wonderful glow that heroin provided him, but things were definitely looking up.

Then one day, while walking home from work, he turned a corner and saw a new poster plastered on the wall of a building. The poster, produced by an antidrug agency, showed all sorts of drug paraphernalia in full color: glassine envelopes with white powder spilling out of them, syringes, needles, a spoon and candle used to heat and dissolve the drug. John was seized with a sudden, intense compulsion to take some heroin. He closed his eyes, trying to will the feeling away, but all he could feel were his churning stomach and his trembling limbs, and all he could think about was getting a fix. He hopped on a bus and went back to his old neighborhood.

hapter 15 discussed mental disorders characterized by maladaptive emotions and thought processes. This chapter considers four more disorders with a physiological basis: autistic disorder, attention-deficit/hyperactivity disorder, stress disorders, and substance abuse disorders.

Autistic Disorder

Description

When a baby is born, the parents normally expect to love and cherish the child and to be loved and cherished in return. Unfortunately, some infants are born with a disorder that impairs their ability to return their parents' affection. The symptoms of **autistic disorder** (often simply referred to as *autism*) include a failure to develop normal social relations with other people, impaired development of communicative ability, and the presence of repetitive, stereotyped behavior. Most people with autistic disorder display cognitive impairments. The syndrome was named and characterized by Kanner (1943), who chose the term (*auto*, "self," *-ism*, "condition") to refer to the child's apparent self-absorption. The reported incidence of autism has increased in the past two decades, but according to Fombonne (2005), evidence indicates that the apparent increase is a result of heightened awareness of the disorder and broadening of the diagnostic criteria. By the way, careful studies have found no evidence that autism is linked to childhood immunization (Thompson et al., 2007; Baird et al., 2008; Hornig et al., 2008).

Autistic disorder is one of several pervasive developmental disorders that have similar symptoms. *Asperger's disorder* is generally less severe, and its symptoms do not include a delay in language development or the presence of important cognitive deficits. The primary symptoms are deficient or absent social interactions and

autistic disorder A chronic disorder whose symptoms include failure to develop normal social relations with other people, impaired development of communicative ability, lack of imaginative ability, and repetitive, stereotyped movements.

477

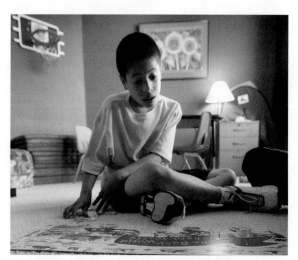

Children with autistic disorders often focus intently on solitary pursuits for long periods of time.

repetitive and stereotyped behaviors along with obsessional interest in narrow subjects. *Rett's disorder* is a genetic neurological syndrome seen in girls that accompanies an arrest of normal brain development that occurs during infancy. This disorder is caused by mutations of a gene on the X chromosome that is expressed in astrocytes but causes abnormalities in neighboring neurons (Ballas et al., 2009; Maezawa et al., 2009). Children with *childhood disintegrative disorder* show normal intellectual and social development and then, some time between the ages of 2 and 10 years, show a severe regression into autism. The prevalence of all forms of pervasive developmental disorders is approximately 60 in 10,000 (Fombonne, 2005).

According to the diagnostic manual of the American Psychiatric Association (*DSM*-IV), a diagnosis of autistic disorder requires the presence of three categories of symptoms: impaired social interactions, absent or deficient communicative abilities, and the presence of stereotyped behaviors. *Social impairments* are the first symptoms to emerge. Infants with autistic disorder do not seem to care whether they are held, or they may arch their backs when picked up, as if they do not want to be held. They do not look or smile at their caregivers. If they are ill, hurt, or tired, they will not look to someone else for comfort. As they get older, they do not enter into social relationships with other children and avoid eye contact with them. They have difficulty predicting other people's behavior or understanding their motivations. In severe cases, autistic people do not even seem to recognize the existence of other people.

The *language development* of people with autism is abnormal or even nonexistent. They often echo what is said to them, and they may refer to themselves as others do—in the second or third person. Autistic people generally show *abnormal interests and behaviors.* For example, they may show stereotyped movements, such as flapping their hand back and forth or rocking back and forth. They may become obsessed with investigating objects, sniffing them, feeling their texture, or moving them back and forth. They may become attached to a particular object and insist on carrying it around with them. They may become preoccupied in lining up objects or in forming patterns with them, oblivious to everything else that is going on around them. They often insist on following precise routines and may become violently upset when they are hindered from doing so. They show no make-believe play and are uninterested in stories that involve fantasy. Although most autistic people are mentally retarded, not all are, and unlike most retarded people, they may be physically adept and graceful. Some have isolated skills, such as the ability to multiply two four-digit numbers very quickly without apparent effort.

Possible Causes

When Kanner first described autism, he suggested that it was of biological origin, but not long afterward, influential clinicians argued that autism was learned. More precisely, it was thought to be taught—by cold, insensitive, distant, demanding, introverted parents. Bettelheim (1967) believed that autism was similar to the apathetic, withdrawn, and hopeless behavior seen in some of the survivors of the Nazi concentration camps of World War II. You can imagine the guilt felt by parents who were told by a mental health professional that they were to blame for their child's pitiful condition. Some professionals saw the existence of autism as evidence for child abuse and advocated that autistic children be removed from their families and placed with foster parents.

Nowadays, researchers and mental health professionals are convinced that autism is caused by biological factors and that parents should be given help and sympathy, not blame. Careful studies have shown that the parents of autistic children are just as warm, sociable, and responsive as other parents (Cox et al., 1975). In addition, parents with one autistic child often raise one or more normal children. If the parents were at fault, we should expect *all* of their offspring to be autistic.

Heritability

Like all the mental disorders described so far, at least some forms of autism appear to be heritable. The best evidence for genetic factors comes from twin studies. These studies indicate that the concordance rate for autism in monozygotic twins is approximately 70 percent, while the rate in dizygotic twins studied so far is approximately 5 percent. The concordance rate for the more broadly defined *autistic spectrum disorders* is 90 percent for monozygotic twins and 10 percent for dizygotic twins (Sebat et al., 2007). Genetic studies indicate that autistic disorder can be caused by a wide variety of mutations, especially those that interfere with neural development and communication (The Autism Genome Project Consortium, 2007; Morrow et al., 2008).

Brain Pathology

The fact that autism is highly heritable is presumptive evidence that the disorder is a result of structural or biochemical abnormalities in the brain. In addition, a variety of medical conditions—especially those that occur during prenatal development—can produce the symptoms of autism. Evidence suggests that approximately 20 percent of all cases of autism have definable biological causes, such as rubella (German measles) during pregnancy; prenatal thalidomide; encephalitis caused by the herpes virus; and tuberous sclerosis, a genetic disorder that causes the formation of benign tumors in many organs, including the brain (DeLong, 1999; Rapin, 1999; Fombonne, 2005).

Evidence obtained in recent years indicates significant abnormalities in the development of the brains of autistic children. Courchesne et al. (2005, 2007) noted that although the autistic brain is, on average, slightly smaller at birth, it begins to grow abnormally quickly, and by 2 to 3 years of age it is about 10 percent larger than a normal brain. Following this early spurt, the growth of the autistic brain slows down, so by adolescence it is only about 1 to 2 percent larger than normal. The regions that appear to be most involved in the functions that are impaired in autism show the greatest growth early in life and the slowest growth between early childhood and adolescence. For example, the frontal cortex and temporal cortex of the autistic brain grow quickly during the first 2 years of life but then show little or no increase in size during the next 4 years, whereas these two regions grow by 20 percent and 17 percent, respectively, in normal brains.

Several studies have found abnormalities in the structure of the higher-order cerebral cortex of the autistic brain, especially those involved in higher-order processes such as communicative functions and interpretation of social stimuli. The unusual features include increased numbers of gyri in the frontal lobes and abnormalities in the number of neurons and in the spacing between them (Casanova, Buxhoeveden, and Gomez, 2003; Levitt et al., 2003). Autistic brains also show abnormalities in white matter. Herbert et al. (2004) found that in the autistic brain, the volume of white matter containing short-range axons was increased but that the volume of white matter containing long-range axons that connect distant regions of the brain was not. Courchesne et al. (2005) suggest that the apparent hyperconnectivity of local regions of the cerebral cortex could account for the exceptional isolated talents and skills shown by some autistics.

Researchers have employed structural and functional imaging methods to investigate the neural basis of the three categories of autistic symptoms. For example, Castelli et al. (2002) showed normal subjects and high-functioning people with autism or Asperger's disorder animations that depicted two triangles interacting in various goal-directed ways (for example, simply chasing or fighting) or in a way that suggested that one triangle was trying to trick or coax the other. For example, one normal subject described an animation in this way: "Triangles cuddling inside the house. Big wanted to persuade little to get out. He didn't want to . . . cuddling again" (p. 1843). People in the autism group were able to accurately describe the goal-directed interactions of the triangles, but they had difficulty accurately describing the "intentions" of a triangle trying to trick or coax the other. Functional imaging during presentation of the animations showed normal activation of early levels of the visual association cortex (the extrastriate cortex), but activation of the superior temporal sulcus (STS) and the medial prefrontal cortex was much lower in members of the autism group. (See *Figure 16.1* and *MyPsychKit 16.1, Inferring Intentions.*) Previous research has shown that the STS plays an important role in detection of stimuli that indicate the actions of another individual (Allison, Puce, and McCarthy, 2000).

The lack of interest in or understanding of other people is reflected in the response of the autistic brain to the sight of the human face. As we saw in Chapter 6, the fusiform face area (FFA), located on a region of the visual association cortex on the base of the brain, is involved in the recognition of individual faces. A functional imaging study by Schultz (2005) found little or no activity in the fusiform face area of autistic adults looking at pictures of human faces. (See *Figure 16.2*.) Autistics are poor at recognizing facial expressions of emotion or the direction of another person's gaze and have low rates of eye contact with other people. It seems likely that the FFA of autistics fails to respond to the sight of the human face because these people spend very little time studying other people's faces and hence do not develop the expertise the rest of us acquire through normal interpersonal interactions.

Baron-Cohen (2002) noted that the behavioral characteristics of people with autistic spectrum disorders appear to be exaggerations of the traits that tend to be associated with males. In fact, the incidence of autistic spectrum disorders is four times more prevalent in males, and that of Asperger's disorder in particular, nine times more prevalent. Baron-Cohen suggested that these disorders may be a reflection of an "extreme male brain." For example, he noted that on average, females are better than males at inferring the thoughts or intentions of others, are more sensitive to facial expressions, are more likely to respond empathetically to the distress of others, and are more likely to share with others and take turns with them. On average, males are less likely to display these characteristics, and they are more likely to compete with their peers, to engage in rough-and-tumble play, and to establish dominance hierarchies. Males also tend to show more interest in toy vehicles, weapons, and building blocks and in pursuits such as engineering, metalworking, and computer programming and are generally better at map reading. In other words, males generally exhibit more interest in working with physical objects and logical systems than with social relations. According to Baron-Cohen, people with autistic spectrum disorders show an exaggerated pattern of masculine interests and behaviors. For example, the lack of interest in other people and an obsession with counting and lining up objects in a row that is seen in many people with autism are seen as extreme examples of masculine traits.

We saw in Chapter 9 that sexual differentiation of the brain is largely controlled by exposure to prenatal androgens. Auyeung et al. (2009) used two tests that measure autistic traits to assess the behavior of normal children

mypsychkit™

Animation 16.1
Inferring Intentions

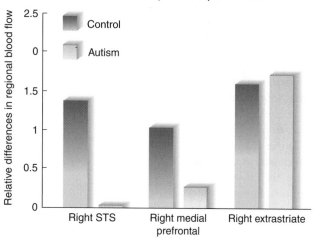

FIGURE 16.1

Inferring Intentions. The graph shows the relative activation of specific brain regions of autistic adults and normal control subjects viewing animations of two triangles moving interactively with implied intentions. STS = superior temporal sulcus.

Regions with Significant Increase in Cerebral Blood Flow

Adapted from Castelli, F., Frith, C., Happé, F., and Frith, U. *Brain*, 2002, *125*, 1839–1849.

whose mothers had undergone amniocentesis (removal of a small amount of amniotic fluid during pregnancy). Amniocentesis normally occurs during the period of peak fetal testosterone secretion, so measurement of testosterone in the amniotic fluid reflects the amount of testosterone to which the fetal brain is exposed. Auyeung and her colleagues found a significant positive correlation between fetal testosterone levels and scores on these tests. The correlation was seen in both males and females separately as well is in the combined group of all children. Even if Baron-Cohen's hypothesis is correct, we cannot conclude that autism is caused by prenatal exposure to excessive amounts of testosterone. An "extreme masculine brain" could be caused by genetic abnormalities that increase the sensitivity of a developing brain to androgens, and there could (and probably are) other causes of autism that have nothing to do with masculinization of the brain.

FIGURE 16.2

The Fusiform Face Area and Autism.   The scans show activation of the fusiform face area of control subjects but not of autistic subjects while looking at pictures of human faces.

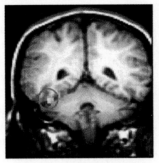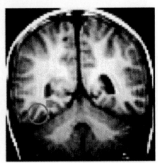

Control   Autistic

Reprinted from *International Journal of Developmental Neuroscience, 23,* Schultz, R. T., Developmental Deficits in Social Perception in Autism: The Role of the Amygdala and Fusiform Face Area, 125–141, Copyright 2005, with permission from Elsevier.

InterimSummary

Autistic Disorder

Autistic disorder occurs in approximately 13 of 10,000 infants. It is characterized by poor or absent social relations and communicative abilities and the presence of repetitive, stereotyped movements. Although autistics are usually, but not always, retarded, they may have a particular, isolated talent. Autistic people have difficulty predicting the behavior of other people or understanding why they act as they do. They tend not to pay attention to other people's faces, as reflected in the lack of activation of the fusiform face area when they do so, and their ability to perceive emotional expressions on other people's faces is impaired.

In the past, clinicians blamed parents for autism, but now it is generally accepted as a disorder with biological roots. Twin studies have shown that autism is highly heritable but that many different genes are responsible for its development. Autism can also be caused by events that interfere with prenatal development, such as prenatal thalidomide or maternal infection with rubella. MRI studies indicate that the brains of babies who become autistic show abnormally rapid growth until the age of 2 to 3 years of age and then grow more slowly than the brains of unaffected children. Regions of the brain involved in higher-order processes such as communicative functions and interpretation of social stimuli develop more quickly in the autistic brain but then fail to continue to develop normally. In addition, long-distance communication between higher-order regions of the brain appears to be impaired. Some characteristics of autism can be seen as exaggerations of behaviors more often seen in males, which has led to the "extreme male brain" hypothesis.

Attention-Deficit/Hyperactivity Disorder

Some children have difficulty concentrating, remaining still, and working on a task. At one time or other, most children exhibit these characteristics, but children with **attention-deficit/hyperactivity disorder (ADHD)** display these symptoms so often that they interfere with the children's ability to learn.

Description

ADHD is the most common behavior disorder that shows itself in childhood. It is usually first discovered in the classroom, where children are expected to sit quietly and pay attention to the teacher or work steadily on a project. Some children's inability to meet these expectations then becomes evident. They have difficulty withholding a response, act without reflecting, often show reckless and impetuous behavior, and let interfering activities intrude into ongoing tasks.

attention-deficit/hyperactivity disorder (ADHD) A disorder characterized by uninhibited responses, lack of sustained attention, and hyperactivity; first shows itself in childhood.

According to the *DSM-IV*, the diagnosis of ADHD requires the presence of six or more of nine symptoms of inattention and six or more of nine symptoms of hyperactivity and impulsivity that have persisted for at least 6 months. Symptoms of inattention include such things as "often had difficulty sustaining attention in tasks of play activities" or "is often easily distracted by extraneous stimuli," and symptoms of hyperactivity and impulsivity include such things as "often runs about or climbs excessively in situations in which it is inappropriate" or "often interrupts or intrudes on others (e.g., butts into conversations or games)" (American Psychiatric Association, 1994, pp. 64–65).

ADHD can be very disruptive of a child's education and that of other children in the same classroom. It is seen in 4 to 5 percent of grade school children. Boys are about ten times more likely than girls to receive a diagnosis of ADHD, but in adulthood the ratio is approximately two to one, which suggests that many girls with this disorder fail to be diagnosed. Because the symptoms can vary—some children's symptoms are primarily those of inattention, some are those of hyperactivity, and some show mixed symptoms—most investigators believe that this disorder has more than one cause. Diagnosis is often difficult, because the symptoms are not well defined. ADHD is often associated with aggression, conduct disorder, learning disabilities, depression, anxiety, and low self-esteem. The most common treatment for ADHD is administration of methylphenidate (Ritalin), a drug that inhibits the reuptake of dopamine.

Possible Causes

There is strong evidence from both family studies and twin studies for hereditary factors that play a role in determining a person's likelihood of developing ADHD. The estimated heritability of ADHD ranges from 75 to 91 percent (Thapar, O'Donovan, and Owen, 2005)

The symptoms of ADHD resemble those produced by damage to the prefrontal cortex: distractibility, forgetfulness, impulsivity, poor planning, and hyperactivity (Aron, Robbins, and Poldrack, 2004). As we saw in Chapter 12, the prefrontal cortex plays a critical role in short-term memory. We use short-term memory to remember what we have just perceived, to remember information that we have just recalled from long-term memory, and to process ("work on") all of this information. For this reason, short-term memory is often referred to as *working memory*. The prefrontal cortex uses working memory to guide thoughts and behavior, regulate attention, monitor the effects of our actions, and organize plans for future actions (Arnsten, 2006). Damage or abnormalities in the neural circuits that perform these functions give rise to the symptoms of ADHD.

As we saw in Chapter 15, the fact that dopamine antagonists were discovered to reduce the positive symptoms of schizophrenia suggested the hypothesis that schizophrenia is caused by an overactivity of dopaminergic transmission. Similarly, the fact that methylphenidate, a dopamine *agonist*, alleviates the symptoms of ADHD has suggested the hypothesis that this disorder is caused by *underactivity* of dopaminergic transmission. We also saw that normal functioning of the prefrontal cortex is impaired by low levels of dopamine receptor stimulation in this region, so the suggestion that abnormalities in dopaminergic transmission play a role in ADHD seem reasonable.

Many studies have shown that the effect of dopamine levels in the prefrontal cortex on the functions of this region follow an inverted U-shaped curve. (See *Figure 16.3*.) Graphs of many behavioral functions have an inverted U shape. For

---

FIGURE 16.3

An Inverted U Curve.   The graph illustrates an inverted (upside-down) U-curve function in which low and high values of the variable on the horizontal axis are associated with low values of the variable on the vertical axis, and moderate values are associated with high values. Presumably, the relation between brain dopamine levels and the symptoms of ADHD follow a function like this one.

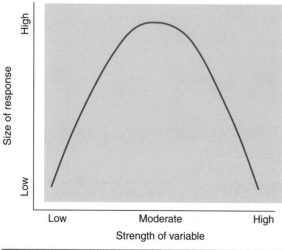

example, moderate levels of motivation increase performance on most tasks, but very low levels fail to induce a person to perform, and very high levels tend to make people nervous and interfere with their performance. The dose-response curve for the effects of methylphenidate also follow an inverted U-shaped function: Doses that are too low are ineffective, and doses that are too high produce increases in activity level that disrupt children's attention and cognition. In fact, a study by Devilbiss and Berridge (2008) found that a moderate dose of methylphenidate increased the responsiveness of neurons in the prefrontal cortex of rats. A high dose of methylphenidate profoundly *suppressed* neural activity.

InterimSummary

Attention-Deficit/Hyperactivity Disorder

Attention-deficit/hyperactivity disorder is the most common behavior disorder that first appears in childhood. Children with ADHD show symptoms of inattention, hyperactivity, and impulsivity. The most common medical treatment is methylphenidate, a dopamine agonist. Family and twin studies indicate a heritable component in this disorder.

Moderate amounts of methylphenidate that decrease the symptoms of ADHD appear to increase the responsiveness of neurons in the prefrontal cortex. Most investigators believe that ADHD is caused by abnormalities in a network of brain structures that include this region.

Stress Disorders

Aversive stimuli can harm people's health. Many of these harmful effects are produced not by the stimuli themselves but by our reactions to them. Walter Cannon, a prominent twentieth-century physiologist, introduced the term **stress** to refer to the physiological reaction caused by the perception of aversive or threatening situations. The physiological responses that accompany the negative emotions prepare us to threaten rivals or fight them or to run away from dangerous situations. Cannon introduced the phrase **fight-or-flight response** to refer to the physiological reactions that prepare us for the strenuous efforts required by fighting or running away. Normally, once we have bluffed or fought with an adversary or run away from a dangerous situation, the threat is over and our physiological condition can return to normal. The fact that the physiological responses may have adverse long-term effects on our health is unimportant as long as the responses are brief. However, sometimes the threatening situations are continuous rather than episodic, producing a more-or-less continuous stress response—and as we will see in the section on posttraumatic stress disorder, sometimes threatening situations are so severe that they trigger responses that can last for months or years.

Physiology of the Stress Response

As we saw in Chapter 10, emotions consist of behavioral, autonomic, and endocrine responses. The latter two components, the autonomic and endocrine responses, are the ones that can have adverse effects on health. (Well, I guess the behavioral components can too—for example, if a person rashly gets into a fight with someone who is much bigger and stronger.) Because threatening situations generally call for vigorous activity, the autonomic and endocrine responses that accompany them are catabolic; that is, they help to mobilize the body's energy resources. The sympathetic branch of the autonomic nervous system is active, and the adrenal glands secrete epinephrine, norepinephrine, and steroid stress hormones. Because the

stress A general, imprecise term that can refer either to a stress response or to a stressor (stressful situation).

fight-or-flight response A species-typical response preparatory to fighting or fleeing; thought to be responsible for some of the deleterious effects of stressful situations on health.

FIGURE 16.4

Control of Secretion of Stress Hormones. The diagram illustrates control of the secretion of glucocorticoids by the adrenal cortex and of catecholamines by the adrenal medulla.

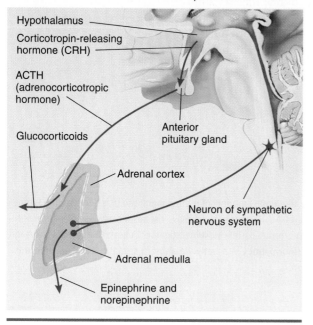

effects of sympathetic activity are similar to those of the adrenal hormones, I will limit my discussion to the hormonal responses.

Epinephrine affects glucose metabolism, causing the nutrients stored in muscles to become available to provide energy for strenuous exercise. Along with norepinephrine, the hormone also increases blood flow to the muscles by increasing the output of the heart. In doing so, it also increases blood pressure, which, over the long term, contributes to cardiovascular disease.

Besides serving as a stress hormone, norepinephrine is (as you know) secreted in the brain as a neurotransmitter. Some of the behavioral and physiological responses produced by aversive stimuli appear to be mediated by noradrenergic neurons. For example, microdialysis studies have found that stressful situations increase the release of norepinephrine in the hypothalamus, frontal cortex, and lateral basal forebrain (Yokoo et al., 1990; Cenci et al., 1992). Presumably, this stress-induced release is controlled by a pathway from the central nucleus of the amygdala to the locus coeruleus, the nucleus of the brain stem that contains NE-secreting neurons.

The other stress-related hormone is *cortisol*, a steroid secreted by the adrenal cortex. Cortisol is called a **glucocorticoid** because it has profound effects on glucose metabolism. In addition, glucocorticoids help to break down protein and convert it to glucose, help to make fats available for energy, increase blood flow, and stimulate behavioral responsiveness, presumably by affecting the brain. They decrease the sensitivity of the gonads to luteinizing hormone (LH), which suppresses the secretion of the sex steroid hormones. In fact, Singer and Zumoff (1992) found that the blood level of testosterone in male hospital residents (doctors, not patients) was severely depressed, presumably because of the stressful work schedule they were obliged to follow. Glucocorticoids have other physiological effects, too, some of which are only poorly understood. Almost every cell in the body contains glucocorticoid receptors, which means that few of them are unaffected by these hormones.

The secretion of glucocorticoids is controlled by neurons in the paraventricular nucleus of the hypothalamus (PVN). The neurons of the PVN secrete a peptide called **corticotropin-releasing hormone (CRH)**, which stimulates the anterior pituitary gland to secrete **adrenocorticotropic hormone (ACTH)**. ACTH enters the general circulation and stimulates the adrenal cortex to secrete glucocorticoids. (See *Figure 16.4.*)

CRH (previously called CRF, or corticotropin-releasing factor) is also secreted within the brain, where it serves as a neuromodulator/neurotransmitter, especially in regions of the limbic system that are involved in emotional responses, such as the periaqueductal gray matter, the locus coeruleus, and the central nucleus of the amygdala. The behavioral effects produced by an injection of CRH into the brain are similar to those produced by aversive situations; thus, some elements of the stress response appear to be produced by the release of CRH by neurons in the brain. For example, intracerebroventricular injection of CRH decreases the amount of time a rat spends in the center of a large open chamber (Britton et al., 1982), enhances the acquisition of a classically conditioned fear response (Cole and Koob, 1988), and increases the startle response elicited by a sudden loud noise (Swerdlow et al., 1986). On the other hand, intracerebroventricular injection of a CRH antagonist *reduces* the anxiety caused by a variety of stressful situations (Kalin, Sherman, and Takahashi, 1988; Heinrichs et al., 1994; Skutella et al., 1994).

glucocorticoid One of a group of hormones of the adrenal cortex that are important in protein and carbohydrate metabolism, secreted especially in times of stress.

corticotropin-releasing hormone (CRH) A hypothalamic hormone that stimulates the anterior pituitary gland to secrete ACTH (adrenocorticotropic hormone).

adrenocorticotropic hormone (ACTH) A hormone released by the anterior pituitary gland in response to CRH; stimulates the adrenal cortex to produce glucocorticoids.

The secretion of glucocorticoids does more than help an animal react to a stressful situation: It helps the animal to survive. If a rat's adrenal glands are removed, the rat becomes much more susceptible to the effects of stress. In fact, a stressful situation that a normal rat would take in its stride might kill one whose adrenal glands have been removed—and physicians know that if an adrenalectomized person is subjected to stressful situations, he or she must be given additional amounts of glucocorticoid (Tyrell and Baxter, 1981).

Health Effects of Long-Term Stress

Many studies of people who have been subjected to stressful situations have found evidence of ill health. For example, survivors of concentration camps, who were obviously subjected to long-term stress, have generally poorer health later in life than other people of the same age (Cohen, 1953). Drivers of subway trains that injure or kill people are more likely to suffer from illnesses several months later (Theorell et al., 1992). Air traffic controllers, especially those who work at busy facilities where the danger of collisions is greatest, show a greater incidence of high blood pressure, which gets worse as they grow older (Cobb and Rose, 1973). (See *Figure 16.5.*) They also are more likely to suffer from ulcers or diabetes.

A pioneer in the study of stress, Hans Selye, suggested that most of the harmful effects of stress were produced by the prolonged secretion of glucocorticoids (Selye, 1976). Although the short-term effects of glucocorticoids are essential, the long-term effects are damaging. These effects include increased blood pressure, damage to muscle tissue, steroid diabetes, infertility, inhibition of growth, inhibition of the inflammatory responses, and suppression of the immune system. High blood pressure can lead to heart attacks and stroke. Inhibition of growth in children who are subjected to prolonged stress prevents them from attaining their full height. Inhibition of the inflammatory response makes it more difficult for the body to heal itself after an injury, and suppression of the immune system makes an individual vulnerable to infections. Long-term administration of steroids to treat inflammatory diseases often produces cognitive deficits and can even lead to *steroid psychosis*, whose symptoms include profound distractibility, anxiety, insomnia, depression, hallucinations, and delusions (Lewis and Smith, 1983; de Kloet, Joëls, and Holsboer, 2005).

The adverse effects of stress on healing were demonstrated in a study by Kiecolt-Glaser et al. (1995), who performed punch biopsy wounds in the subjects' forearms, a harmless procedure that is used often in medical research. The subjects were people who were providing long-term care for relatives with Alzheimer's disease—a situation that is known to cause stress—and control subjects of the same approximate age and family income. The investigators found that healing of the wounds took significantly longer in the caregivers (48.7 days versus 39.3 days). (See *Figure 16.6.*)

Effects of Stress on the Brain

Sapolsky and his colleagues have investigated one rather serious long-term effect of stress: brain damage (Sapolsky, 1992, 1995;

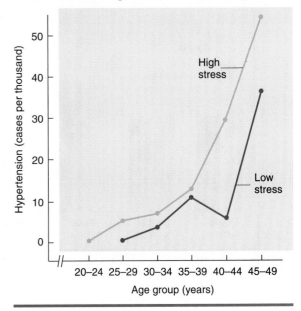

FIGURE 16.5

Stress and Hypertension. The graph shows the incidence of hypertension in various age groups of air traffic controllers at high-stress and low-stress airports.

Based on data from Cobb and Rose, 1973.

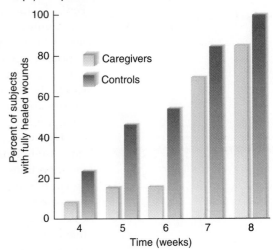

FIGURE 16.6

Stress and Healing of Wounds. The graph shows the percentage of caregivers and control subjects whose wounds had healed as a function of time after the biopsy was performed.

Adapted from Kiecolt-Glaser, J. K., Marucha, P. T., et al. *Lancet*, 1995, *346*, 1194–1196.

FIGURE 16.7

Prenatal Stress and the Amygdala.   The graph shows volumes of nuclei of the amygdala in control rats and rats that had been subjected to prenatal stress.

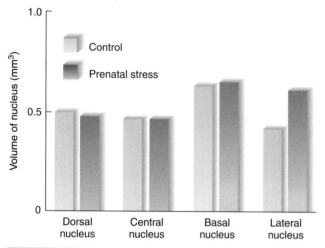

Adapted from Salm, A. K., Pavelko, M., Krouse, E. M., Webster, W., Kraszpulski, M., and Birkle, D. L. *Developmental Brain Research,* 2004, *148,* 159–167.

McEwen and Sapolsky, 1995). As you learned in Chapter 12, the hippocampal formation plays a crucial role in learning and memory, and evidence suggests that one of the causes of memory loss that occurs with aging is degeneration of this brain structure. Research with animals has shown that long-term exposure to glucocorticoids destroys neurons located in field CA1 of the hippocampal formation. Perhaps, then, the stressful stimuli to which people are subjected throughout their lives increase the likelihood of memory problems as they grow older. In fact, Lupien et al. (1996) found that elderly people with elevated blood levels of glucocorticoids learned a maze more slowly than did those with normal levels.

Brunson et al. (2005) confirmed that stress early in life can cause the deterioration of normal hippocampal functions later in life. During the first week after delivery, the investigators placed female rats and their newborn pups in cages with hard floors and only a small amount of nesting material. When the animals were tested at 4 to 5 months of age, their behavior was normal. However, when they were tested at 12 months of age, the investigators observed impaired performance in the Morris water maze and deficient development of long-term potentiation in the hippocampus. They also found dendritic atrophy in the hippocampus, which might have accounted for the impaired spatial learning and synaptic plasticity.

Salm et al. (2004) found that brief episodes of prenatal stress can affect brain development and produce changes that last the animal's lifetime. Once a day during the last week of gestation, they removed pregnant rats from their cage and gave them an injection of a small amount of sterile saline—a procedure that lasted less than 5 minutes. This stress altered the development of their amygdalas. The investigators found that the volume of the lateral nucleus of the amygdala, measured in adulthood, was increased by approximately 30 percent in the animals that sustained prenatal stress. (See *Figure 16.7.*) As previous experiments have shown, prenatal stress increases fearfulness in a novel environment (Ward et al., 2000). Presumably, the increased size of the amygdala contributes to this fearfulness.

A study by Fenoglio, Chen, and Baram (2006) found that experiences that occur during early life can reduce reactivity to stressful situations in adulthood. Fenoglio and her colleagues removed rat pups from their cage, handled them for 15 minutes, and then returned them to their cage. Their mother immediately began licking and grooming the pups. This nurturing behavior activated several regions of the pups' brains, including the central nucleus of the amygdala and the paraventricular nucleus of the hypothalamus, the location of neurons that secrete CRH. The result of this treatment was to reduce the production of CRH in response to stressful stimuli, which conferred a lifelong attenuation of the hormonal stress response.

Uno et al. (1989) found that if long-term stress is intense enough, it can even cause brain damage in young primates. The investigators studied a colony of vervet monkeys housed in a primate center in Kenya. They found that some monkeys died, apparently from stress. Vervet monkeys have a hierarchical society, and monkeys near the bottom of the hierarchy are picked on by the others; thus, they are almost continuously subjected to stress. (Ours is not the only species with social structures that cause a stress reaction in some of its members.) The deceased monkeys had gastric ulcers and enlarged adrenal glands, which are signs of chronic stress—and as Figure 16.8 shows, neurons in the CA1 field of the hippocampal formation were completely destroyed. (See *Figure 16.8.*) Severe stress appears to cause brain damage

FIGURE 16.8

Brain Damage Caused by Stress. The photomicrographs show sections through the hippocampus: (a) a normal monkey and (b) a monkey of low social status subjected to stress. Compare the regions between the arrowheads, which are normally filled with large pyramidal cells.

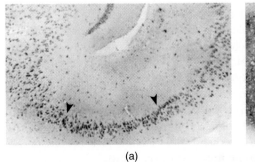
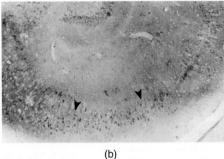

(a)   (b)

From Uno, H., Tarara, R., Else, J. G., et al. *Journal of Neuroscience*, 1989, *9*, 1706–1711. Reprinted by permission of the *Journal of Neuroscience*.

in humans as well; Jensen, Genefke, and Hyldebrandt (1982) found evidence of brain degeneration in CT scans of people who had been subjected to torture.

Several studies have confirmed that the stress of chronic pain has adverse effects on the brain and on cognitive behavior. Apkarian et al. (2004b) found that each year of severe chronic back pain resulted in the loss of 1.3 cm^3 of gray matter in the cerebral cortex, with the greatest reductions seen in the dorsolateral prefrontal cortex. In addition, Apkarian et al. (2004a) found that chronic back pain led to poor performance in a task that has been shown to be affected by lesions of the prefrontal cortex.

Posttraumatic Stress Disorder

The aftermath of tragic and traumatic events such as those that accompany wars and natural disasters often includes psychological symptoms that persist long after the stressful events are over. According to the *DSM-IV*, **posttraumatic stress disorder (PTSD)** is caused by a situation in which a person "experienced, witnessed, or was confronted with an event or events that involved actual or threatened death or serious injury, or a threat to the physical integrity of self or others" that provoked a response that "involved intense fear, helplessness, or horror." The likelihood of developing PTSD is increased if the traumatic event involved danger or violence from other people, such as assault, rape, or wartime experiences (Yehuda and LeDoux, 2007). The symptoms produced by such exposure include recurrent dreams or recollections of the event, feelings that the traumatic event is recurring ("flashback" episodes), and intense psychological distress. These dreams, recollections, or flashback episodes can lead the person to avoid thinking about the traumatic event, which often results in diminished interest in social activities, feelings of detachment from others, suppressed emotional feelings, and a sense that the future is bleak and empty. Particular psychological symptoms include difficulty falling or staying asleep, irritability, outbursts of anger, difficulty in concentrating, and heightened reactions to sudden noises or movements. As this description indicates, people with PTSD have impaired

posttraumatic stress disorder (PTSD) A psychological disorder caused by exposure to a situation of extreme danger and stress; symptoms include recurrent dreams or recollections; can interfere with social activities and cause a feeling of hopelessness.

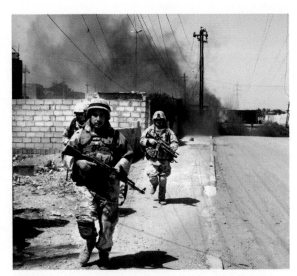

Many American veterans of war grieve the loss of their comrades and relive the horrors experienced during conflict. The experience of wars and other disasters can produce posttraumatic stress disorder in some participants.

FIGURE 16.9

Amygdala and Medial Prefrontal Cortex Activation in PTSD.   The graph shows the activation of the amygdala and medial prefrontal cortex in response to the sight of happy or fearful faces in control subjects and subjects with PTSD.

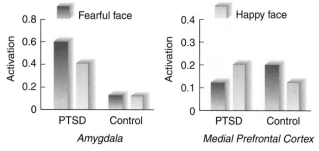

Adapted from Shin, L. M., Wright, C. I., Cannistraro, P. A., et al. *Archives of General Psychiatry*, 2005, *62*, 273–281.

FIGURE 16.10

Role of Desirable and Undesirable Events on Susceptibility to Upper Respiratory Infections. The graph shows the mean percentage change in frequency of undesirable and desirable events during the 10-day period preceding the onset of symptoms of upper respiratory infections.

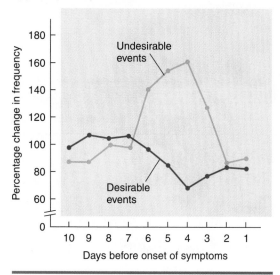

Based on data from Stone, A. A., Reed, B. R., and Neale, J. M. *Journal of Human Stress*, 1987, *13*, 70–74.

mental health functioning. They also tend to have generally poor physical health (Zayfert et al., 2002). Although men are exposed to traumatic events more often than women are, women are more likely to develop PTSD after being exposed to such events (Fullerton et al., 2001).

Evidence from twin studies suggest that genetic factors play a role in a person's susceptibility to develop PTSD. In fact, genetic factors influence not only the likelihood of developing PTSD after being exposed to traumatic events, but also the likelihood that the person will be involved in such an event (Stein et al., 2002). For example, people with a genetic predisposition toward irritability and anger are more likely to be assaulted, and those with a predisposition toward risky behavior are more likely to be involved in accidents.

A few studies have identified several specific genes as possible risk factors for developing PTSD. We are already familiar with one of these genes. As we saw in Chapter 15, the presence of the short allele of the promoter for the 5-HT transporter (5-HTT) gene produces an increased sensitivity to stress and an increased incidence of depression and anxiety disorder. Kilpatrick et al. (2007) studied people living in Florida during the 2004 hurricane season. They found that in people at risk for PTSD (high hurricane exposure and low social support), the presence of the short allele was associated with a 450 percent increase in the incidence of PTSD.

Several studies have found evidence that the amygdala is responsible for emotional reactions in people with PTSD and that the prefrontal cortex plays a role in these reactions in people without PTSD by inhibiting the activity of the amygdala (Rauch, Shin, and Phelps, 2006). For example, a functional imaging study by Shin et al. (2005) found that when shown pictures of faces with fearful expressions, people with PTSD show greater activation of the amygdala and smaller activation of the prefrontal cortex than did people without PTSD. In fact, the symptoms of the people with PTSD were positively correlated with the activation of the amygdala and negatively correlated with the activation of the medial prefrontal cortex. (See *Figure 16.9.*)

Stress and Infectious Diseases

As we have seen, long-term stress can be harmful to one's health and can even result in brain damage. The most important cause of these effects is elevated levels of glucocorticoids, but the high blood pressure caused by epinephrine and norepinephrine also plays a contributing role. In addition, the stress response can impair the functions of the immune system, which protects us from assault from viruses, microbes, fungi, and other types of parasites.

The immune system is one of the most complex systems of the body. Its function is to protect us from infection, and because infectious organisms have developed devious tricks through the process of evolution, our immune system has evolved devious tricks of its own. The immune system derives from white blood cells that develop in the bone marrow and in the thymus gland. Some of the cells roam through the blood or lymphatic system; others reside permanently in one place. Infectious microorganisms have unique proteins on their surfaces, called **antigens**. These proteins serve as the invaders' calling cards, identifying them to the immune system. Through exposure to the microorganisms, the immune system learns to recognize these proteins. (I will not try to explain the mechanism by which this learning takes place.) The result of this learning is the development of special lines of cells that produce specific **antibodies**—proteins that recognize antigens and help to kill the invading microorganism.

Often when a married person dies, his or her spouse dies soon afterward, frequently of an infection. In fact, a wide variety of stress-producing events in a person's life can increase the susceptibility to illness. For example, Glaser et al. (1987) found that medical students were more likely to contract acute infections and to show evidence of suppression of the immune system during the time that final examinations were given.

Stone, Reed, and Neale (1987) attempted to determine whether stressful events in people's daily lives might predispose them to upper respiratory infection. If a person is exposed to a microorganism that might cause such a disease, the symptoms do not occur for several days; that is, there is an incubation period between exposure and signs of the actual illness. Thus, the authors reasoned that if stressful events suppressed the immune system, one might expect to see a higher likelihood of respiratory infections several days after such stress. To test their hypothesis, they asked volunteers to keep a daily record of desirable and undesirable events in their lives over a 12-week period. The volunteers also kept a daily record of any discomfort or symptoms of illness.

The results were as predicted: During the 3- to 5-day period just before showing symptoms of an upper respiratory infection, people experienced an increased number of undesirable events and a decreased number of desirable events in their lives. (See *Figure 16.10*.) Stone et al. (1987) suggested that the effect is caused by decreased production of a particular antibody that is produced by cells in the mucous membranes, including those in the nose, mouth, throat, and lungs. This antibody, IgA (immunoglobulin A), serves as the first defense against infectious microorganisms that enter the nose or mouth. They found that IgA is associated with mood; when a subject is unhappy or depressed, IgA levels are lower than normal. The results suggest that the stress caused by undesirable events may, by suppressing the production of IgA, lead to a rise in the likelihood of upper respiratory infections.

The results of the study by Stone and his colleagues were confirmed by an experiment by Cohen, Tyrrell, and Smith (1991). The investigators found that subjects who were given nasal drops containing cold viruses were much more likely to develop colds if they reported stressful experiences during the past year and if they said they felt threatened, out of control, or overwhelmed by events. (See *Figure 16.11*.)

FIGURE 16.11

Colds and Psychological Stress. The graph shows the percentage of subjects with colds as a function of an index of psychological stress.

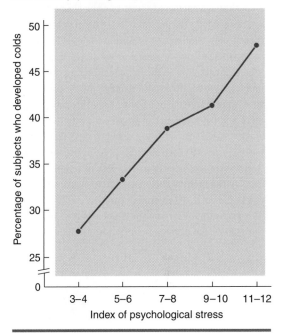

Adapted from Cohen, S., Tyrrell, D. A. J., and Smith, A. P. *New England Journal of Medicine*, 1991, *325*, 606–612.

antigen A protein present on a microorganism that permits the immune system to recognize the microorganism as an invader.

antibody A protein produced by a cell of the immune system that recognizes antigens present on invading microorganisms.

Interim Summary

Stress Disorders

People's emotional reactions to aversive stimuli can harm their health. The stress response, which Cannon called the fight-or-flight response, is useful as a short-term response to threatening stimuli but is harmful in the long term. This response includes increased activity of the sympathetic branch of the autonomic nervous system and increased secretion of hormones by the adrenal gland:

epinephrine, norepinephrine, and glucocorticoids. Corticotropin-releasing hormone, which stimulates the secretion of ACTH by the anterior pituitary gland, is also secreted in the brain, where it elicits some of the emotional responses to stressful situations.

Although increased levels of epinephrine and norepinephrine can raise blood pressure, most of the harm to health comes from glucocorticoids. Prolonged exposure to high levels of these hormones can increase blood pressure, damage muscle tissue, lead to infertility, inhibit growth, inhibit the inflammatory response, and suppress the immune system. It can also damage the hippocampus. Exposure to stress during prenatal or early postnatal life can affect brain development and behavior such as impaired functions of the hippocampus and increased size of the amygdala. These changes appear to predispose animals to react more to stressful situations. In humans, the stress of chronic pain can cause loss of cerebral gray matter, especially in the prefrontal cortex, with accompanying deficits in behaviors that involve the prefrontal cortex.

Exposure to extreme stress can also have long-lasting effects; it can lead to the development of posttraumatic stress disorder. This disorder is associated with memory deficits, poorer health, and a decrease in the size of the hippocampus. Twin studies indicate a hereditary component to susceptibility to PTSD. The prefrontal cortex of people who are resistant to the development of PTSD following severe stress appears to inhibit the amygdala. The prefrontal cortex appears to be hypoactive in people with PTSD.

The immune system consists of white blood cells that develop in the bone marrow or the thymus gland. They produce antibodies that recognize antigens—unique proteins present on the surface of infectious microorganisms. Recognition of these antigens triggers an attack against the invaders. A wide variety of stressful situations have been shown to suppress people's immune system and increase their susceptibility to infectious diseases.

Thought Question

Researchers are puzzled by the fact that glucocorticoids suppress the immune system. Can you think of any potential benefits that come from the fact that our immune system is suppressed during times of danger and stress?

Substance Abuse Disorders

Drug addiction poses a serious problem to our species. Consider the disastrous effects caused by the abuse of one of our oldest drugs, alcohol: automobile accidents, fetal alcohol syndrome, cirrhosis of the liver, Korsakoff's syndrome, increased rate of heart disease, and increased rate of intracerebral hemorrhage. Smoking (addiction to nicotine) greatly increases the chances of dying of lung cancer, heart attack, and stroke; women who smoke give birth to smaller, less healthy babies. Cocaine addiction can cause psychotic behavior, brain damage, and death from overdose; competition for lucrative and illegal markets terrorizes neighborhoods, subverts political and judicial systems, and causes many violent deaths. The use of "designer drugs" exposes users to unknown dangers of untested and often contaminated products, as several people discovered when they acquired Parkinson's disease after taking a synthetic opiate that was tainted with a neurotoxin. Addicts who take their drugs intravenously run a serious risk of contracting AIDS, hepatitis, or other infectious diseases. What makes these drugs so attractive to so many people?

The answer, as you might have predicted from what you have learned about the physiology of reinforcement in Chapter 12, is that all of these substances stimulate brain mechanisms responsible for positive reinforcement. In addition, most of them also reduce or eliminate unpleasant feelings, some of which are produced by the drugs themselves. The immediate consequences of these drugs are more powerful than the realization that in the long term, bad things will happen.

What Is Addiction?

The term *addiction* derives from the Latin word *addicere*, "to sentence." Someone who is addicted to a drug is, in a way, sentenced to a term of involuntary servitude, being obliged to fulfill the demands of his or her drug dependency.

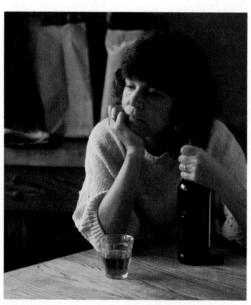

Craving and relapse are important characteristics of substance abuse disorders.

A Little Background

Long ago, people discovered that many substances found in nature—primarily leaves, seeds, and roots of plants but also some animal products—had medicinal qualities. They discovered herbs that helped to prevent infections, that promoted healing, that calmed an upset stomach, that reduced pain, or that helped to provide a night's sleep. They also discovered "recreational drugs": drugs that produced pleasurable effects when eaten, drunk, or smoked. The most universal recreational drug, and perhaps the first one that our ancestors discovered, is ethyl alcohol. Yeast spores are present everywhere, and these microorganisms can feed on sugar solutions and produce alcohol as a by-product. Undoubtedly, people in many different parts of the world discovered the pleasurable effects of drinking liquids that had been left alone for a while, such as the juice that had accumulated in the bottom of a container of fruit. The juice may have become sour and bad-tasting because of the action of bacteria, but the effects of the alcohol encouraged people to experiment, which led to the development of a wide variety of fermented beverages. *Table 16.1* lists the most important addictive drugs and indicates their sites of action.

Positive Reinforcement

Drugs that lead to dependency must first reinforce people's behavior. As we saw in Chapter 12, positive reinforcement refers to the effect that certain stimuli have on the behaviors that preceded them. If, in a particular situation, a behavior is regularly followed by an appetitive stimulus (one that the organism will tend to approach), then that behavior will become more frequent in that situation.

Role in Drug Abuse   The effectiveness of a reinforcing stimulus is greatest if it occurs immediately after a response occurs. If the reinforcing stimulus is delayed, it becomes considerably less effective. The reason for this fact is found by examining the function of instrumental conditioning: learning about the consequences of our own behavior. Normally, causes and effects are closely related in time; we do something, and something happens, good or bad. The consequences of the actions teach us whether to repeat that action, and events that follow a response by more than a few seconds were probably not caused by that response.

An experiment by Logan (1965) illustrates the importance of the immediacy of reinforcement. Logan trained hungry rats to run through a simple maze in which a single passage led to two corridors. At the end of one corridor the rats would find a small piece of food. At the end of the other corridor they would receive much more

TABLE 16.1   Addictive Drugs

Drug	Sites of Action
Ethyl alcohol	NMDA receptor (indirect antagonist); $GABA_A$ receptor (indirect agonist)
Barbiturates	$GABA_A$ receptor (indirect agonist)
Benzodiazepines (tranquilizers)	$GABA_A$ receptor (indirect agonist)
Cannabis (marijuana)	CB_1 cannabinoid receptor (agonist)
Nicotine	Nicotinic ACh receptor (agonist)
Opiates (heroin, morphine, etc.)	μ and δ opiate receptor agonist
Phencyclidine (PCP) and ketamine	NMDA receptor (indirect antagonist)
Cocaine	Blocks reuptake of dopamine (and serotonin and norepinephrine)
Amphetamine	Causes release of dopamine (by running dopamine transporters in reverse)

Adapted from Hyman, S. E., and Malenka, R. C. *Nature Reviews: Neuroscience,* 2001, 2, 695–703.

food, but it would be delivered only after a delay. Although the most intelligent strategy would be to enter the second corridor and wait for the larger amount of food, the rats chose to take the small amount of food that was delivered right away. Immediacy of reinforcement took precedence over quantity.

This phenomenon explains why the most addictive drugs are those that have immediate effects. As we saw in Chapter 4, drug users prefer heroin to morphine not because heroin has a *different* effect, but because it has a more *rapid* effect. In fact, heroin is converted to morphine as soon as it reaches the brain. But because heroin is more lipid soluble, it passes through the blood–brain barrier more rapidly, and its effects on the brain are felt sooner than those of morphine. The most potent reinforcement occurs when drugs produce sudden changes in the activity of the reinforcement mechanism; slow changes are much less reinforcing. A person taking an addictive drug seeks a sudden "rush" produced by a fast-acting drug. (As we will see later, the use of methadone for opiate addiction and nicotine patches for tobacco addiction are based on this phenomenon.)

Neural Mechanisms   As we saw in Chapter 12, all natural reinforcers that have been studied so far (such as food for a hungry animal, water for a thirsty one, or sexual contact) have one physiological effect in common: They cause the release of dopamine in the nucleus accumbens (White, 1996). This effect is not the *only* effect of reinforcing stimuli, and even aversive stimuli can trigger the release of dopamine (Salamone, 1992), but even though there is much that we do not yet understand about the neural basis of reinforcement, the release of dopamine appears to be a *necessary* (but not *sufficient*) condition for positive reinforcement to take place.

Addictive drugs—including amphetamine, cocaine, opiates, nicotine, alcohol, PCP, and cannabis—trigger the release of dopamine in the nucleus accumbens, as measured by microdialysis (Di Chiara, 1995). Different drugs stimulate the release of dopamine in different ways. The details of the ways in which particular drugs interact with the mesolimbic dopaminergic system are described later.

The fact that the reinforcing properties of addictive drugs involve the same brain mechanisms as natural reinforcers indicates that these drugs "hijack" brain mechanisms that normally help us adapt to our environment. It appears that the process of addiction begins in the mesolimbic dopaminergic system and then produces long-term changes in other brain regions that receive input from these neurons (Kauer and Malenka, 2007). The first changes appear to take place in the ventral tegmental area (VTA). Saal et al. (2003) found that a single administration of a variety of addictive drugs (including cocaine, amphetamine, morphine, alcohol, and nicotine) increased the strength of excitatory synapses on dopaminergic neurons in the VTA in mice.

As a result of these changes, increased activation is seen in a variety of regions that receive dopaminergic input from the VTA, including the nucleus accumbens (NAC), located in the ventral striatum. Subsequent changes that are responsible for the compulsive behaviors that characterize addiction occur only after continued use of an addictive drug. The most important of these changes appears to occur in the dorsal striatum: in the caudate nucleus and putamen. We saw in Chapter 12 that the basal ganglia (which includes the dorsal striatum) play a critical role in instrumental conditioning—and the process of addiction involves just that. In fact, a functional imaging study by Volkow et al. (2006) found that when people who were addicted to cocaine watched a video of people smoking cocaine, an increased release of dopamine was seen in the dorsal striatum. These results were similar to what Volkow et al. (2002) saw in a study of hungry people looking at, smelling, and receiving a miniscule taste of appetizing food.

Negative Reinforcement

You have probably heard the old joke in which someone says that the reason he bangs his head against the wall is that "it feels so good when I stop." Of course, that joke is funny (well, mildly amusing) because we know that although no one would act that way, ceasing to bang our head against the wall is certainly better than continuing to do so. If someone else started hitting us on the head and we were able to do something to get them to stop, whatever it was that we did would certainly be reinforced.

A behavior that turns off (or reduces) an aversive stimulus will be reinforced. This phenomenon is known as **negative reinforcement**, and its usefulness is obvious. For example, consider the following scenario: A woman staying in a rented house cannot get to sleep because of the unpleasant screeching noise that the furnace makes. She goes to the basement to discover the source of the noise and finally kicks the side of the oil burner. The noise ceases. The next time the furnace screeches, she immediately goes to the basement and kicks the side of the oil burner. The unpleasant noise (the aversive stimulus) is terminated when the woman kicks the side of the oil burner (the response), so the response is reinforced.

People who abuse some drugs become physically dependent on the drug; that is, they show *tolerance* and *withdrawal symptoms*. As we saw in Chapter 4, **tolerance** is the decreased sensitivity to a drug that comes from its continued use; a user must take larger and larger amounts of the drug for it to be effective. Once a person has taken an opiate regularly enough to develop tolerance, that person will suffer *withdrawal symptoms* if he or she stops taking the drug. **Withdrawal symptoms** are primarily the opposite of the effects of the drug itself. The effects of heroin—euphoria, constipation, and relaxation—lead to the withdrawal effects of dysphoria, cramping and diarrhea, and agitation.

Most investigators believe that tolerance is produced by the body's attempt to compensate for the unusual condition of heroin intoxication. The drug disturbs normal homeostatic mechanisms in the brain, and in reaction these mechanisms begin to produce effects opposite to those of the drug, partially compensating for the disturbance. Because of these compensatory mechanisms, the user must take increasing amounts of heroin to achieve the effects that were produced when he or she first started taking the drug. These mechanisms also account for the symptoms of withdrawal: When the person stops taking the drug, the compensatory mechanisms make themselves felt, unopposed by the action of the drug.

Although positive reinforcement seems to be what provokes drug taking in the first place, reduction of withdrawal effects could certainly play a role in maintaining someone's drug addiction. The withdrawal effects are unpleasant, but as soon as the person takes some of the drug, these effects go away, producing negative reinforcement.

Negative reinforcement could also explain the acquisition of drug addictions under some conditions. If a person is suffering from some unpleasant feelings and then takes a drug that eliminates these feelings, the person's drug-taking behavior is likely to be reinforced. For example, alcohol can relieve feelings of anxiety. If a man finds himself in a situation that arouses anxiety, he might find that having a drink or two makes him feel much better. In fact, people often anticipate this effect and begin drinking before the situation actually occurs.

Craving and Relapse

Why do drug addicts crave drugs? Why does this craving occur even after a long period of abstinence? Even after going for months or years without taking an addictive drug, a former drug addict might sometimes experience intense craving that leads to relapse. Clearly, taking a drug over an extended period of time must produce some long-lasting changes in the brain that increase a person's likelihood of relapsing. Understanding this process might help clinicians to devise therapies that will assist people in breaking their drug dependence once and for all.

One of the ways in which craving has been investigated in laboratory animals is through the *reinstatement model* of drug seeking. Animals are first trained to make a response (for example, pressing a lever) that is reinforced by intravenous injections

negative reinforcement The removal or reduction of an aversive stimulus that is contingent on a particular response, with an attendant increase in the frequency of that response.

tolerance The fact that increasingly large doses of drugs must be taken to achieve a particular effect; caused by compensatory mechanisms that oppose the effect of the drug.

withdrawal symptoms The appearance of symptoms opposite to those produced by a drug when the drug is suddenly no longer taken; caused by the presence of compensatory mechanisms.

FIGURE 16.12

The Reinstatement Procedure, a Measure of Craving.
The graph shows the acquisition of lever pressing for injections of an addictive drug during the self-administration phase, and the extinction of lever pressing when the drug was no longer administered. A "free" shot of the drug or presentation of a cue associated with the drug during acquisition will reinstate responding.

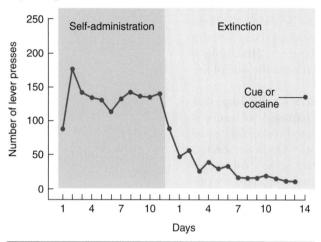

Adapted from Kalivas, P. W., Peters, J., and Knackstedt, L. *Molecular Interventions*, 2006, *6*, 339–344.

of a drug such as cocaine. Next, the response is extinguished by providing injections of a saline solution rather than the drug. Once the animal has stopped responding, the experimenter administers a "free" injection of the drug or presents a stimulus that has been associated with the drug. In response to these stimuli, the animals begin responding at the lever once more (Kalivas, Peters, and Knackstedt, 2006). Presumably, this kind of relapse (reinstatement of a previously extinguished response) is a good model for the craving that motivates drug-seeking behavior in a former addict. (See *Figure 16.12*.)

Not surprisingly, relapses involve activation of the mesolimbic system of dopaminergic neurons. If the nucleus accumbens is inhibited with a direct injection of a drug that blocks neural activity, a "free" shot of cocaine fails to reinstate responding in rats (Grimm and See, 2000; McFarland and Kalivas, 2001).

Functional imaging studies in humans show that drugs of abuse (including cocaine, heroin, and nicotine) or cues associated with them activate several regions of the brain. The cortical regions most often activated include the ACC and orbitofrontal cortex (OFC) and, less often, the insula and dorsolateral prefrontal cortex (Goldstein and Volkow, 2002; Daglish et al., 2003; Brody et al., 2004; Myrick et al., 2004; Wang et al., 2007). For example, Myrick et al. (2004) found that a sip of alcohol and the sight of alcohol-related images increased craving in alcoholic subjects but not control subjects (social drinkers). The NAC, ACC, VTA, and insula were activated in alcoholic subjects, but only the ACC was activated in control subjects. (See *Figure 16.13*.)

As we saw in earlier chapters, the prefrontal cortex plays an important role in executive functions, including planning, evaluation of the consequences of actions, and inhibition of responses when conditions indicate that they would be inappropriate. For example, we saw in Chapter 10 that people with lesions of the medial prefrontal cortex have difficulty inhibiting responses and controlling their emotions. They were also more likely to engage in risky behavior. I'm sure you can see the similarity between this behavior and that of people addicted to drugs. The behavior of

FIGURE 16.13

Craving in Alcoholic People.   This figure shows the activation of the nucleus accumbens (NAC), anterior cingulate cortex (ACC), and ventral tegmental area (VTA) in alcoholic subjects and control subjects who were given a sip of alcohol and were shown alcohol-related images.

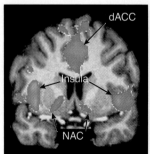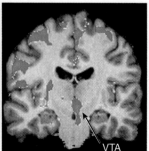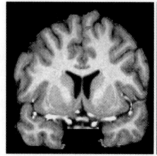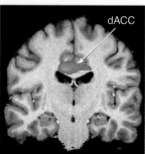

Alcoholics   Controls

Reprinted by permission from Macmillan Publishers Ltd: *Neuropsychopharmacology*, Myrick, H., Anton, R. F., Li, X., et al., Differential brain activity in alcoholics and social drinkers to alcohol cues: Relationship to craving, *29*, 393–402, copyright 2004.

both groups of people is not inhibited by the long-term effects of particular actions, but is dominated by immediate gratification, such as that provided by a drug.

Volkow et al. (2002) found that the activity of the medial prefrontal cortex of cocaine abusers was less active than that of normal subjects during abstinence. In addition, when addicts are performing tasks that normally activate the prefrontal cortex, their medial prefrontal cortex is less activated than that of healthy control subjects, and they perform more poorly on the tasks (Bolla et al., 2004; Garavan and Stout, 2005). In fact, Bolla and her colleagues found that the amount of activation of the medial prefrontal cortex was inversely related to the amount of cocaine that cocaine abusers normally took each week: The lower the brain activity, the more cocaine the person took. (See *Figure 16.14.*)

People with a long history of drug abuse not only show the same deficits on tasks that involve the prefrontal cortex as people with lesions of this region, they also show structural abnormalities of this region. For example, Franklin et al. (2002) reported an average decrease of 5 to 11 percent in the gray matter volume of the superior temporal cortex and various regions of the prefrontal cortex of chronic cocaine abusers.

As we saw in Chapter 15, the negative and cognitive symptoms of schizophrenia appear to be a result of hypofrontality—decreased activity of the prefrontal cortex. These symptoms are very similar to those that accompany long-term drug abuse. In fact, studies have shown a high level of comorbidity of schizophrenia and substance abuse. (*Comorbidity* refers to the simultaneous presence of two or more disorders in the same person.) For example, up to half of all people with schizophrenia have a substance abuse disorder (alcohol or illicit drugs), and 70 to 90 percent are nicotine dependent (Brady and Sinha, 2005). In fact, in the United States, smokers with psychiatric disorders, who constitute approximately 7 percent of the population, consume 34 percent of all cigarettes (Dani and Harris, 2005). Mathalon et al. (2003) found that prefrontal gray matter volumes were 10.1 percent lower in alcoholic patients, 9.0 percent lower in schizophrenic patients, and 15.6 percent lower in patients with both disorders. (See *Figure 16.15.*) These results suggest that abnormalities in the prefrontal cortex may be a common factor in schizophrenia and substance abuse disorders. Whether preexisting abnormalities increase the risk of these disorders or whether the disorders cause the abnormalities has not yet been determined.

Weiser et al. (2004) administered a smoking questionnaire to a random sample of adolescent military recruits each year. Over a 4- to 16-year follow-up period, they found that compared with nonsmokers, the prevalence of hospitalization for schizophrenia was 2.3 times higher in recruits who smoked at least ten cigarettes per day. (See *Figure 16.16.*) These results suggest that abnormalities in the prefrontal cortex may be a common factor in schizophrenia and substance abuse disorders.

The role of the prefrontal cortex in judgment, risk-taking, and control of inappropriate behaviors may explain why adolescents are much more vulnerable to drug addiction than are adults. Adolescence is a time of rapid and profound maturational change in the brain—particularly in the prefrontal cortex. Before these circuits reach their adult form, adolescents are more likely to display increased levels of impulsive, novelty-driven, risky behavior, including experimentation with alcohol, nicotine, and illicit drugs. Addiction in adults most often begins in adolescence or young adulthood. Approximately 50 percent of cases of addiction begin between the ages of 15 and 18, and very few begin after age 20. In addition, early onset of drug-taking is associated with more severe addiction and a greater likelihood of multiple substance abuse (Chambers, Taylor, and Potenza, 2003). Presumably, the

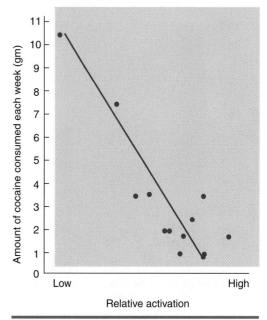

FIGURE 16.14

Cocaine Intake and the Medial Prefrontal Cortex.   The graph shows the relative activation of the medial prefrontal cortex as a function of the amount of cocaine normally taken each week by cocaine abusers.

Adapted from Bolla, K., Ernst, M., Kiehl, K., et al. *Journal of Neuropsychiatry and Clinical Neuroscience,* 2004, *16,* 456–464.

FIGURE 16.15

Alcoholism, Schizophrenia, and Prefrontal Gray Matter.   The graph shows the volume of gray matter in the prefrontal cortex of healthy controls, alcoholic patients, schizophrenic patients, and patients comorbid for both disorders.

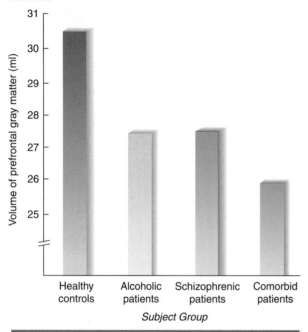

Adapted from Mathalon, D. H., Pfefferbaum, A., Lim, K. O., et al. *Archives of General Psychiatry*, 2003, *60*, 245–252.

final development of neural circuits involved in behavioral control and judgment, along with the maturity that comes from increased experience, help people emerging from adolescence to resist the temptation to abuse drugs. In fact, Tarter et al. (2003) found that 10- to 12-year-old boys who received low scores on tests of behavioral inhibition were more likely to develop substance use disorder by age 19.

As we have just seen, the presence of drug-related stimuli can trigger craving and drug-seeking behavior. In addition, clinicians have long observed that stressful situations can cause former drug addicts to relapse. These effects have also been observed in rats that had previously learned to self-administer cocaine or heroin (Covington and Miczek, 2001). The mechanism that triggers relapse appears to involve the stress-induced release of corticotropin releasing hormone (CRH) in the brain. A study by Hahn, Hopf, and Bonci (2009) found that infusion of CRH caused an enhanced activation of dopaminergic neurons in the ventral tegmental area in mice that had been exposed to cocaine.

Commonly Abused Drugs

People have been known to abuse an enormous variety of drugs, including alcohol, barbiturates, opiates, tobacco, amphetamine, cocaine, cannabis, hallucinogens such as LSD, PCP, volatile solvents such as glues or even gasoline, ether, and nitrous oxide. The pleasure that children often derive from spinning themselves until they become dizzy may even be related to the effects of some of these drugs. Obviously, I cannot hope to discuss all these drugs in any depth and keep this chapter to a reasonable length, so I will restrict my discussion to the most important of them in terms of popularity and potential for addiction. Some drugs, such as caffeine, are both popular and addictive, but because they do not normally cause intoxication, impair health, or interfere with productivity, I will not discuss them here. (Chapter 4 did discuss the behavioral effects and site of action of caffeine.) I will also not discuss the wide variety of hallucinogenic drugs such as LSD or PCP. Although some people enjoy the mind-altering effects of LSD, many people simply find them frightening; in any event, LSD use does not normally lead to addiction. PCP (phencyclidine) acts as an indirect antagonist at the NMDA receptor, which means that its effects overlap with those of alcohol. Rather than devoting space to this drug, I have chosen to say more about alcohol, which is abused far more than any of the hallucinogenic drugs. If you would like to learn more about drugs other than the ones I discuss here, I suggest you consult the suggested readings at the end of this chapter.

Opiates

Opium, derived from a sticky resin produced by the opium poppy, has been eaten and smoked for centuries. Opiate addiction has several high personal and social costs. First, because heroin, the most commonly abused opiate, is an illegal drug in most countries, an addict becomes, by definition, a criminal. Second, because of tolerance, a person must take increasing amounts of the drug to achieve a "high." The habit thus becomes more and more expensive, and the person often turns to crime to obtain enough money to support his or her habit. Third, an opiate addict often uses unsanitary needles; at present, a substantial percentage of people who inject illicit drugs have been exposed in this way to hepatitis or the AIDS virus. Fourth, if the addict is a pregnant woman, her infant will also become dependent on the drug, which easily crosses the placental barrier. The infant must be given opiates right after being born and then weaned off the drug with gradually decreasing doses. Fifth, the uncertainty about the strength of a given batch of heroin makes it possible for a user to receive an unusually large dose of the drug, with possibly fatal consequences.

As we saw earlier, laboratory animals will self-administer opiates. When an opiate is administered systemically, it stimulates opiate receptors located on neurons in various parts of the brain and produces a variety of effects, including analgesia, hypothermia (lowering of body temperature), sedation, and reinforcement. Opiate receptors in the periaqueductal gray matter are primarily responsible for the analgesia, those in the preoptic area are responsible for the hypothermia, those in the mesencephalic reticular formation are responsible for the sedation, and those in the ventral tegmental area and the nucleus accumbens are responsible for the reinforcing effects of opiates.

As we saw earlier, reinforcing stimuli cause the release of dopamine in the nucleus accumbens. Injections of opiates are no exception to this general rule; Wise et al. (1995) found that the level of dopamine in the nucleus accumbens increased by 150 to 300 percent while a rat was pressing a lever that delivered intravenous injections of heroin. Rats will also press a lever that delivers injections of an opiate directly into the ventral tegmental area (Devine and Wise, 1994) or the nucleus accumbens (Goeders, Lane, and Smith, 1984). In other words, injections of opiates into both ends of the mesolimbic dopaminergic system are reinforcing. These findings suggest that the reinforcing effects of opiates are produced by activation of neurons of the mesolimbic system and release of dopamine in the nucleus accumbens.

Stimulant Drugs: Cocaine and Amphetamine

Cocaine and amphetamine have similar behavioral effects, because both act as potent dopamine agonists. However, their sites of action are different. Cocaine binds with and deactivates the dopamine transporter proteins, thus blocking the reuptake of dopamine after it is released by the terminal buttons. Amphetamine also inhibits the reuptake of dopamine, but its most important effect is to directly stimulate the release of dopamine from terminal buttons. *Methamphetamine* is chemically related to amphetamine, but is considerably more potent. Because the effects of cocaine and methamphetamine are so potent and so rapid, they are probably the most effective reinforcers of all available drugs. In fact, if rats or monkeys are given continuous access to a lever that permits them to self-administer cocaine, they often self-inject so much cocaine that they die. Bozarth and Wise (1985) found that rats that self-administered cocaine were almost three times more likely to die than rats that self-administered heroin. (See *Figure 16.17*.)

As we have seen, the mesolimbic dopamine system plays an essential role in all forms of reinforcement. If drugs that block dopamine receptors are injected into the nucleus accumbens, cocaine loses much of its reinforcing effect (McGregor and Roberts, 1993; Caine et al., 1995). In addition, destruction of dopaminergic terminals in the nucleus accumbens with a local injection of 6-HD interferes with the reinforcing effects of both cocaine and amphetamine (Caine and Koob, 1994).

Some evidence suggests that the use of stimulant drugs may have adverse long-term effects on the brain. For example,

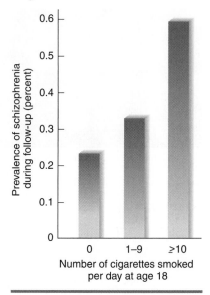

FIGURE 16.16

Smoking and Schizophrenia. The graph shows the prevalence of schizophrenia during a 4- to 16-year follow-up period as a function of number of cigarettes smoked each day at age 18.

Adapted from Weiser, M., Reichenberg, A., Grotto, I., et al. *American Journal of Psychiatry*, 2004, *161*, 1219–1223.

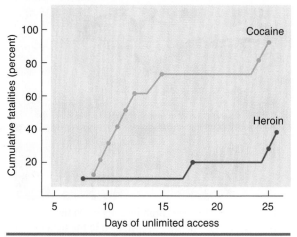

FIGURE 16.17

Cumulative Fatalities of Rats Self-Administering Cocaine or Heroin

Adapted from Bozarth, M. A., and Wise, R. A. *Journal of the American Medical Association*, 1985, *254*, 81–83.

FIGURE 16.18

Dopamine Transporters, Methamphetamine Abuse, and Parkinson's Disease. The scans show concentrations of dopamine transporters from a control subject, a subject who had previously abused methamphetamine, and a subject with Parkinson's disease. Decreased concentrations of dopamine transporters indicate loss of dopaminergic terminals.

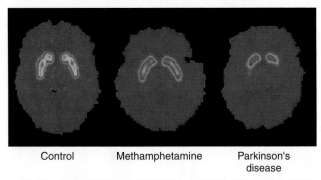

Control   Methamphetamine   Parkinson's disease

From McCann, U. D., Wong, D. F., Yokoi, F., et al. *Journal of Neuroscience*, 1998, *18*, 8417–8422. By permission.

a PET study by McCann et al. (1998) discovered that prior abusers of methamphetamine showed a decrease in the numbers of dopamine transporters in the caudate nucleus and putamen, despite the fact that they had abstained from the drug for approximately 3 years. The decreased number of dopamine transporters suggests that the number of dopaminergic terminals in these regions is diminished. As the authors note, these people might have an increased risk of Parkinson's disease as they get older. (See *Figure 16.18.*) Studies with laboratory animals have also found that methamphetamine can damage terminals of serotonergic axons and trigger death through apoptosis in the cerebral cortex, striatum, and hippocampus (Cadet, Jayanthi, and Deng, 2003).

Nicotine

Nicotine might seem rather tame in comparison to opiates, cocaine, and amphetamine. Nevertheless, nicotine is an addictive drug, and it accounts for more deaths than the so-called "hard" drugs. The combination of nicotine and other substances in tobacco smoke is carcinogenic and leads to cancer of the lungs, mouth, throat, and esophagus. The World Health Organization (WHO, 1997) reported that one-third of the adult population of the world smokes and that smoking is one of the few causes of death that is rising in developing countries. The WHO estimates that 50 percent of the people who begin to smoke as adolescents and continue smoking throughout their lives will die from smoking-related diseases. Investigators estimate that by the year 2015, tobacco will be the largest single health problem worldwide, with 6.4 million deaths per year (Mathers and Loncar, 2006). In fact, tobacco use is the leading cause of preventable death in developed countries (Dani and Harris, 2005). In the United States alone, tobacco addiction kills more than 430,000 people each year (Chou and Narasimhan, 2005). Smoking by pregnant women also has negative effects on the health of their fetuses—apparently worse than those of cocaine (Slotkin, 1998). Unfortunately, approximately 25 percent of pregnant women in the United States expose their fetuses to nicotine.

Although executives of tobacco companies and others whose economic welfare is linked to the production and sale of tobacco products have argued in the past that smoking is a "habit" rather than an "addiction," evidence suggests that the behavior of people who regularly use tobacco is that of compulsive drug users. In a review of the literature, Stolerman and Jarvis (1995) noted that smokers tend to smoke regularly or not at all; few can smoke just a little. Males smoke an average of seventeen cigarettes per day, while females smoke an average of fourteen. Nineteen out of twenty smokers smoke every day, and only 60 out of 3500 smokers questioned smoke fewer than five cigarettes per day. Forty percent of people continue to smoke after having had a laryngectomy (which is usually performed to treat throat cancer). Indeed, physicians have reported that patients with tubes inserted into their tracheas so that they can breathe will sometimes press a cigarette against the opening of these tubes and try to smoke (Hyman and Malenka, 2001). More than 50 percent of heart attack survivors continue to smoke, and about 50 percent of people continue to smoke after submitting to surgery for lung cancer. Of those who attempt to quit smoking by enrolling in a special

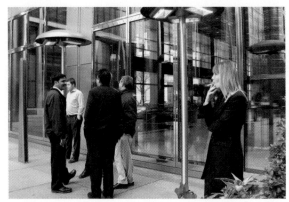

Now that many employers prohibit smoking in the workplace, we have become accustomed to the sight of people outside a building, satisfying their nicotine addictions.

program, 20 percent manage to abstain for 1 year. The record is much poorer for those who try to quit on their own: One-third manage to stop for 1 day, one-fourth for 1 week, but only 4 percent manage to abstain for 6 months. It is difficult to reconcile these figures with the assertion that smoking is merely a "habit" that is pursued for the "pleasure" that it produces.

Ours is not the only species willing to self-administer nicotine; so will laboratory animals (Donny et al., 1995). Nicotine stimulates nicotinic acetylcholine receptors, of course. It also increases the activity of dopaminergic neurons of the mesolimbic system (Mereu et al., 1987) and causes dopamine to be released in the nucleus accumbens (Damsma, Day, and Fibiger, 1989). Figure 16.19 shows the effects of two injections of nicotine or saline on the extracellular dopamine level of the nucleus accumbens, measured by microdialysis. (See *Figure 16.19.*)

Studies have found that the endogenous cannabinoids play a role in the reinforcing effects of nicotine. *Rimonabant*, a drug that blocks cannabinoid CB_1 receptors, blocks the reinforcing effects of nicotine in rats (Cohen, Kodas, and Griebel, 2005), apparently by reducing the release of dopamine in the NAC (De Vries and Schoffelmeer, 2005). As we will see later in this chapter, rimonabant has been used to help prevent relapse in people who are trying to quit smoking.

FIGURE 16.19

Nicotine and Dopamine Release in the Nucleus Accumbens.   The graph shows changes in dopamine concentration in the nucleus accumbens, measured by microdialysis, in response to injections of nicotine or saline. The arrows indicate the time of the injections.

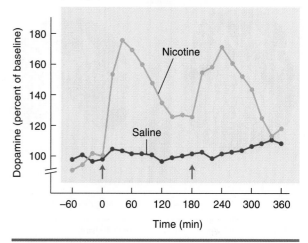

Adapted from Damsma, G., Day, J., and Fibiger, H. C. *European Journal of Pharmacology*, 1989, *168*, 363–368.

Patient N. is a [38-year-old man who] started smoking at the age of 14. At the time of his stroke, he was smoking more than 40 unfiltered cigarettes per day and was enjoying smoking very much. . . . [H]e used to experience frequent urges to smoke, especially upon waking, after eating, when he drank coffee or alcohol, and when he was around other people who were smoking. He often found it difficult to refrain from smoking in situations where it was inappropriate, e.g., at work or when he was sick and bedridden. He was aware of the health risks of smoking before his stroke but was not particularly concerned about those risks. Before his stroke, he had never tried to stop smoking, and he had had no intention of doing so. N. smoked his last cigarette on the evening before his stroke. When asked about his reason for quitting smoking, he stated simply, "I forgot that I was a smoker." When asked to elaborate, he said that he did not forget the fact that he was a smoker but rather that "my body forgot the urge to smoke." He felt no urge to smoke during his hospital stay, even though he had the opportunity to go outside to smoke. His wife was surprised by the fact that he did not want to smoke in the hospital, given the degree of his prior addiction. N. recalled how his roommate in the hospital would frequently go outside to smoke and that he was so disgusted by the smell upon his roommate's return that he asked to change rooms. He volunteered that smoking in his dreams, which used to be pleasurable before his stroke, was now disgusting. N. stated that, although he ultimately came to believe that his stroke was caused in some way by smoking, suffering a stroke was not the reason why he quit. In fact, he did not recall ever making any effort to stop smoking. Instead, it seemed to him that he had spontaneously lost all interest in smoking. When asked whether his stroke might have destroyed some part of his brain . . . that made him want to smoke, he agreed that this was likely to have been the case. (Naqvi et al., 2007, p. 534)

As Naqvi and his colleagues reported (Naqvi et al. 2007; Naqvi and Bechara, 2009), Mr. N. sustained a stroke that damaged his insula. In fact, so did several other patients with insular damage. Naqvi and his colleagues identified nineteen cigarette smokers with damage to the insula and fifty smokers with brain damage that spared this region. Nineteen of the patients had damage to the insula, and twelve of them

FIGURE 16.20

Damage to the Insula and Smoking Cessation.   The diagrams show the regions of the brain (shown in red) where damage was most highly correlated with cessation of smoking.

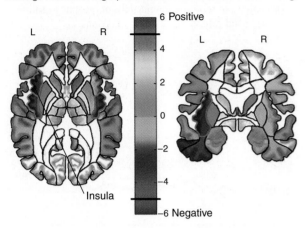

Degree of correlation with smoking cessation

From Naqvi, N. H., Rudrauf, D., Damasio, H., and Bechara, A. *Science*, 2007, *315*, 531–534. Copyright © 2007. Reprinted with permission from AAAS.

"quit smoking easily, immediately, without relapse, and without persistence of the urge to smoke" (p. 531). One patient with insula damage quit smoking but still reported feeling an urge to smoke. Figure 16.20 shows computer-generated images of brain damage that showed a statistically significant correlation with disruption of smoking. As you can see, the insula, which is colored red, showed the highest association with cessation of smoking. (See *Figure 16.20.*) This remarkable finding certainly deserves to be followed up.

One of the deterrents to cessation of smoking is the fact that overeating and weight gain frequently occur when people stop smoking. Jo, Wiedl, and Role (2005) have discovered the apparent cause of this phenomenon. As we saw in Chapter 11, eating and a reduction in metabolic rate are stimulated by the activity of two different types of neurons whose cell bodies are located in the lateral hypothalamus. One of these sets of neurons secretes a peptide called melanocyte-concentrating hormone (MCH). Jo and his colleagues found that nicotinic receptors are located on the terminals of GABAergic neurons in the lateral hypothalamus that form synapses with MCH neurons. When nicotine activates these terminals, the release of GABA is increased, which inhibits MCH neurons, thus suppressing appetite. When people try to quit smoking, they are often discouraged by the fact that the absence of nicotine in their brains releases their MCH neurons from this inhibition, increasing their appetite.

Alcohol

Alcohol has enormous costs to society. A large percentage of deaths and injuries caused by motor vehicle accidents are related to alcohol use, and alcohol contributes to violence and aggression. Chronic alcoholics often lose their jobs, their homes, and their families; many die of cirrhosis of the liver, exposure, or diseases caused by poor living conditions and abuse of their bodies. As we saw in Chapter 14, women who drink during pregnancy run the risk of giving birth to babies with fetal alcohol syndrome, which includes malformation of the head and the brain and accompanying mental retardation. In fact, alcohol consumption by pregnant women is one of the leading causes of mental retardation in the Western world today. Therefore, understanding the physiological and behavioral effects of this drug is an important issue.

At low doses, alcohol produces mild euphoria and has an *anxiolytic* effect; that is, it reduces the discomfort of anxiety. At higher doses, it produces incoordination and sedation. In studies with laboratory animals the anxiolytic effects manifest themselves as a release from the punishing effects of aversive stimuli. For example, if an animal is given electric shocks whenever it makes a particular response (say, one that obtains food or water), it will stop doing so. However, if it is then given some alcohol, it will begin making the response again (Koob et al., 1984). This phenomenon explains why people often do things they normally would not when they have had too much to drink; the alcohol removes the inhibitory effect of social controls on their behavior.

Alcohol produces both positive and negative reinforcement. The positive reinforcement manifests itself as mild euphoria. As we saw earlier, *negative* reinforcement is caused by the termination of an aversive stimulus. If a person feels anxious and uncomfortable, then an anxiolytic drug that relieves this discomfort provides at least a temporary escape from an unpleasant situation.

Alcohol, like other addictive drugs, increases the activity of the dopaminergic neurons of the mesolimbic system and increases the release of dopamine in the nucleus accumbens as measured by microdialysis (Gessa et al., 1985; Imperato and Di Chiara, 1986). The release of dopamine appears to be related to the positive reinforcement that alcohol can produce. An injection of a dopamine antagonist directly into the nucleus accumbens decreases alcohol intake (Samson et al., 1993), as does the injection of a drug into the ventral tegmental area that decreases the activity of the dopaminergic neurons there (Hodge et al., 1993).

Alcohol has two major sites of action in the nervous system, acting as an indirect antagonist at NMDA receptors and an indirect agonist at $GABA_A$ receptors (Chandler, Harris, and Crews, 1998). That is, alcohol enhances the action of GABA at $GABA_A$ receptors and interferes with the transmission of glutamate at NMDA receptors. The anxiolytic effects of a $GABA_A$ agonist are apparently responsible for the negatively reinforcing effects of alcohol. The sedative effect of alcohol also appears to be exerted at the $GABA_A$ receptor. Suzdak et al. (1986) discovered a drug (Ro15–4513) that reverses alcohol intoxication by blocking the alcohol binding site on this receptor. Figure 16.21 shows two rats that received injections of enough alcohol to make them pass out. The one facing us also received an injection of the alcohol antagonist and appears completely sober. (See *Figure 16.21*.)

FIGURE 16.21

Effects of Ro15-4513, an Alcohol Antagonist. Both rats received an injection of alcohol, but the one facing us also received an injection of the alcohol antagonist.

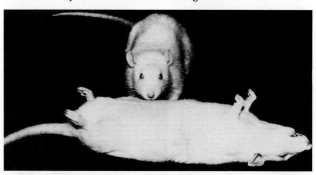

Photograph courtesy of Steven M. Paul, National Institute of Mental Health, Bethesda, Maryland.

This wonder drug has not been put on the market, nor is it likely to be. Although the behavioral effects of alcohol are mediated by their action on $GABA_A$ receptors and NMDA receptors, high doses of alcohol have other, potentially fatal effects on all cells of the body, including destabilization of cell membranes. Thus, people taking some of the alcohol antagonist could then go on to drink themselves to death without becoming drunk in the process. Drug companies naturally fear possible liability suits stemming from such occurrences.

Although the effects of heroin withdrawal have been exaggerated, those produced by alcohol withdrawal are serious and can even be fatal. The increased sensitivity of NMDA receptors as they rebound from the suppressive effect of alcohol can trigger seizures and convulsions. Convulsions caused by alcohol withdrawal are considered to be a medical emergency and are usually treated with an intravenous injection of a benzodiazepine. Liljequist (1991) found that seizures caused by alcohol withdrawal could be prevented by giving mice a drug that blocks NMDA receptors.

I mentioned earlier that opiate receptors appear to be involved in a reinforcement mechanism that does not directly involve dopaminergic neurons. The reinforcing effect of alcohol is at least partly caused by its ability to trigger the release of the endogenous opioids. Several studies have shown that drugs that block opiate receptors also block the reinforcing effects of alcohol in a variety of species, including rats, monkeys, and humans (Altschuler, Phillips, and Feinhandler, 1980; Davidson, Swift, and Fitz, 1996; Reid, 1996). In addition, endogenous opioids may play a role in craving in abstinent alcoholics. Heinz et al. (2005) found that 1 to 3 weeks of abstinence increased the number of μ opiate receptors in the nucleus accumbens. The greater the number of receptors, the more intense the craving was. Presumably, the increased number of μ receptors increased the effects of endogenous opiates on the brain and served as a contributing factor to the craving for alcohol. (See *Figure 16.22.*)

Because naltrexone, a drug that blocks opiate receptors, has become a useful adjunct to treatment of alcoholism, I will discuss this topic further in this chapter.

Cannabis

Another drug that people regularly self-administer—almost exclusively by smoking—is THC, the active ingredient in marijuana. As you learned in Chapter 4, the

FIGURE 16.22

Craving for Alcohol and μ Opiate Receptors.   The PET scans show the presence of μ opiate receptors in the dorsal striatum of detoxified alcoholic patients and healthy control subjects. The graph shows the relative alcohol craving score as a function of relative numbers of μ opiate receptors.

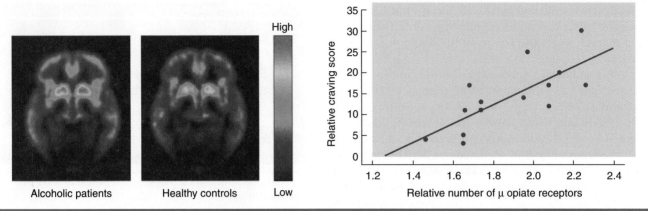

Scans and data points from Heinz, A., Reimold, M., Wrase, J., et al. *Archives of General Psychiatry*, 2005, *62*, 57–64. By permission.

site of action of the endogenous cannabinoids in the brain is the CB$_1$ receptor. Administration of a drug that blocks CB$_1$ receptors abolishes the "high" produced by smoking marijuana (Huestis et al., 2001).

By the way, di Tomaso, Beltramo, and Piomelli (1996) discovered that chocolate contains three anandamide-like chemicals. Whether the existence of these chemicals is related to the great appeal that chocolate has for many people is not yet known. (I suppose that this is the place for a chocoholic joke.)

THC, like other drugs with abuse potential, has a stimulating effect on dopaminergic neurons. A microdialysis study by Chen et al. (1990) found that low doses of THC increased the release of dopamine in the nucleus accumbens. (See *Figure 16.23.*)

FIGURE 16.23

THC and Dopamine Secretion in the Nucleus Accumbens.   The graph shows changes in dopamine concentration in the nucleus accumbens, measured by microdialysis, in response to injections of THC or an inert placebo.

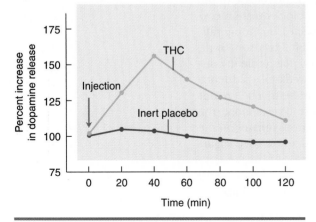

Adapted from Chen, J., Paredes, W., Li, J., et al. *Psychopharmacology*, 1990, *102*, 156–162.

A targeted mutation that blocks the production of CB$_1$ receptors in mice abolishes the reinforcing effect not only of cannabinoids, but also of morphine and heroin (Cossu et al., 2001). This mutation also decreases the reinforcing effects of alcohol and the acquisition of self-administration of cocaine (Houchi et al., 2005; Soria et al., 2005). In addition, as we saw in an earlier subsection, rimonabant, a drug that blocks CB$_1$ receptors, decreases the reinforcing effects of nicotine.

As we saw in Chapter 4, the hippocampus contains a large concentration of THC receptors. Marijuana is known to affect people's memory. Specifically, it impairs their ability to keep track of a particular topic; they frequently lose the thread of a conversation if they are momentarily distracted. Evidence indicates that the drug does so by disrupting the normal functions of the hippocampus, which plays such an important role in memory (Kunos and Batkai, 2001).

Two articles (Moore et al., 2007; Murray et al., 2007) reported a disturbing finding: The incidence of psychotic disorders such as schizophrenia is increased in cannabis users—especially those who have used it frequently. Of course, a correlational study cannot prove the existence of a cause-and-effect relationship. It is possible that people who are more likely to develop psychotic symptoms are also more likely to use cannabis. However, statistical adjustments made by these studies suggest that a cause-and-effect relationship between cannabis use and psychosis cannot be ruled out. The authors, Moore et al. (2007), concluded "that there is now sufficient evidence to warn young people that using cannabis could increase their risk of developing a psychotic illness later in life" (p. 319). This issue certainly deserves further study.

Heredity and Drug Abuse

Not everyone is equally likely to become addicted to a drug. Many people manage to drink alcohol moderately, and most users of potent drugs such as cocaine and heroin use them "recreationally" without becoming dependent on them. Evidence indicates that both genetic and environmental factors play a role in determining a person's likelihood of consuming drugs and of becoming dependent on them. In addition, there are both general factors likelihood of taking and becoming addicted to any of a number of drugs) and specific factors (likelihood of taking and becoming addicted to a particular drug).

A study of male twin pairs (Kendler et al., 2003) found a strong common genetic factor for the use of all categories of drugs and found in addition that shared environmental factors had a stronger effect on use than on abuse. In other words, environment plays a strong role in influencing a person to try a drug and perhaps continue to use it recreationally, but genetics plays a stronger role in determining whether the person becomes addicted.

Goldman, Oroszi, and Ducci (2005) reviewed twin studies that attempted to measure the heritability of various classes of addictive disorders. Heritability (h^2) is the percentage of variability of a trait in a particular population that can be attributed to genetic variability. The average value of h^2 for addiction ranged from approximately 0.4 for hallucinogenic drugs to just over 0.7 for cocaine. As you will see in Figure 16.24, the authors included addiction to gambling, which is not a drug. (See *Figure 16.24*.)

The genetic basis of addiction to alcohol has received more attention than addiction to other drugs. Alcohol consumption is not distributed equally across the population; in the United States, 10 percent of the people drink 50 percent of the alcohol (Heckler, 1983). Many twin studies and adoption studies confirm that the primary reason for this disparity is genetic.

A susceptibility to alcoholism could conceivably be caused by differences in the ability to digest or metabolize alcohol or by differences in the structure or biochemistry of the brain. There is evidence that variability in the gene responsible for the production of alcohol dehydrogenase, an enzyme involved in metabolism of alcohol, plays a role in susceptibility to alcoholism. A particular variant of this gene, which is especially prevalent in eastern Asia, is responsible for a reaction to alcohol intake that most people find aversive and that discourages further drinking (Goldman, Oroszi, and Ducci, 2005). However, most investigators believe that differences in brain physiology—for example, those that control sensitivity to the reinforcing effects of drugs or sensitivity to various environmental stressors—are more likely to play a role.

Investigators have also focused on the possibility that susceptibility to addiction may involve differences in functions of specific neurotransmitter systems. For example, variations in the genes involved in the μ opiate receptor, the $GABA_A$ receptor, and the M_2 muscarinic

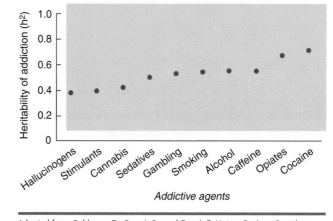

FIGURE 16.24

Heritability (h^2) of Addiction to Specific Addictive Agents

Adapted from Goldman, D., Oroszi, G., and Ducci, F. *Nature Reviews Genetics*, 2005, *6*, 521–532.

acetylcholine receptor have been reported to be associated with the likelihood of alcohol dependence (Edenberg et al., 2004; Wang et al., 2004; Bart et al., 2005).

Therapy for Drug Abuse

There are many reasons for engaging in research on the physiology of drug abuse, including an academic interest in the nature of reinforcement and the pharmacology of psychoactive drugs. However, most researchers entertain the hope that the results of their research will contribute to the development of ways to treat and (better yet) prevent drug abuse in members of our own species. As you well know, the incidence of drug abuse is far too high, so obviously, research has not yet solved the problem. However, real progress has been made.

The most common treatment for opiate addiction is methadone maintenance. Methadone is a potent opiate, just like morphine or heroin. If it were available in a form suitable for injection, it would be abused. (In fact, methadone clinics must control their stock of methadone carefully to prevent it from being stolen and sold to opiate abusers.) Methadone maintenance programs administer the drug to their patients in the form of a liquid, which they must drink in the presence of the personnel supervising this procedure. Because the oral route of administration increases the opiate level in the brain slowly, the drug does not produce a high, the way an injection of heroin will. In addition, because methadone is long-lasting, the patient's opiate receptors remain occupied for a long time, which means that an injection of heroin has little effect. Of course, a very large dose of heroin will displace methadone from opiate receptors and produce a "rush," so the method is not foolproof.

A newer drug, *buprenorphine*, shows promise of being an even better therapeutic agent for opiate addiction than methadone (Vocci, Acri, and Elkashef, 2005). Buprenorphine is a partial agonist for the μ opiate receptor. (You will recall from Chapter 15 that a partial agonist is a drug that has a high affinity for a particular receptor but activates that receptor less than the normal ligand does. This action reduces the effects of a receptor ligand in regions of high concentration and increases it in regions of low concentration, as shown in Figure 15.11.) Buprenorphine blocks the effects of opiates and itself produces only a weak opiate effect. Unlike methadone, it has little value on the illicit drug market. The addition of a small dose of naloxone, a drug that blocks opiate receptors, ensures that the combination drug has no abuse potential—and will, in fact, cause withdrawal symptoms if it is taken by an addict who is currently taking an opiate. A major advantage of buprenorphine, besides its efficacy, is the fact that it can be use in office-based treatment. (See *Figure 16.25.*)

An interesting approach to cocaine addiction is suggested by a study by Carrera et al. (1995), who conjugated cocaine to a foreign protein and managed to stimulate rats' immune systems to develop antibodies to cocaine. The antibodies bound with molecules of cocaine and prevented them from crossing the blood–brain barrier. As a consequence, these "cocaine-immunized" rats were less sensitive to the activating effects of cocaine, and brain levels of cocaine in these animals were lower after an injection of cocaine. Since this study was carried out, animal studies with vaccines against cocaine, heroin, methamphetamine, and nicotine have been carried out, and several human clinical trials with vaccines for cocaine and nicotine have taken

FIGURE 16.25

Buprenorphine as a Treatment for Opiate Addiction. The graph shows the effects of treatment with buprenorphine, buprenorphine + naloxone, and a placebo on opiate craving in recovering opiate addicts.

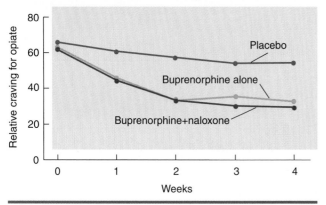

Adapted from Fudala, P. J., Bridge, T. P., Herbert, S., et al. *New England Journal of Medicine*, 2003, *349*, 949–958.

place (Kosten and Owens, 2005; Cornuz et al., 2008). The results of these animal studies and human trials are promising, and more extensive human trials are in progress.

A treatment similar to methadone maintenance has been used as an adjunct to treatment for nicotine addiction. For several years, chewing gum that contains nicotine has been available by prescription, and more recently, transdermal patches that release nicotine through the skin have been marketed. Both methods maintain a sufficiently high level of nicotine in the brain to decrease a person's craving for nicotine. Once the habit of smoking has subsided, the dose of nicotine can be decreased to wean the person from the drug. Carefully controlled studies have shown that nicotine maintenance therapy, and not administration of a placebo, is useful in treatment for nicotine dependence (Stolerman and Jarvis, 1995). However, nicotine maintenance therapy is most effective if it is part of a counseling program.

One of the limitations of treating a smoking addiction with nicotine maintenance is that this procedure does not provide an important non-nicotine component of smoking: the sensations produced by the action of cigarette smoke on the airways. As we saw earlier in this chapter, stimuli associated with the administration of addictive drugs play an important role in sustaining an addictive habit. Smokers who rate the pleasurability of puffs of normal and denicotinized cigarettes within 7 seconds, which is less time than it takes for nicotine to leave the lungs, enter the blood, and reach the brain, reported that puffing denicotinized cigarettes produced equally strong feelings of euphoria and satisfaction and reductions in the urge to smoke. Furthermore, blocking the sensations of cigarette smoke on the airways by inhaling a local anesthetic diminishes smoking satisfaction even though the nicotine still reaches the brain.

Denicotinized cigarettes are not a completely adequate substitute for normal cigarettes, because nicotine itself, not just the other components of smoke, make an important contribution to the sensations felt in the airways. In fact, trimethaphan, a drug that blocks nicotinic receptors in the airways but not in the brain, decreases the sensory effects of smoking and reduces satisfaction. Because trimethaphan does not interfere with the effects of nicotine on the brain, this finding indicates that the central effects of nicotine are not sufficient by themselves to maintain an addiction to nicotine. Instead, the combination of an immediate cue from the sensory effects of cigarette smoke on the airways and a more delayed, and more continuous, effect of nicotine on the brain serves to make smoking so addictive (Naqvi and Bechara, 2005; Rose, 2006).

As we saw earlier in this chapter, studies with laboratory animals have found that the endogenous cannabinoids are involved in the reinforcing effects of nicotine as well as those of marijuana. A recent clinical trial reported that rimonabant, a drug that blocks CB_1 receptors, was effective in helping smokers to quit their habit (Henningfield et al., 2005). One significant benefit of the drug was a decrease in the weight gain that typically accompanies cessation of smoking and often discourages smokers who are trying to quit. As we saw in Chapter 11, the endocannabinoids stimulate eating, apparently by increasing the release of MCH and orexin. Blocking CB_1 receptors abolishes this effect and helps to counteract the effects of withdrawal from nicotine on these neurons.

Another drug, *bupropion*, is an antidepressant drug that serves as a catecholamine reuptake inhibitor. Bupropion has been approved for use in several countries for treating nicotine addiction. Brody et al. (2004) found that smokers treated with bupropion showed less activation of the medial prefrontal cortex and reported less intense craving when they were presented with cigarette-related cues.

Yet another drug, *varenicline*, has been approved for therapeutic use to treat nicotine addiction. Varenicline serves a partial agonist for the nicotinic receptor, just as buprenorphine serves as a partial agonist for the μ-opioid receptor. As a partial nicotinic agonist, varenicline maintains a moderate level of activation of nicotinic receptors but prevents high levels of nicotine from providing excessive levels of

FIGURE 16.26

Varenicline as a Treatment for Smoking. The graph shows the percentage of smokers treated with varenicline, bupropion, or placebo who abstained from cigarette smoking.

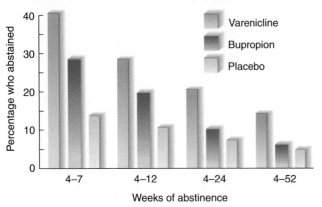

Adapted from Nides, M., Oncken, C., Gonzales, D., et al., *Archives of Internal Medicine*, 2006, *166*, 1561–1568.

stimulation. Figure 16.26 shows the effects of treatment with varenicline and bupropion on the continuous abstinence rates of smokers enrolled in a randomized, double-blind, placebo control study. By the end of the 52-week treatment program, 14.4 percent of the smokers treated with varenicline were still abstinent, compared with 6.3 percent and 4.9 percent for the smokers who received bupropion and placebo. (See *Figure 16.26.*)

As mentioned earlier, several studies have shown that opiate antagonists decrease the reinforcing value of alcohol in a variety of species, including our own. This finding suggests that the reinforcing effect of alcohol—at least in part—is produced by the secretion of endogenous opioids and the activation of opiate receptors in the brain. A study by O'Brien, Volpicelli, and Volpicelli (1996) reported the results of two long-term programs using naltrexone along with more traditional behavioral treatments. Both programs found that administration of naltrexone significantly increased the likelihood of success. As Figure 16.27 shows, naltrexone increased the number of participants who managed to abstain from alcohol. (See *Figure 16.27.*) Currently, many treatment programs are using a sustained-release form of naltrexone to help treat alcoholism, and results with the drug have been encouraging (Kranzler, Modesto-Lowe, and Nuwayser, 1998). Naltrexone may even reduce craving for cigarettes (Vewers, Dhatt, and Tejwani, 1998).

One more drug has shown promise for treatment of alcoholism. As we saw earlier in this chapter, alcohol serves as an indirect agonist at the $GABA_A$ receptor and an indirect antagonist at the NMDA receptor. *Acamprosate*, an NMDA-receptor antagonist that has been used in Europe to treat seizure disorders, was tested for its ability to stop seizures induced by withdrawal from alcohol. The researchers discovered that the drug had an unexpected benefit: Alcoholic patients who received the drug were less likely to start drinking again (Wickelgren, 1998; Buonopane and Petrakis, 2005). Acamprosate has been approved for treatment of alcohol abuse in the United States (Kranzler and Gage, 2008).

FIGURE 16.27

Naltrexone as a Treatment for Alcoholism. The graphs show the mean craving score and proportion of patients who abstained from drinking while receiving naltrexone or a placebo.

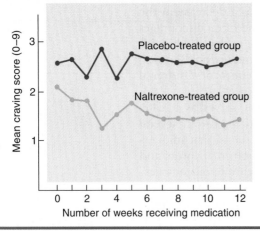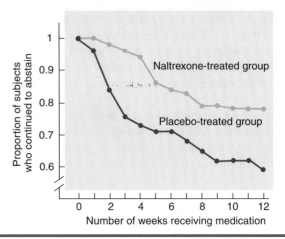

Adapted from O'Brien, C. P., Volpicelli, L. A., and Volpicelli, J. R. *Alcohol*, 1996, *13*, 35–39.

InterimSummary

Substance Abuse Disorders

Addictive drugs are those whose reinforcing effects are so potent that some people who are exposed to them are unable to go for very long without taking the drugs and whose lives become organized around taking them. Positive reinforcement occurs when a behavior is regularly followed by an appetitive stimulus—one that an organism will approach. Addictive drugs produce positive reinforcement; they reinforce drug-taking behavior. Laboratory animals will learn to make responses that result in the delivery of these drugs. The faster a drug produces its effects, the more quickly dependence will be established. All addictive drugs that produce positive reinforcement stimulate the release of dopamine in the nucleus accumbens, a structure that plays an important role in reinforcement. Neural changes that begin in the VTA and NAC eventually involve the dorsal striatum, which plays a critical role in instrumental conditioning.

Negative reinforcement occurs when a behavior is followed by the reduction or termination of an aversive stimulus. If, because of a person's social situation or personality characteristics, he or she feels unhappy or anxious, a drug that reduces these feelings can reinforce drug-taking behavior by means of negative reinforcement. Also, reduction of unpleasant withdrawal symptoms by a dose of the drug undoubtedly plays a role in maintaining drug addictions, but it is not the sole cause of craving.

Craving—the urge to take a drug to which one has become addicted—cannot be completely explained by withdrawal symptoms, because it can occur even after an addict has refrained from taking the drug for a long time. Functional imaging studies find that craving for addictive drugs increases the activity of the ACC, OFC, insula, and dorsolateral prefrontal cortex. Long-term drug abuse is associated with decreased activity of the prefrontal cortex and even with decreased prefrontal gray matter, which may impair people's judgment and ability to inhibit inappropriate responses, such as further drug taking. Schizophrenia is seen in a higher proportion of drug addicts than in the general population. The susceptibility of adolescents to the addictive potential of drugs may be associated with the relative immaturity of the prefrontal cortex. Stressful stimuli can trigger craving and drug-seeking behavior.

Opiates produce analgesia, hypothermia, sedation, and reinforcement. Opiate receptors in the periaqueductal gray matter are responsible for the analgesia, those in the preoptic area for the hypothermia, those in the mesencephalic reticular formation for the sedation, and those in the ventral tegmental area and nucleus accumbens at least partly for the reinforcement. The release of the endogenous opioids may play a role in the reinforcing effects of other addictive drugs such as alcohol.

Cocaine inhibits the reuptake of dopamine by terminal buttons, and amphetamine causes the dopamine transporters in terminal buttons to run in reverse, releasing dopamine from terminal buttons. The reinforcing effects of cocaine and amphetamine are mediated by an increased release of dopamine in the nucleus accumbens. Chronic methamphetamine abuse is associated with reduced numbers of dopaminergic axons and terminals in the striatum (revealed as a decrease in the numbers of dopamine transporters located there).

The status of nicotine as a strongly addictive drug (for both humans and laboratory animals) was long ignored, primarily because it does not cause intoxication and because the ready availability of cigarettes and other tobacco products does not make it necessary for addicts to engage in illegal activities. However, the craving for nicotine is extremely motivating. Nicotine stimulates the release of mesolimbic dopaminergic neurons, and injection of nicotine into the ventral tegmental area is reinforcing. Cannabinoid CB_1 receptors are involved in the reinforcing effect of nicotine as well. Damage to the insula is associated with cessation of smoking, which suggests that this region plays a role in the maintenance of cigarette addiction. Nicotine stimulation of the release of GABA in the lateral hypothalamus decreases the activity of MCH neurons and reduces food intake, which explains why cessation of smoking often leads to weight gain.

Alcohol has positively reinforcing effects and, through its anxiolytic action, has negatively reinforcing effects as well. It serves as an indirect antagonist at NMDA receptors and an indirect agonist at $GABA_A$ receptors. It stimulates the release of dopamine in the nucleus accumbens. Withdrawal from long-term alcohol abuse can lead to seizures, an effect that seems to be caused by withdrawal-induced activation of NMDA receptors. Release of the endogenous opioids also plays a role in the reinforcing effects of alcohol.

The active ingredient in cannabis, THC, stimulates receptors whose natural ligand is anandamide. THC, like other addictive drugs, stimulates the release of dopamine in the nucleus accumbens. The CB_1 receptor is responsible for the physiological and behavioral effects of THC and the endogenous cannabinoids. A targeted mutation against the CB_1 receptor reduces the reinforcing effect of alcohol, cocaine, and the opiates as well as that of the cannabinoids. Blocking CB_1 receptors also decreases the reinforcing effects of nicotine. Cannabinoids produce memory deficits by acting on neurons in the hippocampus. Two disturbing reports indicate that cannabis use is associated with the incidence of schizophrenia.

Most people who are exposed to addictive drugs—even drugs with a high abuse potential—do not become addicts. Evidence suggests that the likelihood of addiction, especially to alcohol and nicotine, is strongly affected by heredity. Drug taking and addiction are affected by general hereditary and environmental factors that apply to all drugs and specific factors that apply to particular drugs.

Although drug abuse is difficult to treat, researchers have developed several useful therapies. Methadone maintenance replaces addiction to heroin by addiction to an opiate that does not produce euphoric effects when administered orally. Buprenorphine, a partial agonist for the μ opioid receptor, reduces craving for opiates.

Because it is not of interest to opiate addicts (especially when it is combined with naltrexone), it can be administered by a physician at an office visit. The development of antibodies to cocaine and nicotine in humans and to several other drugs in rats holds out the possibility that people may some day be immunized against addictive drugs, preventing the entry of the drugs into the brain. Nicotine-containing gum and transdermal patches help smokers to combat their addiction. However, sensations from the airways produced by the presence of cigarette smoke play an important role in addiction, and oral and transdermal administration do not provide these sensations. Rimonabant, a CB_1 receptor antagonist, aids smoking cessation and reduces the likelihood of weight gain. Bupropion, an antidepressant drug, has also been shown to help smokers stop their habit. Varenicline, a partial agonist for the nicotinic receptor, may be even more effective. The most effective pharmacological adjunct to treatment for alcoholism appears to be naltrexone, an opiate receptor blocker that reduces the drug's reinforcing effects. Acamprosate, an NMDA-receptor antagonist, also shows promise in treatment of alcoholism.

A personal note: You are now at the end of the book (as you well know), and you have spent a considerable amount of time reading my words. While working on this book, I have tried to imagine myself talking to someone who is interested in learning something about the physiology of behavior. As I mentioned in the preface, writing is often a lonely activity, and the imaginary audience helped to keep me company. If you would like to turn this communication into a two-way conversation, write to me. My address is given at the end of the preface.

Thought Questions

1. Although executives of tobacco companies used to insist that cigarettes were not addictive and asserted that people smoked simply because of the pleasure the act gave them, research indicates that nicotine is indeed a potent addictive drug. Why do you think it took so long to recognize this fact?

2. In most countries alcohol is legal and marijuana is not. In your opinion, why? What criteria would you use to decide whether a newly discovered drug should be legal or illegal? Danger to health? Effects on fetal development? Effects on behavior? Potential for dependence? If you applied these criteria to various substances in current use, would you have to change the legal status of any of them?

⋮ EPILOGUE   Classically Conditioned Craving

When a person takes heroin, the primary effects of the drug activate homeostatic compensatory mechanisms. These compensatory mechanisms are provided by neural circuits that oppose the effects of the drug. As Siegel (1978) has pointed out, the activation of these compensatory mechanisms is a response that can become classically conditioned to environmental stimuli that are present at the time the drug is taken. The stimuli associated with taking the drug—including the paraphernalia involved in preparing the solution of the drug, the syringe, the needle, the feel of the needle in a vein, and even the sight of companions who are usually present and the room in which the drug is taken—serve as conditional stimuli. The homeostatic compensatory responses provoked by the effects of the drug serve as the unconditional response, which becomes conditioned to the environmental stimuli. Thus, once classical conditioning has taken place, the sight of the conditional stimuli will activate the compensatory mechanisms.

When John, the former addict in the chapter prologue, saw the poster, the sight of the drug paraphernalia acted as a conditional stimulus and elicited the conditional response—the compensatory mechanism. Because he had not taken the drug, he felt only the effect of the compensatory mechanism: dysphoria, agitation, and a strong urge to relieve these symptoms and replace them with feelings of euphoria. He found the urge irresistible.

Experiments with laboratory animals have confirmed that this explanation is correct. For example, Siegel et al. (1982) gave rats daily doses of heroin—always in the same chamber—long enough for tolerance to develop. Then, on the test day, the experimenters gave the rats a large dose of the drug. Some of the animals received the drug in the familiar chamber, while others received it in a new environment. The investigators predicted that the animals receiving the drug in the familiar environment would have some protection from the drug overdose because the stimuli in that environment would produce a classically conditioned compensatory response. Their prediction was correct; almost all of the rats who received the overdose in the new environment died, compared with slightly more than half of the rats injected in the familiar environment. Siegel and his colleagues suggest that when human heroin addicts take the drug in an unfamiliar environment, they too run the risk of death from a drug overdose.

By the way, the story of John that I recounted in the chapter prologue is unlikely to occur nowadays. Because so many heroin addicts trying to break their habit have reported that the sight of drug paraphernalia made it difficult for them to abstain, the agencies trying to combat drug addiction have stopped preparing posters that feature these items.

Key Concepts

AUTISTIC DISORDER

1. Autistic disorder is characterized by poor or absent social relations, communicative abilities, and imaginative abilities and the presence of repetitive, purposeless movements.
2. Although autism used to be blamed on poor parenting behavior, it is now recognized that the disorder is caused by hereditary factors or events that interfere with prenatal development.

ATTENTION-DEFICIT/HYPERACTIVITY DISORDER

3. Attention-deficit/hyperactivity disorder (ADHD) shows up in childhood, and is characterized by difficulty concentrating, remaining still, and working on a task. Children with ADHD also have difficulty withholding a response, act without reflecting, often show reckless and impetuous behavior, and let interfering activities intrude into ongoing tasks.
4. ADHD is treated by dopamine agonists such as methylphenidate (Ritalin). The disorder may be caused by abnormalities in the brain's reinforcement mechanisms, which result in a steeper delay of reinforcement gradient. Evidence suggests the presence of abnormalities in the prefrontal cortex and caudate nucleus.

STRESS DISORDERS

5. The stress response consists of the physiological components of an emotional response to threatening stimuli. The long-term effects of these responses—particularly of the secretion of the glucocorticoids—can damage a person's health. Stress-related secretion of catecholamines may be a factor in the development of cardiovascular disease.

6. Stress can suppress the immune system, primarily through the secretion of glucocorticoids and therefore can make a person more susceptible to infections.

SUBSTANCE ABUSE DISORDERS

7. All addictive substances studied so far—including opiates, cocaine, amphetamine, nicotine, marijuana, and alcohol—have been shown to cause the release of dopamine in the nucleus accumbens.
8. Although chronic intake of opiates causes tolerance and leads to withdrawal symptoms, these phenomena are not responsible for addiction, which is caused by the ability of these drugs to activate dopaminergic mechanisms of reinforcement.
9. Craving and relapse may occur because taking addictive drugs for an extended period of time causes abnormalities in the nucleus accumbens and prefrontal cortex that impair judgment and the ability to withhold inappropriate behaviors.
10. Alcohol has two sites of action: It serves as an indirect agonist at the $GABA_A$ receptor and an indirect antagonist at the NMDA receptor.
11. Research indicates that the susceptibility to drug abuse is strongly influenced by heredity. Binging and steady alcohol drinking appear to caused by different mechanisms.
12. Physiological therapy for drug addiction includes methadone and buprenorphine (a partial agonist for the μ opiate receptor) for opiate addiction, nicotine maintenance therapy (nicotine chewing gum or skin patches) or bupropion (an antidepressant drug) for addiction to nicotine, and naltrexone (an opiate receptor blocker) or acamprosate (an NMDA-receptor antagonist) for alcoholism.

Suggested Readings

Autism Genome Project Consortium. Mapping autism risk loci using genetic linkage and chromosomal rearrangements. *Nature Genetics*, 2007, *39*, 319–328.

Bush, G., Valera, E. M., and Seidman, L. J. Functional neuroimaging of attention-deficit/hyperactivity disorder: A review and suggested future directions. *Biological Psychiatry*, 2005, *57*, 1273–1284.

Chambers, R. A., Taylor, J. R., and Potenza, M. N. Developmental neurocircuitry of motivation in adolescence: A critical period of addiction vulnerability. *American Journal of Psychiatry*, 2003, *160*, 1041–1052.

Chao, J., and Nestler, E. J. Molecular neurobiology of drug addiction. *Annual Review of Medicine*, 2004, *55*, 113–132.

Charmandari, E., Tsigos, C., and Chrousos, G. Endocrinology of the stress response. *Annual Review of Physiology*, 2005, *67*, 259–284.

Courchesne, E., Pierce, K., Schumann, C. M., Redcay, E., Buckwalter, J. A., Kennedy, D. P., and Morgan, J. Mapping early brain development in autism. *Neuron*, 2007, *56*, 399–413.

Ducci, F., and Goldman, D. Genetic approaches to addiction: Genes and alcohol. *Addiction*, 2008, *103*, 1414–1428.

Hyman, S. E., Malenka, R. C., and Nestler, E. J. Neural mechanisms of addiction: The role of reward-related learning and memory. *Annual Review of Neuroscience*, 2006, *29*, 565–598.

Kalivas, P. W., and O'Brien, C. Drug addiction as a pathology of staged neuroplasticity. *Neuropsychopharmacology*, 2008, *33*, 166–180.

Kauer, J. A., and Malenka, R. C. Synaptic plasticity and addiction. *Nature Reviews: Neuroscience*, 2007, *8*, 844–858.

Muhle, R., Trentacoste, S. V., and Rapin, I. The genetics of autism. *Pediatrics*, 2004, *113*, e472–e486.

Vocci, F. J., Acri, J., and Elkashef, A. Medication development for addictive disorders: The state of the science. *American Journal of Psychiatry*, 2005, *162*, 1432–1440.

Yehuda, R., and LeDoux, J. Response variation following trauma: A translational neuroscience approach to understanding PTSD. *Neuron*, 2007, *56*, 19–32.

Additional Resources

Visit www.mypsychkit.com for additional review and practice of the material covered in this chapter. Within MyPsychKit, you can take practice tests and receive a customized study plan to help you review. Dozens of animations, tutorials, and Web links are also available. You can even review using the interactive electronic version of this textbook. You will need to register for MyPsychKit. See www.mypsychkit.com for complete details.

References

Abelson, J. L., Curtis, G. C., Sagher, O., et al. Deep brain stimulation for refractory obsessive-compulsive disorder. *Biological Psychiatry*, 2005, *57*, 510–516.

Abercrombie, H. C., Schaefer, S. M., Larson, C. L., et al. Metabolic rate in the right amygdala predicts negative affect in depressed patients. *Neuroreport*, 1998, *9*, 3301–3307.

Adams, D. B., Gold, A. R., and Burt, A. D. Rise in female-initiated sexual activity at ovulation and its suppression by oral contraceptives. *New England Journal of Medicine*, 1978, *299*, 1145–1150.

Adey, W. R., Bors, E., and Porter, R. W. EEG sleep patterns after high cervical lesions in man. *Archives of Neurology*, 1968, *19*, 377–383.

Adler, C. M., Malhotra, A. K., Elman, I., et al. Comparison of ketamine-induced thought disorder in healthy volunteers and thought disorder in schizophrenia. *American Journal of Psychiatry*, 1999, *156*, 1646–1649.

Adolphs, R., Damasio, H., Tranel, D., et al. A Role for somatosensory cortices in the visual recognition of emotion as revealed by three-dimensional lesion mapping. *Journal of Neuroscience*, 2000, *20*, 2683–2690.

Adolphs, R., and Tranel, D. Intact recognition of emotional prosody following amygdala damage. *Neuropsychologia*, 1999, *37*, 1285–1292.

Adolphs, R., Tranel, D., Damasio, H., and Damasio, A. Fear and the human amygdala. *Journal of Neuroscience*, 1995, *15*, 5879–5891.

Adolphs, R., Tranel, D., Damasio, H., and Damasio, A. Impaired recognition of emotion in facial expressions following bilateral damage to the human amygdala. *Nature*, 1994, *372*, 669–672.

Advokat, C., and Kutlesic, V. Pharmacotherapy of the eating disorders: A commentary. *Neuroscience and Biobehavioral Reviews*, 1995, *19*, 59–66.

Agarwal, N., Pacher, P., Tegeder, I., et al. Cannabinoids mediate analgesia largely via peripheral type 1 cannabinoid receptors in nociceptors. *Nature Neuroscience*, 2007, *10*, 870–879.

Aharon, L., Etcoff, N., Ariely, D., et al. Beautiful faces have variable reward value: fMRI and behavioral evidence. *Neuron*, 2001, *32*, 537–551.

Alain, C., He, Y., and Grady, C. The contribution of the inferior parietal lobe to auditory spatial working memory. *Journal of Cognitive Neuroscience*, 2008, *20*, 285–295.

Alexander, G. M. An evolutionary perspective of sex-typed toy preferences: Pink, blue, and the brain. *Archives of Sexual Behavior*, 2003, *32*, 7–14.

Alexander, G. M., and Hines, M. Sex differences in response to children's toys in non-human primates (*Cercopithecus aethiops sabaeus*). *Evolution and Human Behavior*, 2002, *23*, 467–479.

Alexander, M. P., Fischer, R. S., and Friedman, R. Lesion localization in apractic agraphia. *Archives of Neurology*, 1992, *49*, 246–251.

Alirezaei, M., Watry, D. D., Flynn, C. F., et al. Human immunodeficiency virus-1/surface glycoprotein 120 induces apoptosis through RNA-activated protein kinase signaling in neurons. *Journal of Neuroscience*, 2007, *27*, 11047–11055.

Alkire, M. T., Haier, R. J., Fallon, J. H., and Cahill, L. Hippocampal, but not amygdala, activity at encoding correlates with long-term, free recall of nonemotional information. *Proceedings of the National Academy of Sciences, USA*, 1998, *95*, 14506–14510.

Allen, L. S., and Gorski, R. A. Sexual orientation and the size of the anterior commissure in the human brain. *Proceedings of the National Academy of Sciences, USA*, 1992, *89*, 7199–7202.

Allison, T., Puce, A., and McCarthy, G. Social perception from visual cues: Role of the STS region. *Trends in Cognitive Science*, 2000, *4*, 267–278.

Altschuler, H. L., Phillips, P. E., and Feinhandler, D. A. Alterations of ethanol self-administration by naltrexone. *Life Sciences*, 1980, *26*, 679–688.

Amaral, D. G. The amygdala, social behavior, and danger detection. *Annals of the New York Academy of Sciences*, 2003, *1000*, 337–347.

Amaral, D. G., Price, J. L., Pitkänen, A., and Carmichael, S. T. Anatomical organization of the primate amygdaloid complex. In *The Amygdala: Neurobiological Aspects of Emotion, Memory, and Mental Dysfunction*, edited by J. P. Aggleton. New York: Wiley-Liss, 1992.

American Psychiatric Association. *Diagnostic and Statistical Manual of Mental Disorders*, 4th ed. Washington, DC: American Psychiatric Association, 1994.

Anand, B. K., and Brobeck, J. R. Hypothalamic control of food intake in rats and cats. *Yale Journal of Biology and Medicine*, 1951, *24*, 123–140.

Ancoli-Israel, S., and Roth, T. Characteristics of insomnia in the United States: Results of the 1991 National Sleep Foundation survey. *Sleep*, 1999, *22*, S347–S353.

Anderson, A. K., and Phelps, E. A. Expression without recognition: Contributions of the human amygdala to emotional communication. *Psychological Science*, 2000, *11*, 106–111.

Anderson, A. K., and Phelps, E. A. Intact recognition of vocal expressions of fear following bilateral lesions of the human amygdala. *Neuroreport*, 1998, *9*, 3607–3613.

Anderson, S., Barrash, J., Bechara, A., and Tranel, D. Impairments of emotion and real-world complex behavior following childhood- or adult-onset damage to ventromedial prefrontal cortex. *Journal of the International Neuropsychological Society*, 2006, *12*, 224–235.

Annese, J., Gazzaniga, M. S., and Toga, A. W. Localization of the human cortical visual area MT based on computer aided histological analysis. *Cerebral Cortex*, 2005, *15*, 1044–1053.

Anonymous. Effects of sexual activity on beard growth in man. *Nature*, 1970, *226*, 867–870.

Apkarian, A. V., Sosa, Y., Krauss, B. R., et al. Chronic pain patients are impaired on an emotional decision-making task. *Pain*, 2004a, *108*, 129–136.

Apkarian, A. V., Sosa, Y., Sonty, S., et al. Chronic back pain is associated with decreased prefrontal and thalamic gray matter density. *Journal of Neuroscience*, 2004b, *24*, 10410–10415.

Arancio, O., Kandel, E. R., and Hawkins, R. D. Activity-dependent long-term enhancement of transmitter release by presynaptic 3′,5′-cyclic GMP in cultured hippocampal neurons. *Nature*, 1995, *376*, 74–80.

Arendt, J., Deacon, S., English, J., et al. Melatonin and adjustment to phase-shift. *Journal of Sleep Research*, 1995, *4*, 74–79.

Ariyasu, H., Takaya, K., Tagami, T., et al. Stomach is a major source of circulating ghrelin, and feeding state determines plasma ghrelin-like immunoreactivity levels in humans. *Journal of Clinical Endocrinology and Metabolism*, 2001, *86*, 4753–4758.

Arnason, B. G. Immunologic therapy of multiple sclerosis. *Annual Review of Medicine*, 1999, *50*, 291–302.

Arnott, S. T., Binns, M. A., Grady, C. L., and Alain, C. Assessing the auditory dual-pathway model in humans. *Neuroimage*, 2004, *22*, 401–408.

Arnsten, A. F. T. Fundamentals of attention-deficit/hyperactivity disorder: Circuits and pathways. *Journal of Clinical Psychiatry*, 2006, *67* (Suppl. 8), 7–12.

Aron, A. R., Robbins, T. W., and Poldrack, R. A. Inhibition and the right inferior frontal cortex. *Trends in Cognitive Science*, 2004, *8*, 170–177.

Aronson, B. D., Bell-Pedersen, D., Block, G. D., et al. Circadian rhythms. *Brain Research Reviews*, 1993, *18*, 315–333.

Arora, S., and Anubhuti. Role of neuropeptides in appetite regulation and obesity—A review. *Neuropeptides*, 2006, *40*, 375–401.

Aschoff, J. Circadian rhythms: General features and endocrinological aspects. In *Endocrine Rhythms*, edited by D. T. Krieger. New York: Raven Press, 1979.

Asnis, G. M., Hameedi, F. A., Goddard, A. W., et al. Fluvoxamine in the treatment of panic disorder: A multi-center, double-blind, placebo-controlled study in outpatients. *Psychiatry Research*, 2001, *103*, 1–14.

Astafiev, S. V., Shulman, G. L., Stanley, C. M., et al. Functional organization of human intraparietal and frontal cortex for attending, looking, and pointing. *Journal of Neuroscience*, 2003, *23*, 4689–4699.

Aston-Jones, G., and Bloom, F. E. Activity of norepinephrine-containing locus coeruleus neurons in behaving rats anticipates fluctuations in the sleep-waking cycle. *Journal of Neuroscience*, 1981, *1*, 876–886.

Aston-Jones, G., Rajkowski, J., Kubiak, P., and Alexinsky, T. Locus coeruleus neurons in monkey are selectively activated by attended cues in a vigilance task. *Journal of Neuroscience*, 1994, *14*, 4467–4480.

Attia, E., Haiman, C., Walsh, T., and Flater, S. T. Does fluoxetine augment the inpatient treatment of anorexia nervosa? *American Journal of Psychiatry*, 1998, *155*, 548–551.

Auerbach, J., Geller, V., Lezer, S., et al. Dopamine D4 receptor (D4DR) and serotonin transporter promoter (5-HTTLPR) polymorphisms in the determination of temperament in 2-month-old infants. *Molecular Psychiatry*, 1999, *4*, 369–373.

Autism Genome Project Consortium, The. Mapping autism risk loci using genetic linkage and chromosomal rearrangements. *Nature Genetics*, 2007, *39*, 319–328.

Auyeung, B., Baron-Cohen, S., Ashwin, E., et al. Fetal testosterone and autistic traits. *British Journal of Psychology*, 2009, *100*, 1–22.

Avenet, P., and Lindemann, B. Perspectives of taste reception. *Journal of Membrane Biology*, 1989, *112*, 1–8.

Avila, M. T., Weiler, M. A., Lahti, A. C., et al. Effects of ketamine on leading saccades during smooth-pursuit eye movements may implicate cerebellar dysfunction in schizophrenia. *American Journal of Psychiatry*, 2002, *159*, 1490–1496.

Ayala, R., Shu, T., and Tsai, L.-H. Trekking across the brain: The journal of neuronal migration. *Cell*, 2007, *128*, 29–43.

Aziz-Zadeh, L., Cattaneo, L., Rochat, M., and Rizzolatti, G. Covert speech arrest induced by rTMS over both motor and nonmotor left hemisphere frontal sites. *Journal of Cognitive Neuroscience*, 2005, *17*, 928–938.

Baddeley, A. D. Memory: Verbal and visual subsystems of working memory. *Current Biology*, 1993, *3*, 563–565.

Bagatell, C. J., Heiman, J. R., Rivier, J. E., and Bremner, W. J. Effects of endogenous testosterone and estradiol on sexual behavior in normal young men. *Journal of Clinical Endocrinology and Metabolism*, 1994, *7*, 211–216.

Bagnasco, M., Tulipano, G., Melis, M. R., et al. Endogenous ghrelin is an orexigenic peptide acting in the arcuate nucleus in response to fasting. *Regulatory Peptides*, 2003, *28*, 161–167.

Bai, F. L., Yamano, M., Shiotani, Y., et al. An arcuato-paraventricular and-dorsomedial hypothalamic neuropeptide Y-containing system which lacks noradrenaline in the rat. *Brain Research*, 1985, *331*, 172–175.

Bailey, C. H., and Kandel, E. R. Synaptic remodeling, synaptic growth and the storage of long-term memory in *Aplysia*. *Progress in Brain Research*, 2008, *169*, 179–198.

Bailey, J. M., and Pillard, R. C. A genetic study of male sexual orientation. *Archives of General Psychiatry*, 1991, *48*, 1089–1096.

Bailey, J. M., Pillard, R. C., Neale, M. C., and Agyei, Y. Heritable factors influence sexual orientation in women. *Archives of General Psychiatry*, 1993, *50*, 217–223.

Baird, G., Pickles, A., Simonoff, E., et al. Measles vaccination and antibody response in autism spectrum disorders. *Archives of Disease in Childhood*, 2008, *93*, 832–837.

Bak, T. H., O'Donovan, D. G., Xuereb, J. H., et al. Selective impairment of verb processing associated with pathological changes in Brodman areas 44 and 45 in the motor neurone disease-dementia-aphasia syndrome. *Brain*, 2001, *124*, 103–120.

Ballantine, H. T., Bouckoms, A. J., Thomas, E. K., and Giriunas, I. E. Treatment of psychiatric illness by stereotactic cingulotomy. *Biological Psychiatry*, 1987, *22*, 807–819.

Ballas, N., Lioy, D. T., Grunseich, C., and Mandel, G. Non-cell autonomous influence of MeCP2-deficient glia on neuronal dendritic morphology. *Nature Neuroscience*, 2009, *12*, 311–317.

Bandell, M., Macpherson, L. J., and Patapoutian, A. From chills to chilis: Mechanisms for thermosensation and chemesthesis via thermoTRPs. *Current Opinion in Neurobiology*, 2007, *17*, 490–497.

Barber, T. X. Responding to "hypnotic" suggestions: An introspective report. *American Journal of Clinical Hypnosis*, 1975, *18*, 6–22.

Barclay, C. D., Cutting, J. E., and Kozlowski, L. T. Temporal and spatial factors in gait perception that influence gender recognition. *Perception and Psychophysics*, 1978, *23*, 145–152.

Bard, F., Cannon, C., Barbour, R., et al. Peripherally administered antibodies against amyloid beta-peptide enter the central nervous system and reduce pathology in a mouse model of Alzheimer disease. *Nature Medicine*, 2000, *6*, 916–919.

Baron-Cohen, S. The extreme male brain theory of autism. *Trends in Cognitive Sciences*, 2002, *6*, 248–254.

Bart, G., Kreek, M. J., Ott, J., et al. Increased attributable risk related to a functional μ-opioid receptor gene polymorphism in association with alcohol dependence in central Sweden. *Neuropsychopharmacology*, 2005, *30*, 417–422.

Bartels, A., and Zeki, S. The neural correlates of maternal and romantic love. *Neuroimage*, 2004, *21*, 1155–1166.

Bartels, A., and Zeki, S. The neural basis of romantic love. *Neuroreport*, 2000, *27*, 3829–3834.

Bartness, T. J., Powers, J. B., Hastings, M. H., et al. The timed infusion paradigm for melatonin delivery: What has it taught us about the melatonin signal, its reception, and the photoperiodic control of seasonal responses? *Journal of Pineal Research*, 1993, *15*, 161–190.

Basheer, R., Strecker, R. E., Thakkar, M. M., and McCarley, R. W. Adenosine and sleep–wake regulation. *Progress in Neurobiology*, 2004, *73*, 379–396.

Batterham, R. L., Cowley, M. A., Small, C. J., et al. Gut hormone PYY$_{3-36}$ physiologically inhibits food intake. *Nature*, 2002, *418*, 650–654.

Batterham, R. L., ffytche, D. H., Rosenthal, J. M., et al. PYY modulation of cortical and hypothalamic brain areas predicts feeding behaviour in humans. *Nature*, 2007, *450*, 106–109.

Bautista, D. M., Jordt, S.-E., Nikai, T., et al. TRPA1 mediates the inflammatory actions of environmental irritants and proalgesic agents. *Cell*, 2006, *124*, 1269–1282.

Bayley, P. J., Frascino, J. C., and Squire, L. R. Robust habit learning in the absence of awareness and independent of the medial temporal lobe. *Nature*, 2005, *436*, 550–553.

Beamer, W., Bermant, G., and Clegg, M. T. Copulatory behaviour of the ram, Ovis aries. II. Factors affecting copulatory satiation. *Animal Behavior*, 1969, *17*, 706–711.

Bear, O., and Fedio, P. Qualitative analysis of interictal behavior in temporal lobe epilepsy. *Archives of Neurology*, 1977, *34*, 454–467.

Beauvois, M. F., and Dérouesné, J. Lexical or orthographic dysgraphia. *Brain*, 1981, *104*, 21–45.

Beauvois, M. F., and Dérouesné, J. Phonological alexia: Three dissociations. *Journal of Neurology, Neurosurgery and Psychiatry*, 1979, *42*, 1115–1124.

Bechara, A., Tranel, D., Damasio, H., et al. Double dissociation of conditioning and declarative knowledge relative to the amygdala and hippocampus in humans. *Science*, 1995, *269*, 1115–1118.

Beckstead, R. M., Morse, J. R., and Norgren, R. The nucleus of the solitary tract in the monkey: Projections to the thalamus and brainstem nuclei. *Journal of Comparative Neurology*, 1980, *190*, 259–282.

Beidler, L. M. Physiological properties of mammalian taste receptors. In *Taste and Smell in Vertebrates*, edited by G. E. W. Wolstenholme. London: J. &A. Churchill, 1970.

Bell, A. P., Weinberg, M. S., and Hammersmith, S. K. *Sexual Preference: Its Development in Men and Women*. Bloomington: Indiana University Press, 1981.

Bell, A. P., and Weinberg, M. S. *Homosexualities: A Study of Diversity Among Men and Women*, New York: Simon and Schuster, 1978.

Benchenane, K., López-Atalaya, J. P., Fernández-Monreal, M., et al. Equivocal roles of tissue-type plasminogen activator in stroke-induced injury. *Trends in Neuroscience*, 2004, *27*, 155–160.

Benedetti, F., Arduino, C., and Amanzio, M. Somatotopic activation of opioid systems by target-directed expectations of analgesia. *Journal of Neuroscience*, 1999, *19*, 3639–3648.

Benington, J. H., Kodali, S. K., and Heller, H. C. Monoaminergic and cholinergic modulation of REM-sleep timing in rats. *Brain Research*, 1995, *681*, 141–146.

Bennett, D. A., Wilson, R. S., Schneider, J. A., et al. Education modifies the relation of AD pathology to level of cognitive function in older persons. *Neurology*, 2003, *60*, 1909–1915.

Bensimon, G., Lacomblez, L., and Meininger, V. A controlled trial of riluzole in amyotrophic lateral sclerosis. ALS/Riluzole Study Group. *New England Journal of Medicine*, 1994, *330*, 585–591.

Benson, D. F., Djenderedjian, A., Miller, B. L., et al. Neural basis of confabulation. *Neurology*, 1996, *46*, 1239–1243.

Ben-Tovim, D. I. Eating disorders: Outcome, prevention, and treatment of eating disorders. *Current Opinion in Psychiatry*, 2003, *16*, 65–69.

Berkovic, S. F., Mulley, J. C., Scheffer, I. E., and Petrou, S. Human epilepsies: Interaction of genetic and acquired factors. *Trends in Neurosciences*, 2006, *29*, 391–397.

Bermant, G., and Davidson, J. M. *Biological Bases of Sexual Behavior*. New York: Harper & Row, 1974.

Berson, D. M., Dunn, F. A., and Takao, M. Phototransduction by retinal ganglion cells that set the circadian clock. *Science*, 2002, *295*, 1070–1073.

Berthier, M., Kulisevsky, J., Gironell, A., and Heras, J. A. Obsessive-compulsive disorder associated with brain lesions: Clinical phenomenology, cognitive function, and anatomic correlates. *Neurology*, 1996, *47*, 353–361.

Bertolini, A., Ferrari, A., Ottani, A., et al. Paracetamol: New vistas of an old drug. *CNS Drug Review*, 2006, *12*, 250–275.

Best, P. J., White, A. M., and Minai, A. Spatial processing in the brain: The activity of hippocampal place cells. *Annual Review of Neuroscience*, 2001, *24*, 459–486.

Bettelheim, B. *The Empty Fortress*. New York: Free Press, 1967.

Billings, L. M., Green, K. N., McGaugh, J. L., and LaFerla, F. M. Learning decreases Aβ*56 and tau pathology and ameliorates behavioral decline in 3xTg-AD mice. *Journal of Neuroscience*, 2007, *27*, 751–761.

Bisiach, E., and Luzzatti, C. Unilateral neglect of representational space. *Cortex*, 1978, *14*, 129–133.

Bittel, D. C., and Butler, M. G. Prader-Willi syndrome: Clinical genetics, cytogenetics and molecular biology. *Expert Reviews in Molecular Medicine*, 2005, *7*, 1–20.

Blanchard, R. Fraternal birth order and the maternal immune hypothesis of male homosexuality. *Hormones and Behavior*, 2001, *40*, 105–114.

Blaustein, J. D., and Olster, D. H. Gonadal steroid hormone receptors and social behaviors. In *Advances in Comparative and Environmental Physiology, Vol. 3*, edited by J. Balthazart. Berlin: Springer-Verlag, 1989.

Blest, A. D. The function of eyespot patterns in insects. *Behaviour*, 1957, *11*, 209–256.

Bleuler, E. *Dementia Praecox of the Group of Schizophrenia*, 1911. Translated by J. Zinkin. New York: International Universities Press, 1911/1950.

Bliss, T. V., and Lømo, T. Long-lasting potentiation of synaptic transmission in the dentate area of the anaesthetized rabbit following stimulation of the perforant path. *Journal of Physiology*, 1973, *232*, 331–356.

Blundell, J. E., and Halford, J. C. G. Serotonin and appetite regulation: Implications for the pharmacological treatment of obesity. *CNS Drugs*, 1998, *9*, 473–495.

Bodner, S. M., Morshed, S. A., and Peterson, B. S. The question of PANDAS in adults. *Biological Psychiatry*, 2001, *49*, 807–810.

Boeve, B. F., Silber, M. H., Saper, C. B., et al. Pathophysiology of REM sleep behaviour disorder and relevance to neurodegenerative disease. *Brain*, 2007, *130*, 2770–2788.

Bogaert, A. F. Biological versus nonbiological older brothers and men's sexual orientation. *Proceedings of the National Academy of Sciences, USA*, 2006, *103*, 10771–10774.

Bohbot, V. D., Lerch, J., Thorndycraft, B., et al. Gray matter differences correlate with spontaneous strategies in a human virtual navigation task. *Journal of Neuroscience*, 2007, *27*, 10078–10083.

Bolla, K., Ernst, M., Kiehl, K., et al. Prefrontal cortical dysfunction in abstinent cocaine abusers. *Journal of Neuropsychiatry and Clinical Neuroscience*, 2004, *16*, 456–464.

Bolwig, T. G., Woldbye, D. P., and Mikkelsen, J. D. Electroconvulsive therapy as an anticonvulsant: A possible role of neuropeptide Y (NPY). *Journal of ECT*, 1999, *15*, 93–101.

Bonnin, A., Torii, M., Wang, L., et al. Serotonin modulates the response of embryonic thalamocortical axons to netrin-1. *Nature Neuroscience*, 2007, *10*, 588–597.

Boodman, S. G. Hungry in the dark: Some sleepeaters don't wake up for their strange nighttime binges. *Washington Post*, Sept. 7, 2004, HE01.

Born, R. T., and Tootell, R. B. H. Spatial frequency tuning of single units in macaque supragranular striate cortex. *Proceedings of the National Academy of Sciences, USA*, 1991, *88*, 7066–7070.

Borod, J. C., Koff, E., Yecker, S., et al. Facial asymmetry during emotional expression: Gender, valence, and measurement technique. *Neuropsychologia*, 1998, *36*, 1209–1215.

Bossy-Wetzel, E., Schwarzenbacher, R., and Lipton, S. A. Molecular pathways to neurodegeneration. *Nature Medicine*, 2004, *10*, S2–S9.

Bouchard, C., Tremblay, A., Despres, J. P., et al. The response to long-term overfeeding in identical twins. *New England Journal of Medicine*, 1990, *322*, 1477–1482.

Boulos, Z., Campbell, S. S., Lewy, A. J., et al. Light treatment for sleep disorders: Consensus report. 7: Jet-lag. *Journal of Biological Rhythms*, 1995, *10*, 167–176.

Bourne, J., and Harris, K. M. Do thin spines learn to be mushroom spines that remember? *Current Opinion in Neurobiology*, 2007, *17*, 381–386.

Bouton, M. E., and King, D. A. Contextual control of the extinction of conditioned fear: Tests for the associative value of the context. *Journal of Experimental Psychology: Animal Behavior Processes*, 1983, *9*, 248–265.

Bouvier, S. E., and Engel, S. A. Behavioral deficits and cortical damage loci in cerebral achromatopsia. *Cerebral Cortex*, 2006, *16*, 183–191.

Boynton, R. M. *Human Color Vision*. New York: Holt, Rinehart and Winston, 1979.

Bozarth, M. A., and Wise, R. A. Toxicity associated with long-term intravenous heroin and cocaine self-administration in the rat. *Journal of the American Medical Association*, 1985, *254*, 81–83.

Bradbury, M. W. B. *The Concept of a Blood-Brain Barrier*. New York: John Wiley & Sons, 1979.

Brady, K. T., and Sinha, R. Co-occurring mental and substance use disorders: The neurobiological effects of chronic stress. *American Journal of Psychiatry*, 2005, *162*, 1483–1493.

Bray, G. A. Drug treatment of obesity. *American Journal of Clinical Nutrition*, 1992, *55*, 538S–544S.

Bray, G. A., Nielsen, S. J., and Popkin, B. M. Consumption of high-fructose corn syrup in beverages may play a role in the epidemic of obesity. *American Journal of Clinical Nutrition*, 2004, *79*, 537–543.

Breedlove, S. M. Sexual differentiation of the human nervous system. *Annual Review of Psychology*, 1994, *45*, 389–418.

Breedlove, S. M. Sexual differentiation of the brain and behavior. In *Behavioral Endocrinology*, edited by J. B. Becker, S. M. Breedlove, and D. Crews. Cambridge, Mass.: MIT Press, 1992.

Brennan, P. A., and Keverne, E. B. Something in the air? New insights into mammalian pheromones. *Current Biology*, 2004, *14*, R81–R89.

Brewer, J. B., Zhao, Z., Desmond, J. E., et al. Making memories: Brain activity that predicts how well visual experience will be remembered. *Science*, 1998, *281*, 1185–1187.

Brickner, R. M. *The Intellectual Functions of the Frontal Lobe: A Study Based Upon Observations of a Man After Partial Frontal Lobectomy*. New York: Macmillan, 1936.

Bridges, R. S., DiBiase, R., Loundes, D. D., and Doherty, P. C. Prolactin stimulation of maternal behavior in female rats. *Science*, 1985, *227*, 782–784.

Britten, K. H., and van Wezel, R. J. Electrical microstimulation of cortical area MST biases heading perception in monkeys. *Nature Neuroscience*, 1998, *1*, 59–63.

Britton, D. R., Koob, G. F., Rivier, J., and Vale, W. Intraventricular corticotropin-releasing factor enhances behavioral effects of novelty. *Life Sciences*, 1982, *31*, 363–367.

Broberger, C., de Lecea, L., Sutcliffe, J. G., and Hökfelt, T. Hypocretin/orexin- and melanin-concentrating hormone-expressing cells form distinct populations in the rodent lateral hypothalamus: Relationship to the neuropeptide Y and agouti gene-related protein systems. *Journal of Comparative Neurology*, 1998, *402*, 460–474.

Broca, P. Remarques sur le siège de la faculté du langage articulé, suivies d'une observation d'aphemie (perte de la parole). *Bulletin de la Société Anatomique (Paris)*, 1861, *36*, 330–357.

Brody, A. L., Mandelkern, M. A., Lee, G., et al. Attenuation of cue-induced cigarette craving and anterior cingulate cortex activation in bupropion-treated smokers: A preliminary study. *Psychiatry Research*, 2004, *130*, 269–281.

Brolin, R. E. Bariatric surgery and long-term control of morbid obesity. *Journal of the American Medical Association*, 2002, *288*, 2793–2796.

Brown, A. M., Tekkök, S. B., and Ransom, B. R. Energy transfer from astrocytes to axons: The role of CNS glycogen. *Neurochemistry International*, 2004, *45*, 529–536.

Brown, A. S. Prenatal infection as a risk factor for schizophrenia. *Schizophrenia bulletin*, 2006, *32*, 200–202.

Brown, A. S., Hooton, J., Schaefer, C. A., et al. Elevated maternal interleukin-8 levels and risk of schizophrenia in adult offspring. *American Journal of Psychiatry*, 2004, *161*, 889–895.

Brown, R. E., Stevens, D. R., and Haas, H. L. The physiology of brain histamine. *Progress in Neurobiology*, 2001, *63*, 637–672.

Brown, S., Ingham, R. J., Ingham, J. C., et al. Stuttered and fluent speech production: An ALE meta-analysis of functional neuroimaging studies. *Human Brain Mapping*, 2005, *25*, 105–117.

Brown, T. H., Ganong, A. H., Kairiss, E. W., et al. Long-term potentiation in two synaptic systems of the hippocampal brain slice. In *Neural Models of Plasticity: Experimental and Theoretical Approaches*, edited by J. H. Byrne and W. O. Berry. San Diego: Academic Press, 1989.

Brownell, H. H., Michel, D., Powelson, J., and Gardner, H. Surprise but not coherence: Sensitivity to verbal humor in right-hemisphere patients. *Brain and Language*, 1983, *18*, 20–27.

Brownell, H. H., Simpson, T. L., Bihrle, A. M., et al. Appreciation of metaphoric alternative word meanings by left and right brain-damaged patients. *Neuropsychologia*, 1990, *28*, 173–184.

Brownell, W. E., Bader, C. R., Bertrand, D., and de-Ribaupierre, Y. Evoked mechanical responses of isolated cochlear outer hair cells. *Science*, 1985, *227*, 194–196.

Brozowski, T. J., Brown, R. M., Rosvold, H. E., and Goldman, P. S. Cognitive deficit caused by regional depletion of dopamine in prefrontal cortex of rhesus monkey. *Science*, 1979, *205*, 929–932.

Bruce, H. M. A block to pregnancy in the mouse caused by proximity of strange males. *Journal of Reproduction and Fertility*, 1960a, *1*, 96–103.

Bruce, H. M. Further observations of pregnancy block in mice caused by proximity of strange males. *Journal of Reproduction and Fertility*, 1960b, *2*, 311–312.

Bruijn, L. I., Miller, T. M., and Cleveland, D. W. Unraveling the mechanisms involved in motor neuron degeneration in ALS. *Annual Review of Neuroscience*, 2004, *27*, 723–749.

Brüning, J. C., Gautam, D., Burks, D. J., et al. Role of brain insulin receptor in control of body weight and reproduction. *Science*, 2000, *289*, 2122–2125.

Brunson, K. L., Kramár, E., Lin, B., et al. Mechanisms of late-onset cognitive decline after early-life stress. *Journal of Neuroscience*, 2005, *25*, 9328–9338.

Buccino, G., Riggio, L., Melli, G., et al. Listening to action-related sentences modulates the activity of the motor system: A combined TMS and behavioral study. *Cognitive Brain Research*, 2005, *24*, 355–363.

Buchsbaum, M. S., Gillin, J. C., Wu, J., et al. Regional cerebral glucose metabolic rate in human sleep assessed by positron emission tomography. *Life Sciences*, 1989, *45*, 1349–1356.

Buck, L. Information coding in the vertebrate olfactory system. *Annual Review of Neuroscience*, 1996, *19*, 517–544.

Buck, L., and Axel, R. A novel multigene family may encode odorant receptors: A molecular basis for odor recognition. *Cell*, 1991, *65*, 175–187.

Buffalo, E. A., Bellgowan, P. S. F., and Martin, A. The hippocampus and the surrounding cortex play different roles in memory. Poster presented at the meeting of the Organization for Human Brain Mapping, Budapest, 2004. (www.meetingassistant.com/ohbm/FORMATTED/CategoryAbstracts/cat6.html)

Buggy, J., Hoffman, W. E., Phillips, M. I., et al. Osmosensitivity of rat third ventricle and interactions with angiotensin. *American Journal of Physiology*, 1979, *236*, R75–R82.

Bullivant, S. B., Sellergren, S. A., Stern, K., et al. Women's sexual experience during the menstrual cycle: Identification of the sexual phase by noninvasive measurement of luteinizing hormone. *Journal of Sex Research*, 2004, *41*, 82–93.

Bunyard, L. B., Katzel, L. I., Busby-Whitehead, M. J., et al. Energy requirements of middle-aged men are modifiable by physical activity. *American Journal of Clinical Nutrition*, 1998, *68*, 1136–1142.

Buonopane, A., and Petrakis, I. L. Pharmacotherapy of alcohol use disorders. *Substance Use and Misuse*, 2005, *40*, 2001–2020.

Buxbaum, L. J., Glosser, G., and Coslett, H. B. Impaired face and word recognition without object agnosia. *Neuropsychologia*, 1999, *37*, 41–50.

Byne, W., Tobet, S., Mattiace, L. A., et al. The interstitial nuclei of the human anterior hypothalamus: An investigation of variation with sex, sexual orientation, and HIV status. *Hormones and Behavior*, 2001, *40*, 85–92.

Cabanac, M., and Lafrance, L. Facial consummatory responses in rats support the ponderostat hypothesis. *Physiology and Behavior*, 1991, *50*, 179–183.

Cadet, J. L., Jayanthi, S., and Deng, X. Speed kills: Cellular and molecular bases of methamphetamine-induced nerve terminal degeneration and neuronal apoptosis. *FASEB Journal*, 2003, *17*, 1775–1788.

Caine, S. B., Heinrichs, S. C., Coffin, V. L., and Koob, G. F. Effects of the dopamine D-1 antagonist SCH 23390 microinjected into the accumbens, amygdala or striatum on cocaine self-administration in the rat. *Brain Research*, 1995, *692*, 47–56.

Caine, S. B., and Koob, G. F. Effects of mesolimbic dopamine depletion on responding maintained by cocaine and food. *Journal of the Experimental Analysis of Behavior*, 1994, *61*, 213–221.

Calder, A. J., Young, A. W., Rowland, D., et al. Facial emotion recognition after bilateral amygdala damage: Differentially severe impairment of fear. *Cognitive Neuropsychology*, 1996, *13*, 699–745.

Campeau, S., Hayward, M. D., Hope, B. T., et al. Induction of the c-fos proto-oncogene in rat amygdala during unconditioned and conditioned fear. *Brain Research*, 1991, *565*, 349–352.

Camperio-Ciani, A., Corna, F., and Capiluppi, C. Evidence for maternally inherited factors favouring male homosexuality and promoting female fecundity. *Proceedings of the Royal Society of London B*, 2004, *271*, 2217–2221.

Campfield, L. A., Smith, F. J., Guisez, Y., Devos, R., and Burn, P. Recombinant mouse ob protein: Evidence for a peripheral signal linking adiposity and central neural networks. *Science*, 1995, *269*, 546–549.

Cannon, M., Jones, P. B., and Murray, R. M. Obstetric complications and schizophrenia: Historical and meta-analytic review. *American Journal of Psychiatry*, 2002, *159*, 1080–1092.

Cannon, M., Jones, P., Gilvarry, C., et al. Premorbid social functioning in schizophrenia and bipolar disorder: Similarities and differences. *American Journal of Psychiatry*, 1997, *154*, 1544–1550.

Carr, D. B., and Sesack, S. R. Projections from the rat prefrontal cortex to the ventral tegmental area: Target specificity in the synaptic associations with mesoaccumbens and mesocortical neurons. *Journal of Neuroscience*, 2000, *20*, 3864–3873.

Carrera, M. R., Ashley, J. A., Parsons, L. H., et al. Suppression of psychoactive effects of cocaine by active immunization. *Nature*, 1995, *378*, 727–730.

Carroll, R. C., Lissin, D. V., von Zastrow, M., et al. Rapid redistribution of glutamate receptors contributes to long-term depression in hippocampal cultures. *Nature Neuroscience*, 1999, *2*, 454–460.

Carter, C. S. Hormonal influences on human sexual behavior. In *Behavioral Endocrinology*, edited by J. B. Becker, S. M. Breedlove, and D. Crews. Cambridge, Mass.: MIT Press, 1992.

Casanova, M. F., Buxhoeveden, D., and Gomez, J. Disruption in the inhibitory architecture of the cell minicolumn: Implications for autism. *Neuroscientist*, 2003, *9*, 496–507.

Caspi, A., Sugden, K., Moffitt, T. E., et al. Influence of life stress on depression: Moderation by a polymorphism in the 5-HTT gene. *Science*, 2003, *301*, 386–389.

Castelli, F., Frith, C., Happé, F., and Frith, U. Autism, Asperger syndrome and brain mechanisms for the attribution of mental states to animated shapes. *Brain*, 2002, *125*, 1839–1849.

Catani, M., Jones, D. K., and ffytche, D. H. Perisylvian language networks of the human brain. *Annals of Neurology*, 2005, *57*, 8–16.

Caterina, M. J., Leffler, A., Malmberg, A. B., et al. Impaired nociception and pain sensation in mice lacking the capsaicin receptor. *Science*, 2000, *288*, 306–313.

Cavaco, S., Anderson, S. W., Allen, J. S., et al. The scope of preserved procedural memory in amnesia. *Brain*, 2004, *127*, 1863–1867.

Cenci, M. A., Kalen, P., Mandel, R. J., and Bjoerklund, A. Regional differences in the regulation of dopamine and noradrenaline release in medial frontal cortex, nucleus accumbens and caudate-putamen: A microdialysis study in the rat. *Brain Research*, 1992, *581*, 217–228.

Cerletti, U., and Bini, L. Electric shock treatment. *Bollettino ed Atti della Accademia Medica di Roma*, 1938, *64*, 36.

Chambers, R. A., Taylor, J. R., and Potenza, M. N. Developmental neurocircuitry of motivation in adolescence: A critical period of addiction vulnerability. *American Journal of Psychiatry*, 2003, *160*, 1041–1052.

Chan, J. L., Mun, E. C., Stoyneva, V., et al. Peptide YY levels are elevated after gastric bypass surgery. *Obesity*, 2006, *14*, 194–198.

Chandler, L. J., Harris, R. A., and Crews, F. T. Ethanol tolerance and synaptic plasticity. *Trends in Pharmacological Science*, 1998, *19*, 491–495.

Chatterjee, S., and Callaway, E. M. Parallel colour-opponent pathways to primary visual cortex. *Nature*, 2003, *426*, 668–671.

Chemelli, R. M., Willie, J. T., Sinton, C. M., et al. Narcolepsy in orexin knockout mice: Molecular genetics of sleep regulation. *Cell*, 1999, *98*, 437–451.

Chen, J., Paredes, W., Li, J., et al. Delta⁹-tetrahydrocannabinol produces naloxone-blockable enhancement of presynaptic basal dopamine efflux in nucleus accumbens of conscious, freely-moving rats as measured by intracerebral microdialysis. *Psychopharmacology*, 1990, *102*, 156–162.

Chen, Y. W., and Dilsaver, S. C. Lifetime rates of suicide attempts among subjects with bipolar and unipolar disorders relative to subjects with other axis I disorders. *Biological Psychiatry*, 1996, *39*, 896–899.

Chenn, A., and Walsh, C. A. Regulation of cerebral cortical size by control of cell cycle exit in neural precursors. *Science*, 2002, *297*, 365–369.

Cho, M. M., DeVries, A. C., Williams, J. R., and Carter, C. S. The effects of oxytocin and vasopressin on partner preferences in male and female prairie voles (*Microtus ochrogaster*). *Behavioral Neuroscience*, 1999, *113*, 1071–1079.

Chou, I-H., and Narasimhan, K. Neurobiology of addiction. *Nature Neuroscience*, 2005, *8*, 1427.

Chou, T. C., Bjorkum, A. A., Gaus, S. E., et al. Afferents to the ventrolateral preoptic nucleus. *Journal of Neuroscience*, 2002, *22*, 977–990.

Chubb, J. E., Bradshaw, N. J., Soares, D. C., et al. The DISC locus in psychiatric illness. *Molecular Psychiatry*, 2008, *13*, 36–64.

Clark, J. T., Kalra, P. S., Crowley, W. R., and Kalra, S. P. Neuropeptide Y and human pancreatic polypeptide stimulates feeding behavior in rats. *Endocrinology*, 1984, *115*, 427–429.

Cnattingius, S., Hultman, C. M., Dahl, M., and Sparen, P. Very preterm birth, birth trauma, and the risk of anorexia nervosa among girls. *Archives of General Psychiatry*, 1999, *56*, 634–638.

Cobb, S., and Rose, R. M. Hypertension, peptic ulcer, and diabetes in air traffic controllers. *Journal of the American Medical Association*, 1973, *224*, 489–492.

Coccaro, E. F., and Kavoussi, R. J. Fluoxetine and impulsive aggressive behavior in personality-disordered subjects. *Archives of General Psychiatry*, 1997, *54*, 1081–1088.

Cohen, C., Kodas, E., and Griebel, G. CB₁ receptor antagonists for the treatment of nicotine addiction. *Pharmacology, Biochemistry and Behavior*, 2005, *81*, 387–395.

Cohen, E. A. *Human Behavior in the Concentration Camp.* New York: W. W. Norton, 1953.

Cohen, S., Tyrrell, D. A. J., and Smith, A. P. Psychological stress and susceptibility to the common cold. *New England Journal of Medicine*, 1991, *325*, 606–612.

Cohen-Bendehan, C. C., van de Beek, C., and Berenbaum, S. A. Prenatal sex hormone effects on child and adult sex-typed behavior:

Methods and findings. *Neuroscience and Biobehavioral Reviews*, 2005, *47*, 230–237.

Colapinto, J. *As Nature Made Him: The Boy Who Was Raised as a Girl.* New York: HarperCollins, 2000.

Cole, B. J., and Koob, G. F. Propranolol antagonizes the enhanced conditioned fear produced by corticotropin releasing factor. *Journal of Pharmacology and Experimental Therapeutics*, 1988, *247*, 901–910.

Collaborative Research Group. A novel gene containing a trinucleotide repeat that is expanded and unstable on Huntington's disease chromosomes. *Cell*, 1993, *72*, 971–983.

Connellan, J., Baron-Cohen, S., Wheelwright, S., et al. Sex differences in human neonatal social perception. *Infant Behavior and Development*, 2000, *23*, 113–118.

Conway, B. R., Moeller, S., and Tsao, D. Y. Specialized color modules in macaque extrastriate cortex. *Neuron*, 2007, *56*, 560–573.

Coolen, L. M., Allard, J., Truitt, W. A., and McKenna, K. E. Central regulation of ejaculation. *Physiology and Behavior*, 2004, *83*, 203–215.

Coolen, L. M., and Wood, R. I. Testosterone stimulation of the medial preoptic area and medial amygdala in the control of male hamster sexual behavior: Redundancy without amplification. *Behavioural Brain Research*, 1999, *98*, 143–153.

Cooper, J. A. A mechanism for inside-out lamination in the neocortex. *Trends in Neurosciences*, 2008, *31*, 113–119.

Coover, G. D., Murison, R., and Jellestad, F. K. Subtotal lesions of the amygdala: The rostral central nucleus in passive avoidance and ulceration. *Physiology and Behavior*, 1992, *51*, 795–803.

Copeland, B. J., and Pillsbury, H. C. Cochlear implantation for the treatment of deafness. *Annual Review of Medicine*, 2004, *55*, 157–167.

Corey, D. P., Garcia-Añoveros, J., Holt, J. R., et al. TRPA1 is a candidate for the mechanosensitive transduction channel of vertebrate hair cells. *Nature*, 2004, *432*, 723–730.

Corkin, S., Amaral, D. G., González, R. G., et al. H. M.'s medial temporal lobe lesion: Findings from magnetic resonance imaging. *Journal of Neuroscience*, 1997, *17*, 3964–3979.

Corkin, S., Sullivan, E. V., Twitchell, T. E., and Grove, E. The amnesic patient H. M.: Clinical observations and test performance 28 years after operation. *Society for Neuroscience Abstracts*, 1981, *7*, 235.

Cornuz, J., Zwahlen, S., Jungi, W. G., et al. A vaccine against nicotine for smoking cessation: A randomized controlled trial. *PLoS One*, 2008, *3*, e2547.

Cossu, G., Ledent, C., Fattore, L., et al. Cannabinoid CB₁ receptor knockout mice fail to self-administer morphine but not other drugs of abuse. *Behavioural Brain Research*, 2001, *118*, 61–65.

Cotman, C. W., Berchtold, N. C., and Christie, L.-A. Exercise builds brain health: Key roles of growth factor cascades and inflammation. *Trends in Neuroscience*, 2007, *30*, 464–472.

Cottingham, S. L., and Pfaff, D. Interconnectedness of steroid hormone-binding neuron: Existence and implications. *Current Topics in Neuroendocrinology*, 1986, *7*, 223–249.

Courchesne, E., Pierce, K., Schumann, C. M., et al. Mapping early brain development in autism. *Neuron*, 2007, *56*, 399–413.

Courchesne, E., Redcay, E., Morgan, J. T., and Kennedy, D. P. Autism at the beginning: Microstructural and growth abnormalities underlying the cognitive and behavioral phenotype of autism. *Development and Psychopathology*, 2005, *17*, 577–597.

Court, J., Bergh, C., and Södersten, P. Mandometer treatment of Australian patients with eating disorders. *Medical Journal of Australia*, 2008, *288*, 120–121.

Covington, H. E., and Miczek, K. A. Repeated social-defeat stress, cocaine or morphine: Effects on behavioral sensitization and intravenous cocain self-administration "binges." *Psychopharmacology*, 2001, *158*, 388–398.

Cox, A., Rutter, M., Newman, S., and Bartak, L. A comparative study of infantile autism and specific developmental language disorders. I. Parental characteristics. *British Journal of Psychiatry*, 1975, *126*, 146–159.

Cox, J. J., Reimann, F., Nicholas, A. K., et al. An SCN9A channelopathy causes congenital inability to experience pain. *Nature*, 2006, *444*, 894–898.

Crane, G. E. Iproniazid (Marsilid) phosphate, a therapeutic agent for mental disorders and debilitating diseases. *Psychiatry Research Reports*, 1957, *8*, 142–152.

Creese, I., Burt, D. R., and Snyder, S. H. Dopamine receptor binding predicts clinical and pharmacological potencies of antischizophrenic drugs. *Science*, 1976, *192*, 481–483.

Crow, T. J. How and why genetic linkage has not solved the problem of psychosis: Review and hypothesis. *American Journal of Psychiatry*, 2007, *164*, 13–21.

Cubelli, R. A selective deficit for writing vowels in acquired dysgraphia. *Nature*, 1991, *353*, 258–260.

Culham, J. C., and Kanwisher, N. Neuroimaging of cognitive functions in human parietal cortex. *Current Opinion in Neurobiology*, 2001, *11*, 157–163.

Culotta, E., and Koshland, D. E. NO news is good news. *Science*, 1992, *258*, 1862–1865.

Czerniczyniec, A., Bustamante, J., and Arnaiz-Lores, S. Improvement of mouse brain mitochondrial function after deprenyl treatment. *Neuroscience*, 2007, *144*, 685–693.

Czisch, M., Wehrle, R., Kaufmann, C., et al. Functional MRI during sleep: BOLD signal decreases and their electrophysiological correlates. *European Journal of Neuroscience*, 2004, *20*, 566–574.

Daban, C., Martinez-Aran, A., Cruz, N., and Vieta, E. Safety and efficacy of vagus nerve stimulation in treatment-resistant depression. A systematic review. *Journal of Affective Disorders*, 2008, *110*, 1–15.

Daglish, M. R., Weinstein, A., Malizia, A. L., et al. Functional connectivity analysis of the neural circuits of opiate craving: "More" rather than "different"? *NeuroImage*, 2003, *20*, 1964–1970.

Damasio, A. R., and Damasio, H. Hemianopia, hemiachromatopsia, and the mechanisms of alexia. *Cortex*, 1986, *22*, 161–169.

Damasio, A. R., and Damasio, H. The anatomic basis of pure alexia. *Neurology*, 1983, *33*, 1573–1583.

Damasio, A. R., Grabowski, T. J., Bechara, A., et al. Subcortical and cortical brain activity during the feeling of self-generated emotions. *Nature Neuroscience*, 2000, *3*, 1049–1056.

Damasio, A. R., and Tranel, D. Nouns and verbs are retrieved with differentially distributed neural systems. *Proceedings of the National Academy of Sciences, USA*, 1993, *90*, 4957–4960.

Damasio, A. R., Yamada, T., Damasio, H., et al. Central achromatopsia: Behavioral, anatomic, and physiologic aspects. *Neurology*, 1980, *30*, 1064–1071.

Damasio, H. Neuroimaging contributions to the understanding of aphasia. In *Handbook of Neuropsychology, Vol. 2*, edited by F. Boller and J. Grafman. Amsterdam: Elsevier, 1989.

Damasio, H., and Damasio, A. R. The anatomical basis of conduction aphasia. *Brain*, 1980, *103*, 337–350.

Damasio, H., Eslinger, P., and Adams, H. P. Aphasia following basal ganglia lesions: New evidence. *Seminars in Neurology*, 1984, *4*, 151–161.

Damasio, H., Grabowski, T., Frank, R., et al. The return of Phineas Gage: Clues about the brain from the skull of a famous patient. *Science*, 1994, *264*, 1102–1105.

Damsma, G., Day, J., and Fibiger, H. C. Lack of tolerance to nicotine-induced dopamine release in the nucleus accumbens. *European Journal of Pharmacology*, 1989, *168*, 363–368.

Dani, J. A., and Harris, R. A. Nicotine addiction and comorbidity with alcohol abuse and mental illness. Nature *Neuroscience*, 2005, *8*, 1465–1470.

Daniele, A., Giustolisi, L., Silveri, M. C., et al. Evidence for a possible neuroanatomical basis for lexical processing of nouns and verbs. *Neuropsychologia*, 1994, *32*, 1325–1341.

Daniels, D., Miselis, R. R., and Flanagan-Cato, L. M. Central neuronal circuit innervating the lordosis-producing muscles defined by transneuronal transport of pseudorabies virus. *Journal of Neuroscience*, 1999, *19*, 2823–2833.

Darwin, C. *The Expression of the Emotions in Man and Animals*. Chicago: University of Chicago Press, 1872/1965.

Davidson, D., Swift, R., and Fitz, E. Naltrexone increases the latency to drink alcohol in social drinkers. *Alcoholism: Clinical and Experimental Research*, 1996, *20*, 732–739.

Davis, J. O., Phelps, J. A., and Bracha, H. S. Prenatal development of monozygotic twins and concordance for schizophrenia. *Schizophrenia Bulletin*, 1995, *21*, 357–366.

Davis, M. The role of the amygdala in fear-potentiated startle: Implications for animal models of anxiety. *Trends in Pharmacological Sciences*, 1992, *13*, 35–41.

Daw, N. W. Colour-coded ganglion cells in the goldfish retina: Extension of their receptive fields by means of new stimuli. *Journal of Physiology (London)*, 1968, *197*, 567–592.

Dawson, T. M., and Dawson, V. L. Molecular pathways of neurodegeneration in Parkinson's disease. *Science*, 2003, *302*, 819–822.

Deacon, S., and Arendt, J. Adapting to phase shifts. I. An experimental model for jet lag and shift work. *Physiology and Behavior*, 1996, *59*, 665–673.

Dealberto, M. J. Why are immigrants at increased risk for psychosis? Vitamin D insufficiency, epigenetic mechanisms, or both? *Medical Hypotheses*, 2007, *68*, 259–267.

Dean, P. Effects of inferotemporal lesions on the behavior of monkeys. *Psychological Bulletin*, 1976, *83*, 41–71.

Debanne, D., Gähwiler, B. H., and Thompson, S. M. Asynchronous pre- and postsynaptic activity induces associative long-term depression in area CA$_1$ of the rat hippocampus in vitro. *Proceedings of the National Academy of Sciences, USA*. 1994, *91*, 1148–1152.

Debiec, J., LeDoux, J. E., and Nader, K. Cellular and systems reconsolidation in the hippocampus. *Neuron*, 2002, *36*, 527–538.

Deffenbacher, K. E., Kenyon, J. B., Hoover, D. M., et al. Refinement of the 6p21.3 quantitative trait locus influencing dyslexia: Linkage and association analysis. *Human Genetics*, 2004, *115*, 128–138.

de Gelder, B. Towards the neurobiology of emotional body language. *Nature Reviews: Neuroscience*, 2006, *7*, 242–249.

Dejerine, J. Contribution à l'étude anatomo-pathologique et clinique des différentes variétés de cécité verbale. *Comptes Rendus des Séances de la Société de Biologie et de Ses Filiales*, 1892, *4*, 61–90.

De Jonge, F. H., Louwerse, A. L., Ooms, M. P., et al. Lesions of the SDN-POA inhibit sexual behavior of male Wistar rats. *Brain Research Bulletin*, 1989, *23*, 483–492.

de Kloet, E. R., Joëls, M., and Holsboer, F. Stress and the brain: From adaptation to disease. *Nature Reviews: Neuroscience*, 2005, *6*, 463–475.

Del Cerro, M. C. R., Izquierdo, M. A. P., Rosenblatt, J. S., et al. Brain 2-deoxyglucose levels related to maternal behavior-inducing stimuli in the rat. *Brain Research*, 1995, *696*, 213–220.

Delgado, P. L., Charney, D. S., Price, L. H., et al. Serotonin function and the mechanism of antidepressant action: Reversal of antidepressant induced remission by rapid depletion of plasma tryptophan. *Archives of General Psychiatry*, 1990, *47*, 411–418.

DeLoache, J. S., Uttal, D. H., and Rosengren, K. S. Scale errors offer evidence for a perception-action dissociation early in life. *Science*, 2004, *304*, 1027–1029.

DeLong, G. R. Autism: New data suggest a new hypothesis. *Neurology*, 1999, *52*, 911–916.

Dement, W. C. The effect of dream deprivation. *Science*, 1960, *131*, 1705–1707.

Démonet, J.-F., Taylor, M. J., and Chaix, Y. Developmental dyslexia. *Lancet*, 2004, *363*, 1451–1460.

De Ocampo, J., Foldvary, N., Dinner, D. S., and Golish, J. *Sleep Medicine*, 2002, *3*, 525–526.

Deol, M. S., and Gluecksohn-Waelsch, S. The role of inner hair cells in hearing. *Nature*, 1979, *278*, 250–252.

Dérouesné, J., and Beauvois, M. F. Phonological processing in reading: Data from alexia. *Journal of Neurology, Neurosurgery, and Psychiatry*, 1979, *42*, 1125–1132.

De Strooper, B. Aph-1, Pen-2, and nicastrin with presenilin generate an active γ-secretase complex. *Neuron*, 2003, *38*, 9–12.

Deutsch, J. A., and Gonzalez, M. F. Gastric nutrient content signals satiety. *Behavioral and Neural Biology*, 1980, *30*, 113–116.

De Valois, R. L., Albrecht, D. G., and Thorell, L. Cortical cells: Bar detectors or spatial frequency filters? In *Frontiers in Visual Science*, edited by S. J. Cool and E. L. Smith. Berlin: Springer-Verlag, 1978.

De Valois, R. L., and De Valois, K. K. *Spatial Vision*. New York: Oxford University Press, 1988.

Devane, W. A., Hanus, L., Breuer, A., et al. Isolation and structure of a brain constituent that binds to the cannabinoid receptor. *Science*, 1992, *258*, 1946–1949.

Devilbiss, D. M., and Berridge, C. W. Cognition-enhancing doses of methylphenidate preferentially increase prefrontal cortex neuronal responsiveness. *Biological Psychiatry*, 2008, *64*, 626–635.

Devine, D. P., and Wise, R. A. Self-administration of morphine, DAMGO, and DPDPE into the ventral tegmental area of rats. *Journal of Neuroscience*, 1994, *14*, 1978–1984.

De Vries, T. J., and Schoffelmeer, A. N. M. Cannabinoid CB$_1$ receptors control conditioned drug seeking. *Trends in Pharmacological Sciences*, 2005, *26*, 420–426.

Diamond, M., and Sigmundson, H. K. Sex reassignment at birth: Long-term review and clinical implications. *Archives of Pediatric and Adolescent Medicine*, 1997, *151*, 298–304.

Di Chiara, G. The role of dopamine in drug abuse viewed from the perspective of its role in motivation. *Drug and Alcohol Dependency*, 1995, *38*, 95–137.

DiFiglia, M., Sena-Esteves, M., Chase, K., et al. Therapeutic silencing of mutant huntingtin with siRNA attenuates striatal and cortical neuropathology and behavioral deficits. *Proceedings of the National Academy of Sciences, USA*, 2007, *104*, 17204–17209.

Dijk, D. J., Boulos, Z., Eastman, C. I., et al. Light treatment for sleep disorders: Consensus report. 2. Basic properties of circadian physiology and sleep regulation. *Journal of Biological Rhythms*, 1995, *10*, 113–125.

Di Marzo, V., and Matias, I. Endocannabinoid control of food intake and energy balance. *Nature Neuroscience*, 2005, *8*, 585–589.

di Tomaso, E., Beltramo, M., and Piomelli, D. Brain cannabinoids in chocolate. *Nature*, 1996, *382*, 677–678.

Doetsch, F., and Hen, R. Young and excitable: The function of new neurons in the adult mammalian brain. *Current Opinion in Neuroscience*, 2005, *15*, 121–128.

Domschke, K., Stevens, S., Beck, B., et al. Blushing propensity in social anxiety disorder: Influence of serotonin transporter gene variation. *Journal of Neural Transmission*, 2009, *116*, 663–666.

Donny, E. C., Caggiula, A. R., Knopf, S., and Brown, C. Nicotine self-administration in rats. *Psychopharmacology*, 1995, *122*, 390–394.

Dorries, K. M., Adkins, R. E., and Halpern, B. P. Sensitivity and behavioral responses to the pheromone androsteneone are not mediated by the vomeronasal organ in domestic pigs. *Brain, Behavior, and Evolution*, 1997, *49*, 53–62.

Doty, R. L. Olfaction. *Annual Review of Psychology*, 2001, *52*, 423–452.

Dougherty, D. D., Baie, L., Gosgrove, G. R., et al. Prospective long-term follow-up of 44 patients who received cingulotomy for treatment-refractory obsessive-compulsive disorder. *American Journal of Psychiatry*, 2002, *159*, 269–275.

Douglass, J., McKinzie, A. A., and Couceyro, P. PCR differential display identifies a rat brain mRNA that is transcriptionally regulated by cocaine and amphetamine. *Journal of Neuroscience*, 1995, *15*, 2471–2481.

Downing, P. E., Chan, A. W.-Y., Peelen, M. V., et al. Domain specificity in visual cortex. *Cerebral Cortex*, 2006, *16*, 1453–1461.

Drake, C. L., Roehrs, T., Richardson, G., et al. Shift work sleep disorder: Prevalence and consequences beyond that of symptomatic day workers. *Sleep*, 2004, *27*, 1453–1462.

Drevets, W. C. Neuroimaging and neuropathological studies of depression: implications for the cognitive-emotional features of mood disorders. *Current Opinions in Neurobiology*, 2001, *11*, 240–249.

Drevets, W. C. Functional anatomical abnormalities in limbic and prefrontal cortical structures in major depression. *Progress in Brain Research*, 2000, *126*, 413–431.

Drevets, W. C., Price, J. L., Simpson, J. R., et al. Subgenual prefrontal cortex abnormalities in mood disorders. *Nature*, 1997, *386*, 824–827.

Drevets, W. C., Videen, T. O., Price, J. L., et al. A functional anatomical study of unipolar depression. *Journal of Neuroscience*, 1992, *12*, 3628–3641.

Dube, M. G., Kalra, S. P., and Kalra, P. S. Food intake elicited by central administration of orexins/hypocretins: Identification of hypothalamic sites of action. *Brain Research*, 1999, *842*, 473–477.

Duchenne, G.-B. *The Mechanism of Human Facial Expression* (translated by R. A. Cuthbertson). Cambridge, U.K.: Cambridge University Press, 1990. (Original work published 1862.)

Dukelow, S. P., DeSouza, J. F., Culham, J. C., et al. Distinguishing subregions of the human MT+ complex using visual fields and pursuit eye movements. *Journal of Neurophysiology*, 2001, *86*, 1991–2000.

Dunn, A. L., Trivedi, M. H., Kampert, J. B., et al. Exercise treatment for depression: Efficacy and dose response. *American Journal of Preventive Medicine*, 2005, *28*, 1–8.

Durie, D. J. Sleep in animals. In *Psychopharmacology of Sleep*, edited by D. Wheatley. New York: Raven Press, 1981.

Eastman, C. I., Boulos, Z., Terman, M., et al. Light treatment for sleep disorders: Consensus report. VI. Shift work. *Journal of Biological Rhythms*, 1995, *10*, 157–164.

Eaton, W. W., Kessler, R. C., Wittchen, H. U., and Magee, W. J. Panic and panic disorder in the United States. *American Journal of Psychiatry*, 1994, *151*, 413–420.

Eaton, W. W., Mortensen, P. B., and Frydenberg, M. Obstetric factors, urbanization and psychosis. *Schizophrenia Research*, 2000, *43*, 117–123.

Ebisawa, T., Uchiyama, M., Kajimura, N., et al. Association of structural polymorphisms in the human period3 gene with delayed sleep phase syndrome. *EMBRO Reports*, 2001, *2*, 342–346.

Eden, G. F., and Zeffiro, T. A. Neural systems affected in developmental dyslexia revealed by functional neuroimaging. *Neuron*, 1998, *21*, 279–282.

Edenberg, H. J., Dick, D. M., Xuei, X., et al. Variations in *GABRA2*, encoding the α2 subunit of the GABA$_A$ receptor, are associated with alcohol dependence and with brain oscillations. *American Journal of Human Genetics*, 2004, *74*, 705–714.

Edwards, D. P., Purpura, K. P., and Kaplan, E. Contrast sensitivity and spatial-frequency response of primate cortical neurons in and around the cytochrome oxidase blobs. *Vision Research*, 1995, *35*, 1501–1523.

Egan, G., Silk, T., Zamarripa, F., et al. Neural correlates of the emergence of consciousness of thirst. *Proceedings of the National Academy of Sciences, USA*, 2003, *100*, 15241–15246.

Ehrsson, H. H., Spence, C., and Passingham, R. E. That's my hand! Activity in premotor cortex reflects feeling of ownership of a limb. *Science*, 2004, *305*, 875–877.

Ehrsson, H. H., Wiech, K., Weiskopf, N., et al. Threatening a rubber hand that you feel is yours elicits a cortical anxiety response. *Proceedings of the National Academy of Sciences, USA*, 2007, *104*, 9828–9833.

Eichenbaum, H., Otto, T., and Cohen, N. J. The hippocampus: What does it do? *Behavioral and Neural Biology*, 1992, *57*, 2–36.

Eichenbaum, H., Stewart, C., and Morris, R. G. M. Hippocampal representation in spatial learning. *Journal of Neuroscience*, 1990, *10*, 331–339.

Ekman, P. Facial expressions of emotion: An old controversy and new findings. *Philosophical Transactions of the Royal Society of London* [*B*], 1992, *335*, 63–69.

Ekman, P. *The Face of Man: Expressions of Universal Emotions in a New Guinea Village.* New York: Garland STPM Press, 1980.

Ekman, P., and Davidson, R. J. Voluntary smiling changes regional brain activity. *Psychological Science*, 1993, *4*, 342–345.

Ekman, P., and Friesen, W. V. Constants across cultures in the face and emotion. *Journal of Personality and Social Psychology*, 1971, *17*, 124–129.

Ekman, P., Levenson, R. W., and Friesen, W. V. Autonomic nervous system activity distinguished between emotions. *Science*, 1983, *221*, 1208–1210.

El Mansari, M., and Blier, P. In vivo electrophysiological characterization of 5-HT receptors in the guinea pig head of caudate nucleus and orbitofrontal cortex. *Neuropharmacology*, 1997, *36*, 577–588.

El Mansari, M., Sakai, K., and Jouvet, M. Unitary characteristics of presumptive cholinergic tegmental neurons during the sleep-waking cycle in freely moving cats. *Experimental Brain Research*, 1989, *76*, 519–529.

Elbert, T., Pantev, C., Wienbruch, C., et al. Increased cortical representation of the fingers of the left hand in string players. *Science*, 1995, *270*, 305–307.

Elias, C. F., Lee, C., Kelly, J., et al. Leptin activates hypothalamic CART neurons projecting to the spinal cord. *Neuron*, 1998b, *21*, 1375–1385.

Elias, C. F., Saper, C. B., Maratos-Flier, E., et al. Chemically defined projections linking the mediobasal hypothalamus and the lateral hypothalamic area. *Journal of Comparative Neurology*, 1998a, *402*, 442–459.

Elmquist, J. K., Elias, C. F., and Saper, C. B. From lesions to leptin: Hypothalamic control of food intake and body weight. *Neuron*, 1999, *22*, 221–232.

Elsworth, J. D., Jentsch, J. D., Morrow, B. A., et al. Clozapine normalizes prefrontal cortex dopamine transmission in monkeys subchronically exposed to phencyclidine. *Neuropsychopharmacology*, 2008, *33*, 491–496.

Emmorey, K., Mehta, S., and Grabowski, T. J. The neural correlates of sign versus word production. *NeuroImage*, 2007, *36*, 202–208.

Eslinger, P. J., and Damasio, A. R. Severe disturbance of higher cognition after bilateral frontal lobe ablation: Patient EVR. *Neurology*, 1985, *35*, 1731–1741.

Fadiga, L., Craighero, L., Buccino, G., and Rizzolatti, G. Speech listening specifically modulates the excitability of tongue muscles: A TMS study. *European Journal of Neuroscience*, 2002, *15*, 399–402.

Farina, C., Weber, M. S., Meinl, E., et al. Glatiramer acetate in multiple sclerosis: Update on potential mechanisms of action. *Lancet Neurology*, 2005, *4*, 567–575.

Farlow, M., Murrell, J., Ghetti, B., et al. Clinical characteristics in a kindred with early-onset Alzheimer's-disease and their linkage to a GfiT change at position-2149 of amyloid precursor protein gene. *Neurology*, 1994, *44*, 105–111.

Farooqi, I. S., and O'Rahilly, S. Monogenic obesity in humans. *Annual Review of Medicine*, 2005, *56*, 443–458.

Feder, H. H. Estrous cyclicity in mammals. In *Neuroendocrinology of Reproduction*, edited by N. T. Adler. New York: Plenum Press, 1981.

Feinle, C., Grundy, D., and Read, N. W. Effects of duodenal nutrients on sensory and motor responses of the human stomach to distension. *American Journal of Physiology*, 1997, *273*, G721–726.

Fenoglio, K. A., Chen, Y., and Baram, T. Z. Neuroplasticity of the hypothalamic-pituitary-adrenal axis early in life requires recurrent recruitment of stress-regulation brain regions. *Journal of Neuroscience*, 2006, *26*, 2434–2442.

Fernandez, F., Morishita, W., Zuniga, E., et al. Pharmacotherapy for cognitive impairment in a mouse model of Down syndrome. *Nature Neuroscience*, 2007, *10*, 411–413.

Fernandez-Ruiz, J., Wang, J., Aigner, T. G., and Mishkin, M. Visual habit formation in monkeys with neurotoxic lesions of the ventrocaudal neostriatum. *Proceedings of the National Academy of Sciences, USA*, 2001, *98*, 4196–4201.

Ferris, C. F., Kulkarni, P., Sullivan, J. M., et al. Pup suckling is more rewarding than cocaine: Evidence from functional magnetic resonance imaging and three-dimensional computational analysis. *Journal of Neuroscience*, 2005, *25*, 149–156.

Fettiplace, R., and Hackney, C. M. The sensory and motor roles of auditory hair cells. *Nature Reviews: Neuroscience*, 2006, *7*, 19–29.

Fibiger, H. C. The dopamine hypothesis of schizophrenia and mood disorders: Contradictions and speculations. In *The Mesolimbic Dopamine System: From Motivation to Action*, edited by P. Willner and J. Scheel-Krüger. Chichester, England: John Wiley & Sons, 1991.

Field, T., Woodson, R., Greenberg, R., and Cohen, D. Discrimination and imitation of facial expressions in neonates. *Science*, 1982, *218*, 179–181.

Fieve, R. R. The clinical effects of lithium treatment. *Trends in Neurosciences*, 1979, *2*, 66–68.

Finger, S. *Origins of Neuroscience: A History of Explorations into Brain Function*. New York: Oxford University Press, 1994.

Fisher, C., Gross, J., and Zuch, J. Cycle of penile erection synchronous with dreaming (REM) sleep: Preliminary report. *Archives of General Psychiatry*, 1965, *12*, 29–45.

Fiske, A. P., and Haslam, N. Is obsessive-compulsive disorder a pathology of the human disposition to perform socially meaningful rituals? Evidence of similar content. *Journal of Nervous and Mental Disease*, 1997, *185*, 211–222.

Fitzgerald, P. Repetitive transcranial magnetic stimulation and electroconvulsive therapy: Complementary or competitive therapeutic options in depression? *Australas Psychiatry*, 2004, *12*, 234–238.

Fitzpatrick, D., Itoh, K., and Diamond, I. T. The laminar organization of the lateral geniculate body and the striate cortex in the squirrel monkey (*Saimiri sciureus*). *Journal of Neuroscience*, 1983, *3*, 673–702.

Fitzsimons, J. T., and Moore-Gillon, M. J. Drinking and antidiuresis in response to reductions in venous return in the dog: Neural and endocrine mechanisms. *Journal of Physiology (London)*, 1980, *308*, 403–416.

Flaum, M., and Andreasen, N. C. Diagnostic criteria for schizophrenia and related disorders: Options for DNS-IV. *Schizophrenia Bulletin*, 1990, *17*, 27–49.

Flock, A. Physiological properties of sensory hairs in the ear. In *Psychophysics and Physiology of Hearing*, edited by E. F. Evans and J. P. Wilson. London: Academic Press, 1977.

Flum, D. R., Salem, L., Elrod, J. A. B., et al. Early mortality among Medicare beneficiaries undergoing bariatric surgical procedures. *Journal of the American Medical Association*, 2005, *294*, 1903–1908.

Flynn, F. W., and Grill, H. J. Insulin elicits ingestion in decerebrate rats. *Science*, 1983, *221*, 188–190.

Fombonne, E. Epidemiology of autistic disorder and other pervasive developmental disorders. *Journal of Clinical Psychiatry*, 2005, *66* (Suppl. 10), 3–8.

Fontaine, D., Mattei, V., Borg, M., et al. Effect of subthalamic nucleus stimulation on obsessive-compulsive disorder in a patient with Parkinson disease: Case report. *Journal of Neurosurgery*, 2004, *100*, 1084–1086.

Forno, L. S. Neuropathology of Parkinson's disease. *Journal of Neuropathology and Experimental Neurology*, 1996, *55*, 259–272.

Foundas, A. L., Bollich, A. M., Feldman, J., et al. Aberrant auditory processing and atypical planum temporale in developmental stuttering. *Neurology*, 2004, *63*, 1640–1646.

Fowler, J. S., Logan, J., Wang, G. J., and Volkow, N. D. Monoamine oxidase and cigarette smoking. *Neurotoxicology*, 2003, *24*, 75–82.

Franklin, T. R., Acton, P. D., Maldjian, J. A., et al. Decreased gray matter concentration in the insular, orbitofrontal, cingulate, and temporal cortices of cocaine patients. *Biological Psychiatry*, 2002, *51*, 134–142.

Freed, C. R. Will embryonic stem cells be a useful source of dopamine neurons for transplant into patients with Parkinson's disease? *Proceedings of the National Academy of Sciences, USA*, 2002, *99*, 1755–1757.

Freedman, M. S., Lucas, R. J., Soni, B., et al. Regulation of mammalian circadian behavior by non-rod, non-cone, ocular photoreceptors. *Science*, 1999, *284*, 502–504.

Frey, S. H., Vinton, D., Norlund, R., and Grafton, S. T. Cortical topography of human anterior intraparietal cortex active during visually guided grasping. *Cognitive Brain Research*, 2005, *23*, 397–405.

Fried, I., Katz, A., McCarthy, G., et al. Functional organization of human supplementary motor cortex studied by electrical stimulation. *Journal of Neuroscience*, 1991, *11*, 3656–3666.

Friedman, M. I., and Bruno, J. P. Exchange of water during lactation. *Science*, 1976, *191*, 409–410.

Friedman, M. I., Horn, C. C., and Ji, H. Peripheral signals in the control of feeding behavior. *Chemical Senses*, 2005, *30* (Suppl. 1), i182–i183.

Fry, J. M. Treatment modalities for narcolepsy. *Neurology*, 1998, *50*, S43–S48.

Fukuwatari, T., Shibata, K., Igushi, K., et al. Role of gustation in the recognition of oleate and triolein in anomic rats. *Physiology and Behavior*, 2003, *78*, 579–583.

Fuller, P. M., Saper, C. B., and Lu, J. The pontine REM switch: Past and present. *Journal of Physiology*, 2007, *584*, 735–741.

Fullerton, C. S., Ursano, R. J., Epstein, R. S., et al. Gender differences in posttraumatic stress disorder after motor vehicle accidents. *American Journal of Psychiatry*, 2001, *158*, 1485–1491.

Fulton, J. F. *Functional Localization in Relation to Frontal Lobotomy*. New York: Oxford University Press, 1949.

Furmark, T., Tillfors, M., Garpenstrand, H., et al. Serotonin transporter polymorphism related to amygdala excitability and symptom severity in patients with social phobia. *Neuroscience Letters*, 2004, *362*, 189–192.

Gaillard, R., Naccache, L., Pinel, P., et al. Direct intracranial, fmri, and lesion evidence for the causal role of left inferotemporal cortex in reading. *Neuron*, 2006, *50*, 191–204.

Galen. *De Usu Partium*. Translated by M. T. May. Ithaca, NY: Cornell University Press, 1968.

Gallassi, R., Morreale, A., Montagna, P., et al. Fatal familial insomnia: Behavioral and cognitive features. *Neurology*, 1996, *46*, 935–939.

Gallese, V., Fadiga, L., Fogassi, L., and Rizzolatti, G. Action recognition in the premotor cortex. *Brain*, 1996, *119*, 593–609.

Garavan, H., and Stout, J. C. Neurocognitive insights into substance abuse. *Trends in Cognitive Sciences*, 2005, *9*, 195–201.

Garcia-Velasco, J., and Mondragon, M. The incidence of the vomeronasal organ in 1000 human subjects and its possible clinical significance. *Journal of Steroid Biochemistry and Molecular Biology*, 1991, *39*, 561–563.

Gardner, H., Brownell, H. H., Wapner, W., and Michelow, D. Missing the point: The role of the right hemisphere in the processing of complex linguistic materials. In *Cognitive Processing in the Right Hemisphere*, edited by E. Pericman. New York: Academic Press, 1983.

Gariano, R. F., and Groves, P. M. Burst firing induced in midbrain dopamine neurons by stimulation of the medial prefrontal and anterior cingulate cortices. *Brain Research*, 1988, *462*, 194–198.

Garriga-Canut, M., Schoenike, B., Qazi, R., et al. 2-Deoxy-D-glucose reduces epilepsy progression by NRSF-CtBP-dependent metabolic regulation of chromatin structure. *Nature Neuroscience*, 2006, *9*, 1382–1387.

Gaspar, P., Cases, O., and Maroteaux, L. The developmental role of serotonin: News from mouse molecular genetics. *Nature Reviews: Neuroscience*, 2003, *4*, 1002–1012.

Gazzaniga, M. Forty-five years of split-brain research and still going strong. *Nature Reviews: Neuroscience*, 2005, *6*, 653–659.

Gazzaniga, M. S., and LeDoux, J. E. *The Integrated Mind*. New York: Plenum Press, 1978.

Gentilucci, M. Grasp observation influences speech production. *European Journal of Neuroscience*, 2003, *17*, 179–184.

George, M. S., Parekh, P. I., Rosinsky, N., et al. Understanding emotional prosody activates right hemisphere regions. *Archives of Neurology*, 1996, *53*, 665–670.

Gerashchenko, D., Blanco-Centurion, C., Greco, M. A., and Shiromani, P. J. Effects of lateral hypothalamic lesion with the neurotoxin hypocretin-2-saporin on sleep in Long-Evans rats. *Neuroscience*, 2003, *116*, 223–235.

Gerashchenko, D., Kohls, M. D., Greco, M., et al. Hypocretin-2-saporin lesions of the lateral hypothalamus produce narcoleptic-like sleep behavior in the rat. *Journal of Neuroscience*, 2001, *21*, 7273–7283.

Gerbino, L., Oleshansky, M., and Gershon, S. Clinical use and mode of action of lithium. In *Psychopharmacology: A Generation of Progress*, edited by M. A. Lipton, A. DiMascio, and K. F. Killam. New York: Raven Press, 1978.

Gerhand, S. Routes to reading: A report of a non-semantic reader with equivalent performance on regular and exception words. *Neuropsychologia*, 2001, *39*, 1473–1484.

Gershon, E. S., Bunney, W. E., Leckman, J., et al. The inheritance of affective disorders: A review of data and hypotheses. *Behavior Genetics*, 1976, *6*, 227–261.

Geschwind, N., Quadfasel, F. A., and Segarra, J. M. Isolation of the speech area. *Neuropsychologia*, 1968, *6*, 327–340.

Gessa, G. L., Muntoni, F., Collu, M., et al. Low doses of ethanol activate dopaminergic neurons in the ventral tegmental area. *Brain Research*, 1985, *348*, 201–204.

Getz, L. L., and Carter, C. S. Prairie-vole partnerships. *American Scientist*, 1996, *84*, 55–62.

Ghilardi, J. R., Röhrich, H., Lindsay, T. H., et al. Selective blockade of the capsaicin receptor TRPV1 attenuates bone cancer pain. *Journal of Neuroscience*, 2005, *25*, 3126–3131.

Gibbs, J., Young, R. C., and Smith, G. P. Cholecystokinin decreases food intake in rats. *Journal of Comparative and Physiological Psychology*, 1973, *84*, 488–495.

Giedd, J. N., Rapoport, J. L., Garvey, M. A., et al. MRI assessment of children with obsessive-compulsive disorder or tics associated with streptococcal infection. *American Journal of Psychiatry*, 2000, *157*, 281–283.

Giedd, J. N., Rapoport, J. L., Kruesi, M. J. P., et al. Sydenham's chorea: Magnetic resonance imaging of the basal ganglia. *Neurology*, 1995, *45*, 2199–2202.

Gillespie, P. G. Molecular machinery of auditory and vestibular transduction. *Current Opinion in Neurobiology*, 1995, *5*, 449–455.

Gillette, M. U., and McArthur, A. J. Circadian actions of melatonin at the suprachiasmatic nucleus. *Behavioural Brain Research*, 1995, *73*, 135–139.

Glaser, R., Rice, J., Sheridan, J., Post, A., et al. Stress-related immune suppression: Health implications. *Brain, Behavior, and Immunity*, 1987, *1*, 7–20.

Glaum, S. R., Hara, M., Bindokas, V. P., et al. Leptin, the obese gene product, rapidly modulates synaptic transmission in the hypothalamus. *Molecular Pharmacology*, 1996, *50*, 230–235.

Gloor, P., Olivier, A., Quesney, L. F., et al. The role of the limbic system in experiential phenomena of temporal lobe epilepsy. *Annals of Neurology*, 1982, *12*, 129–144.

Goddard, G. V. Development of epileptic seizures through brain stimulation at low intensity. *Nature*, 1967, *214*, 1020–1021.

Godfrey, P. A., Malnic, B., and Buck, L. The mouse olfactory receptor gene family. *Proceedings of the National Academy of Sciences, USA*, 2004, *101*, 2156–2161.

Goeders, N. E., Lane, J. D., and Smith, J. E. Self-administration of methionine enkephalin into the nucleus accumbens. *Pharmacology, Biochemistry, and Behavior*, 1984, *20*, 451–455.

Goedert, M. Alpha-synuclein and neurodegenerative diseases. *Nature Review Neuroscience*, 2001, *2*, 492–501.

Goldberg, R. F., Perfetti, C. A., and Schneider, W. Perceptual knowledge retrieval activates sensory brain regions. *Journal of Neuroscience*, 2006, *26*, 4917–4921.

Goldman, D., Oroszi, G., and Ducci, F. The genetics of addictions: Uncovering the genes. *Nature Reviews Genetics*, 2005, *6*, 521–532.

Goldstein, J. M., Seidman, L. J., Horton, N. J., et al. Normal sexual dimorphism of the adult human brain assessed by *in vivo* magnetic resonance imaging. *Cerebral Cortex*, 2001, *11*, 490–497.

Goldstein, R. A., and Volkow, N. D. Drug addiction and its underlying neurobiological basis: Neuroimaging evidence for the involvement of the frontal cortex. *American Journal of Psychiatry*, 2002, *159*, 1642–1652.

Goodale, M. A., Meenan, J. P., Bülthoff, H. H., et al. Separate neural pathways for the visual analysis of object shape in perception and prehension. *Current Biology*, 1994, *4*, 604–610.

Goodale, M. A., and Milner, A. D. Separate visual pathways for perception and action. *Trends in Neuroscience*, 1992, *15*, 20–25.

Goodale, M. A., and Westwood, D. A. An evolving view of duplex vision: Separate by interacting cortical pathways for perception and action. *Current Opinion in Neurobiology*, 2004, *14*, 203–211.

Goodglass, H., and Kaplan, E. *Assessment of Aphasia and Related Disorders*. Philadelphia: Lea & Febiger, 1972.

Gooren, L. The biology of human psychosexual differentiation. *Hormones and Behavior*, 2006, *50*, 589–601.

Gordon, H. W., and Sperry, R. Lateralization of olfactory perception in the surgically separated hemispheres in man. *Neuropsychologia*, 1969, *7*, 111–120.

Gorski, R. A., Gordon, J. H., Shryne, J. E., and Southam, A. M. Evidence for a morphological sex difference within the medial preoptic area of the rat brain. *Brain Research*, 1978, *148*, 333–346.

Gosselin, N., Peretz, I., Noulhiane, M., et al. Impaired recognition of scary music following unilateral temporal lobe excision. *Brain*, 2005, *128*, 628–640.

Gottesman, I. I., and Shields, J. *Schizophrenia: The Epigenetic Puzzle*. New York: Cambridge University Press, 1982.

Gould, E., Beylin, A., Tanapat, P., et al. Learning enhances adult neurogenesis in the hippocampal formation. *Nature Neuroscience*, 1999, *2*, 260–265.

Gouras, P. Identification of cone mechanisms in monkey ganglion cells. *Journal of Physiology*, 1968, *199*, 533–538.

Grafton, S. T., Waters, C., Sutton, J., et al. Pallidotomy increases activity of motor association cortex in Parkinson's disease: A positron emission tomographic study. *Annals of Neurology*, 1995, *37*, 776–783.

Graybiel, A. M. Basal ganglia: New therapeutic approaches to Parkinson's disease. *Current Biology*, 1996, *6*, 368–371.

Greene, J. D., Sommerville, R. B., Nystrom, L. E., et al. An fMRI investigation of emotional engagement in moral judgment. *Science*, 2001, *293*, 2105–2108.

Grelotti, D. J., Gauthier, I., and Schultz, R. T. Social interest and the development of cortical face specialization: What autism teaches us about face processing. *Developmental Psychobiology*, 2002, *40*, 213–225.

Grill, H. J., and Kaplan, J. M. Caudal brainstem participates in the distributed neural control of feeding. In *Handbook of Behavioral Neurobiology, Vol. 10: Neurobiology of Food and Fluid Intake*, edited by E. Stricker. New York: Plenum Press, 1990.

Grill-Spector, K., Knouf, N., and Kanwisher, N. The fusiform face area subserves face perception, not generic within-category identification. *Nature Neuroscience*, 2004, *7*, 555–561.

Grill-Spector, K., and Malach, R. The human visual cortex. *Annual Review of Neuroscience*, 2004, *27*, 649–677.

Grimm, J. W., and See, R. E. Dissociation of primary and secondary reward-relevant limbic nuclei in an animal model of relapse. *Neuropsychopharmacology*, 2000, *22*, 473–479.

Gross, C. G. Visual functions of inferotemporal cortex. In *Handbook of Sensory Physiology, Vol. 7: Central Processing of Visual Information*, edited by R. Jung. Berlin: Springer-Verlag, 1973.

Grossman, E. D., and Blake, R. Brain activity evoked by inverted and imagined biological motion. *Vision Research*, 2001, *41*, 1475–1482.

Grossman, E. D., Donnelly, M., Price, R., et al. Brain areas involved in perception of biological motion. *Journal of Cognitive Neuroscience*, 2000, *12*, 711–720.

Groves, D. A., and Brown, V. J. Vagal nerve stimulation: A review of its applications and potential mechanisms that mediate its clinical effects. *Neuroscience and Biobehavioral Reviews*, 2005, *29*, 493–500.

Grunhaus, L., Shipley, J. E., Eiser, A., et al. Sleep-onset rapid eye movement after electroconvulsive therapy is more frequent in patients who respond less well to electroconvulsive therapy. *Biological Psychiatry*, 1997, *42*, 191–200.

Grunze, H. Reevaluating therapies for bipolar depression, *Journal of Clinical Psychiatry*, 2005, *66* (Suppl. 5), 17–25.

Guehl, D., Benazzouz, A., Aouizerate, B., et al. Neuronal correlates of obsessions in the caudate nucleus. *Biological Psychiatry*, 2008, *63*, 557–562.

Guilleminault, C., Wilson, R. A., and Dement, W. C. A study on cataplexy. *Archives of Neurology*, 1974, *31*, 255–261.

Gurd, J. M., and Marshall, J. C. Cognition: Righting reading. *Current Biology*, 1993, *3*, 593–595.

Gurin, B., Owens, S., Okuyama, T., et al. Effect of physical training and its cessation on percent fat and bone density of children with obesity. *Obesity Research*, 1999, *7*, 208–214.

Gvilia, I., Xu, F., McGinty, D., and Szymusiak, R. Homeostatic regulation of sleep: A role for preoptic area neurons. *Journal of Neuroscience*, 2006, *26*, 9426–9433.

Habib, M. The neurological basis of developmental dyslexia: An overview and working hypothesis. *Brain*, 2000, *123*, 2373–2399.

Hacke, W., Albers, G., Al-Rawi, Y., et al. The desmoteplase in acute ischemic stroke trial (DIAS): A phase II MRI-based 9-hour window acute stroke thrombolysis trial with intravenous desmoteplase. *Stroke*, 2005, *36*, 66–73.

Hadjikhani, N., and de Gelder, B. Seeing fearful body expressions activates the fusiform cortex and amygdala. *Current Biology*, 2003, *13*, 2201–2205.

Hadjikhani, N., Liu, A. K., Dale, A. M., et al. Retinotopy and color sensitivity in human visual cortical area V8. *Nature Neuroscience*, 1998, *1*, 235–241.

Hague, S. M., Klaffke, S., and Bandmann, O. Neurodegenerative disorders: Parkinson's disease and Huntington's disease. *Journal of Neurology, Neurosurgery, and Psychiatry*, 2005, *76*, 1058–1063.

Hahn, J., Hopf, F. W., and Bonci, A. Chronic cocaine enhances corticotropin-releasing factor-dependent potentiation of excitatory transmission in ventral tegmental area dopamine neurons. *Journal of Neuroscience*, 2009, *29*, 6535–6544.

Hahn, T. M., Breininger, J. F., Baskin, D. G., and Schwartz, M. W. Coexpression of Agrp and NPY in fasting-activated hypothalamic neurons. *Nature Neuroscience*, 1998, *1*, 271–272.

Hainer, V., Stunkard, A., Kunesova, M., et al. A twin study of weight loss and metabolic efficiency. *International Journal of Obesity and Related Metabolic Disorders*, 2001, *25*, 533–537.

Hajak, G., Clarenbach, P., Fischer, W., et al. Effects of hypnotics on sleep quality and daytime well-being: Data from a comparative multicentre study in outpatients with insomnia. *European Psychiatry*, 1995, *10* (Suppl. 3), 173S–179S.

Halaas, J. L., Gajiwala, K. D., Maffei, M., et al. Weight-reducing effects of the plasma protein encoded by the obese gene. *Science*, 1995, *269*, 543–546.

Halassa, M. M., Florian, C., Fellin, T., et al. Astrocytic modulation of sleep homeostasis and cognitive consequences of sleep loss. *Neuron,* 2009, *61,* 213–219.

Haley, J. E., Wilcox, G. L., and Chapman, P. F. The role of nitric oxide in hippocampal long-term potentiation. *Neuron,* 1992, *8,* 211–216.

Halgren, E., Walter, R. D., Cherlow, D. G., and Crandall, P. E. Mental phenomena evoked by electrical stimulation of the human hippocampal formation and amygdala. *Brain,* 1978, *101,* 83–117.

Halpern, M. The organization and function of the vomeronasal system. *Annual Review of Neuroscience,* 1987, *10,* 325–362.

Hamet, P., and Tremblay, J. Genetics and genomics of depression. *Metabolism: Clinical and Experimental,* 2005, *54,* 10–15.

Hanna, G. L., Veenstra-VanderWeele, J., Cox, N. J., et al. Genome-wide linkage analysis of families with obsessive-compulsive disorder ascertained through pediatric probands. *American Journal of Medical Genetics,* 2002, *114,* 541–552.

Hardy, J. Amyloid, the presinilins and Alzheimer's disease. *Trends in Neuroscience,* 1997, *4,* 154–159.

Hariri, A. R., Drabant, B. A., Munoz, K. E., et al. A susceptibility gene for affective disorders and the response of the human amygdala. *Archives of General Psychiatry,* 2005, *62,* 146–152.

Hariri, A. R., Mattay, V. S., Tessitore, A., et al. Serotonin transporter genetic variation and the response of the human amygdala. *Science,* 2002, *297,* 400–403.

Harrison, Y., and Horne, J. A. One night of sleep loss impairs innovative thinking and flexible decision-making. *Organizational Behavior and Human Decision Processes,* 1999, *78,* 128–145.

Hattar, S., Liao, H.-W., Takao, M., et al. Melanopsin-containing retinal ganglion cells: Architecture, projections, and intrinsic photosensitivity. *Science,* 2002, *295,* 1065–1070.

Haug, H.-J. Prediction of sleep deprivation outcome by diurnal variation of mood. *Biological Psychiatry,* 1992, *31,* 271–278.

Hauk, O., Johnsrude, I., and Pulvermüller, F. Somatotopic representation of action words in human motor and premotor cortex. *Neuron,* 2004, *41,* 301–307.

Hebb, D. O. *The Organization of Behaviour.* New York: Wiley-Interscience, 1949.

Heckler, M. M. *Fifth Special Report to the U.S. Congress on Alcohol and Health.* Washington, DC: U.S. Government Printing Office, 1983.

Heffner, H. E., and Heffner, R. S. Role of primate auditory cortex in hearing. In *Comparative Perception, Vol. II: Complex Signals,* edited by W. C. Stebbins and M. A. Berkley. New York: John Wiley & Sons, 1990.

Heilman, K. M., Watson, R. T., and Bowers, D. Affective disorders associated with hemispheric disease. In *Neuropsychology of Human Emotion,* edited by K. M. Heilman and P. Satz. New York: Guilford Press, 1983.

Heimer, L., and Larsson, K. Impairment of mating behavior in male rats following lesions in the preoptic-anterior hypothalamic continuum. *Brain Research,* 1966/1967, *3,* 248–263.

Heinrichs, S. C., Menzaghi, F., Pich, E. M., et al. Anti-stress action of a corticotropin-releasing factor antagonist on behavioral reactivity to stressors of varying type and intensity. *Neuropsychopharmacology,* 1994, *11,* 179–186.

Heinz, A., Reimold, M., Wrase, J., et al. Correlation of stable elevations in striatal μ-opioid receptor availability in detoxified alcoholic patients with alcohol craving. *Archives of General Psychiatry,* 2005, *62,* 57–64.

Helenius, P., Uutela, K., and Hari, R. Auditory stream segregation in dyslexic adults. *Brain,* 1999, *122,* 907–913.

Hellhammer, D. H., Hubert, W., and Schurmeyer, T. Changes in saliva testosterone after psychological stimulation in men. *Psychoneuroendocrinology,* 1985, *10,* 77–81.

Helmuth, L. Dyslexia: Same brains, different languages. *Science,* 2001, *291,* 2064–2065.

Hendrickson, A. E., Wagoner, N., and Cowan, W. M. Autoradiographic and electron microscopic study of retino-hypothalamic connections. *Zeitschrift für Zellforschung und Mikroskopische Anatomie,* 1972, *125,* 1–26.

Hendry, S. H. C., and Yoshioka, T. A neurochemically distinct third channel in the cacaque dorsal lateral geniculare nucleus. *Science,* 1994, *264,* 575–577.

Henke, P. G. The telencephalic limbic system and experimental gastric pathology: A review. *Neuroscience and Biobehavioral Reviews,* 1982, *6,* 381–390.

Henningfield, J. E., Fant, R. V., Buchhalter, A. R., and Stitzer, M. L. Pharmacotherapy for nicotine dependence. *CA: A Cancer Journal for Clinicians,* 2005, *55,* 281–299.

Henry, M. L., Beeson, P. M., Stark, A. J., and Rapcsak, S. Z. The role of left perisylvian cortical regions in spelling. *Brain and Language,* 2007, *100,* 44–52.

Herbert, M. R., Ziegler, D. A., Makris, N., et al. Localization of white matter volume increase in autism and developmental language disorder. *Annals of Neurology,* 2004, *55,* 530–540.

Hetherington, A. W., and Ranson, S. W. Hypothalamic lesions and adiposity in the rat. *Anatomical Record,* 1942, *78,* 149–172.

Hettema, J. M., Neale, M. C., and Kendler, K. S. A review and meta-analysis of the genetic epidemiology of anxiety disorders. *American Journal of Psychiatry,* 2001, *158,* 1568–1578.

Hetz, C., Russelakis-Carneiro, M., Maundrell, K., et al. Caspase-12 and endoplasmic reticulum stress mediate neurotoxicity of pathological prion protein. *The EMBO Journal,* 2003, *22,* 5435–5445.

Heuser, J. E. Synaptic vesicle exocytosis revealed in quick-frozen frog neuromuscular junctions treated with 4-aminopyridine and given a single electrical shock. In *Society for Neuroscience Symposia, Vol. II,* edited by W. M. Cowan and J. A. Ferrendelli. Bethesda, Md.: Society for Neuroscience, 1977.

Heuser, J. E., Reese, T. S., Dennis, M. J., et al. Synaptic vesicle exocytosis captured by quick freezing and correlated with quantal transmitter release. *Journal of Cell Biology,* 1979, *81,* 275–300.

Heywood, C. A., and Kentridge, R. W. Achromatopsia, color vision, and cortex. *Neurology Clinics of North America,* 2003, *21,* 483–500.

Hickok, G., Bellugi, U., and Klima, E. S. The neurobiology of sign language and its implications for the neural basis of language. *Nature,* 1996, *381,* 699–702.

Hill, J. O., Wyatt, H. R., Reed, G. W., and Peters, J. C. Obesity and the environment: Where do we go from here? *Science,* 2003, *299,* 853–855.

Hill, J. P., Hauptman, J., Anderson, J., et al. Orlistat, a lipase inhibitor, for weight maintenance after conventional dieting: A 1-year study. *American Journal of Clinical Nutrition,* 1999, *69,* 1108–1116.

Hillebrand, J. J. G., de Rijke, C. E., Brakkee, J. H., et al. Voluntary access to a warm plate reduces hyperactivity in activity-based anorexia. *Physiology and Behavior,* 2005, *85,* 151–157.

Hobson, J. A. *The Dreaming Brain.* New York: Basic Books, 1988.

Hochberg, L. R., Serruya, M. D., Friehs, G. M., et al. Neuronal ensemble control of prosthetic devices by a human with tetraplegia. *Nature,* 2006, *442,* 164–171.

Hock, C., Konietzko, U., Streffer, J. R., et al. Antibodies against β-amyloid slow cognitive decline in Alzheimer's disease. *Neuron,* 2003, *38,* 547–554.

Hodge, C. W., Haraguchi, M., Erickson, H., and Samson, H. H. Ventral tegmental microinjections of quinpirole decrease ethanol and sucrose-reinforced responding. *Alcohol: Clinical and Experimental Research,* 1993, *17,* 370–375.

Hoeft, F., Meyler, A., Hernandez, A., et al. Functional and morphometric brain dissociation between dyslexia and reading ability. *Proceedings of the National Academy of Sciences, USA,* 2007, *104,* 4234–4239.

Hohman, G. W. Some effects of spinal cord lesions on experienced emotional feelings. *Psychophysiology,* 1966, *3,* 143–156.

Holden, C. The violence of the lambs. *Science,* 2000, *289,* 580–581.

Hollander, E., Schiffman, E., Cohen, B., et al. Signs of central nervous system dysfunction in obsessive-compulsive disorder. *Archives of General Psychiatry,* 1990, *47,* 27–32.

Holstege, G., Georgiadis, J. R., Paans, A. M. J., et al. Brain activation during human male ejaculation. *Journal of Neuroscience,* 2003b, *23,* 9185–9193.

Holstege, G., Reinders, A. A. T., Panns, A. M. J., et al. Brain activation during female sexual orgasm. Program No. 727.7, *2003 Abstract Viewer/Itinerary Planner.* Washington, DC: Society for Neuroscience, 2003a.

Honda, T., Tabata, H., and Nakajima, K. Cellular and molecular mechanisms of neuronal migration in neocortical development. *Seminars in Cell & Developmental Biology,* 2003, *14,* 169–174.

Hopf, H. C., Mueller-Forell, W., and Hopf, N. J. Localization of emotional and volitional facial paresis. *Neurology,* 1992, *42,* 1918–1923.

Hoppe, C. Controlling epilepsy. *Scientific American Mind,* 2006, *17,* 62–67.

Horne, J. A. A review of the biological effects of total sleep deprivation in man. *Biological Psychology,* 1978, *7,* 55–102.

Hornig, M., Briese, T., Buie, T., et al. Lack of association between measles virus vaccine and autism with enteropathy: A case-control study. *PLoS One,* 2008, *3,* e3140.

Horowitz, R. M., and Gentili, B. Dihydrochalcone sweeteners. In *Symposium: Sweeteners*, edited by G. E. Inglett. Westport, Conn.: Avi Publishing, 1974.

Horton, J. C., and Hubel, D. H. Cytochrome oxidase stain preferentially labels intersection of ocular dominance and vertical orientation columns in macaque striate cortex. *Society for Neuroscience Abstracts*, 1980, *6*, 315.

Houchi, H., Babovic, D., Pierrefiche, O., et al. CB1 receptor knockout mice display reduced ethanol-induced conditioned place preference and increased striatal dopamine D2 receptors. *Neuropsychopharmacology*, 2005, *30*, 339–340.

Howell, S., Westergaard, G., Hoos, B., et al. Serotonergic influences on life-history outcomes in free-ranging male rhesus macaques. *American Journal of Primatology*, 2007, *69*, 851–865.

Hubel, D. H., and Wiesel, T. N. Brain mechanisms of vision. *Scientific American*, 1979, *241*, 150–162.

Hubel, D. H., and Wiesel, T. N. Functional architecture of macaque monkey visual cortex. *Proceedings of the Royal Society of London*, 1977, *198*, 1–59.

Hublin, C. Narcolepsy: Current drug-treatment options. *CNS Drugs*, 1996, *5*, 426–436.

Hublin, C., Kaprio, J., Partinen, M., et al. Prevalence and genetics of sleepwalking: A population-based twin study. *Neurology*, 1997, *48*, 177–181.

Hudspeth, A. J., and Gillespie, P. G. Pulling springs to tune transduction: Adaptation by hair cells. *Neuron*, 1994, *12*, 1–9.

Huestis, M. A., Gorelick, D. A., Heishman, S. J., et al. Blockade of effects of smoked marijuana by the CB1-selective cannabinoid receptor antagonist SR131716. *Archives of General Psychiatry*, 2001, *58*, 322–328.

Hughes, J., Smith, T. W., Kosterlitz, H. W., et al. Identification of two related pentapeptides from the brain with potent opiate agonist activity. *Nature*, 1975, *258*, 577–579.

Hull, E., and Dominguez, J. M. Sexual behavior in male rodents. *Hormones and Behavior*, 2007, *52*, 45–55.

Hulshoff-Pol, H. E., Schnack, H. G., Bertens, M. G., et al. Volume changes in gray matter in patients with schizophrenia. *American Journal of Psychiatry*, 2002, *159*, 244–250.

Humphrey, A. L., and Hendrickson, A. E. Radial zones of high metabolic activity in squirrel monkey striate cortex. *Society for Neuroscience Abstracts*, 1980, *6*, 315.

Hungs, M., and Mignot, E. Hypocretin/orexin, sleep and narcolepsy. *Bioessays*, 2001, *23*, 397–408.

Hunt, D. M., Dulai, K. S., Cowing, J. A., et al. Molecular evolution of trichromacy in primates. *Vision Research*, 1998, *38*, 3299–3306.

Hussey, E., and Safford, A. Perception of facial expression in somatosensory cortex supports simulationist models. *Journal of Neuroscience*, 2009, *29*, 301–302.

Hyman, S. E., and Malenka, R. C. Addiction and the brain: The neurobiology of compulsion and its persistence. *Nature Reviews: Neuroscience*, 2001, *2*, 695–703.

Iacoboni, M., Woods, R. P., Brass, M., et al. Cortical mechanisms of human imitation. *Science*, 1999, *286*, 2526–2528.

Iaria, G., Petrides, M., Dagher, et al. Cognitive strategies dependent on the hippocampus and caudate nucleus in human navigation: Variability and change with practice. *Journal of Neuroscience*, 2003, *23*, 5945–5952.

Ibuka, N., and Kawamura, H. Loss of circadian rhythm in sleep-wakefulness cycle in the rat by suprachiasmatic nucleus lesions. *Brain Research*, 1975, *96*, 76–81.

Iggo, A., and Andres, K. H. Morphology of cutaneous receptors. *Annual Review of Neuroscience*, 1982, *5*, 1–32.

Imperato, A., and Di Chiara, G. Preferential stimulation of dopamine-release in the accumbens of freely moving rats by ethanol. *Journal of Pharmacology and Experimental Therapeutics*, 1986, *239*, 219–228.

Inoue, M., Koyanagi, T., Nakahara, H., et al. Functional development of human eye movement in utero assessed quantitatively with real time ultrasound. *American Journal of Obstetrics and Gynecology*, 1986, *155*, 170–174.

Insel, T. R. A neurobiological basis of social attachment. *American Journal of Psychiatry*, 1997, *154*, 726–735.

Insel, T. R., Wang, Z. X., and Ferris, C. F. Patterns of brain vasopressin receptor distribution associated with social organization in microtine rodents. *Journal of Neuroscience*, 1994, *14*, 5381–5392.

Isoldi, K. K., and Aronne, L. J. The challenge of treating obesity: The endocannabinoid system as a potential target. *Journal of the American Dietetic Association*, 2008, *108*, 823–831.

Iversen, L. Cannabis and the brain. *Brain*, 2003, *126*, 1252–1270.

Iwata, M. Kanji versus Kana: Neuropsychological correlates of the Japanese writing system. *Trends in Neurosciences*, 1984, *7*, 290–293.

Izard, C. E. *The Face of Emotion*. New York: Appleton-Century-Crofts, 1971.

Jackson, M. E., Frost, A. S., and Moghaddam, B. Stimulation of prefrontal cortex at physiologically relevant frequencies inhibits dopamine release in the nucleus accumbens. *Journal of Neurochemistry*, 2001, *78*, 920–923.

Jacob, S., and McClintock, M. K. Psychological state and mood effects of steroidal chemosignals in women and men. *Hormones and Behavior*, 2000, *37*, 57–78.

Jacobs, B. L., and McGinty, D. J. Participation of the amygdala in complex stimulus recognition and behavioral inhibition: Evidence from unit studies. *Brain Research*, 1972, *36*, 431–436.

Jacobs, G. H. Primate photopigments and primate color vision. *Proceedings of the National Academy of Sciences, USA*, 1996, *93*, 577–581.

Jacobsen, C. F., Wolfe, J. B., and Jackson, T. A. An experimental analysis of the functions of the frontal association areas in primates. *Journal of Nervous and Mental Disorders*, 1935, *82*, 1–14.

Jakobson, L. S., Archibald, Y. M., Carey, D., and Goodale, M. A. A kinematic analysis of reaching and grasping movements in a patient recovering from optic ataxia. *Neuropsychologia*, 1991, *29*, 803–809.

James, T. W., Culham, J., Humphrey, G. K., et al. Ventral occipital lesions impair object recognition but not object-directed grasping: An fMRI study. *Brain*, 2003, *126*, 2463–2475.

James, W. What is an emotion? *Mind*, 1884, *9*, 188–205.

Jaramillo, F. Signal transduction in hair cells and its regulation by calcium. *Neuron*, 1995, *15*, 1227–1230.

Javitt, D. C. Glycine transport inhibitors and the treatment of schizophrenia. *Biological Psychiatry*, 2008, *63*, 6–8.

Jaynes, J. The problem of animate motion in the seventeenth century. *Journal of the History of Ideas*, 1970, *6*, 219–234.

Jensen, T., Genefke, I., and Hyldebrandt, N. Cerebral atrophy in young torture victims. *New England Journal of Medicine*, 1982, *307*, 1341.

Jentsch, J. D., Redmond, D. E., Elsworth, J. D., et al. Enduring cognitive deficits and cortical dopamine dysfunction in monkeys after long-term administration of phencyclidine. *Science*, 1997, *277*, 953–955.

Jentsch, J. D., Tran, A., Taylor, J. R., and Roth, R. H. Prefrontal cortical involvement in phencyclidine-induced activation of the mesolimbic dopamine system: Behavioral and neurochemical evidence. *Psychopharmacology*, 1998, *138*, 89–95.

Jessberger, S., and Kempermann, G. Adultborn hippocampal neurons mature into activity-dependent responsiveness. *European Journal of Neuroscience*, 2003, *18*, 2707–2712.

Jeste, D. V., Del Carmen, R., Lohr, J. B., and Wyatt, R. J. Did schizophrenia exist before the eighteenth century? *Comprehensive Psychiatry*, 1985, *26*, 493–503.

Jha, S. K., Coleman, T., and Frank, M. G. Sleep and sleep regulation in the ferret (*Mustela putorius furo*). *Behavioural Brain Research*, 2006, *172*, 106–113.

Jo, Y.-H., Wiedl, D., and Role, L. W. Cholinergic modulation of appetite-related synapses in mouse lateral hypothalamic slice. *Journal of Neuroscience*, 2005, *25*, 11133–11144.

Jobard, G., Crivello, F., and Tzourio-Mazoyer, N. Evaluation of the dual route theory of reading: A metaanalysis of 35 neuroimaging studies. *NeuroImage*, 2003, *20*, 693–712.

Jobst, E. E., Enriori, P. J., and Cowley, M. A. The electrophysiology of feeding circuits. *Trends in Endocrinology and Metabolism*, 2004, *15*, 488–499.

Johansson, G. Visual perception of biological motion and a model for its analysis. *Perception and Psychophysics*, 1973, *14*, 201–211.

Johnson, M. K., Kim, J. K., and Risse, G. Do alcoholic Korsakoff's syndrome patients acquire affective reactions? *Journal of Experimental Psychology: Learning, Memory, and Cognition*, 1985, *11*, 22–36.

Johnson, M. K., and Raye, C. L. False memories and confabulation. *Trends in Cognitive Sciences*, 1998, *2*, 137–145.

Jones, B. E. Influence of the brainstem reticular formation, including intrinsic monoaminergic and cholinergic neurons, on forebrain mechanisms of sleep and waking. In *The Diencephalon and Sleep*, edited by M. Mancia and G. Marini. New York: Raven Press, 1990.

Jones, S. S., Collins, K., and Hong, H.-W. An audience effect on smile production in 10-

month-old infants. *Psychological Science*, 1991, *2*, 45–49.

Jornales, V. E., Jakob, M., Zamani, A., and Vaina, L. M. Deficits on complex motion perception, spatial discrimination and eye-movements in a patient with bilateral occipital-parietal lesions. *Investigative Ophthalmology and Visual Science*, 1997, *38*, S72.

Jouvet, M. The role of monoamines and acetylcholine-containing neurons in the regulation of the sleep-waking cycle. *Ergebnisse der Physiologie*, 1972, *64*, 166–307.

Jouvet-Mounier, D., Astic, L., and Lacote, D. Ontogenesis of the states of sleep in rat, cat, and guinea pig during the first postnatal month. *Developmental Psychobiology*, 1970, *2*, 216–239.

Kalin, N. H., Sherman, J. E., and Takahashi, L. K. Antagonism of endogenous CRG systems attenuates stress-induced freezing behavior in rats. *Brain Research*, 1988, *457*, 130–135.

Kalivas, P. W., Peters, J., and Knackstedt, L. Animal models and brain circuits in drug addiction. *Molecular Interventions*, 2006, *6*, 339–344.

Kanner, L. Autistic disturbances of affective contact. *The Nervous Child*, 1943, *2*, 217–250.

Kaplitt, M. G., Feigin, A., Tang, C., et al. Safety and tolerability of gene therapy with an adeno-associated virus (AAV) borne GAD gene for Parkinson's disease: An open label, phase I trial. *Lancet*, 2007, *369*, 2097–2105.

Kapp, B. S., Frysinger, R. C., Gallagher, M., and Haselton, J. R. Amygdala central nucleus lesions: Effect on heart rate conditioning in the rabbit. *Physiology and Behavior*, 1979, *23*, 1109–1117.

Karacan, I., Salis, P. J., and Williams, R. L. The role of the sleep laboratory in diagnosis and treatment of impotence. In *Sleep Disorders: Diagnosis and Treatment*, edited by R. J. Williams and I. Karacan. New York: John Wiley & Sons, 1978.

Karacan, I., Williams, R. L., Finley, W. W., and Hursch, C. J. The effects of naps on nocturnal sleep: Influence on the need for stage 1 REM and stage 4 sleep. *Biological Psychiatry*, 1970, *2*, 391–399.

Karlson, P., and Luscher, M. "Pheromones": A new term for a class of biologically active substances. *Nature*, 1959, *183*, 55–56.

Kaspar, B. K., Lladó, J., Sherkat, N., et al. Retrograde viral delivery of IGF-1 prolongs survival in a mouse ALS model. *Science*, 2003, *301*, 839–842.

Katanoda, K., Yoshikawa, K., and Sugishita, M. A functional MRI study on the neural substrates for writing. *Human Brain Mapping*, 2001, *13*, 34–42.

Kauer, J. A., and Malenka, R. C. Synaptic plasticity and addiction. *Nature Reviews: Neuroscience*, 2007, *8*, 844–858.

Kawauchi, H., Kawazoe, I., Tsubokawa, M., et al. Characterization of melanin-concentrating hormone in chum salmon pituitaries. *Nature*, 1983, *305*, 321–323.

Kaye, W. H., Nagata, T., Weltzin, T. E., et al. Double-blind placebo-controlled administration of fluoxetine in restricting- and restricting-purging-type anorexia nervosa. *Biological Psychiatry*, 2001, *49*, 644–652.

Kelso, S. R., Ganong, A. H., and Brown, T. H. Hebbian synapses in hippocampus. *Proceedings of the National Academy of Sciences, USA*, 1986, *83*, 5326–5330.

Kempermann, G., Wiskott, L., and Gage, F. H. Functional significance of adult neurogenesis. *Current Opinion in Neurobiology*, 2004, *13*, 186–191.

Kendell, R. E., and Adams, W. Unexplained fluctuations in the risk for schizophrenia by month and year of birth. *British Journal of Psychiatry*, 1991, *158*, 758–763.

Kendler, K. S., Jacobson, K. C., Prescott, C. A., and Neale, M. C. Specificity of genetic and environmental risk factors for use and abuse/dependency of cannabis, cocaine, hallucinogens, sedatives, stimulants, and opiates in male twins. *American Journal of Psychiatry*, 2003, *160*, 687–695.

Kertesz, A. Anatomy of jargon. In *Jargonaphasia*, edited by J. Brown. New York: Academic Press, 1981.

Kessler, R. C., Berglund, P., Demler, O., et al. The epidemiology of major depressive disorder: Results from the National Comorbidity Survey Replication (NCS-R). *JAMA*, 2003, *289*, 3095–3105.

Kessler, R. C., Chiu, W. T., Jin, R., et al. The epidemiology of panic attacks, panic disorder, and agoraphobia in the National Comorbidity Survey Replication. *Archives of General Psychiatry*, 2006, *63*, 415–424.

Kety, S. S., Rosenthal, D., Wender, P. H., and Schulsinger, K. F. The types and prevalence of mental illness in the biological and adoptive families of adopted schizophrenics. In *The Transmission of Schizophrenia*, edited by D. Rosenthal and S. S. Kety. New York: Pergamon Press, 1968.

Kety, S. S., Wender, P. H., Jacobsen, B., et al. Mental illness in the biological and adoptive relatives of schizophrenic adoptees: Replication of the Copenhagen Study in the rest of Denmark. *Archives of General Psychiatry*, 1994, *51*, 442–455.

Keyes, A., Brozek, J., Henschel, A., et al. *The Biology of Human Starvation*. Minneapolis: University of Minnesota Press, 1950.

Khateb, A., Fort, P., Pegna, A., et al. Cholinergic nucleus basalis neurons are excited by histamine in vitro. *Neuroscience*, 1995, *69*, 495–506.

Kiang, N. Y.-S. *Discharge Patterns of Single Fibers in the Cat's Auditory Nerve*. Cambridge, Mass.: MIT Press, 1965.

Kiecolt-Glaser, J. K., Marucha, P. T., Malarkey, W. B., et al. Slowing of wound healing by psychological stress. *Lancet*, 1995, *346*, 1194–1196.

Kihlstrom, J. F. Hypnosis. *Annual Review of Psychology*, 1985, *36*, 385–418.

Kilpatrick, D. G., Koenen, K. C., Ruggiero, K. J., et al. The serotonin transporter genotype and social support and moderation of posttraumatic stress disorder and depression in hurricane-exposed adults. *American Journal of Psychiatry*, 2007, *164*, 1693–1699.

Kinnamon, S. C., and Cummings, T. A. Chemosensory transduction mechanisms in taste. *Annual Review of Physiology*, 1992, *54*, 715–731.

Kirkpatrick, B., Kim, J. W., and Insel, T. R. Limbic system fos expression associated with paternal behavior. *Brain Research*, 1994, *658*, 112–118.

Kirwan, C. B., Bayley, P. J., Galván, V. V., and Squire, L. R. Detailed recollection of remote autobiographical memory after damage to the medial temporal lobe. *Proceedings of the*

National Academy of Sciences, USA, 2008, *105*, 2676–2680.

Kitada, T., Asakawa, S., Hattori, N., et al. Mutations in the parkin gene cause autosomal recessive juvenile parkinsonism. *Nature*, 1998, *392*, 605–608.

Klaur, J., Zhao, Z., Klein, G. M., et al. The neurotoxicity of tissue plasminogen activator? *Journal of Cerebral Blood Flow and Metabolism*, 2004, *24*, 945–963.

Klein, D. A., and Walsh, B. T. Eating disorders: Clinical features and pathophysiology. *Physiology and Behavior*, 2004, *81*, 359–374.

Klunk, W. E., Engler, H., Nordberg, A., et al. Imaging the pathology of Alzheimer's disease: Amyloid-imaging with positron emission tomography. *Neuroimaging Clinics of North America*, 2003, *13*, 781–789.

Knebelmann, B., Boussin, L., Guerrier, D., et al. Anti-Muellerian hormone Bruxelles: A nonsense mutation associated with the persistent Muellerian duct syndrome. *Proceedings of the National Academy of Sciences, USA*, 1991, *88*, 3767–3771.

Knecht, S., Drager, B., Deppe, M., et al. Handedness and hemispheric language dominance in healthy humans. *Brain*, 2000, *123*, 2512–2518.

Knutson, B., Adams, C. M., Fong, G. W., and Hommer, D. Anticipation of increasing monetary reward selectively recruits nucleus accumbens. *Journal of Neuroscience*, 2001, *21*, RC159 (1–5).

Knutson, B., and Adcock, R. A. Remembrance of rewards past. *Neuron*, 2005, *45*, 331–332.

Koenigs, M., Young, L., Adolphs, R., et al. Damage to the prefrontal cortex increases utilitarian moral judgments. *Nature*, 2007, *446*, 908–911.

Kojima, M., Hosoda, H., Date, Y., et al. Ghrelin is a growth-hormone–releasing acylated peptide from stomach. *Nature*, 1999, *402*, 656–660.

Komisaruk, B. R., and Larsson, K. Suppression of a spinal and a cranial nerve reflex by vaginal or rectal probing in rats. *Brain Research*, 1971, *35*, 231–235.

Komisaruk, B. R., and Steinman, J. L. Genital stimulation as a trigger for neuroendocrine and behavioral control of reproduction. *Annals of the New York Academy of Sciences*, 1987, *474*, 64–75.

Kong, J., Shepel, N., Holden, C. P., et al. Brain glycogen decreases with increased periods of wakefulness: Implications for homeostatic drive to sleep. *Journal of Neuroscience*, 2002, *22*, 5581–5587.

Koob, G. F., Thatcher-Britton, K., Britton, D., et al. Destruction of the locus coeruleus or the dorsal NE bundle does not alter the release of punished responding by ethanol and chlordiazepoxide. *Physiology and Behavior*, 1984, *33*, 479–485.

Koopman, P. Gonad development: Signals for sex. *Current Biology*, 2001, *11*, R481–R483.

Koroshetz, W. J., and Moskowitz, M. A. Emerging treatments for stroke in humans. *Trends in Pharmacological Sciences*, 1996, *17*, 227–233.

Kortegaard, L. S., Hoerder, K., Joergensen, J., et al. A preliminary population-based twin study of self-reported eating disorder. *Psychological Medicine*, 2001, *31*, 361–365.

Kosten, T., and Owens, S. M. Immunotherapy for the treatment of drug abuse. *Phar-*

macology and Therapeutics, 2005, *108*, 76–85.

Kourtzi, A., and Kanwisher, N. Activation in human MT/MST by static images with implied motion. *Journal of Cognitive Neuroscience*, 2000, *12*, 48–55.

Kovács, G., Vogels, R., and Orban, G. A. Selectivity of macaque inferior temporal neurons for partially occluded shapes. *Journal of Neuroscience*, 1995, *15*, 1984–1997.

Koylu, E. O., Couceyro, P. R., Lambert, P. D., and Kuhar, M. J. Cocaine- and amphetamine-regulated transcript peptide immunohistochemical localization in the rat brain. *Journal of Comparative Neurology*, 1998, *391*, 115–132.

Kozlowski, L. T., and Cutting, J. E. Recognizing the sex of a walker from a dynamic point-light display. *Perception and Psychophysics*, 1977, *21*, 575–580.

Kramer, F. M., Jeffery, R. W., Forster, J. L., and Snell, M. K. Long-term follow-up of behavioral treatment for obesity: Patterns of weight regain among men and women. *International journal of Obesity*, 1989, *13*, 123–136.

Kranzler, H. R., and Gage, A. Acamprosate efficacy in alcohol-dependent patients: summary of results from three pivotal trials. *American Journal on Addictions*, 2008, *17*, 70–76.

Kranzler, H. R., Modesto-Lowe, V., and Nuwayser, E. S. Sustained-release naltrexone for alcoholism treatment: A preliminary study. *Alcoholism: Clinical and Experimental Research*, 1998, *22*, 1074–1079.

Kraut, R. E., and Johnston, R. Social and emotional messages of smiling: An ethological approach. *Journal of Personality and Social Psychology*, 1979, *37*, 1539–1553.

Kress, M., and Zeilhofer, H. U. Capsaicin, protons and heat: New excitement about nociceptors. *Trends in Pharmacological Science*, 1999, *20*, 112–118.

Kristensen, P., Judge, M. E., Thim, L., et al. Hypothalamic CART is a new anorectic peptide regulated by leptin. *Nature*, 1998, *393*, 72–76.

Krolak-Salmon, P., Hénaff, M.-A., Vighetto, A., et al. Early amygdala reaction to fear spreading in occipital, temporal, and frontal cortex: A depth electrode ERP study in human. *Neuron*, 2004, *42*, 665–676.

Kuffler, S. W. Discharge patterns and functional organization of mammalian retina. *Journal of Neurophysiology*, 1953, *16*, 37–68.

Kuffler, S. W. Neurons in the retina: Organization, inhibition and excitation problems. *Cold Spring Harbor Symposium on Quantitative Biology*, 1952, *17*, 281–292.

Kumar, M. J., and Andersen, J. K. Perspectives on MAO-B in aging and neurological disease: Where do we go from here? *Molecular Neurobiology*, 2004, *30*, 77–89.

Kunos, G., and Batkai, S. Novel physiologic functions of endocannabinoids as revealed through the use of mutant mice. *Neurochemical Research*, 2001, *26*, 1015–1021.

Kupfer, D. J. REM latency: A psychobiologic marker for primary depressive disease. *Biological Psychiatry*, 1976, *11*, 159–174.

Kurihara, K. Recent progress in taste receptor mechanisms. In *Umami: A Basic Taste*, edited by Y. Kawamura and M. R. Kare. New York: Dekker, 1987.

Kushner, M. G., Kim, S. W., Donahue, C., et al. D-cycloserine augmented exposure therapy for obsessive-compulsive disorder. *Biological Psychiatry*, 2007, *62*, 835–838.

LaBar, K. S., LeDoux, J. E., Spencer, D. D., and Phelps, E. A. Impaired fear conditioning following unilateral temporal lobectomy in humans. *Journal of Neuroscience*, 1995, *15*, 6846–6855.

Lahti, A. C., Weiler, M. A., Michaelidis, T., et al. Effects of ketamine in normal and schizophrenic volunteers. *Neuropsychopharmacology*, 2001, *25*, 455–467.

Lai, E. C., Jankovic, J., Krauss, J. K., et al. Long-term efficacy of posteroventral pallidotomy in the treatment of Parkinson's disease. *Neurology*, 2000, *55*, 1218–1222.

Lange, C. G. *Über Gemüthsbewegungen*. Leipzig, East Germany: T. Thomas, 1887.

Langston, J. W., and Ballard, P. Parkinsonism induced by 1-methyl-4-phenyl-1,2,3,6-tetrahydropyridine (MPTP): Implications for treatment and the pathogenesis of Parkinson's disease. *Canadian Journal of Neurological Science*, 1984, *11* (1 Suppl.), 160–165.

Langston, J. W., Ballard, P., Tetrud, J., and Irwin, I. Chronic parkinsonism in humans due to a product of meperidine-analog synthesis. *Science*, 1983, *219*, 979–980.

Larson, P. S. Deep brain stimulation for psychiatric disorders. *Neurotherapeutics*, 2008, *5*, 50–58.

Laugerette, F., Passilly-Degrace, P., Patris, B., et al. *Journal of Clinical Investigation*, 2005, *115*, 3177–3184.

Lavoie, B., and Parent, A. Immunohistochemical study of the serotoninergic innervation of the basal ganglia in the squirrel monkey. *Journal of Comparative Neurology*, 1990, *299*, 1–16.

Lavond, D. G., Kim, J. J., and Thompson, R. F. Mammalian brain substrates of aversive classical conditioning. *Annual Review of Psychology*, 1993, *44*, 317–342.

Lê, S., Cardebat, D., Boulanouar, K., et al. Seeing, since childhood, without ventral stream: A behavioural study. *Brain*, 2002, *125*, 58–74.

LeDoux, J. E. Brain mechanisms of emotion and emotional learning. *Current Opinion in Neurobiology*, 1992, *2*, 191–197.

LeDoux, J. E. Emotion circuits in the brain. *Annual Review of Neuroscience*, 2000, *23*, 155–184.

LeDoux, J. E., Sakaguchi, A., and Reis, D. J. Subcortical efferent projections of the medial geniculate nucleus mediate emotional responses conditioned to acoustic stimuli. *Journal of Neuroscience*, 1984, *4*, 683–698.

Lee, A. K., and Wilson, M. A. Memory of sequential experience in the hippocampus during slow wave sleep. *Neuron*, 2002, *36*, 1183–1194.

Lee, A. W., and Brown, R. E. Comparison of medial preoptic, amygdala, and nucleus accumbens lesions on parental behavior in California mice (*Peromyscus californicus*). *Physiology and Behavior*, 2007, *92*, 617–628.

Lee, M. S., Lee, H. Y., Lee, H. J., and Ryu, S. H. Serotonin transporter promoter gene polymorphism and long-term outcome of antidepressant treatment. *Psychiatric Genetics*, 2004, *14*, 111–115.

Le Grand, R., Mondloch, C. J., Maurer, D., and Brent, H. P. Early visual experience and face processing. *Nature*, 2001, *410*, 890.

Lehman, M. N., Silver, R., Gladstone, W. R., et al. Circadian rhythmicity restored by neural transplant: Immunocytochemical characterization with the host brain. *Journal of Neuroscience*, 1987, *7*, 1626–1638.

Lehn, H., Steffenach, H.-A., van Strien, N. M., et al. A specific role of the human hippocampus in recall of temporal sequences. *Journal of Neuroscience*, 2009, *29*, 3475–3484.

Leibenluft, E., and Wehr, T. A. Is sleep deprivation useful in the treatment of depression? *American Journal of Psychiatry*, 1992, *149*, 159–168.

Leonard, H. L., Lenane, M. C., Swedo, et al. Tics and Tourette's disorder: a 2- to 7-year follow-up of 54 obsessive-compulsive children. *American Journal of Psychiatry*, 1992, *149*, 1244–1251.

Leonard, C. M., Rolls, E. T., Wilson, F. A. W., and Baylis, G. C. Neurons in the amygdala of the monkey with responses selective for faces. *Behavioral Brain Research*, 1985, *15*, 159–176.

Lesch, K. P., and Mossner, R. Genetically driven variation in serotonin uptake: Is there a link to affective spectrum, neurodevelopmental, and neurodegenerative disorders? *Biological Psychiatry*, 1988, *44*, 179–192.

Lesné, S., Ali, C., Bagriel, C., et al. NMDA receptor activation inhibits α-secretase and promotes neuronal amyloid-β production. *Journal of Neuroscience*, 2005, *25*, 9367–9377.

Lesser, R. Selective preservation of oral spelling without semantics in a case of multi-infarct dementia. *Cortex*, 1989, *25*, 239–250.

LeVay, S. A difference in hypothalamic structure between heterosexual and homosexual men. *Science*, 1991, *253*, 1034–1037.

Levenson, R. W., Ekman, P., and Friesen, W. V. Voluntary facial action generates emotion-specific autonomic nervous system activity. *Psychophysiology*, 1990, *27*, 363–384.

Levitt, J. G., Blanton, R. E., Smalley, S., et al. Cortical sulcal maps in autism. *Cerebral Cortex*, 2003, *13*, 728–735.

Levy, R. M., and Bredesen, D. E. Controversies in HIV-related central nervous system disease: Neuropsychological aspects of HIV-1 infection. In *AIDS Clinical Review 1989*, edited by P. Volberding, and M. A. Jacobson. New York: Marcel Dekker, 1989.

Lewin, R. Big first scored with nerve diseases. *Science*, 1989, *245*, 467–468.

Lewis, D. A., and Smith, R. E. Steroid-induced psychiatric syndromes: A report of 14 cases and a review of the literature. *Journal of the Affective Disorders*, 1983, *5*, 19–32.

Lewy, A. K., Lefler, B. J., Emens, J. S., and Bauer, V. K. The circadian basis of winter depression. *Proceedings of the National Academy of Sciences, USA*, 2006, *103*, 7414–7419.

Li, S.-H., Lam, S., Cheng, A. L., and Li, X.-J. Intranuclear huntingtin increases the expression of caspase-1 and induces apoptosis. *Human Molecular Genetics*, 2000, *9*, 2859–2867.

Li, X., Li, W., Wang, H., et al. Pseudogenization of a sweet-receptor gene accounts for cats' indifference toward sugar. *PLoS Genetics*, 2005, *1*, 27–35.

Lidberg, L., Asberg, M., and Sundqvist-Stensman, U. B. 5-Hydroxyindoleacetic acid levels in attempted suicides who have killed their children. *Lancet*, 1984, *2*, 928.

Lidberg, L., Tuck, J. R., Asberg, M., et al. Homicide, suicide and CSF 5-HIAA. *Acta Psychiatrica Scandanavica*, 1985, *71*, 230–236.

Lieberman, J. A. Dopamine partial agonists: A new class of antipsychotic. *CNS Drugs*, 2004, *18*, 251–267.

Liepert, J., Bauder, H., Wolfgang, H. R., et al. Treatment-induced cortical reorganization after stroke in humans. *Stroke*, 2000, *31*, 1210–1216.

Liljequist, S. The competitive NMDA receptor antagonist, CGP 39551, inhibits ethanol withdrawal seizures. *European Journal of Pharmacology*, 1991, *192*, 197–198.

Lim, M. M., and Young, L. F. Vasopressin-dependent neuronal circuits underlying pair bond formation in the monogamous prairie vole. *Neuroscience*. 2004, *125*, 35–45.

Lin, J. S., Sakai, K., and Jouvet, M. Evidence for histaminergic arousal mechanisms in the hypothalamus of cat. *Neuropharmacology*, 1998, *27*, 111–122.

Lin, L., Faraco, J., Li, R., et al. The sleep disorder canine narcolepsy is caused by a mutation in the hypocretin (orexin) receptor 2. *Cell*, 1999, *98*, 365–376.

Lindgren, A. C., Barkeling, B., Hägg, A., et al. Eating behavior in Prader-Willi syndrome, normal weight, and obese control groups. *Journal of Pediatrics*, 2000, *137*, 50–55.

Links, J. M., Zubieta, J. K., Meltzer, C. G., et al. Influence of spatially heterogenous background activity on "hot object" quantitation in brain emission computed tomography. *Journal of Computer Assisted Tomography*, 1996, *20*, 680–687.

Liotti, M., Mayberg, H. S., McGinnis, S., et al. Unmasking disease-specific cerebral blood flow abnormalities: Mood challenge in patients with remitted unipolar depression. *American Journal of Psychiatry*, 2002, *159*, 1830–1840.

Liu, C., Zhang, W.-T., Tang, Y.-Y., et al. The visual word form area: Evidence from an fMRI study of implicit processing of Chinese characters. *NeuroImage*, 2008, *40*, 1350–1361.

Livingstone, M. S., and Hubel, D. H. Psychophysical evidence for separate channels for the perception of form, color, movement, and depth. *Journal of Neuroscience*, 1987, *7*, 3416–3468.

Livingstone, M. S., and Hubel, D. H. Anatomy and physiology of a color system in the primate visual cortex. *Journal of Neuroscience*, 1984, *4*, 309–356.

Lledo, P. M., Hjelmstad, G. O., Mukherji, S., et al. Calcium/calmodulin-dependent kinase II and long-term potentiation enhance synaptic transmission by the same mechanism. *Proceedings of the National Academy of Sciences, USA*, 1995, *92*, 11175–11179.

Logan, F. A. Decision making by rats: Delay versus amount of reward. *Journal of Comparative and Physiological Psychology*, 1965, *59*, 1–12.

Lømo, T. Frequency potentiation of excitatory synaptic activity in the dentate area of the hippocampal formation. *Acta Physiologica Scandinavica*, 1966, *68* (Suppl. 227), 128.

Lozano, A. M., Mayberg, H. S., Giacobbe, P., et al. Subcallosal cingulate gyrus deep brain stimulation for treatment-resistant depression. *Biological Psychiatry*, 2008, *64*, 461–467.

Lu, J., Greco, M. A., Shiromani, P., and Saper, C. B. Effect of lesions of the ventrolateral preoptic nucleus on NREM and REM sleep. *Journal of Neuroscience*, 2000, *20*, 3830–3842.

Lu, J., Sherman, D., Devor, M., and Saper, C. B. A putative flip-flop switch for control of REM sleep. *Nature*, 2006, *441*, 589–594.

Lu, J., Zhang, Y.-H., Chou, T. C., et al. Contrasting effects of ibotenate lesions of the paraventricular nucleus and subparaventricular zone on sleep-wake cycle and temperature regulation. *Journal of Neuroscience*, 2001, *21*, 4864–4874.

Ludwig, D. S., Tritos, N. A., Mastaitis, J. W., et al. Melanin-concentrating hormone overexpression in transgenic mice leads to obesity and insulin resistance. *Journal of Clinical Investigation*, 2001, *107*, 379–386.

Luo, M., Fee, M. S., and Katz, L. C. Encoding pheromonal signals in the accessory olfactory bulb of behaving mice. *Science*, 2003, *299*, 1196–1201.

Lupien, S., Lecours, A. R., Schwartz, G., et al. Longitudinal study of basal cortisol levels in healthy elderly subjects: Evidence for subgroups. *Neurobiology of Aging*, 1996, *17*, 95–105.

Luppi, P. H., Gervasoni, D., Verret, L., et al. Paradoxical (REM) sleep genesis: the switch from an aminergic-cholinergic to a GABAergic-glutamatergic hypothesis. *Journal of Physiology* (*Paris*), 2007, *100*, 271–283.

Lüscher, C., Xia, H., Beattie, E. C., et al. Role of AMPA receptor cycling in synaptic transmission and plasticity. *Neuron*, 1999, *24*, 649–658.

Luukinen, H., Viramo, P., Herala, M., et al. Fall-related brain injuries and the risk of dementia in elderly people: A population-based study. *European Journal of Neurology*, 2005, *12*, 85–92.

Luzzi, S., Pucci, E., Di Bella, P., and Piccirilli, M. Topographical disorientation consequent to amnesia of spatial location in a patient with right parahippocampal damage. *Cortex*, 2000, *36*, 427–434.

Lynch, G., Larson, J., Kelso, S., et al. Intracellular injections of EGTA block induction of long-term potentiation. *Nature*, 1984, *305*, 719–721.

Lytton, W. W., and Brust, J. C. M. Direct dyslexia: Preserved oral reading of real words in Wernicke's aphasia. *Brain*, 1989, *112*, 583–594.

Ma, W., Miao, Z., and Novotny, M. Induction of estrus in grouped female mice (*Mus domesticus*) by synthetic analogs of preputial gland constituents. *Chemical Senses*, 1999, *24*, 289–293.

MacDonald, A. W., Carter, C. S., Kerns, J. G., et al. Specificity of prefrontal dysfunction and context processing deficits to schizophrenia in never-medicated patients with first-episode psychosis. *American Journal of Psychiatry*, 2005, *162*, 475–484.

MacLean, H. E., Warne, G. L., and Zajac, J. D. Defects of androgen receptor function: From sex reversal to motor-neuron disease. *Molecular and Cellular Endocrinology*, 1995, *112*, 133–141.

MacLean, P. D. Psychosomatic disease and the "visceral brain": Recent developments bearing on the Papez theory of emotion. *Psychosomatic Medicine*, 1949, *11*, 338–353.

Madden, P. A. F., Heath, A. C., Rosenthal, N. E., and Martin, N. G. Seasonal changes in mood and behavior: The role of genetic factors. *Archives of General Psychiatry*, 1996, *53*, 47–55.

Maezawa, I., Swanberg, S., Harvey, D., et al. Rett syndrome astrocytes are abnormal and spread MeCP2 deficiency through gap junctions. *Journal of Neuroscience*, 2009, *29*, 6061–5061.

Maggard, M. A., Shugarman, L. R., Suttorp, M., et al. Meta-analysis: Surgical treatment of obesity. *Annals of Internal Medicine*, 2005, *142*, 547–559.

Magistretti, P. J., Pellerin, L., Rothman, D. L., and Shulman, R. G. Energy on demand. *Science*, 1999, *283*, 496–497.

Maguire, E. A., Frackowiak, R. S. J., and Frith, C. D. Recalling routes around London: Activation of the right hippocampus in taxi drivers. *Journal of Neuroscience*, 1997, *17*, 7103–7110.

Maguire, E. A., Gadian, D. G., Johnsrude, I. S., et al. Navigation-related structural change in the hippocampi of taxi drivers. *Proceedings of the National Academy of Sciences, USA*, 2000, *97*, 4398–4403.

Mahley, R. W., and Rall, S. C. Apolipoprotein E: Far more than a lipid transport protein. *Annual Review of Genomics and Human Genetics*, 2000, *1*, 507–537.

Mahowald, M. W., and Schenck, C. H. Insights from studying human sleep disorders. *Nature*, 2005, *437*, 1279–1285.

Maj, M. Organic mental disorders in HIV-1 infection. *AIDS*, 1990, *4*, 831–840.

Mak, G. K., Enwere, E. K., Gregg, C., et al. Male pheromone-stimulated neurogenesis in the adult female brain: Possible role in mating behavior. *Nature Neuroscience*, 2007, *10*, 1003–1011.

Málaga-Trillo, E., Solis, G. P., Schrock, Y., et al. Regulation of embryonic cell adhesion by the prion protein. *PLoS Biology*, 2009, *7*, 0576–0590.

Mallucci, G., Dickinson, A., Linehan, J., et al. Depleting neuronal PrP in prion infections prevents disease and reverses spongiosis. *Science*, 2003, *302*, 871–874.

Malnic, B., Godfrey, P. A., and Buck, L. B. The human olfactory receptor gene family. *Proceedings of the National Academy of Sciences, USA*, 2004, *101*, 2584–2589.

Malnic, B., Hirono, J., Sato, T., and Buck, L. B. Combinatorial receptor codes for odors. *Cell*, 1999, *96*, 713–723.

Malsbury, C. W. Facilitation of male rat copulatory behavior by electrical stimulation of the medial preoptic area. *Physiology and Behavior*, 1971, *7*, 797–805.

Manji, H. K., Moore, G. J., and Chen, G. Bipolar disorder: Leads from the molecular and cellular mechanisms of action of mood stabilisers. *British Journal of Psychiatry*, 2001, *178* (Suppl. 41), S107–S109.

Manley, R. S., O'Brien, K. M., and Samuels, S. Fitness instructors' recognition of eating disorders and attendant ethical/liability issued. *Eating Disorders*, 2008, *16*, 103–116.

Mao-Draayer, Y., and Panitch, H. Alexia without agraphia in multiple sclerosis: Case report with magnetic resonance imaging localization. *Multiple Sclerosis*, 2004, *10*, 705–707.

Maquet, P. Sleep function(s) and cerebral metabolism. *Behavioural Brain Research*, 1995, *69*, 75–83.

Maquet, P., Dive, D., Salmon, E., et al. Cerebral glucose utilization during sleep-wake cycle in man determined by positron emission tomography and [18F]2-fluro-2-deoxy-D-glucose method. *Brain Research*, 1990, *413*, 136–143.

Maret, G., Testa, B., Jenner, P., et al. The MPTP story: MAO activates tetrahydropyridine derivatives to toxins causing parkinsonism. *Drug Metabolism Review*, 1990, *22*, 291–332.

Margolin, D. I., and Goodman-Schulman, R. Oral and written spelling impairments. In *Cognitive Neuropsychology in Clinical Practice*, edited by D. I. Margolin. New York: Oxford University Press, 1992.

Margolin, D. I., Marcel, A. J., and Carlson, N. R. Common mechanisms in dysnomia and post-semantic surface dyslexia: Processing deficits and selective attention. In *Surface Dyslexia: Neuropsychological and Cognitive Studies of Phonological Reading*, edited by M. Coltheart. London: Lawrence Erlbaum Associates, 1985.

Margolin, D. I., and Walker, J. A. Personal communication, 1981.

Marrocco, R. T., Witte, E. A., and Davidson, M. C. Arousal systems. *Current Opinion in Neurobiology*, 1994, *4*, 166–170.

Marrosu, F., Portas, C., Mascia, M. S., et al. Microdialysis measurement of cortical and hippocampal acetylcholine release during sleep–wake cycle in freely moving cats. *Brain Research*, 1995, *671*, 329–332.

Marshall, L., and Born, J. The contribution of sleep to hippocampus-dependent memory consolidation. *Trends in Cognitive Science*, 2007, *11*, 442–450.

Marson, L., and McKenna, K. E. A role for 5-hydroxytryptamine in descending inhibition of spinal sexual reflexes. *Experimental Brain Research*, 1992, *88*, 313–320.

Martin, K. C., and Zukin, R. S. RNA trafficking and local protein synthesis in dendrites: An overview. *Journal of Neuroscience*, 2006, *26*, 7131–7134.

Martinez, M., Campion, D., Babron, M. C., and Clergetdarpous, F. Is a single mutation at the same locus responsible for all affected cases in a large Alzheimer pedigree (Fad4)? *Genetic Epidemiology*, 1993, *10*, 431–435.

Martins, I. J., Hone, E., Foster, J. K., et al. Apolipoprotein E, cholesterol metabolism, diabetes, and the convergence of risk factors for Alzheimer's disease and cardiovascular disease. *Molecular Psychiatry*, 2006, *11*, 721–736.

Mas, M. Neurobiological correlates of masculine sexual behavior. *Neuroscience and Biobehavioral Reviews*, 1995, *19*, 261–277.

Masland, R. H. Neuronal diversity in the retina. *Current Opinion in Neurobiology*, 2001, *11*, 431–436.

Mathalon, D. H., Pfefferbaum, A., Lim, K. O., et al. Compounded brain volume deficits in schizophrenia-alcoholism comorbidity. *Archives of General Psychiatry*, 2003, *60*, 245–252.

Mathers, C. D., and Loncar, D. Projections of global mortality and burden of disease from 2002 to 2030. *PLoS Medicine*, 2006, *3*, e442.

Mathis, C. A., Klunk, W. E., Price, J. C., and DeKosky, S. T. Imaging technology for neurodegerative diseases. *Archives of Neurology*, 2005, *62*, 196–200.

Matsuda, L. A., Lolait, S. J., Brownstein, M. J., et al. Structure of a cannabinoid receptor and functional expression of the cloned cDNA. *Nature*, 1990, *346*, 561–564.

Matsumoto, D., and Willingham, B. Spontaneous facial expressions of emotion of congenitally and noncongenitally blind individuals. *Journal of Personality and Social Psychology*, 2009, *96*, 1–10.

Matsunami, H., Montmayeur, J.-P., and Buck, L. B. A family of candidate taste receptors in human and mouse. *Nature*, 2000, *404*, 601–604.

Mattson, M. P., Haughey, N. J., and Nath, A. Cell death in HIV dementia. *Cell Death and Differentiation*, 2005, *12*, 893–904.

Maviel, T., Durkin, T. P., Menzaghi, F., and Bontempi, B. Sites of neocortical reorganization critical for remote spatial memory. *Science*, 2004, *305*, 96–99.

Mayberg, H. S., Lozano, A. M., Voon, V., et al. Deep brain stimulation for treatment-resistant depression. *Neuron*, 2005, *45*, 651–660.

Mayers, A. G., and Baldwin, D. S. Antidepressants and their effect on sleep. *Human Psychopharmacology*, 2005, *20*, 533–559.

McCandliss, B. D., Cohen, L., and Dehaene, S. The visual word form area: Expertise for reading in the fusiform gyrus. *Trends in Cognitive Science*, 2003, *7*, 293–299.

McCann, U. D., Wong, D. F., Yokoi, F., et al. Reduced striatal dopamine transporter density in abstinent methamphetamine and methcathinone users: Evidence from positron emission tomography studies with [11C]WIN-35,428. *Journal of Neuroscience*, 1998, *18*, 8417–8422.

McCarley, R. W., and Hobson, J. A. The form of dreams and the biology of sleep. In *Handbook of Dreams: Research, Theory, and Applications*, edited by B. Wolman. New York: Van Nostrand Reinhold, 1979.

McClintock, M. K. Menstrual synchrony and suppression. *Nature*, 1971, *229*, 244–245.

McClintock, M. K., and Adler, N. T. The role of the female during copulation in wild and domestic Norway rats (*Rattus norvegicus*). *Behaviour*, 1978, *67*, 67–96.

McCormick, D. A. Neurotransmitter actions in the thalamus and cerebral cortex. *Journal of Clinical Neurophysiology*, 1992, *9*, 212–223.

McEwen, B. S., and Sapolsky, R. M. Stress and cognitive function. *Current Biology*, 1995, *5*, 205–216.

McFarland, K., and Kalivas, P. W. The circuitry mediating cocaine-induced reinstatement of drug-seeking behavior. *Journal of Neuroscience*, 2001, *21*, 8655–8663.

McGregor, A., and Roberts, D. C. S. Dopaminergic antagonism within the nucleus accumbens or the amygdala produces differential effects on intravenous cocaine self-administration under fixed and progressive ratio schedules of reinforcement. *Brain Research*, 1993, *624*, 245–252.

McHugh, T. J., Blum, K. I., Tsien, J. Z., et al. Impaired hippocampal representation of space in CA1-specific NMDAR1 knockout mice. *Cell*, 1996, *87*, 1339–1349.

Mednick, S. A., Machon, R. A., and Huttunen, M. O. An update on the Helsinki influenza project. *Archives of General Psychiatry*, 1990, *47*, 292.

Mednick, S., Nakayama, K., and Stickgold, R. Sleep-dependent learning: A nap is as good as a night. *Nature Neuroscience*, 2003, *6*, 697–698.

Meeren, H. K., van Heijnsbergen, C. C., and de Gelder, B. Rapid perceptual integration of facial expression and emotional body language. *Proceedings of the National Academy of Science*, 2005, *102*, 16518–16523.

Melzak, R. Phantom limbs. *Scientific American*, 1992, *266(4)*, 120–126.

Menon, V., and Desmond, J. E. Left superior parietal cortex involvement in writing: Integrating fMRI with lesion evidence. *Cognitive Brain Research*, 2001, *12*, 337–340.

Meredith, M. Chronic recording of vomeronasal pump activation in awake behaving hamsters. *Physiology and Behavior*, 1994, *56*, 345–354.

Meredith, M., and O'Connell, R. J. Efferent control of stimulus access to the hamster vomeronasal organ. *Journal of Physiology*, 1979, *286*, 301–316.

Mereu, G., Yoon, K.-W. P., Boi, V., et al. Preferential stimulation of ventral tegmental area dopaminergic neurons by nicotine. *European Journal of Pharmacology*, 1987, *141*, 395–400.

Merikangas, K. R., and Low, N. C. Genetic epidemiology of anxiety disorders. *Handbook of Experimental Pharmacology*, 2005, *169*, 163–179.

Mesulam, M.-M. Patterns in behavioral neuroanatomy: Association areas, the limbic system, and hemispheric specialization. In *Principles of Behavioral Neurology*, edited by M.-M. Mesulam. Philadelphia: F. A. Davis, 1985.

Meyer, M., Alter, K., Friederici, A. D., et al. FMRI reveals brain regions mediating slow prosodic modulations in spoken sentences. *Human Brain Mapping*, 2002, *17*, 73–88.

Meyer-Bahlburg, H. F. L. Gender identity outcome in female-raised 46, XY persons with penile agenesis, cloacal exstrophy of the bladder, or penile ablation. *Archives of Sexual Behavior*, 2005, *34*, 423–438.

Meyer-Bahlburg, H. F. L. Psychoendocrine research on sexual orientation. Current status and future options. *Progress in Brain Research*, 1984, *63*, 375–398.

Michel, L., Derkinderen, P., Laplaud, D., et al. Emotional facial palsy following striato-capsular infarction. *Journal of Neurology, Neurosurgery, and Psychiatry*, 2008, *79*, 193–194.

Mignot, E. Genetic and familial aspects of narcolepsy. *Neurology*, 1998, *50*, S16–S22.

Mileykovskiy, B. Y., Kiyashchenko, L. I., and Siegel, J. M. Behavioral correlates of activity in identified hypocretin/orexin neurons. *Neuron*, 2005, *46*, 787–798.

Miller, N. E. Understanding the use of animals in behavioral research: Some critical issues. *Annals of the New York Academy of Sciences*, 1983, *406*, 113–118.

Milner, A. D., Perrett, D. I., Johnston, R. S., and Benson, P. J. Perception and action in "visual form agnosia." *Brain*, 1991, *114*, 405–428.

Milner, B. Memory and the temporal regions of the brain. In *Biology of Memory*, edited by K. H. Pribram and D. E. Broadbent. New York: Academic Press, 1970.

Milner, B., Corkin, S., and Teuber, H.-L. Further analysis of the hippocampal amnesic syndrome: 14-year follow-up study of H. M. *Neuropsychologia*, 1968, *6*, 317–338.

Mindus, P., Rasmussen, S. A., and Lindquist, C. Neurosurgical treatment for refractory obsessive-compulsive disorder: Implications for understanding frontal lobe function. *Journal of Neuropsychiatry and Clinical Neurosciences*, 1994, *6*, 467–477.

Mishkin, M. Visual mechanisms beyond the striate cortex. In *Frontiers in Physiological Psychology*, edited by R. W. Russell. New York: Academic Press, 1966.

Mitchell, J. D., Wokke, J. H., and Borasio, G. D. Recombinant human insulin-like growth factor I (rhIGF-I) for amyotrophic lateral sclerosis/motor neuron disease. *Cochrane Database of Systematic Reviews*, 2007, Oct. 17(4): CD002064.

Mitchell, J. E. Psychopharmacology of eating disorders. *Annals of the New York Academy of Sciences*, 1989, *575*, 41–49.

Mitchell, P. B., and Loo, C. K. Transcranial magnetic stimulation for depression. *The Australian and New Zealand Journal of Psychiatry*, 2006, *40*, 379–380.

Mitler, M. M. Evaluation of treatment with stimulants in narcolepsy. *Sleep*, 1994, *17*, S103–S106.

Moghaddam, B., and Bunney, B. S. Differential effect of cocaine on extracellular dopamine levels in rat medial prefrontal cortex and nucleus accumbens: Comparison to amphetamine. *Synapse*, 1989, *4*, 156–161.

Mollon, J. D. "Tho' she kneel'd in that place where they grew...": The uses and origins of primate colour vision. *Journal of Experimental Biology*, 1989, *146*, 21–38.

Mombaerts, P. Molecular biology of odorant receptors in vertebrates. *Annual Review of Neuroscience*, 1999, *22*, 487–510.

Money, J., and Ehrhardt, A. *Man & Woman, Boy & Girl*. Baltimore: Johns Hopkins University Press, 1972.

Monk, C. S., Telzer, E. H., Mogg, K., et al. Amygdala and ventrolateral prefrontal cortex activation to masked angry faces in children and adolescents with generalized anxiety disorder. *Archives of General Psychiatry*, 2008, *65*, 568–576.

Monsonego, A., and Weiner, H. L. Immunotherapeutic approaches to Alzheimer's disease. *Science*, 2003, *302*, 834–838.

Montagna, P., Gambetti, P., Cortelli, P., and Lugaresi, E. Familial and sporadic fatal insomnia. *The Lancet Neurology*, 2003, *2*, 167–176.

Moore, D. J., West, A. B., Dawson, V. L., and Dawson, T. M. Molecular pathophysiology of Parkinson's Disease. *Annual Review of Neuroscience*, 2005, *28*, 57–87.

Moore, G. J., Bebchuk, J. M., Wilds, I. B., et al. Lithium-induced increase in human brain grey matter. *Lancet*, 2000, *356*, 1241–1242.

Moore, R. Y., and Eichler, V. B. Loss of a circadian adrenal corticosterone rhythm following suprachiasmatic lesions in the rat. *Brain Research*, 1972, *42*, 201–206.

Moore, R. Y., Speh, J. C., and Leak, R. K. Suprachiasmatic nucleus organization. *Cell Tissue Research*, 2002, *309*, 89–98.

Moore, T. H. M., Zummit, S., Lingford-Hughes, A., et al. Cannabis use and risk of psychotic or affective mental health outcomes: A systematic review. *Lancet*, 2007, *370*, 319–328.

Moran, T. H., Shnayder, L., Hostetler, A. M., and McHugh, P. R. Pylorectomy reduces the satiety action of cholecystokinin. *American Journal of Physiology*, 1989, *255*, R1059–R1063.

Morgenthaler, T. I., and Silber, M. H. Amnestic sleep-related eating disorder associated with zolpidem. *Sleep Medicine*, 2002, *3*, 323–327.

Morris, J. A., Gobrogge, K. L., Jordan, C. L., and Breedlove, S. M. Brain aromatase: Dyed-in-the-wool homosexuality. *Endocrinology*, 2004, *145*, 475–477.

Morris, J. S., Frith, C. D., Perrett, D. I., et al. A differential neural response in the human amygdala to fearful and happy facial expressions. *Nature*, 1996, *383*, 812–815.

Morris, N. M., Udry, J. R., Khan-Dawood, F., and Dawood, M. Y. Marital sex frequency and midcycle female testosterone. *Archives of Sexual Behavior*, 1987, *16*, 27–37.

Morris, R. G. M., Garrud, P., Rawlins, J. N. P., and O'Keefe, J. Place navigation impaired in rats with hippocampal lesions. *Nature*, 1982, *297*, 681–683.

Morrow, E. M., Yoo, S.-Y., Flkavell, S. W., et al. Identifying autism loci and genes by tracing recent shared ancestry. *Science*, 2008, *321*, 218–223.

Moscovitch, M., and Olds, J. Asymmetries in emotional facial expressions and their possible relation to hemispheric specialization. *Neuropsychologia*, 1982, *20*, 71–81.

Mueser, K. T., and McGurk, S. R. Schizophrenia. *The Lancet*, 2004, *363*, 2063–2072.

Mukhametov, L. M. Sleep in marine mammals. In *Sleep Mechanisms*, edited by A. A. Borbély and J. L. Valatx. Munich: Springer-Verlag, 1984.

Murray, R. M., Morrison, P. D., Henquet, C., and Di Forti, M. Cannabis, the mind and society: The hash realities. *Nature Reviews: Neuroscience*, 2007, *8*, 885–895.

Murray, S. O., Boyaci, H., and Kersten, D. The representation of perceived angular size in human primary visual cortex. *Nature Neuroscience*, 2006, *9*, 429–434.

Murre, J. M. J., Graham, K. S., and Hodges, J. R. Semantic dementia: Relevance to connectionist models of long-term memory. *Brain*, 2001, *124*, 647–675.

Myrick, H., Anton, R. F., Li, X., et al. Differential brain activity in alcoholics and social drinkers to alcohol cues: Relationship to craving. *Neuropsychopharmacology*, 2004, *29*, 393–402.

Nadeau, S. E. Impaired grammar with normal fluency and phonology. *Brain*, 1988, *111*, 1111–1137.

Nader, K. Memory traces unbound. *Trends in Neuroscience*, 2003, *26*, 65–72.

Nader, K., Majidishad, P., Amorapanth, P., and LeDoux, J. E. Damage to the lateral and central, but not other, amygdaloid nuclei prevents the acquisition of auditory fear conditioning. *Learning and Memory*, 2001, *8*, 156–163.

Naeser, M. A., Palumbo, C. L., Helm-Estabrooks, N., et al. Severe nonfluency in aphasia. Role of the medial subcallosal fasciculus and other white matter pathways in recovery of spontaneous speech. *Brain*, 1989, *112*, 1–38.

Nägerl, U. V., Köstinger, G., Anderson, J. C., et al. Protracted synaptogenesis after activity-dependent spinogenesis in hippocampal neurons. *Journal of Neuroscience*, 2007, *27*, 8149–8156.

Najjar, M. Zolpidem and amnestic sleep related eating disorder. *Journal of Clinical Sleep Medicine*, 2007, *15*, 637–638.

Nakahara, D., Ozaki, N., Miura, Y., et al. Increased dopamine and serotonin metabolism in rat nucleus accumbens produced by intracranial self-stimulation of medial forebrain bundle as measured by in vivo microdialysis. *Brain Research*, 1989, *495*, 178–181.

Nakazato, M., Mauakami, N., Date, Y., et al. A role for ghrelin in the central regulation of feeding. *Nature*, 2001, *409*, 194–198.

Nambu, T., Sakurai, T., Mizukami, K., et al. Distribution of orexin neurons in the adult rat brain. *Brain Research*, 1999, *827*, 243–260.

Naqvi, N. H., and Bechara, A. The hidden island of addiction: The insula. *Trends in Neuroscience*, 2009, *32*, 56–57.

Naqvi, N. H., and Bechara, A. The airway sensory impact of nicotine contributes to the conditioned reinforcing effects of individual puffs from cigarettes. *Pharmacology, Biochemistry and Behavior*, 2005, *81*, 821–829.

Naqvi, N. H., Rudrauf, D., Damasio, H., and Bechara, A. Damage to the insula disrupts addiction to cigarette smoking. *Science*, 2007, *315*, 531–534.

Nathans, J. The evolution and physiology of human color vision: Insights from molecular genetic studies of visual pigments. *Neuron*, 1999, *24*, 299–312.

Nauta, W. J. H. Some efferent connections of the prefrontal cortex in the monkey. In *The Frontal Granular Cortex and Behavior*, edited by J. M. Warren and K. Akert. New York: McGraw-Hill, 1964.

Nazir, T. A., Jacobs, A. M., and O'Regan, J. K. Letter legibility and visual word recognition. *Memory and Cognition*, 1998, *26*, 810–821.

Nef, P., Hermansborgmeyer, I., Artierespin, H., et al. Spatial pattern of receptor expression in the olfactory epithelium. *Proceedings of the National Academy of Sciences, USA*, 1992, *89*, 8948–8952.

Nergårdh, R., Ammar, A., Brodin, U., et al. Neuropeptide Y facilitates activity-based anorexia. *Psychoneuroendocrinology*, 2007, *32*, 493–502.

Neumann, K., Preibisch, C., Euler, H. A., et al. Cortical plasticity associated with stuttering therapy. *Journal of Fluency Disorders*, 2005, *30*, 23–39.

New, A. S., Buchsbaum, M. S., Hazlett, E. A., et al. Fluoxetine increases relative metabolic rate in prefrontal cortex in impulsive aggression. *Psychopharmacology*, 2004, *176*, 451–458.

Nichelli, P., Grafman, J., Pietrini, P., et al. Where the brain appreciates the moral of a story. *NeuroReport*, 1995, *6*, 2309–2313.

Nicholl, C. S., and Russell, R. M. Analysis of animal rights literature reveals the underlying motives of the movement: Ammunition for counter offensive by scientists. *Endocrinology*, 1990, *127*, 985–989.

Nicoll, J. A. R., Wilkinson, D., Holmes, C., et al. Neuropathology of human Alzheimer disease after immunization with amyloid-β peptide: A case report. *Nature Medicine*, 2003, *9*, 448–452.

Nielsen, S. J., Siega-Ritz, A. M., and Popkin, B. M. Trends in energy intake in U.S. between 1977 and 1996: Similar shifts seen across age groups. *Obesity Research*, 2002, *10*, 370–378.

Nikolic, W. V., Bai, Y., Obregon, D., et al. Transcutaneous β-amyloid immunization reduces cerebral β-amyloid deposits without T cell infiltration and microhemorrhage. *Proceedings of the National Academy of Sciences, USA*, 2007, *104*, 2507–2512.

Nilius, B., Owsianik, G., Voets, T., and Peters, J. A. Transient receptor potential cation channels in disease. *Physiological Review*, 2007, *87*, 165–217.

NINDS. Tissue plasminogen activator for acute ischemic stroke. The National Institute of Neurological Disorders and Stroke RT-PA stroke study group. *New England Journal of Medicine*, 1995, *333*, 1189–1191.

Nishino, S. Clinical and neurobiological aspects of narcolepsy. *Sleep Medicine*, 2007, *8*, 373–399.

Nishino, S., Ripley, B., Overeem, S., et al. Hypocretin (orexin) deficiency in human narcolepsy. *Lancet*, 2000, *355*, 39–40.

Nobler, M. S., Oquendo, M. A., Kegeles, L. S., et al. Deceased regional brain metabolism after ECT. *American Journal of Psychiatry*, 2001, *158*, 305–308.

Norgren, R., and Grill, H. Brain-stem control of ingestive behavior. In *The Physiological Mechanisms of Motivation*, edited by D. W. Pfaff. New York: Springer-Verlag, 1982.

Normandin, J., and Murphy, A. Z. Nucleus paragigantocellularis afferents in male and female rats: Organization, gonadal steroid receptor expression, and activation during sexual behavior. *Journal of Comparative Neurology*, 2008, *508*, 771–794.

Novin, D., VanderWeele, D. A., and Rezek, M. Hepatic-portal 2-deoxy-D-glucose infusion causes eating: Evidence for peripheral glucoreceptors. *Science*, 1973, *181*, 858–860.

Novotny, M. V., Ma, W., Wiesler, D., and Zidek, L. Positive identification of the puberty-accelerating pheromone of the house mouse: The volatile ligands associating with the major urinary protein. *Proceedings of the Royal Society of London [B]*, 1999, *266*, 2017–2022.

Numan, M. Medial preoptic area and maternal behavior in the female rat. *Journal of Comparative and Physiological Psychology*, 1974, *87*, 746–759.

Numan, M., and Numan, M. J. Projection sites of medial preoptic area and ventral bed nucleus of the stria terminalis neurons that express Fos during maternal behavior in female rats. *Journal of Neuroendocrinology*, 1997, *9*, 369–384.

Numan, M., and Smith, H. G. Maternal behavior in rats: Evidence for the involvement of

preoptic projections to the ventral tegmental area. *Behavioral Neuroscience*, 1984, *98*, 712–727.

Nutt, D. J., Glue, P., Lawson, C. W., and Wilson, S. Flumazenil provocation of panic attacks: Evidence for altered benzodiazepine receptor sensitivity in panic disorders. *Archives of General Psychiatry*, 1990, *47*, 917–925.

O'Brien, C. P., Volpicelli, L. A., and Volpicelli, J. R. Naltrexone in the treatment of alcoholism: A clinical review. *Alcohol*, 1996, *13*, 35–39.

O'Connor, M., Walbridge, M., Sandson, T., and Alexander, M. A neuropsychological analysis of Capgras syndrome. *Neuropsychiatry, Neuropsychology, and Behavioral Neurology*, 1996, *9*, 265–271.

O'Keefe, J., and Bouma, H. Complex sensory properties of certain amygadala units in the freely moving cat. *Experimental Neurology*, 1969, *23*, 384–398.

O'Keefe, J., and Dostrovsky, T. The hippocampus as a spatial map: Preliminary evidence from unit activity in the freely moving rat. *Brain Research*, 1971, *34*, 171–175.

Oaknin, S., Rodriguez del Castillo, A., Guerra, M., et al. Change in forebrain Na, K-ATPase activity and serum hormone levels during sexual behavior in male rats. *Physiology and Behavior*, 1989, *45*, 407–410.

Oberman, L. M., Winkielman, P., and Ramachandran, V. S. Face to face: Blocking facial mimicry can selectively impair recognition of emotional expressions. *Social Neuroscience*, 2007, *2*, 167–178.

Obler, L. K., and Gjerlow, K. *Language and the Brain*. Cambridge, U.K.: Cambridge University Press, 1999.

Oertel, D., and Young, E. D. What's a cerebellar circuit doing in the auditory system? *Trends in Neuroscience*, 2004, *27*, 104–110.

Ogawa, S., Olazabal, U. E., Parhar, I. S., and Pfaff, D. W. Effects of intrahypothalamic administration of antisense DNA for progesterone receptor mRNA on reproductive behavior and progesterone receptor immunoreactivity in female rat. *Journal of Neuroscience*, 1994, *14*, 1766–1774.

Ogden, C. L., Carroll, M. D., and Flegal, K. M. Epidemiologic trends in overweight and obesity. *Endocrinology and Metabolism Clinics of North America*, 2003, *32*, 741–760.

Olanow, C. W., Goetz, C. G., Kordower, J. H., et al. A double-blind controlled trial of bilateral fetal nigral transplantation in Parkinson's disease. *Annals of Neurology*, 2003, *54*, 403–414.

Olausson, H., Lamarre, Y., Backlund, H., et al. Unmyelinated Tactical afferents signal touch and project to insular cortex. *Nature Neuroscience*, 2002, *5*, 900–904.

Olausson, H., Lamarre, Y., Backlund, H., et al. Unihemispheric sleep deprivation in bottlenose dolphins. *Journal of Sleep Research*, 1992, *1*, 40–44.

Olds, J. Commentary. In *Brain Stimulation and Motivation*, edited by E. S. Valenstein. Glenview, Ill.: Scott, Foresman, 1973.

Oleksenko, A. I., Mukhametov, L. M., Polyakova, I. G., et al. Unihemispheric sleep deprivation in bottlenose dolphins. *Journal of Sleep Research*, 1992, *1*, 40–44.

Omura, K., Tsukamoto, T., Kotani, Y., et al.

Neural correlates of phoneme-to-grapheme conversion. *Neuroreport*, 2004, *15*, 949–953.

Opitz, B., and Friederici, A. D. Neural basis of processing sequential and hierarchical syntactic structures. *Human Brain Mapping*, 2007, *28*, 585–592.

Opitz, B., and Friederici, A. D. Interactions of the hippocampal system and the prefrontal cortex in learning language-like rules. *NeuroImage*, 2003, *19*, 1730–1737.

Otsuki, M., Soma, Y., Arai, T., et al. Pure apraxic agraphia with abnormal writing stroke sequences: Report of a Japanese patient with a left superior parietal haemorrhage. *Journal of Neurology, Neurosurgery, and Psychiatry*, 1999, *66*, 233–237.

Overduin, J., Frayo, R. S., Grill, H. J., et al. Role of the duodenum and macronutrient type in ghrelin regulation. *Endocrinology*, 2005, *146*, 845–850.

Packard, M. G., and Teather, L. A. Double dissociation of hippocampal and dorsal-striatal memory systems by posttraining intracerebral injections of 2-amino-5-phosphonopentanoic acid. *Behavioral Neuroscience*, 1997, *111*, 543–551.

Padberg, F., and Moller, H. J. Repetitive transcranial magnetic stimulation: Does it have potential in the treatment of depression? *CNS Drugs*, 2003, *17*, 383–403.

Pallast, E. G. M., Jongbloet, P. H., Straatman, H. M., and Zeilhuis, G. A. Excess of seasonality of births among patients with schizophrenia and seasonal ovopathy. *Schizophrenia Bulletin*, 1994, *20*, 269–276.

Papadimitriou, G. N., Christodoulou, G. N., Katsouyanni, K., and Stefanis, C. N. Therapy and prevention of affective illness by total sleep deprivation. *Journal of the Affective Disorders*, 1993, *27*, 107–116.

Papez, J. W. A proposed mechanism of emotion. *Archives of Neurology and Psychiatry*, 1937, *38*, 725–744.

Pardo, J. V., Sheikh, S. A., Schwindt, G. C., et al. Chronic vagus nerve stimulation for treatment-resistant depression decreases resting ventromedial prefrontal glucose metabolism. *NeuroImage*, 2008, *42*, 879–889.

Paré, D., Quirk, G. J., and LeDoux, J. E. New vistas on amygdala networks in conditioned fear. *Journal of Neurophysiology*, 2004, *92*, 1–9.

Pascoe, J. P., and Kapp, B. S. Electrophysiological characteristics of amygaloid central nucleus neurons during Pavlovian fear conditioning in the rabbit. *Behavioural Brain Research*, 1985, *16*, 117–133.

Pasterski, V. L., Geffner, M. E., Brain, C., et al. Prenatal hormones and postnatal socialization by parents as determinants of male-typical toy play in girls with congenital adrenal hyperplasia. *Child Development*, 2005, *76*, 264–278.

Pattatucci, A. M. L., and Hamer, D. H. Development and familiality of sexual orientation in females. *Behavior Genetics*, 1995, *25*, 407–420.

Paulesu, E., Démonet, J.-F., Fazio, F., et al. Dyslexia: Cultural diversity and biological unity. *Science*, 2001, *291*, 2165–2167.

Paulus, M. P., Feinstein, J. S., Castillo, G., et al. Dose-dependent decrease of activation in bilateral amygdala and insula by lorazepam during emotion during emotion processing.

Archives of General Psychiatry, 2005, *62*, 282–288.

Pavlov, I. *Conditioned Reflexes.* London: Oxford University Press, 1927.

Peck, B. K., and Vanderwolf, C. H. Effects of raphe stimulation on hippocampal and neocortical activity and behaviour. *Brain Research*, 1991, *568*, 244–252.

Pedersen-Bjergaard, U., Host, U., Kelbaek, H., et al. Influence of meal composition on postprandial peripheral plasma concentrations of vasoactive peptides in man. *Scandinavian Journal of Clinical and Laboratory Investigation*, 1996, *56*, 497–503.

Peigneux, P., Laureys, S., Fuchs, S., et al. Are spatial memories strengthened in the human hippocampus during slow wave sleep? *Neuron*, 2004, *44*, 535–545.

Pelleymounter, M. A., Cullen, M. J., Baker, M. B., et al. Effects of the obese gene product on body weight regulation in ob/ob mice. *Science*, 1995, *269*, 540–543.

Pelphrey, K. A., Morris, J. P., Michelich, C. R., et al. Functional anatomy of biological motion perception in posterior temporal cortex: An fMRI study of eye, mouth and hand movements. *Cerebral Cortex*, 2005, *15*, 1866–1876.

Penfield, W., and Perot, P. The brain's record of auditory and visual experience: A final summary and discussion. *Brain*, 1963, *86*, 595–697.

Pereira, A. C., Huddleston, D. E., Brickman, A. M., et al. In *in vivo* correlate of exercise-induced neurogenesis in the adult dentate gyrus. *Proceedings of the National Academy of Sciences, USA*, 2007, *104*, 5638–5643.

Peretz, I., Blood, A. J., Penhune, V., and Zatorre, R. Cortical deafness to dissonance. *Brain*, 2001, *124*, 928–940.

Peretz, I., Gagnon, L., and Bouchard, B. Music and emotion: Perceptual determinants, immediacy, and isolation after brain damage. *Cognition*, 1998, *68*, 111–141.

Peretz, I., and Zatorre, R. J. Brain organization for music processing. *Annual Review of Psychology*, 2005, *56*, 89–114.

Pert, C. B., Snowman, A. M., and Snyder, S. H. Localization of opiate receptor binding in presynaptic membranes of rat brain. *Brain Research*, 1974, *70*, 184–188.

Petre-Quadens, O., and De Lee, C. Eye movement frequencies and related paradoxical sleep cycles: Developmental changes. *Chronobiologia*, 1974, *1*, 347–355.

Pettito, L. A., Zatorre, R. J., Gauna, K., et al. Speech-like cerebral activity in profoundly deaf people processing signed languages: Implications for the neural basis of human language. *Proceedings of the National Academy of Sciences, USA*, 2000, *97*, 13961–13966.

Peuskens, H., Sunaert, S., Dupont, P., et al. Human brain regions involved in heading estimation. *Journal of Neuroscience*, 2001, *21*, 2451–2461.

Peyron, R., Laurent, B., and Garcia-Larrea, L. Functional imaging of brain responses to pain. A review and meta-analysis. *Neurophysiology Clinics*, 2000, *30*, 263–288.

Pezawas, L., Meyer-Linderberg, A., Drabant, E. M., et al. 5-HTTLPR polymorphism impacts human cingulate-amygdala interactions: A genetic susceptibility mechanism for depression. *Nature Neuroscience*, 2005, *8*, 828–834.

Pfaff, D. W., and Sakuma, Y. Deficit in the lordosis reflex of female rats caused by lesions in the ventromedial nucleus of the hypothalamus. *Journal of Physiology*, 1979, *288*, 203–210.

Pfaus, J. G., Kleopoulos, S. P., Mobbs, C. V., et al. Sexual stimulation activates c-fos within estrogen-concentrating regions of the female rat forebrain. *Brain Research*, 1993, *624*, 253–267.

Phelps, E. A., Delgado, M. R., Nearing, K. I., and LeDoux, J. E. Extinction learning in humans: Role of the amygdala and vmPFC. *Neuron*, 2004, *43*, 897–905.

Phelps, E. A., O'Connor, K. J., Gatenby, J. C., et al. Activation of the left amygdala to a cognitive representation of fear. *Nature Neuroscience*, 2001, *4*, 437–441.

Phiel, C. J., and Klein, P. S. Molecular targets of lithium action. *Annual Review of Pharmacology and Toxicology*, 2001, *41*, 789–813.

Phillips, A. G., Coury, A., Fiorino, D., et al. Self-stimulation of the ventral tegmental area enhances dopamine release in the nucleus accumbens: A microdialysis study. *Annals of the New York Academy of Sciences*, 1992, *654*, 199–206.

Phillips, D. P., and Farmer, M. E. Acquired word deafness, and the temporal grain of sound representation in the primary auditory cortex. *Behavioural Brain Research*, 1990, *40*, 85–94.

Phillips, M. I., and Felix, D. Specific angiotensin II receptive neurons in the cat subfornical organ. *Brain Research*, 1976, *109*, 531–540.

Piccirillo, J. F., Duntley, S., and Schotland, H. Obstructive sleep apnea. *Journal of the American Medical Association*, 2000, *284*, 1492–1494.

Pickles, J. O., and Corey, D. P. Mechanoelectrical transduction by hair cells. *Trends in Neuroscience*, 1992, *15*, 254–259.

Pijl, S., and Schwarz, D. W. F. Intonation of musical intervals by deaf subjects stimulated with single bipolar cochlear implant electrodes. *Hearing Research*, 1995a, *89*, 203–211.

Pijl, S., and Schwarz, D. W. F. Melody recognition and musical interval perception by deaf subjects stimulated with electrical pulse trains through single cochlear implant electrodes. *Journal of the Acoustical Society of America*, 1995b, *98*, 886–895.

Pike, K. M., Walsh, B. T., Vitousek, K., et al. Cognitive behavior therapy in the posthospitalization treatment of anorexia nervosa. *American Journal of Psychiatry*, 2003, *160*, 2046–2049.

Pitcher, D., Garrido, L., Walsh, V., and Duchaine, B. C. Transcranial magnetic stimulation disrupts the perception and embodiment of facial expressions. *Journal of Neuroscience*, 2008, *28*, 8929–8933.

Pitkänen, A., Savander, V., and LeDoux, J. E. Organization of intra-amygdaloid circuits: An emerging framework for understanding functions of the amygdala. *Trends in Neuroscience*, 1997, *20*, 517–523.

Pleim, E. T., and Barfield, R. J. Progesterone versus estrogen facilitation of female sexual behavior by intracranial administration to female rats. *Hormones and Behavior*, 1988, *22*, 150–159.

Pobric, G., Jefferies, E., and Lambon Ralph, M. A. Anterior temporal lobes mediate semantic representation: Mimicking semantic dementia by using rTMS in normal participants. *Proceedings of the National Academy of Sciences, USA*, 2007, *104*, 20137–20141.

Poeppel, D. Pure word deafness and the bilateral processing of the speech code. *Cognitive Science*, 2001, *25*, 679–693.

Poggio, G. F., and Poggio, T. The analysis of stereopsis. *Annual Review of Neuroscience*, 1984, *7*, 379–412.

Polymeropoulos, M. H., Higgins, J. J., Golbe, L. I., et al. Mapping of a gene for Parkinson's disease to chromosome 4q21–q23. *Science*, 1996, *274*, 1197–1199.

Pomp, D., and Nielsen, M. K. Quantitative genetics of energy balance: Lessons from animal models. *Obesity Research*, 1999, *7*, 106–110.

Pompili, M., Mancinelli, I., Girardi, P., et al. Suicide in anorexia nervosa: A meta-analysis. *International Journal of Eating Disorders*, 2004, *36*, 99–103.

Popova, N. K. From genes to aggressive behavior: The role of serotonergic system. *BioEssays*, 2006, *28*, 495–503.

Porkka-Heiskanen, T., Strecker, R. E., and McCarley, R. W. Brain site-specificity of extracellular adenosine concentration changes during sleep deprivation and spontaneous sleep: An *in vivo* microdialysis study. *Neuroscience*, 2000, *99*, 507–517.

Porter, J., Craven, B., Khan, R. M., et al. Mechanisms of scent-tracking in humans. *Nature Neuroscience*, 2007, *10*, 27–29.

Powers, J. B., and Winans, S. S. Vomeronasal organ: Critical role in mediating sexual behavior of the male hamster. *Science*, 1975, *187*, 961–963.

Price, D. B. Psychological and neural mechanisms of the affective dimension of pain. *Science*, 2000, *288*, 1769–1772.

Price, D. L., and Sisodia, S. S. Mutant genes in familial Alzheimer's disease and transgenic models. *Annual Review of Neuroscience*, 1998, *21*, 479–505.

Price, L. H., and Heninger, G. R. Drug therapy: Lithium in the treatment of mood disorders. *New England Journal of Medicine*, 1994, *331*, 591–598.

Pritchard, T. C., Hamilton, R. B., Morse, J. R., and Norgren, R. Projections of thalamic gustatory and lingual areas in the monkey, *Macaca fascicularis*. *Journal of Comparative Neurology*, 1986, *244*, 213–228.

Provencio, I., Rodriguez, I. R., Jiang, G., et al. A novel human opsin in the inner retinal. *Journal of Neuroscience*, 2000, *20*, 600–605.

Prusiner, S. B. Novel proteinaceous infectious particles cause scrapie. *Science*, 1982, *216*, 136–144.

Qu, D., Ludwig, D. S., Gammeltoft, S., et al. A role for melanin concentrating hormone in the central regulation of feeding behaviour. *Nature*, 1996, *380*, 243–247.

Quillen, E. W., Keil, L. C., and Reid, I. A. Effects of baroreceptor denervation on endocrine and drinking responses to caval constriction in dogs. *American Journal of Physiology*, 1990, *259*, R619–R626.

Quirk, G. J. Memory for extinction of conditioned fear is long-lasting and persists following spontaneous recovery. *Learning and Memory*, 2002, *9*, 402–407.

Quirk, G. J., Garcia, R., and González-Lima, F. Prefrontal mechanisms in extinction of conditioned fear. *Biological Psychiatry*, 2006, *60*, 337–343.

Quirk, G. J., Repa, J. C., and LeDoux, J. E. Fear conditioning enhances short-latency auditory responses of lateral amygdala neurons: Parallel recordings in the freely behaving rat. *Neuron*, 1995, *15*, 1029–1039.

Raine, A., Lencz, T., Bihrle, S., et al. Reduced prefrontal gray matter volume and reduced autonomic activity in antisocial personality disorder. *Archives of General Psychiatry*, 2002, *57*, 119–127.

Raine, A., Meloy, J. R., Bihrle, S., et al. Reduced prefrontal and increased subcortical brain functioning assessed using positron emission tomography in predatory and affective murderers. *Behavioral Science and the Law*, 1998, *16*, 319–332.

Rainville, P., Duncan, G. H., Price, D. D., et al. Pain affect encoded in human anterior cingulate but not somaatosensory cortex. *Science*, 1997, *277*, 968–971.

Rakic, P. A small step for the cell, a giant leap for mankind: a hypothesis of neocortical expansion during evolution. *Trends in Neuroscience*, 1995, *18*, 383–388.

Rakic, P. Specification of cerebral cortical areas. *Science*, 1988, *241*, 170–176.

Ralph, M. R., and Lehman, M. N. Transplantation: A new tool in the analysis of the mammalian hypothalamic circadian pacemaker. *Trends in Neuroscience*, 1991, *14*, 362–366.

Ramakrishnan, K., and Scheid, D. C. Treatment options for insomnia. *American Family Physician*, 2007, *76*, 517–526.

Ramesh, V., Thakkar, M. M., Strecker, R. E., et al. Wakefulness-inducing effects of histamine in the basal forebrain of freely moving rats. *Behavioural Brain Research*, 2004, *152*, 271–278.

Ramirez, I. Why do sugars taste good? *Neuroscience and Biobehavioral Reviews*, 1990, *14*, 125–134.

Ramus, F., Rosen, S., Dakin, S. C., et al. Theories of developmental dyslexia: Insights from a multiple case study of dyslexic adults. *Brain*, 2003, *126*, 841–865.

Rapin, I. Autism in search of a home in the brain. *Neurology*, 1999, *52*, 902–904.

Rapoport, J. L. Recent advances in obsessive-compulsive disorder. *Neuropsychopharmacology*, 1991, *5*, 1–10.

Rapoport, J. L., Ryland, D. H., and Kriete, M. Drug treatment of canine acral lick: An animal model of obsessive-compulsive disorder. *Archives of General Psychiatry*, 1992, *49*, 517–521.

Rasmusson, D. D., Clow, K., and Szerb, J. C. Modification of neocortical acetylcholine release and electroencephalogram desynchronization due to brain stem stimulation by drugs applied to the basal forebrain. *Neuroscience*, 1994, *60*, 665–677.

Rattenborg, N. C., Lima, S. L., and Amlaner, C. J. Facultative control of avian unihemispheric sleep under the risk of predation. *Behavioural Brain Research*, 1999, *105*, 163–172.

Rauch, S. L., Shin, L. M., and Phelps, E. A. Neurocircuitry models of posttraumatic stress disorder and extinction: Human neuroimaging research—Past, present, and future. *Biological Psychiatry*, 2006, *60*, 376–382.

Rauschecker, J. P., and Tian, B. Mechanisms and streams for processing of "what" and "where" in auditory cortex. *Proceedings of the National Academy of Sciences, USA*, 2000, *97*, 11800–11806.

Ravussin, E., Valencia, M. E., Esparza, J., et al. Effects of traditional lifestyle on obesity in Pima Indians. *Diabetes Care*, 1994, *17*, 1067–1074.

Raymond, C. R. LTP forms 1, 2, and 3: Different mechanisms for the "long" in long-term potentiation. *Trends in Neuroscience*, 2007, *30*, 167–175.

Reber, P. J., and Squire, L. R. Encapsulation of implicit and explicit memory in sequence learning. *Journal of Cognitive Neuroscience*, 1998, *10*, 248–263.

Recer, P. Study: English is a factor in dyslexia. Washington, DC: Associated Press, 16 March 2001.

Reddrop, C., Moldrich, R. X., Beart, P. M., et al. Vampire bat salivary plasminogen activator (desmoteplase) inhibits tissue-type plasminogen activator-induced potentiation of excitotoxic injury. *Stroke*, 2005, *36*, 1241–1246.

Redmond, D. E., Bjugstad, K. B., Teng, Y. D., et al. Behavioral improvement in a primate Parkinson's model is associated with multiple homeostatic effects of human neural stem cells. *Proceedings of the National Academy of Sciences, USA*, 2007, *104*, 12175–12180.

Reed, C. L., Caselli, R. J., and Farah, M. J. Tactile agnosia: Underlying impairment and implications for normal tactile object recognition. *Brain*, 1996, *119*, 875–888.

Regan, B. C., Julliot, C., Simmen, B., et al. Fruits, foliage and the evolution of primate colour vision. *Philosophical Transactions of the Royal Society of London* [B], 2001, *356*, 229–283.

Reid, L. D. Endogenous opioids and alcohol dependence: Opioid alkaloids and the propensity to drink alcoholic beverages. *Alcohol*, 1996, *13*, 5–11.

Reinehr, T., Roth, C. L., Schernthaner, G. H., et al. Peptide YY and glucagon-like peptide-1 in morbidly obese patients before and after surgically induced weight loss. *Obesity Surgery*, 2007, *17*, 1571–1577.

Reiner, W. G. Gender identity and sex-of-rearing in children with disorders of sexual differentiation. *Journal of Pediatric Endocrinology and Metabolism*, 2005, *18*, 549–553.

Reppert, S. M., and Weaver, D. R. Molecular analysis of mammalian circadian rhythms. *Annual Review of Physiology*, 2001, *63*, 647–676.

Ressler, K. J., and Mayberg, H. S. Targeting abnormal neural circuits in mood and anxiety disorders: From the laboratory to the clinic. *Nature Neuroscience*, 2007, *10*, 1116–1124.

Ressler, K. J., Sullivan, S. L., and Buck, L. A molecular dissection of spatial patterning in the olfactory system. *Current Opinion in Neurobiology*, 1994, *4*, 588–596.

Rétey, J. V., Adam, M., Honegger, E., et al. A functional genetic variation of adenosine deaminase affects the duration and intensity of deep sleep in humans. *Proceedings of the National Academy of Sciences, USA*, 2005, *102*, 15676–15681.

Rhees, R. W., Shryne, J. E., and Gorski, R. A. Onset of the hormone-sensitive perinatal period for sexual differentiation of the sexually dimorphic nucleus of the preoptic area in female rats. *Journal of Neurobiology*, 1990a, *21*, 781–786.

Rhees, R. W., Shryne, J. E., and Gorski, R. A. Termination of the hormone-sensitive period for differentiation of the sexually dimorphic nucleus of the preoptic area in male and female rats. *Developmental Brain Research*, 1990b, *52*, 17–23.

Rho, J. M. Can reducing sugar retard kindling? *Epilepsy Currents*, 2008, *8*, 83–84.

Rhodes, R. A., Murthy, N. B., Dresner, M. A., et al. Human 5-HT transporter availability predicts amygdala reactivity in vivo. *Journal of Neuroscience*, 2007, *27*, 9233–9237.

Riemann, D., Wiegand, M., and Berger, M. Are there predictors for sleep deprivation response in depressive patients? *Biological Psychiatry*, 1991, *29*, 707–710.

Rijntjes, M., Dettmers, C., Buchel, C., et al. A blueprint for movement: Functional and anatomical representations in the human motor system. *Journal of Neuroscience*, 1999, *19*, 8043–8048.

Rimmele, U., Hediger, K., Heinrichs, M., and Klaver, P. Oxytocin makes a face in memory familiar. *Journal of Neuroscience*, 2009, *29*, 38–42.

Ritter, R. C., Brenner, L., and Yox, D. P. Participation of vagal sensory neurons in putative satiety signals from the upper gastrointestinal tract. In *Neuroanatomy and Physiology of Abdominal Vagal Afferents*, edited by S. Ritter, R. C. Ritter, and C. D. Barnes. Boca Raton, Fla.: CRC Press, 1992.

Ritter, S., Dinh, T. T., and Friedman, M. I. Induction of Fos-like immunoreactivity (Fos-li) and stimulation of feeding by 2,5-anhydro-D-mannitol (2,5-AM) require the vagus nerve. *Brain Research*, 1994, *646*, 53–64.

Ritter, S., and Taylor, J. S. Vagal sensory neurons are required for lipoprivic but not glucoprivic feeding in rats. *American Journal of Physiology*, 1990, *258*, R1395–R1401.

Ritter, S., Dinh, T. T., and Zhang, Y. Localization of hindbrain glucoreceptive sites controlling food intake and blood glucose. *Brain Research*, 2000, *856*, 37–47.

Rizzolatti, R., Fogassi, L., and Gallese, V. Neurophysiological mechanisms underlying the understanding and imitation of action. *Nature Reviews: Neuroscience*, 2001, *2*, 661–670.

Robbins, L. N., Helzer, J. E., Weissman, M. M., et al. Lifetime prevalence of specific psychiatric disorders in three sites. *Archives of General Psychiatry*, 1984, *41*, 949–958.

Roberts, S. C., Havlicek, J., Flegr, J., et al. Female facial attractiveness increases during the fertile phase of the menstrual cycle. *Biology Letters*, 2004, *271*, S270–S272.

Robertson, G. S., Pfaus, J. G., Atkinson, L. J., et al. Sexual behavior increases c-fos expression in the forebrain of the male rat. *Brain Research*, 1991, *564*, 352–357.

Robinson, D., Wu, H., Munne, R. A., et al. Reduced caudate nucleus volume in obsessive-compulsive disorder. *Archives of General Psychiatry*, 1995, *52*, 393–398.

Rodrigues, S. M., Schafe, G. E., and LeDoux, J. E. Molecular mechanisms underlying emotional learning and memory in the lateral amygdala. *Neuron*, 2004, *44*, 75–91.

Rodrigues, S. M., Schafe, G. E., and LeDoux, J. E. Intra-amygdala blockade of the NR2B subunit of the NMDA receptor disrupts the acquisition but not the expression of fear conditioning. *Journal of Neuroscience*, 2001, *21*, 6889–6896.

Roeltgen, D. P., Rothi, L. H., and Heilman, K. M. Linguistic semantic apraphia: A dissociation of the lexical spelling system from semantics. *Brain and Language*, 1986, *27*, 257–280.

Roffwarg, H. P., Muzio, J. N., and Dement, W. C. Ontogenetic development of human sleep-dream cycle. *Science*, 1966, *152*, 604–619.

Rogawski, M. A., and Wenk, G. L. The neuropharmacological basis for the use of memantine in the treatment of Alzheimer's disease. *CNS Drug Reviews*, 2003, *9*, 275–308.

Rogers, T. T., Hocking, J., Noppeney, U., et al. Anterior temporal cortex and semantic memory: Reconciling findings from neuropsychology and functional imaging. *Cognitive, Affective, and Behavioral Neuroscience*, 2006, *6*, 201–213.

Rolls, E. T. Feeding and reward. In *The Neural Basis of Feeding and Reward*, edited by B. G. Hobel and D. Novin. Brunswick, Me.: Haer Institute, 1982.

Rolls, E. T., and Baylis, G. C. Size and contrast have only small effects on the responses to faces of neurons in the cortex of the superior temporal sulcus of the monkey. *Experimental Brain Research*, 1986, *65*, 38–48.

Rolls, E. T., Murzi, E., Yaxley, S., et al. *Brain Research*, 1986, *368*, 79–86.

Rolls, E. T., Yaxley, S., and Sienkiewicz, Z. J. Gustatory responses of single neurons in the orbitofrontal cortex of the macaque monkey. *Journal of Neurophysiology*, 1990, *64*, 1055–1066.

Romanovsky, A. A. Thermoregulation: Some concepts have changed. Functional architecture of the thermoregulatory system. *American Journal of Physiology*, 2007, *292*, R37–R46.

Rose, J. E. Nicotine and nonnicotine factors in cigarette addiction. *Psychopharmacology*, 2006, *184*, 274–285.

Rosenblatt, J. S., Hazelwood, S., and Poole, J. Maternal behavior in male rats: Effects of medial preoptic area lesions and presence of maternal aggression. *Hormones and Behavior*, 1996, *30*, 201–215.

Rosenthal, D. A program of research on heredity in schizophrenia. *Behavioral Science*, 1971, *16*, 191–201.

Rosenthal, N. E., Sack, D. A., Gillin, C., et al. Seasonal affective disorder: A description of the syndrome and preliminary findings with light therapy. *Archives of General Psychiatry*, 1984, *41*, 72–80.

Rosenthal, N. E., Sack, D. A., James, S. P., et al. Seasonal affective disorder and phototherapy. *Annals of the New York Academy of Sciences*, 1985, *453*, 260–269.

Roses, A. D. A model for susceptibility polymorphisms for complex diseases: Apolipoprotein E and Alzheimer disease. *Neurogenetics*, 1997, *1*, 3–11.

Rubin, B. S., and Barfield, R. J. Priming of estrous responsiveness by implants of 17B-estradiol in the ventromedial hypothalamic nucleus of female rats. *Endocrinology*, 1980, *106*, 504–509.

Rubin, L. L., and Staddon, J. M. The cell biology of the blood–brain barrier. *Annual Review of Neuroscience*, 1999, *22*, 11–28.

Rück, C., Karlsson, A., Steele, J. D., et al. Capsulotomy for obsessive-compulsive disorder. *Archives of General Psychiatry*, 2008, *65*, 914–922.

Rumpel, S., LeDoux, J., Zador, A., and Malinow, R. Postsynaptic receptor trafficking underlying a form of associative learning. *Science*, 2005, *308*, 83–88.

Russchen, F. T., Amaral, D. G., and Price, J. L. The afferent connections of the substantia innominata in the monkey, *Macaca fascicularis*. *Journal of Comparative Neurology*, 1986, *242*, 1–27.

Russell, G. F. M., and Treasure, J. The modern history of anorexia nervosa: An interpretation of why the illness has changed. *Annals of the New York Academy of Sciences*, 1989, *575*, 13–30.

Russell, M. J., Switz, G. M., and Thompson, K. Olfactory influences on the human menstrual cycle. *Pharmacology, Biochemistry and Behavior*, 1980, *13*, 737–738.

Ryback, R. S., and Lewis, O. F. Effects of prolonged bed rest on EEG sleep patterns in young, healthy volunteers. *Electroencephalography and Clinical Neurophysiology*, 1971, *31*, 395–399.

Saal, D., Dong, Y., Bonci, A., and Malenka, R. C. Drugs of abuse and stress trigger a common synaptic adaptation in dopamine neurons. *Neuron*, 2003, *37*, 577–582.

Sachar, E. J., and Baron, M. The biology of affective disorders. *Annual Review of Neuroscience*, 1979, *2*, 505–518.

Sackeim, H. A. Lateral asymmetry in bodily response to hypnotic suggestion. *Biological Psychiatry*, 1982, *17*, 437–447.

Sackeim, H. A., Decina, P., Prohovnik, I., et al. Anticonvulsant and antidepressant properties of electroconvulsive therapy: A proposed mechanism of action. *Biological Psychiatry*, 1983, *18*, 1301–1310.

Sackeim, H. A., and Gur, R. C. Lateral asymmetry in intensity of emotional expression. *Neuropsychologia*, 1978, *16*, 473–482.

Sackeim, H. A., Paulus, D., and Weiman, A. L. Classroom seating and hypnotic susceptibility. *Journal of Abnormal Psychology*, 1979, *88*, 81–84.

Saffran, E. M., Marin, O. S. M., and Yeni-Komshian, G. H. An analysis of speech perception in word deafness. *Brain and Language*, 1976, *3*, 209–228.

Saffran, E. M., Schwartz, M. F., and Marin, O. S. M. Evidence from aphasia: Isolating the components of a production model. In *Language Production*, edited by B. Butterworth. London: Academic Press, 1980.

Sahay, A., and Hen, R. Adult hippocampal neurogenesis in depression. *Nature Neuroscience*, 2007, *10*, 1110–1115.

Sahu, A., Kalra, P. S., and Kalra, S. P. Food deprivation and ingestion induce reciprocal changes in neuropeptide Y concentrations in the paraventricular nucleus. *Peptides*, 1988, *9*, 83–86.

Sakai, F., Meyer, J. S., Karacan, I., et al. Normal human sleep: Regional cerebral haemodynamics. *Annals of Neurology*, 1979, *7*, 471–478.

Sakuma, Y., and Pfaff, D. W. Convergent effects of lordosis-relevant somatosensory and hypothalamic influences on central gray cells in the rat mesencephalon. *Experimental Neurology*, 1980a, *70*, 269–281.

Sakuma, Y., and Pfaff, D. W. Excitability of female rat central gray cells with medullary projections: Changes produced by hypothalamic stimulation and estrogen treatment. *Journal of Neurophysiology*, 1980b, *44*, 1012–1023.

Sakuma, Y., and Pfaff, D. W. Facilitation of female reproductive behavior from mesencephalic central grey in the rat. *American Journal of Physiology*, 1979a, *237*, R279–R284.

Sakuma, Y., and Pfaff, D. W. Mesencephalic mechanisms for integration of female reproductive behavior in the rat. *American Journal of Physiology*, 1979b, *237*, R285–R290.

Sakurai, T. The neural circuit of orexin (hypocretin): Maintaining sleep and wakefulness. *Nature Reviews: Neuroscience*, 2007, *8*, 171–181.

Sakurai, T., Amemiya, A., Ishii, M., et al. Orexins and orexin receptors: A family of hypothalamic neuropeptides and G protein-coupled receptors that regulate feeding behavior. *Cell*, 1998, *20*, 573–585.

Sakurai, Y., Ichikawa, Y., and Mannen, T. Pure alexia from a posterior occipital lesion. *Neurology*, 2001, *56*, 778–781.

Sakurai, Y., Momose, T., Iwata, M., et al. Different cortical activity in reading of Kanji words, Kana words and Kana nonwords. *Cognitive Brain Research*, 2000, *9*, 111–115.

Sakurai, Y., Sakai, K., Sakuta, M., and Iwata, M. Naming difficulties in alexia with agraphia for kanji after a left posterior inferior temporal lesion. *Journal of Neurology, Neurosurgery, and Psychiatry*, 1994, *57*, 609–613.

Salamone, J. D. Complex motor and sensorimotor function of striatal and accumbens dopamine: Involvement in instrumental behavior processes. *Psychopharmacology*, 1992, *107*, 160–174.

Salas, J. C. T., Iwasaki, H., Jodo, E., et al. Penile erection and micturition events triggered by electrical stimulation of the mesopontine tegmental area. *American Journal of Physiology*, 2007, *294*, R102–R111.

Salm, A. K., Pavelko, M., Krouse, E. M., et al. Lateral amygdaloid nucleus expansion in adult rats is associated with exposure to prenatal stress. *Developmental Brain Research*, 2004, *148*, 159–167.

Salmelin, R., Schnitzler, A., Schmitz, F., and Freund, H. J. Single word reading in developmental stutterers and fluent speakers. *Brain*, 2000, *123*, 1184–1202.

Samson, H. H., Hodge, C. W., Tolliver, G. A., and Haraguchi, M. Effect of dopamine agonists and antagonists on ethanol reinforced behavior: The involvement of the nucleus accumbens. *Brain Research Bulletin*, 1993, *30*, 133–141.

Sanacora, G., Mason, G. F., Rothman, D. L., et al. Increased cortical GABA concentrations in depressed patients receiving ECT. *American Journal of Psychiatry*, 2003, *160*, 577–579.

Saper, C. B., Chou, T. C., and Scammell, T. E. The sleep switch: Hypothalamic control of sleep and wakefulness. *Trends in Neurosciences*, 2001, *24*, 726–731.

Saper, C. B., Scammell, T. E., and Lu, J. Hypothalamic regulation of sleep and circadian rhythms. *Nature*, 2005, *437*, 1257–1263.

Sapolsky, R. M. Is impaired neurogenesis relevant to the affective symptoms of depression? *Biological Psychiatry*, 2004, *56*, 137–139.

Sapolsky, R. M. Social subordinance as a marker of hypercortisolism: Some unexpected subtleties. *Annals of the New York Academy of Sciences*, 1995, *771*, 626–639.

Sapolsky, R. M. Stress, the Aging Brain and the Mechanisms of Neuron Death. Cambridge, Mass.: MIT Press, 1992.

Savic, I., Berglund, H., Gulyas, B., and Roland, P. Smelling of odorous sex hormone-like compounds causes sex-differentiated hypothalamic activations in humans. *Neuron*, 2001, *31*, 661–668.

Savic, I., Berglund, H., and Lindström, P. Brain response to putative pheromones in homosexual men. *Proceedings of the National Academy of Sciences, USA*, 2005, *102*, 7356–7361.

Sawaguchi, T., and Goldman-Rakic, P. S. The role of D1-dopamine receptor in working memory: Local injections of dopamine antagonists into the prefrontal cortex of rhesus monkeys performing an oculomotor delayed-response task. *Journal of Neurophysiology*, 1994, *71*, 515–528.

Sawchenko, P. E. Toward a new neurobiology of energy balance, appetite, and obesity: The anatomist weigh in. *Journal of Comparative Neurology*, 1998, *402*, 435–441.

Saxena, S., Brody, A. L., Schwartz, J. M., and Baxter, L. R. Neuroimaging and frontal-subcortical circuitry in obsessive-compulsive disorder. *British Journal of Psychiatry*, 1998, *173*, 26–37.

Scammell, T. E., Gerashchenko, D. Y., Mochizuki, T., et al. An adenosine A2a agonist increases sleep and induces Fos in ventrolateral preoptic neurons. *Neuroscience*, 2001, *107*, 653–663.

Scarpace, P. J., Matheny, M., Moore, R. L., and Kumar, M. V. Modulation of uncoupling protein 2 and uncoupling protein 3: Regulation by denervation, leptin and retinoic acid treatment. *Journal of Endocrinology*, 2000, *164*, 331–337.

Schafe, G. E., Bauer, E. P., Rosis, S., et al. Memory consolidation of Pavlovian fear conditioning requires nitric oxide signaling in the lateral amygdala. *European Journal of Neuroscience*, 2005, *22*, 201–211.

Schafe, G. E. Doyère, V., and LeDoux, J. E. Tracking the fear engram: The lateral amygdala is an essential locus of fear memory storage. *Journal of Neuroscience*, 2005, *25*, 10010–10015.

Schaller, G., Schmidt, A., Pleiner, J., et al. Plasma ghrelin concentrations are not regulated by glucose or insulin: A double-blind, placebo-controlled crossover clamp study. *Diabetes*, 2003, *52*, 16–20.

Schein, S. J., and Desimone, R. Spectral properties of V4 neurons in the macaque. *Journal of Neuroscience*, 1990, *10*, 3369–3389.

Schenck, C. H., Bundlie, S. R., Ettinger, M. G., and Mahowald, M. W. Chronic behavioral disorders of human REM sleep: A new category of parasomnia. *Sleep*, 1986, *9*, 293–308.

Schenck, C. H., Hurwitz, T. D., Bundlie, S. R., and Mahowald, M. W. Sleep-related eating disorders: Polysomnographic correlates of a heterogeneous syndrome distinct from daytime eating disorders. *Sleep*, 1991, *14*, 419–431.

Schenck, C. H., Hurwitz, T. D., and Mahowald, M. W. REM-sleep behavior disorder: An update on a series of 96 patients and a review of the world literature. *Journal of Sleep Research*, 1993, *2*, 224–231.

Schenck, C. H., and Mahowald, M. W. Motor dyscontrol in narcolepsy: Rapid-eye-movement (REM) sleep without atonia and REM sleep behavior disorder. *Annals of Neurology*, 1992, *32*, 3–10.

Schenk, D., Barbour, R., Dunn, W., et al. Immunization with amyloid-beta attenuates Alzheimer-disease-like pathology in the PDAPPmouse. *Nature*, 1999, 400, 173–177.

Schenkein, J., and Montagna, P. Self management of fatal familial insomnia. Part 1: What is FFI? *Medscape General Medicine*, 2006a, *8*, 65.

Schenkein, J., and Montagna, P. Self management of fatal familial insomnia. Part 2: Case Report. *Medscape General Medicine*, 2006b, *8*, 66.

Scherschlicht, R., Polc, P., Schneeberger, J., et al. Selective suppression of rapid eye movement sleep (REMS) in cats by typical and atypical antidepressants. In *Typical and Atypical Antidepressants: Molecular Mechanisms*, edited by E. Costa and G. Racagni. New York: Raven Press, 1982.

Schiffman, J., Ekstrom, M., LaBrie, J., et al. Minor physical anomalies and schizophrenia spectrum disorders: A prospective investigation. *American Journal of Psychiatry*, 2002, *159*, 238–243.

Schiffman, J., Walker, E., Ekstrom, M., et al. Childhood videotaped social and neuromotor precursors of schizophrenia: A prospective investigation, *American Journal of Psychiatry*, 2004, *161*, 2021–2027.

Schiller, P. H., and Malpeli, J. G. Properties and tectal projections of monkey retinal ganglion cells. *Journal of Neurophysiology*, 1977, *40*, 428–445.

Schmid, D., Held, K., Ising, M., et al. Ghrelin stimulates appetite, imagination of food, GH, ACTH, and cortisol, but does not affect leptin in normal controls. *Neuropsychopharmacology*, 2005, *30*, 1187–1192.

Schmidt, M. H., Valatx, J.-L., Sakai, K., et al. Role of the lateral preoptic area in sleep-related erectile mechanisms and sleep generation in the rat. *Journal of Neuroscience*, 2000, *20*, 6640–6647.

Schmidt-Hieber, C., Jonas, P., and Bischofberger, J. Enhanced synaptic plasticity in newly generated granule cells of the adult hippocampus. *Nature*, 2004, *429*, 184–187.

Schneider, B., Muller, M. J., and Philipp, M. Mortality in affective disorders. *Journal of the Affective Disorders*, 2001, *65*, 263–274.

Schneider, P., Scherg, M., Dosch, H. G., et al. Morphology of Heschl's gyrus reflects enhanced activation in the auditory cortex of musicians. *Nature Neuroscience*, 2002, *5*, 688–694.

Schnider, A. Spontaneous confabulation and the adaptation of thought to ongoing reality. *Nature Reviews Neuroscience*, 2003, *4*, 662–671.

Schoenfeld, M. A., Neuer, G., Tempelmann, C., et al. Functional magnetic resonance tomography correlates of taste perception in the human primary taste cortex. *Neuroscience*, 2004, *127*, 347–353.

Schrauwen, P., Xia, J., Bogardus, C., et al. Skeletal muscle uncoupling protein 3 expression is a determinant of energy expenditure in Pima Indians. *Diabetes*, 1999, *48*, 146–149.

Schultz, R. T. Developmental deficits in social perception in autism: The role of the amygdala and fusiform face area. *International Journal of Developmental Neuroscience*, 2005, *23*, 125–141.

Schulz, G. M., Varga, M., Jeffires, K., et al. Functional neuroanatomy of human vocalization: An $H_2^{15}O$ PET study. *Cerebral Cortex*, 2005, *15*, 1835–1847.

Schwartz, M. F., Marin, O. S. M., and Saffran, E. M. Dissociations of language function in dementia: A case study. *Brain and Language*, 1979, *7*, 277–306.

Schwartz, M. F., Saffran, E. M., and Marin, O. S. M. The word order problem in agrammatism. I. Comprehension. *Brain and Language*, 1980, *10*, 249–262.

Schwartz, S., Ponz, A., Poryazova, R., et al. Abnormal activity in hypothalamus and amygdala during humour processing in human narcolepsy with cataplexy. *Brain*, 2008, *131*, 514–522.

Schwartz, W. J., and Gainer, H. Suprachiasmatic nucleus: Use of ^{14}C-labelled deoxyglucose uptake as a functional marker. *Science*, 1977, *197*, 1089–1091.

Schwarzlose, R. F., Baker, C. I., and Kanwisher, N. Separate face and body selectivity on the fusiform gyrus. *Journal of Neuroscience*, 2005, *25*, 11055–11059.

Scott, K. The sweet and the bitter of mammalian taste. *Current Opinions in Neurobiology*, 2004, *14*, 423–427.

Scott, S. K., Blank, E. C., Rosen, S., and Wise, R. J. S. Identification of a pathway for intelligible speech in the left temporal lobe. *Brain*, 2000, *123*, 2400–2406.

Scott, T. R., and Plata-Salaman, C. R. Coding of taste quality. In *Smell and Taste in Health and Disease*, edited by T. N. Getchell. New York: Raven Press, 1991.

Scoville, W. B., and Milner, B. Loss of recent memory after bilateral hippocampal lesions. *Journal of Neurology, Neurosurgery and Psychiatry*, 1957, *20*, 11–21.

Sebat, J., Lakshmi, B., Malhotra, D., et al. Strong association of de novo copy number mutations with autism. *Science*, 2007, *316*, 445–449.

Selye, H. *The Stress of Life*. New York: McGraw-Hill, 1976.

Sforza, E., Montagna, P., Tinuper, P., et al. Sleep-wake cycle abnormalities in fatal familial insomnia: Evidence of the role of the thalamus in sleep regulation. *Electroencephalography and Clinical Neurophysiology*, 1995, *94*, 398–405.

Shallice, T. Phonological agraphia and the lexical route in writing. *Brain*, 1981, *104*, 413–429.

Sham, P. C., O'Callaghan, E., Takei, N., et al. Schizophrenia following pre-natal exposure to influenza epidemics between 1939 and

1960. *British Journal of Psychiatry*, 1992, *160*, 461–466.

Shannon, R. V. Understanding hearing through deafness. *Proceedings of the National Academy of Sciences, USA*, 2007, *104*, 6883–6884.

Shapiro, L. E., Leonard, C. M., Sessions, C. E., et al. Comparative neuroanatomy of the sexually dimorphic hypothalamus in monogamous and polygamous voles. *Brain Research*, 1991, *541*, 232–240.

Sharp, D. J., Scott, S. K., and Wise, R. J. S. Retrieving meaning after temporal lobe infarction: The role of the basal language area. *Annals of Neurology*, 2004, *56*, 836–846.

Shaywitz, B. A., Shaywitz, S. E., Pugh, K. R., et al. Disruption of posterior brain systems for reading in children with developmental dyslexia. *Biological Psychiatry*, 2002, *52*, 101–110.

Shearman, L. P., Sriram, S., Weaver, D. R., et al. Interacting molecular loops in the mammalian circadian clock. *Science*, 2000, *288*, 1013–1019.

Shen, K., and Meyer, T. Dynamic control of CaMKII translocation and localization in hippocampal neurons by NMDA stimulation. *Science*, 1999, *284*, 162–166.

Shenton, M. E., Dickey, C. C., Frumin, M., and McCarley, R. W. A review of MRI findings in schizophrenia. *Schizophrenia Research*, 2001, *49*, 1–52.

Shepherd, G. M. Discrimination of molecular signals by the olfactory receptor neuron. *Neuron*, 1994, *13*, 771–790.

Sher, A. E. Surgery for obstructive sleep apnea. *Progress in Clinical Biology Research*, 1990, *345*, 407–415.

Sherin, J. E., Elmquist, J. K., Torrealba, F., and Saper, C. B. Innervation of histaminergic tuberomammillary neurons by GABAergic and galaninergic neurons in the ventrolateral preoptic nucleus of the rat. *Journal of Neuroscience*, 1998, *18*, 4705–4721.

Shi, S.-H., Hayashi, Y., Petralia, R. S., et al. Rapid spine delivery and redistribution of AMPA receptors after synaptic NMDA receptor activation. *Science*, 1999, *284*, 1811–1816.

Shim, S. S., Hammonds, M. D., and Kee, B. S. Potentiation of the NMDA receptor in the treatment of schizophrenia: Focused on the glycine site. *European Archives of Psychiatry and Clinical Neuroscience*, 2008, *258*, 16–27.

Shimada, M., Tritos, N. A., Lowell, B. B., et al. Mice lacking melanin-concentrating hormone are hypophagic and lean. *Nature*, 1998, *396*, 670–674.

Shimura, T., Yamamoto, T., and Shimokochi, M. The medial preoptic area is involved in both sexual arousal and performance in male rats: Re-evaluation of neuron activity in freely moving animals. *Brain Research*, 1994, *640*, 215–222.

Shin, L. M., Wright, C. I., Cannistraro, P. A., et al. A functional magnetic resonance imaging study of amygdala and medial prefrontal cortex responses to overtly presented fearful faces in posttraumatic stress disorder. *Archives of General Psychiatry*, 2005, *62*, 273–281.

Shipley, M. T., and Ennis, M. Functional organization of the olfactory system. *Journal of Neurobiology*, 1996, *30*, 123–176.

Shoulson, I., Oakes, D., Fahn, S., et al. Parkinson Study Group. Impact of sustained deprenyl (selegiline) in levodopa-treated Parkinson's disease: A randomized placebo-controlled extension of the deprenyl and tocopherol antioxidative therapy of parkinsonism trial. *Annals of Neurology*, 2002, *51*, 604–612.

Shuto, Y., Shibasaki, T., Otagiri, A., et al. Hypothalamic growth hormone secretagogue receptor regulates growth hormone secretion, feeding, and adiposity. *Journal of Clinical Investigation*, 2002, *109*, 1429–1436.

Sidman, M., Stoddard, L. T., and Mohr, J. P. Some additional quantitative observations of immediate memory in a patient with bilateral hippocampal lesions. *Neuropsychologia*, 1968, *6*, 245–254.

Siegel, J. Clues to the functions of mammalian sleep. *Nature*, 2005, *437*, 1264–1271.

Siegel, R. M., and Andersen, R. A. Motion perceptual deficits following ibotenic acid lesions of the middle temporal area (MT) in the behaving monkey. *Society for Neuroscience Abstracts*, 1986, *12*, 1183.

Siegel, S. A. Pavlovian conditioning analysis of morphine tolerance. In *Behavioral Tolerance: Research and Treatment Implications*, edited by N. A. Krasnegor. Washington, DC: NIDA Research Monographs, 1978.

Siegel, S., Hinson, R. E., Krank, M. D., and McCully, J. Heroin "overdose" death: Contribution of drug-associated environmental cues. *Science*, 1982, *216*, 436–437.

Siegle, G. J., Carter, C. S., and Thase, M. E. Use of fMRI to predict recovery from unipolar depression with cognitive behavior therapy. *American Journal of Psychiatry*, 2006, *163*, 735–738.

Silva, A. J., Stevens, C. F., Tonegawa, S., and Wang, Y. Deficient hippocampal long-term potentiation in-calcium-calmodulin kinase II mutant mice. *Science*, 1992, *257*, 201–206.

Silver, J. M., Shin, C., and McNamara, J. O. Antiepileptogenic effects of conventional anticonvulsants in the kindling model of epilepsy. *Annals of Neurology*, 1991, *29*, 356–363.

Silver, R., LeSauter, J., Tresco, P. A., and Lehman, M. N. A diffusible coupling signal from the transplanted suprachiasmatic nucleus controlling circadian locomotor rhythms. *Nature*, 1996, *382*, 810–813.

Silveri, M. C. Peripheral aspects of writing can be differentially affected by sensorial and attentional defect: Evidence from a patient with afferent dysgraphia and case dissociation. *Cortex*, 1996, *32*, 155–172.

Simpson, J. B., Epstein, A. N., and Camardo, J. S. The localization of dipsogenic receptors for angiotensin II in the subfornical organ. *Journal of Comparative and Physiological Psychology*, 1978, *92*, 581–608.

Simuni, T., Jaggi, J. L., Mulholland, H., et al. Bilateral stimulation of the subthalamic nucleus in patients with Parkinson disease: A study of efficacy and safety. *Journal of Neurosurgery*, 2002, *96*, 666–672.

Sinclair, A. H., Berta, P., Palmer, M. S., et al. A gene from the human sex-determining region encodes a protein with homology to a conserved DNA-binding motif. *Nature*, 1990, *346*, 240–244.

Sindelar, D. K., Ste. Marie, L., Miura, G. I., et al. Neuropeptide Y is required for hyperphagic feeding in response to neuroglucopenia. *Endocrinology*, 2004, *145*, 3363–3368.

Singer, C., and Weiner, W. J. Male sexual dysfunction. *Neurologist*, 1996, *2*, 119–129.

Singer, F., and Zumoff, B. Subnormal serum testosterone levels in male internal medicine residents. *Steroids*, 1992, *57*, 86–89.

Singer, T., Seymour, B., O'Doherty, J., et al. Empathy for pain involves the affective but not sensory components of pain. *Science*, 2004, *303*, 1157–1162.

Singh, D., and Bronstad, P. M. Female body odour is a potential cue to ovulation. *Proceedings of the Royal Society of London B*, 2001, *268*, 797–801.

Sinha, S. R., and Kossoff, E. H. The ketogenic diet. *Neurologist*, 2005, *11*, 161–170.

Sipos, M. L., and Nyby, J. G. Concurrent androgenic stimulation of the ventral tegmental area and medial preoptic area: Synergistic effects on male-typical reproductive behaviors in house mice. *Brain Research*, 1996, *729*, 29–44.

Skaggs, W. E., and McNaughton, B. L. Spatial firing properties of hippocampal CA$_1$ populations in an environment containing two visually identical regions. *Journal of Neuroscience*, 1998, *18*, 8455–8466.

Skene, D. J., Lockley, S. W., and Arendt, J. Melatonin in circadian sleep disorders in the blind. *Biological Signals and Receptors*, 1999, *8*, 90–95.

Skutella, T., Criswell, H., Moy, S., et al. Corticotropin-releasing hormone (CRH) antisense oligodeoxynucleotide induces anxiolytic effects in rat. *Neuroreport*, 1994, *5*, 2181–2185.

Slotkin, T. A. Fetal nicotine or cocaine exposure: Which one is worse? *Journal of Pharmacology and Experimental Therapeutics*, 1998, *22*, 521–527.

Smith, G. P. Animal models of human eating disorders. *Annals of the New York Academy of Sciences*, 1989, *16*, 219–237.

Smith, G. P., Gibbs, J., and Kulkosky, P. J. Relationships between brain-gut peptides and neurons in the control of food intake. In *The Neural Basis of Feeding and Reward*, edited by B. G. Hoebel and D. Novin. Brunswick, Me.: Haer Institute, 1982.

Smith, M. J. Sex determination: Turning on sex. *Current Biology*, 1994, *4*, 1003–1005.

Snyder, B. J., and Olanow, C. W. Stem cell treatment for Parkinson's disease: An update for 2005. *Current Opinion in Neurobiology*, 2005, *18*, 376–385.

Snyder, L. H., Batista, A. P., and Andersen, R. A. Intention-related activity in the posterior parietal cortex: A review. *Vision Research*, 2000, *40*, 1433–1441.

Snyder, S. H. *Madness and the Brain*. New York: McGraw-Hill, 1974.

Soares, J. C., and Gershon, S. The lithium ion: A foundation for psychopharmacological specificity. *Neuropsychopharmacology*, 1998, *19*, 167–182.

Södersten, P., Bergh, C., and Zandian, M. Understanding eating disorders. *Hormones and Behavior*, 2006, *50*, 572–578.

Solyom, L., Turnbull, I. M., and Wilensky, M. A case of self-inflicted leucotomy. *British Journal of Psychiatry*, 1987, *151*, 855–857.

Soria, G., Mendizabal, V., Rourino, C., et al. Lack of CB$_1$ cannabinoid receptor impairs cocaine self-administration. *Neuropsychopharmacology*, 2005, *30*, 1670–1680.

Sormani, M. P., Bruzzi, P., Comi, G., and Filippi, M. The distribution of the magnetic resonance imaging response to glatiramer acetate in multiple sclerosis. *Multiple Sclerosis*, 2005, *11*, 447–449.

Sotillo, M., Carretié, L., Hinojosa, J. A., et al. Neural activity associated with metaphor comprehension: Spatial analysis. *Neuroscience Letters*, 2005, *373*, 5–9.

Soto, C. Unfolding the role of protein misfolding in neurodegenerative diseases. *Nature Review Neuroscience*, 2003, *4*, 49–60.

Sotthibundhu, A., Sykes, A. M., Fox, B., et al. β-Amyloid$_{1-42}$ induces neuronal death through the p75 neurotrophin receptor. *Journal of Neuroscience*, 2008, *28*, 3941–3946.

Speelman, J. D., Schuurman, R., de Bie, R. M., et al. A. Stereotactic neurosurgery for tremor. *Movement Disorders*, 2002, *17*, S84–S88.

Sperry, R. W. Brain bisection and consciousness. In *Brain and Conscious Experience*, edited by J. Eccles. New York: Springer-Verlag, 1966.

Spiers, H. J., Maguire, E. A., and Burgess, N. Hippocampal amnesia. *Neurocase*, 2001, *7*, 357–382.

Squire, L. R. Memory and the hippocampus: A synthesis from findings with rats, monkeys, and humans. *Psychological Review*, 1992, *99*, 195–231.

Squire, L. R. Stable impairment in remote memory following electroconvulsive therapy. *Neuropsychologia*, 1974, *13*, 51–58.

Squire, L. R., and Bayley, P. J. The neuroscience of remote memory. *Current Opinion in Neurobiology*, 2007, *17*, 185–196.

Squire, L. R., Shimamura, A. P., and Amaral, D. G. Memory and the hippocampus. In *Neural Models of Plasticity: Experimental and Theoretical Approaches*, edited by J. H. Byrne and W. O. Berry. San Diego: Academic Press, 1989.

St. George-Hyslop, P. H., Tanzi, R. E., Polinsky, R. J., et al. The genetic defect causing familial Alzheimer's disease maps on chromosome 21. *Science*, 1987, *235*, 885–890.

Stahl, S. M., Grady, M. M., Moret, C., and Briley, M. SNRIs: Their pharmacology, clinical efficacy, and tolerability in comparison with other classes of antidepressants. *CNS Spectrums*, 2005, *10*, 732–747.

Stanislavsky, C. *An Actor Prepares*. New York: Theater Arts/Routledge, 1936.

Starkey, S. J., Walker, M. P., Beresford, I. J. M., and Hagan, R. M. Modulation of the rat suprachiasmatic circadian clock by melatonin in-vitro. *Neuroreport*, 1995, *6*, 1947–1951.

Steele, A. D., Emsley, J. G., Ozdinler, P. H., et al. Prion protein (PrPc) positively regulates neural precursor proliferation during developmental and adult mammalian neurogenesis. *Proceedings of the National Academy of Sciences, USA*, 2006, *203*, 3416–3421.

Steeves, J. K. E., Humphrey, G. K., Culham, J. C., et al. Behavioral and neuroimaging evidence for a contribution of color and texture information to scene classification in a patient with visual form agnosia. *Journal of Cognitive Neuroscience*, 2004, *16*, 955–965.

Stefanacci, L., and Amaral, D. G. Topographic organization of cortical inputs to the lateral nucleus of the macaque monkey amygdala: A retrograde tracing study. *Journal of Comparative Neurology*, 2000, *22*, 52–79.

Stefanatos, G. A., Gershkoff, A., and Madigan, S. On pure word deafness, temporal processing, and the left hemisphere. *Journal of the International Neuropsychological Society*, 2005, *11*, 456–470.

Stein, M. B., Jang, K. L., Taylor, S., et al. Genetic and environmental influences on trauma exposure and posttraumatic stress disorder symptoms: A twin study. *American Journal of Psychiatry*, 2002, *159*, 1675–1681.

Stein, M. B., Simmons, A. N., Feinstein, J. S., and Paulus, M. P. Increased amygdala and insula activation during emotion processing in anxiety-prone subjects. *American Journal of Psychiatry*, 2007, *164*, 318–327.

Stein, M. B., and Uhde, T. W. The biology of anxiety disorders. In American Psychiatric Press Textbook of Psychopharmacology. Washington, DC: American Psychiatric Press, 1995.

Steinhausen, H. C. The outcome of anorexia nervosa in the 20th century. *American Journal of Psychiatry*, 2002, *159*, 1284–1293.

Steininger, R. L., Alam, M. N., Szymusiak, R., and McGinty, D. State dependent discharge of ruberomammillary neurons in the rat hypothalamus. *Sleep Research*, 1996, *25*, 28.

Stephan, F. K., and Nuñez, A. A. Elimination of circadian rhythms in drinking activity, sleep, and temperature by isolation of the suprachiasmatic nuclei. *Behavioral Biology*, 1977, *20*, 1–16.

Stephan, F. K., and Zucker, I. Circadian rhythms in drinking behavior and locomotor activity of rats are eliminated by hypothalamic lesion. *Proceedings of the National Academy of Sciences, USA*, 1972, *69*, 1583–1586.

Steriade, M. Arousal: Revisiting the reticular activating system. *Science*, 1996, *272*, 225–226.

Stevens, J. R. Neurology and neuropathology of schizophrenia. In *Schizophrenia as a Brain Disease*, edited by F. A. Henn and H. A. Nasrallah. New York: Oxford University Press, 1982.

Stinson, D., and Thompson, C. Clinical experience with phototherapy. *Journal of the Affective Disorders*, 1990, *18*, 129–135.

Stolerman, I. P., and Jarvis, M. J. The scientific case that nicotine is addictive. *Psychopharmacology*, 1995, *117*, 2–10.

Stone, A. A., Reed, B. R., and Neale, J. M. Changes in daily event frequency precede episodes of physical symptoms. *Journal of Human Stress*, 1987, *13*, 70–74.

Stowers, L., Holy, T. E., Meister, M., et al. Loss of sex discrimination of male-male aggression in mice deficient for TRP2. *Science*, 2002, *295*, 1493–1500.

Strange, P. G. Antipsychotic drug action: Antagonism, inverse agonism or partial agonism. *Trends in Pharmacological Science*, 2008, *29*, 314–321.

Sturgis, J. D., and Bridges, R. S. N-methyl-DL-aspartic acid lesions of the medial preoptic area disrupt ongoing parental behavior in male rats. *Physiology and Behavior*, 1997, *62*, 305–310.

Styron, W. *Darkness Visible: A Memoir of Madness*. New York: Random House, 1990.

Sulik, K. K. Genesis of alcohol-induced craniofacial dysmorphism. *Experimental Biology and Medicine*, 2005, *230*, 366–375.

Sun, Y., Ahmed, S., and Smith, R. G. Deletion of ghrelin impairs neither growth nor appetite. *Molecular and Cellular Biology*, 2003, *23*, 7973–7981.

Sun, Y., Wang, P., Zheng, H., and Smith, R. G. Ghrelin stimulation of growth hormone release and appetite is mediated through the growth hormone secretagogue receptor. *Proceedings of the National Academy of Sciences, USA*, 2004, *101*, 4679–4684.

Suntsova, N., Guzman-Marin, R., Kumar, S., et al. The median preoptic nucleus reciprocally modulates activity of arousal-related and sleep-related neurons in the perifornical lateral hypothalamus. *Journal of Neuroscience*, 2007, *27*, 1616–1630.

Suzdak, P. D., Glowa, J. R., Crawley, J. N., et al. A selective imidazobenzodiazepine antagonist of ethanol in the rat. *Science*, 1986, *234*, 1243–1247.

Suzuki, W. A., and Amaral, D. G. Functional neuroanatomy of the medial temporal lobe memory system. *Cortex*, 2004, *40*, 220–222.

Swaab, D. F., Gooren, L. J. G., and Hofman, M. A. Brain research, gender, and sexual orientation. *Journal of Homosexuality*, 1995, *28*, 283–301.

Swaab, D. F., and Hofman, M. A. An enlarged suprachiasmatic nucleus in homosexual men. *Brain Research*, 1990, *537*, 141–148.

Sweet, W. H. Participant in brain stimulation in behaving subjects. Neurosciences Research Program Workshop, 1966.

Swerdlow, N. R., Geyer, M. A., Vale, W. W., and Koob, G. F. Corticotropin-releasing factor potentiates acoustic startle in rats: Blockade by chlordiazepoxide. *Psychopharmacology*, 1986, *88*, 147–152.

Szuba, M. P., Baxter, L. R., and Fairbanks, L. A. Effects of partial sleep deprivation on the diurnal variation of mood and motor activity in major depression. *Biological Psychiatry*, 1991, *30*, 817–829.

Takahashi, L. K. Hormonal regulation of sociosexual behavior in female mammals. *Neuroscience and Biobehavioral Reviews*, 1990, *14*, 403–413.

Takahashi, Y. K., Nagayma, S., and Mori, K. Detection and masking of spoiled food smells by odor maps in the olfactory bulb. *Journal of Neuroscience*, 2004, *24*, 8690–8694.

Takashima, A., Petersson, K. M., Rutters, F., et al. Declarative memory consolidation in humans: A prospective functional magnetic resonance imaging study. *Proceedings of the National Academy of Sciences, USA*, 2006, *103*, 756–761.

Tan, L. H., Laird, A. R., Li, K., and Fox, P. T. Neuroanatomical correlates of phonological processing of Chinese characters and alphabetic words: A meta-analysis. *Human Brain Mapping*, 2005, *25*, 83–91.

Tan, T. M. M., Vanderpump, M., Khoo, B., et al. Somatostatin infusion lowers plasma ghrelin without reducing appetite in adults with Prader-Willi syndrome. *Journal of Clinical Endocrinology and Metabolism*, 2004, *89*, 4162–4165.

Tanner, C. M. The role of environmental toxins in the etiology of Parkinson's disease. *Trends in Neuroscience*, 1989, *12*, 49–54.

Tarter, R. E., Kirisci, L., Mezzich, A., et al. Neurobehavioral disinhibition in childhood predicts early age at onset of substance use disorder. *American Journal of Psychiatry*, 2003, *160*, 1078–1085.

Taub, E., Uswatte, F., King, D. K., et al. A placebo-controlled trial of constraint-induced movement therapy for upper extremity after stroke. *Stroke*, 2006, *37*, 1045–1049.

Tavera-Mendoza, L. E., and White, J. H. Cell defenses and the sunshine vitamin. *Scientific American*, 2007, *297(5)*, 62–72.

Teitelbaum, P., and Stellar, E. Recovery from the failure to eat produced by hypothalamic lesions. *Science*, 1954, *120*, 894–895.

Terenius, L., and Wahlström, A. Morphine-like ligand for opiate receptors in human CSF. *Life Sciences*, 1975, *16*, 1759–1764.

Terman, M. Evolving applications of light therapy. *Sleep Medicine Reviews*, 2007, *11*, 497–507.

Terry, R. D., and Davies, P. Dementia of the Alzheimer type. *Annual Review of Neuroscience*, 1980, *3*, 77–96.

Tetel, M. J., Getzinger, M. J., and Blaustein, J. D. Fos expression in the rat brain following vaginal-cervical stimulation by mating and manual probing. *Journal of Neuroendocrinology*, 1993, *5*, 397–404.

Tetrud, J. W., and Langston, J. W. The effect of deprenyl (Selegiline) on the natural history of Parkinson's disease. *Science*, 1989, *245*, 519–522.

Thaker, G. K., and Carpenter, W. T. Advances in schizophrenia. *Nature Medicine*, 2001, *7*, 667–671.

Thapar, A., O'Donovan, M., and Owen, M. J. The genetics of attention deficit hyperactivity disorder. *Human Molecular Genetics*, 2005, *14*, R275–R282.

Thase, M. E. Treatment issues related to sleep and depression. *Journal of Clinical Psychiatry*, 2000, *61*, 46–50.

Theorell, T., Leymann, H., Jodko, M., et al. "Person under train" incidents: Medical consequences for subway drivers. *Psychosomatic Medicine*, 1992, *54*, 480–488.

Thiels, E., Xie, X. P., Yeckel, M. F., et al. NMDA receptor-dependent LTD in different subfields of hippocampus in vivo and in vitro. *Hippocampus*, 1996, *6*, 43–51.

Thomas, C., Avidan, G., Humphreys, K., et al. Reduced structural connectivity in ventral visual cortex in congenital prosopagnosia. *Nature Neuroscience*, 2009, *12*, 29–31.

Thompson, S. M., Fortunato, C., McKinney, R. A., et al. Mechanisms underlying the neuropathological consequences of epileptic activity in the rat hippocampus in vitro. *Journal of Comparative Neurology*, 1996, *372*, 515–528.

Thompson, W. W., Price, C., Goodson, B., et al. Early thimerosal exposure and neuropsychological outcomes at 7 to 10 years. *New England Journal of Medicine*, 2007, *357*, 1281–1292.

Thomson, J. J. *Rights, Restitution, and Risk: Essays in Moral Theory*. Cambridge, MA: Harvard University Press, 1986.

Thuy, D. H. D., Matsuo, K., Nakamura, K., et al. Implicit and explicit processing of kanji and kana words and non-words studied with fMRI. *Neuroimage*, 2004, *23*, 878–889.

Toh, K. L., Jones, C. R., He, Y., et al. An h*Per2* phosphorylation site mutation in familial advanced sleep phase syndrome. *Science*, 2001, *291*, 1040–1043.

Tootell, R. B. H., Tsao, D., and Vanduffel, W. Neuroimaging weighs in: Humans meet macaques in "primate" visual cortex. *Journal of Neuroscience*, 2003, *23*, 3981–3989.

Topper, R., Kosinski, C., and Mull, M. Volitional type of facial palsy associated with pontine ischemia. *Journal of Neurology, Neurosurgery, and Psychiatry*, 1995, *58*, 732–734.

Tordoff, M. G., and Friedman, M. I. Hepatic control of feeding: Effect of glucose, fructose, and mannitol. *American Journal of Physiology*, 1988, *254*, R969–R976.

Tracy, J. L., and Robbins, R. W. The automaticity of emotion recognition. *Emotion*, 2008, *8*, 81–95.

Triarhou, L. C. The percipient observations of Constantin von Economo on encephalitis lethargica and sleep disruption and their lasting impact on contemporary sleep research. *Brain Research Bulletin*, 2006, *69*, 244–258.

Trulson, M. E., and Jacobs, B. L. Raphe unit activity in freely moving cats: Correlation with level of behavioral arousal. *Brain Research*, 1979, *163*, 135–150.

Tsacopoulos, M., and Magistretti, P. J. Metabolic coupling between glia and neurons. *Journal of Neuroscience*, 1996, *16*, 877–885.

Tsao, D. Y., Vanduffel, W., Sasaki, Y., et al. Stereopsis activates V3A and caudal intraparietal areas in macaques and humans. *Neuron*, 2003, *39*, 555–568.

Tschöp, M., Smiley, D. L., and Heiman, M. L. Ghrelin induces adiposity in rodents. *Nature*, 2000, *407*, 908–913.

Tsien, J. Z., Huerta, P. T., and Tonegawa, S. The essential role of hippocampal CA1 NMDA receptor-dependent synaptic plasticity in spatial memory. *Cell*, 1996, *87*, 1327–1338.

Tsuang, M. T., Gilbertson, M. W., and Faraone, S. V. The genetics of schizophrenia: Current knowledge and future directions. *Schizophrenia Research*, 1991, *4*, 157–171.

Tucker, M. A., Hirota, Y., Wamsley, E. J., et al. A daytime nap containing solely non-REM sleep enhances declarative but not procedural memory. *Neurobiology of Learning and Memory*, 2006, *86*, 241–247.

Turner, S. M., Beidel, D. C., and Nathan, R. S. Biological factors in obsessive-compulsive disorders. *Psychological Bulletin*, 1985, *97*, 430–450.

Tyrell, J. B., and Baxter, J. D. Glucocorticoid therapy. In *Endocrinology and Metabolism*, edited by P. Felig, J. D. Baxter, A. E. Broadus, and L. A. Frohman. New York: McGraw-Hill, 1981.

Unger, J., McNeill, T. H., Moxley, R. T., et al. Distribution of insulin receptor-like immunoreactivity in the rat forebrain. *Neuroscience*, 1989, *31*, 143–157.

Ungerleider, L. G., and Mishkin, M. Two cortical visual systems. In *Analysis of Visual Behavior*, edited by D. J. Ingle, M. A. Goodale, and R. J. W. Mansfield. Cambridge, Mass.: MIT Press, 1982.

Uno, H., Tarara, R., Else, J. G., et al. Hippocampal damage associated with prolonged and fatal stress in primates. *Journal of Neuroscience*, 1989, *9*, 1705–1711.

Urban, P. P., Wicht, S., Marx, J., Mitrovic, S., et al. Isolated voluntary facial paresis due to pontine ischemia. *Neurology*, 1998, *50*, 1859–1862.

Urgesi, C., Berlucchi, G., and Aglioti, S. M. Magnetic stimulation of extrastriate body area impairs visual processing of nonfacial body parts. *Current Biology*, 2004, *13*, 2130–2134.

Vaina, L. M. Complex motion perception and its deficits. *Current Opinion in Neurobiology*, 1998, *8*, 494–502.

Valenstein, E. S. *Great and Desperate Cures: The Rise and Decline of Psychosurgery and Other Radical Treatments for Mental Illness*. New York: Basic Books, 1986.

Valenza, N., Ptak, R., Zimine, I., et al. Dissociated active and passive tactile shape recognition: A case study of pure tactile apraxia. *Brain*, 2001, *124*, 2287–2298.

Vandenbergh, J. G., Whitsett, J. M., and Lombardi, J. R. Partial isolation of a pheromone accelerating puberty in female mice. *Journal of Reproductive Fertility*, 1975, *43*, 515–523.

Vandenbulcke, M., Peeters, R., Fannes, K., and Vandenberghe, R. Knowledge of visual attributes in the right hemisphere. *Nature Neuroscience*, 2006, *9*, 964–970.

Van den Top, M., Lee, K., Whyment, A. D., et al. Orexigen-sensitive NPY/AGRP pacemaker neurons in the hypothalamic arcuate nucleus. *Nature Neuroscience*, 2004, *7*, 493–494.

van der Lee, S., and Boot, L. M. Spontaneous pseudopregnancy in mice. *Acta Physiologica et Pharmacologica Neerlandica*, 1955, *4*, 442–444.

Vanderwolf, C. H. The electrocorticogam in relation to physiology and behavior: A new analysis. *Electroencephalography and Clinical Neurophysiology*, 1992, *82*, 165–175.

Van Gelder, R. N., Herzog, E. D., Schwartz, W. J., and Taghert, P. H. Circadian rhythms: In the loop at last. *Science*, 2003, *300*, 1534–1535.

Van Goozen, S., Wiegant, V., Endert, E., et al. Psychoendrocrinological assessments of the menstrual cycle: The relationship between hormones, sexuality, and mood. *Archives of Sexual Behavior*, 1997, *26*, 359–382.

Van Leengoed, E., Kerker, E., and Swanson, H. H. Inhibition of post-partum maternal behaviour in the rat by injecting an oxytocin antagonist into the cerebral ventricles. *Journal of Endocrinology*, 1987, *112*, 275–282.

Vassar, R., Ngai, J., and Axel, R. Spatial segregation of odorant receptor expression in the mammalian olfactory epithelium. *Cell*, 1993, *74*, 309–318.

Veldman, B. A., Wijn, A. M., Knoers, N., et al. Genetic and environmental risk factors in Parkinson's disease. *Clinical Neurology and Neurosurgery*, 1998, *100*, 15–26.

Vergnes, M., Depaulis, A., Boehrer, A., and Kempf, E. Selective increase of offensive behavior in the rat following intrahypothalamic 5,7-DHT-induced serotonin depletion. *Brain Research*, 1988, *29*, 85–91.

Verney, E. B. The antidiuretic hormone and the factors which determine its release. *Proceedings of the Royal Society of London [B]*, 1947, *135*, 25–106.

Vewers, M. E., Dhatt, R., and Tejwani, G. A. Naltrexone administration affects ad libitum smoking behavior. *Psychopharmacology*, 1998, *140*, 185–190.

Vgontzas, A. N., and Kales, A. Sleep and its disorders. *Annual Review of Medicine*, 1999, *50*, 387–400.

Vikingstad, E. M., Cao, Y., Thomas, A. J., et al. Language hemispheric dominance in patients with congenital lesions of eloquent brain. *Neurosurgery*, 2000, *47*, 562–570.

Vinckier, F., Dehaene, S., Jobert, A., et al. Hierarchical coding of letter strings in the ventral stream: Dissecting the inner organization of the visual word-form system. *Neurons*, 2007, *55*, 143–156.

Virkkunen, M., De Jong, J., Bartko, J., and Linnoila, M. Psychobiological concomitants of history of suicide attempts among violent offenders and impulsive fire setters. *Archives of General Psychiatry*, 1989, *46*, 604–606.

Vocci, F. J., Acri, J., and Elkashef, A. Medical development for addictive disorders: The state of the science. *American Journal of Psychiatry*, 2005, *162*, 1431–1440.

Vogel, G. W., Buffenstein, A., Minter, K., and Hennessey, A. Drug effects on REM sleep and on endogenous depression. *Neuroscience and Biobehavioral Reviews*, 1990, *14*, 49–63.

Vogel, G. W., Thurmond, A., Gibbons, P., et al. REM sleep reduction effects on depression syndromes. *Archives of General Psychiatry*, 1975, *32*, 765–777.

Vogel, G. W., Vogel, F., McAbee, R. S., and Thurmond, A. J. Improvement of depression by REM sleep deprivation: New findings and a theory. *Archives of General Psychiatry*, 1980, *37*, 247–253.

Volkow, N. D., Wang, G.-J., Fowler, J. S., et al. "Nonhedonic" food motivation in humans involves dopamine in the dorsal striatum and methyl phenidate amplifies this effect. *Synapse*, 2002, *44*, 175–180.

Volkow, N. D., Wang, G.-J., Telang, F., et al. Cocaine cues and dopamine in dorsal striatum: Mechanism of craving in cocaine addiction. *Journal of Neuroscience*, 2006, *26*, 6583–6588.

Volpe, B. T., LeDoux, J. E., and Gazzaniga, M. S. Information processing of visual stimuli in an "extinguished" field. *Nature*, 1979, *282*, 722–724.

Wada, H., Inagaki, N., Itowi, N., and Yamatodani, A. Histaminergic neuron systems in the brain: Distribution and possible functions. *Brain Research Bulletin*, 1991, *27*, 367–370.

Wallen, K. Sex and context: Hormones and primate sexual motivation. *Hormones and Behavior*, 2001, *40*, 339–357.

Wallen, K. Desire and ability: Hormones and the regulation of female sexual behavior. *Neuroscience and Biobehavioral Reviews*, 1990, *14*, 233–241.

Wallen, K., Eisler, J. A., Tannenbaum, P. L., et al. Antide (Nal-Lys GnRH antagonist) suppression of pituitary-testicular function and sexual behavior in group-living rhesus monkeys. *Physiology and Behavior*, 1991, *50*, 429–435.

Walsh, B. T., and Devlin, M. J. Eating disorders: Progress and problems. *Science*, 1998, *280*, 1387–1390.

Walsh, T., McClellan, J. M., McCarthy, S. E., et al. Rare structural variants disrupt multiple genes in Neurodevelopmental pathways in schizophrenia. *Science*, 2008, *320*, 539–543.

Walsh, V., Carden, D., Butler, S. R., and Kulikowski, J. J. The effects of V4 lesions on the visual abilities of macaques: Hue discrimination and color constancy. *Behavioural Brain Research*, 1993, *53*, 51–62.

Walters, E. E., and Kendler, K. S. Anorexia nervosa and anorexic-like syndromes in a population-based female twin sample. *American Journal of Psychiatry*, 1995, *152*, 64–71.

Wandell, B. A., Dumoulin, S. O., and Brewer, A. A. Visual field maps in human cortex. *Neuron*, 2007, *56*, 366–383.

Wang, G. J., Hinrichs, A. L., Stock, H., et al. Evidence of common and specific genetic effects: Association of the muscarinic acetylcholine receptor M2 (CHRM2) gene with alcohol dependence and major depressive syndrome. *Human Molecular Genetics*, 2004, *13*, 1903–1911.

Wang, Z., Faith, M., Patterson, F., et al. Neural substrates of abstinence-induced cigarette cravings in chronic smokers. *Journal of Neuroscience*, 2007, *27*, 14035–14040.

Ward, H. E., Johnson, E. A., Salm, A. K., and Birkle, D. L. Effects of prenatal stress on defensive withdrawal behavior and corticotrophin releasing factor systems in rat brain. *Physiology and Behavior*, 2000, *70*, 359–366.

Warne, G. L., and Zajac, J. D. Disorders of sexual differentiation. *Endocrinology and Metabolism Clinics of North America*, 1998, *27*, 945–967.

Watkins, K. E., Dronkers, N. F., and Vargha-Khadem, F. Behavioural analysis of an inherited speech and language disorder: Comparison with acquired aphasia. *Brain*, 2002, *125*, 452–464.

Watkins, K. E., Smith, S. M., Davis, S., and Howell, P. Structural and functional abnormalities of the motor system in developmental stuttering. *Brain*, 2008, *131*, 50–59.

Watkins, K. E., Vargha-Khadem, F., Ashburner, J., et al. MRI analysis of an inherited speech and language disorder: Structural brain abnormalities. *Brain*, 2002, *125*, 465–478.

Wattendorf, D. J., and Muenke, M. Prader-Willi syndrome. *American Family Physician*, 2005, *72*, 827–830.

Weinberger, D. R. Schizophrenia and the frontal lobe. *Trends in Neurosciences*, 1988, *11*, 367–370.

Weinberger, D. R., and Wyatt, R. J. Brain morphology in schizophrenia: *In vivo* studies. In *Schizophrenia as a Brain Disease*, edited by F. A. Henn and H. A. Nasrallah. New York: Oxford University Press, 1982.

Weiner, R. D., and Krystal, A. D. The present use of electroconvulsive therapy. *Annual Review of Medicine*, 1994, *45*, 273–281.

Weiser, M., Reichenberg, A., Grotto, I., et al. Higher rates of cigarette smoking in male adolescents before the onset of schizophrenia: A historical-prospective cohort study. *American Journal of Psychiatry*, 2004, *161*, 1219–1223.

Wernicke, C. *Der Aphasische Symptomenkomplex*. Breslau, Poland: Cohn & Weigert, 1874.

Whalen, P. J., Rauch, S. L., Etcoff, N. L., et al. Masked presentations of emotional facial expressions modulate amygdala activity without explicit knowledge. *Journal of Neuroscience*, 1998, *18*, 411–418.

Whipple, B., and Komisaruk, B. R. Analgesia produced in women by genital self-stimulation. *Journal of Sex Research*, 1988, *24*, 130–140.

White, F. J. Synaptic regulation of mesocorticolimbic dopamine neurons. *Annual Review of Neuroscience*, 1996, *19*, 405–436.

White, J. Autonomic discharge from stimulation of the hypothalamus in man. *Association for Research in Nervous and Mental Disorders*, 1940, *20*, 854–863.

Whiteside, S. P., Port, J. D., and Abramowitz, J. S. A meta-analysis of functional neuroimaging in obsessive-compulsive disorder. *Psychiatry Research: Neuroimaging*, 2004, *132*, 69–79.

Whitten, W. K. Occurrence of anestrus in mice caged in groups. *Journal of Endocrinology*, 1959, *18*, 102–107.

WHO. *Tobacco or Health, a Global Status Report*. Geneva, Switzerland: World Health Organization Publications, 1997.

Wickelgren, I. Drug may suppress the craving for nicotine. *Science*, 1998, *282*, 1797–1798.

Wiesner, B. P., and Sheard, N. *Maternal Behaviour in the Rat*. London: Oliver and Brody, 1933.

Wigren, H.-K., Schepens, M., Matto, V., et al. Glutamatergic stimulation of the basal forebrain elevates extracellular adenosine and increases the subsequent sleep. *Neuroscience*, 2007, *147*, 811–823.

Wilensky, A. E., Schafe, G. E., and LeDoux, J. E. Functional inactivation of the amygdala before but not after auditory fear conditioning prevents memory formation. *Journal of Neuroscience*, 1999, *19*, RC48 (1–5).

Wilhelmus, M. M. M., Otte-Höller, I., Davis, J., et al. Apolipoprotein E genotype regulates amyloid-β cytotoxicity. *Journal of Neuroscience*, 2005, *25*, 3621–3627.

Willesen, M. G., Kristensen, P., and Romer, J. Co-localization of growth hormone secretagogue receptor and NPY mRNA in the arcuate nucleus of the rat. *Neuroendocrinology*, 1999, *70*, 306–316.

Williams, J. R., Insel, T. R., Harbaugh, C. R., and Carter, C. S. Oxytocin centrally administered facilitates formation of a partner preference in female prairie voles (*Microtus ochrogaster*). *Journal of Neuroendocrinology*, 1994, *6*, 247–250.

Williams, Z. M., and Eskandar, E. N. Selective enhancement of associative learning by microstimulation of the anterior caudate. *Nature Neuroscience*, 2006, *9*, 562–568.

Willour, V. L., Shugart, Y. Y., Samuels, J., et al. Replication study supports evidence for linkage to 9p24 in obsessive-compulsive disorder. *American Journal of Medical Genetics*, 2004, *75*, 508–513.

Wilson, B. E., Meyer, G. E., Cleveland, J. C., and Weigle, D. S. Identification of candidate genes for a factor regulating body weight in primates. *American Journal of Physiology*, 1990, *259*, R1149–R1155.

Winans, E. Aripiprazole. *American Journal of Health-System Pharmacy*, 2003, *60*, 2437–2445.

Winans, S. S., and Powers, J. B. Olfactory and vomeronasal deafferentation of male hamsters: Histological and behavioral analyses. *Brain Research*, 1977, *126*, 325–344.

Wirz-Justice, A., Graw, P., Kraeuchi, K., et al. 'Natural' light treatment of seasonal affective disorder. *Journal of Affective Disorders*, 1996, *37*, 109–120.

Wirz-Justice, A., and Van den Hoofdakker, R. H. Sleep deprivation in depression: what do we know, where do we go? *Biological Psychiatry*, 1999, *46*, 445–453.

Wise, M. S. Narcolepsy and other disorders of excessive sleepiness. *Medical Clinics of North America*, 2004, *99*, 597–610.

Wise, R. A. Dopamine, learning, and motivation. *Nature Reviews: Neuroscience*, 2004, *5*, 483–494.

Wise, R. A., Leone, P., Rivest, R., and Leeb, K. Elevations of nucleus accumbens dopamine and DOPAC levels during intravenous heroin self-administration. *Synapse*, 1995, *21*, 140–148.

Wise, S. P., and Rapoport, J. L. Obsessive compulsive disorder: Is it a basal ganglia dysfunction? *Psychopharmacology Bulletin*, 1988, *24*, 380–384.

Wissinger, B., and Sharpe, L. T. New aspects of an old theme: The genetic basis of human color vision. *American Journal of Human Genetics*, 1998, *63*, 1257–1262.

Wolfe, P. A., Cobb, J. L., and D'Agostino, R. B. In *Stroke: Pathophysiology, Diagnosis, and Management*, edited by H. J. M. Barnett, B. M. Stein, J. P. Mohr, and F. M. Yatsu. New York: Churchill Livingstone, 1992.

Wolpaw, J. R., and McFarland, D. J. Control of a two-dimensional movement signal by a noninvasive brain–computer interface in humans. *Proceedings of the National Academy of Sciences, USA*, 2004, *101*, 17849–17854.

Wong-Riley, M. T. Personal communication, 1978. Cited by Livingstone, M. S., and Hubel, D. H. Thalamic inputs to cytochrome oxidase-rich regions in monkey visual cortex. *Proceedings of the National Academy of Sciences, USA*, 1982, *79*, 6098–6101.

Wood, E. R., Dudchenko, P. A., Robitsek, R. J., and Eichenbaum, H. Hippocampal neurons encode information about different types of memory episodes occurring in the same location. *Neuron*, 2000, *27*, 623–633.

Wood, R. I., and Newman, S. W. Mating activates androgen receptor-containing neurons in chemosensory pathways of the male Syrian hamster brain. *Brain Research*, 1993, *614*, 65–77.

Woodhead, G. J., Mutch, C. A., Olson, E. C., and Chenn, A. Cell-autonomous β-catenin signaling regulates cortical precursor proliferation. *Journal of Neuroscience*, 2006, *26*, 12620–12630.

Woodruff-Pak, D. S. Eyeblink classical conditioning in H. M.: Delay and trace paradigms. *Behavioral Neuroscience*, 1993, *107*, 911–925.

Woods, B. T. Is schizophrenia a progressive neurodevelopmental disorder? Toward a unitary pathogenetic mechanism. *American Journal of Psychiatry*, 1998, *155*, 1661–1670.

Woods, S. C., Lotter, E. C., McKay, L. D., and Porte, D. Chronic intracerebroventricular infusion of insulin reduces food intake and body weight of baboons. *Nature*, 1979, *282*, 503–505.

Woodworth, R. S., and Schlosberg, H. *Experimental Psychology*. New York: Holt, Rinehart and Winston, 1954.

Wu, J. C., and Bunney, W. E. The biological basis of an antidepressant response to sleep deprivation and relapse: Review and hypothesis. *American Journal of Psychiatry*, 1990, *147*, 14–21.

Wyart, C., Webster, W. W., Chen, J. H., et al. Smelling a single component of male sweat alters levels of cortisol in women. *Journal of Neuroscience*, 2007, *27*, 1261–1265.

Wynne, K., Stanley, S., McGowan, B., and Bloom, S. Appetite control. *Journal of Endocrinology*, 2005, *184*, 291–318.

Wysocki, C. J. Neurobehavioral evidence for the involvement of the vomeronasal system in mammalian reproduction. *Neuroscience and Biobehavioral Reviews*, 1979, *3*, 301–341.

Yadav, J. S., Wholey, M. H., Kuntz, R. E., et al. Protected carotid-artery stenting versus endarterectomy in high-risk patients. *New England Journal of Medicine*, 2004, *351*, 1493–1501.

Yamanaka, A., Beuckmann, C. T., Willie, J. T., et al. Hypothalamic orexin neurons regulate arousal according to energy balance in mice. *Neuron*, 2003, *38*, 701–713.

Yamasaki, T., Taniwaki, T., Tobimatsu, S., et al. Electrophysiological correlates of associative visual agnosia lesioned in the ventral pathway. *Journal of Neurological Science*, 2004, *221*, 53–60.

Yan, L., and Silver, R. Resetting the brain clock: Time course and localization of mPER1 and mPER2 protein expression in suprachiasmatic nucleus during phase shifts. *European Journal of Neuroscience*, 2004, *19*, 1105–1109.

Yang, T., and Maunsell, J. H. R. The effect of perceptual learning on neuronal responses in monkey visual area V4. *Journal of Neuroscience*, 2004, *24*, 1617–1626.

Yehuda, R., and LeDoux, J. Response variation following trauma: A translational neuroscience approach to understanding PTSD. *Neuron*, 2007, *56*, 19–32.

Yokoo, H., Tanaka, M., Yoshida, M., et al. Direct evidence of conditioned fear-elicited enhancement of noradrenaline release in the rat hypothalamus assessed by intracranial microdialysis. *Brain Research*, 1990, *536*, 305–308.

Yost, W. A. Auditory image perception and analysis: The basis for hearing. *Hearing Research*, 1991, *56*, 8–18.

Young, A. W., Aggleton, J. P., Hellawell, D. J., et al. Face processing impairments after amygdalotomy. *Brain*, 1995, *118*, 15–24.

Youngren, K. D., Inglis, F. M., Pivirotto, P. J., et al. Clozapine preferentially increases dopamine release in the rhesus monkey prefrontal cortex compared with the caudate nucleus. *Neuropsychopharmacology*, 1999, *20*, 403–412.

Zandian, M., Ioakimidis, I., Bergh, C., and Södersten, P. Cause and treatment of anorexia nervosa. *Physiology and Behavior*, 2007, *92*, 293–290.

Zayfert, C., Dums, A. R., Ferguson, R. J., and Hegel, M. T. Health functioning impairments associated with posttraumatic stress disorder, anxiety disorders, and depression. *Journal of Nervous and Mental Disease*, 2002, *190*, 233–240.

Zeki, S. The representation of colours in the cerebral cortex. *Nature*, 1980, *284*, 412–418.

Zeki, S., Aglioti, S., McKeefry, D., and Berlucchi, G. The neurological basis of conscious color perception in a blind patient. *Proceedings of the National Academy of Sciences, USA*, 1999, *96*, 13594–13596.

Zeki, S., and Marini, L. Three cortical stages of colour processing in the human brain. *Brain*, 1998, *121*, 1669–1685.

Zeki, S., and Shipp, S. The functional logic of cortical connections. *Nature*, 1988, *335*, 311–317.

Zenner, H.-P., Zimmermann, U., and Schmitt, U. Reversible contraction of isolated mammalian cochlear hair cells. *Hearing Research*, 1985, *18*, 127–133.

Zentner, M., and Kagan, J. Infants' perception of consonance and dissonance in music. *Infant Behavior and Development*, 1998, *21*, 483–492.

Zhong, C.-B., and Liljenquist, K. Washing away your sins: Threatened morality and physical cleansing. *Science*, 2006, *313*, 1451–1452.

Zigman, J. M., Nakano, Y., Coppari, R., et al. Mice lacking ghrelin receptors resist the development of diet-induced obesity. *Journal of Clinical Investigation*, 2005, *115*, 3564–3572.

Zihl, J., Von Cramon, D., Mai, N., and Schmid, C. Disturbance of movement vision after bilateral posterior brain damage. Further evidence and follow up observations. *Brain*, 1991, *114*, 2235–2252.

Zorrilla, E. P., Iwasaki, S., Moss, J. A., et al. Vaccination against weight gain. *Proceedings of the National Academy of Sciences, USA*, 2006, *103*, 12961–12962.

Zubieta, J.-K., Bueller, J. A., Jackson, L. R., et al. Placebo effects mediated by endogenous opioid activity on μ-opioid receptors. *Journal of Neuroscience*, 2005, *25*, 7754–7762.

Name Index

Subject Index

Page references in **bold** refer to definitions; references in *italic* refer to figures *f* and tables *t*.

Photo Credits

p. 1, © ORNL/Photo Researchers, Inc.; p. 3, © AJPhoto/Photo Researchers, Inc.; p. 6, Photo courtesy of the author; p. 11, Figure 1.9, photo courtesy of the author; p. 17, © Srulik Haramaty/Phototake ; p. 24, © Thomas Deerinck, NCMIR/Photo Researchers, Inc.; p. 33, © Jeff Greenberg/The Image Works; p. 40, © Lisa Poole/AP Images; p. 56, Anatomical Travelogue/Photo Researchers, Inc.; p. 75, © David Parker/Photo Researchers, Inc.; p. 79, © Rolfo Rolf Brenner/Getty Images; p. 88, © LUSH PIX/AGE Fotostock; p. 100, © Scott Camazine/Photo Researchers, Inc.; p. 101, © Herbert Zettl/zefa/Corbis; p. 115, © Lawrence Migdale/Photo Researchers; p. 121, Figure 5.7, photo courtesy of the author; p. 142, © Michael Schwartz/The Image Works; p. 146, © Reuters/CORBIS; p. 148, C3748 Juergen Effner/dpa/Corbis; p. 155, © Michael Fogden/Animas Animals; p. 171, © Rudi Von Brief/PhotoEdit; p. 177, © Thomas Schmidt/Getty Images; p. 195, © STOCK4B-RF/Getty Images Royalty Free; p. 202, © Robert Harding Picture Library/AGE Fotostock; p. 212, © Kate Mitchell/Corbis; p. 223, © Francois Gohier/Photo Researchers, Inc.; p. 240, © Alex Farnsworth/The Image Works; p. 244, © LWA/Getty Images; p. 257, © Kelly-Mooney Photography/Corbis; p. 270, © Tom McHugh/Photo Researchers, Inc.; p. 275, © COMSTOCK Images/AGE Fotostock; p. 283, © Song Zhenping/XinHua/Xinhua Press/Corbis; p. 284, © Photograph by Jack and Beverly Wilgus.; p. 301, © Ableimages/Getty Images; p. 312, © Barnabas Kindersley/Dorling Kindersley; p. 324, © Robin Nelson/PhotoEdit; p. 330, © AGE fotostock/SuperStock; p. 336, © Stan Carroll/The Commercial Appeal /Landov; p. 349, © Kevin Dodge/Corbis; p. 354, © Joe Bator/Corbis; p. 362, Corbis Royalty Free; p. 377, © Scott Barrow/Corbis; p. 379, © Jetta Productions/Getty Images; p. 400, © Jed & Kaoru Share/Corbis; p. 410, © Klaus Rose/dpa /Landov; p. 417, © Paul Conklin/PhotoEdit; p. 423, © Mika/zefa/Corbis; p. 442, © Photolibrary; p. 448, © Keith Bedford/Reuters/Corbis; p. 465, © John Griffin/The Image Works; p. 476, © David White/Alamy; p. 478, © Michael Macor/The Chronicle/Corbis; p. 487, Petty Officer 2nd Class Samuel C. Peterson/Reuters/Corbis; p. 490, © David Young-Wolff/Getty Images; p. 498, © Gianni Muratore/Alamy Images